Chinese Medicine Liberation: Inner Documents

Chinese Medicine Liberation: Inner Documents
Y. Seidman
Editors, co-authors: Zac Patterson, Lois Nethery
Published by: Hunyuan Group Inc.
Greenwich, Connecticut, USA
Email: info@hunyuan.org
Website: http://www.chineseclassics.org

ISBN: 978-0-9891679-3-2
Library of Congress Control Number: 2015902417
1st Edition (March, 2015)
Printed in the United States of America

Images: Original images of China in the early 1900s were generously provided by the family of Geneviève le Goff. Please see "Acknowledgements" in the back of this book for further information.

"The Liberation of Chinese Medicine

After the establishment of the People's Republic of China, under the leadership of the brilliant leader chairman Mao, the three grand health policies were put forth: Chinese and Western medicine must unite; prevention is the focus; and gearing towards workers, peasants and soldiers.

Chinese medicine advanced studies schools and specialty advanced classes were established. These remolded Chinese medicine and cultivated Chinese medicine. Other Chinese medicine research organizations were also established. They researched Chinese medicine and, at last, Chinese medicine could free itself.

It stripped itself from the feudal smelting and from the capitalist shackles. It strode towards the great path of a scientific new China, a scientific medicine."[1]

[1] *Beijing Chinese Medicine* (periodical), 1952 June 15th (1st volume 3rd publication)

Contents

Preface

At first I started this book like any other history book, producing a narrative with analysis, as is customary. But with time I realized that a better objective, that specifically reaches to the Chinese medicine community, is to present historical reality as it unfolded. This is to say, I wanted to create a genuine feel for readers what it was like in that time: how did practitioners feel in the 1930s when Chinese medicine fought for its survival against Western medicine? How did they feel when they encountered, used and were used by the modern Republic? What was it like for Chinese medicine practitioners when the Communists dictated medical practice primarily from ideological grounds?

The plan then was to collect documents and significant book excerpts that had been influential in their time, translated with only short commentaries, thus allowing readers to assess for themselves. This collection reveals a clear narrative of the struggles, successes and disappointments of everyday Chinese medicine practitioners living and practicing during those changing times. More importantly, they expose the reasons behind, and methodology for, transforming the old Chinese medicine into a modern system. What happened in the transformation of Chinese medicine in the past is something that we—contemporary practitioners—should not only know but also use to evaluate our direction going forward. This discussion is not *about* Chinese medicine—we *are* Chinese medicine!

I call these documents the "Inner Documents", symbolizing the revealing of secrets that others don't get to see. These influential articles and books have long been forgotten in China and were hardly known in the West. Modern Chinese medicine (branded as "TCM") comes from standardized textbooks—books culminating from numerous twists and turns during the 20th century. These "inner documents" show the TCM evolution (or, as some suggest, "revolution") and may prove an enlightening discovery for our profession.

As this discovery unfolds, we find that once upon a time in China, during the Republic years, were "The Great Debates" between modern scientific medicine and Chinese medicine. Then in Communist China, TCM was standardized and merged by force with Western medicine. In the West, however, it does not flow especially well with Western medicine—outside of China, medical doctors aren't impelled to accept Chinese medicine. The Republic's great debates between Western and Chinese medicine practitioners are our treasure house—a valuable starting place for both co-existing successfully with Western medicine and constructing a more effective life medicine.

I am a practitioner of Chinese medicine and, with that, my ability to present a complete history with all its facts is limited. I am greatly in debt to historians of Chinese medicine who dedicate their lives to bring us more facts from the lost pages of history. Especially, I would like to acknowledge the historian Sean Hsiang-lin Lei 雷祥麟, whose research of modern Chinese medicine history I find enlightening. His recent book, *Neither Donkey nor Horse: Medicine in the Struggle over China's Modernity* (Chicago: The University of Chicago Press, 2014), narrates the modern history of Chinese medicine since the late nineteenth century and thereby provides a helpful framework for contextualizing many of the historical documents collected in this book.

I believe that Chinese medicine has a bright future. Knowing the mayhem that took place in 20th century Chinese medicine during China's series of massive political upheavals allows us to know and develop Chinese medicine in the 21st century. Instead of being led blindfolded we can stride ahead with a clear vision.

In Connecticut

February 9th, 2015

Yaron Seidman

Foreword

As a historian who has spent more than a decade on historical documents pertaining to the recent past of Chinese medicine, I was deeply moved to find that Yaron Seidman and his team have translated almost one thousand pages of them into English. In his preface to this book, Seidman briefly tell us what motivated him as a clinical practitioner to take on this unusual task.

What he has gleaned from these "inner documents" are surprising historical facts that, if used effectively, can help bring about a liberating development of Chinese medicine. Since in the preface he does not provide any concrete case to elaborate this vision, I invite anyone with curiosity about these facts and their liberating potential to read the following statement and ask him- or herself two questions: When and why did practitioners of Chinese medicine make such a radical statement? How could thousands of statements like this have influenced the contents of Chinese medicine as taught and practiced around the world at this time?

> While Chinese and Western understandings are different and have their own drawbacks and strengths, there is no way that both are simultaneously true. Some people... suggest a compromise formula, saying that Western medicine is good at anatomy but Chinese medicine is good at qi-transformation. ...We should know that one specific disease is a specific thing. Therefore, there is only one understanding that can be true 真是 (zhenshi). There is no way that both understandings can be simultaneously true.

This statement was made by Lu Yuanlei 陸淵雷 (1894–1955) in 1932, in response to an assignment by the quasi-official Institute of National Medicine to formulate a set of guidelines for the task of "scientizing" Chinese medicine—the task that the Republican government demanded of this institute and the very rationale for founding it in the first place. Before delving into substantive issues, Lu outlined five principles as indisputable points of departure for this task, and the above-cited statement stood out to be the principle that generated the most heated debates at that time.[2]

[2] Note from the book's authors: For the Great Debates of the era, see pp. 374–583; for Tan Cizhong's counter argument to Lu Yuanlei and summary of Lu's five points, see pp. 542–553; A letter from Mr. Lu, see p. 487; for an excerpt from Lu's official proposal, see p. 340

While this statement might sound self-evident or even naïve to us, it was the first time that some practitioners of Chinese medicine began embracing the zero-sum game of scientific realism. To highlight the historic status of this decision, Lu took as his target the famous contrast between Chinese qi-transformation and Western anatomy, thereby pitting his own position against that of Tang Zonghai 唐宗海 (1851–1908), the late Qing physician who had coined the precursor of this contrast in the early 1890s and the widely acclaimed founder of the School of Converging Chinese and Western medicine (Zhongxiyi huitong 中西醫匯通). Instead of treating these two concepts as incommensurable, however, Tang had used it to create communication and even convergence between the two styles of medicine. Not knowing the mono-theistic conceptions of truth, reality and science, Tang would have had a hard time comprehending why "there is no way that both understandings can be simultaneously true." To abolish once and for all the kind of non-modernist syncretism represented by Tang and his followers, Lu insisted on imposing this principle as the indisputable foundation for creating a nationally unified, scientized Chinese medicine.

I have basically answered the first question I posed above, about when and why Chinese medicine practitioners began embracing the Modernist idea that there exists only one reality, one science and one truth (zhenshi). I believe that it is Yaron's intention to invite you, the reader, to answer the second question, concerning the effects of this situation for contemporary Chinese medicine developments, for yourself, not with the help of a historian's narrative but with the original documents prepared in this collection. By allowing the reader to engage directly with these crucial debates and struggles, whose results have given shape to a modern Chinese medicine but have been made invisible in TCM textbooks, these documents open up the valuable possibilities to rethink these historic decisions and to reshape the future of Chinese medicine.

25th January 2015

Sean Hsiang-lin Lei 雷祥麟

Associate research fellow, Institute of Modern History, Academia Sinica, Taiwan

Associate professor, Institute of Science, Technology, and Society, National Yang-Ming University

Research notes

History is not my thing. I know people who are passionately interested in history—they love to read historical books, they love to visit museums and they truly are able to get a sense of a kind of living experience from inert relics and documents. I admire their ability to be able to apply the imagination in this way. For me, when I'm in contact with any kind of historical presentation—whether it's a book or a documentary or a museum exhibition—there's a niggling feeling of "but what else?" For example, a re-creation of a farmhouse kitchen from the 1800s—there's the fireplace, the pots, the rustic furniture—but what about the people who lived there? What about the egg shells and potato peelings, the mixed smells of soup and animal dung, children squabbling in the corner, the wife pregnant again, illiterate, the relentless cold of the dirt floor in winter? We can never really know what they felt. We can only get hints and then, with our own imagination, mixed in with our own experience in these modern times, we somehow fill in the gaps. If it's clear that history is part make-believe then I am OK with that. It's when historical accounts are presented as solid truth, however, that I believe we can become led astray.

What happens when we become led astray is that we lose contact with our own innate felt sense of truth. This is permissible, perhaps, if the historical narrative in question is on a mundane topic. When the historical narrative is about medicine, however, and the audience is made up of those who practice medicine, then the narrative will best serve the audience if it can lead them back to this felt sense that connects with their deeper instinct. However, the challenge—the ongoing challenge—is to allow our sense of certainty to become a little destabilized. This is the path of development as a practitioner-scholar, a path we need to walk if we are not to fall backwards. Patients will always bless us with the unknown—gaps in our knowledge or new information that doesn't sit well within our clinical framework. If we "pretend to know" then immediately we are shut off from an opportunity to grow in our practice. On the other hand, if we can sit with this uncertainty, opening ourselves a little to the unknown, then we can gradually become familiar with a wider range of phenomena. This expands the terrain upon which we can move about. This feeling of uncertainty, if used purposefully, therefore can lead to greater freedom. The beneficiaries, of course, are our patients. When we can become comfortable and familiar with a wider terrain, while being open to further uncertainty, they gain both from our knowledge and the natural humility that this process engenders.

This feeling of going astray was an undercurrent in my practice but I had no way to articulate it until I heard Dr Yaron Seidman present his Hunyuan approach. This was a very uncomfortable encounter with uncertainty. I simultaneously felt immense relief that my niggling feeling about modern Chinese medicine practice had a basis to it, but at the same time the proposed solution, as Dr Seidman had developed for his own practice and has been sharing with other practitioners for several years, was so unfamiliar that I was left, for a moment in time, with nothing. Fortunately there was a lot of clinical support and access to learning materials and I was able to traverse the terrain quickly enough to gain a foothold, learning through several channels simultaneously—clinical application, studying classical quotes, developing "Xin Fa" or Heart method, researching nuances of ancient characters and becoming acquainted with select herbs in a new and satisfying way. Explaining the principle to patients was often, and continues to be, an important way to develop. The more we can use everyday language and lived experience to explain Chinese medicine to our patients, the deeper they grasp the process and become participants and, with their often illuminating and insightful feedback, the more we can learn for ourselves.

Medicine will never be a fixed entity. We move in the realm of the imperfect. Even if we could finally stave off all disease, we are still within our human life cycle—there is birth and growth, maturity and old age—and that is the path of each individual, practitioner and patient alike. Perhaps the ancients were onto something—chasing the treatment of symptoms, we are always on the run. Standing still and seeing phenomena for what they are, how they come into being and how they decline and what persists throughout these transformations—if we can research *this*, what does it mean for medicine?

When I enrolled in Chinese medicine school, I'd expected to be exposed to these kinds of grand mysteries, the wisdom of the East and so on. Certainly it was a good education, and seeing things through a new perspective is always beneficial to stay supple and glimpse our own assumptions and ignorance. Many of the methods and treatments were effective. But what was missing was this deeper level of enquiry, seeking the root of things, in order to enhance medicine, to enhance life.

In these pages we can become the "outer circle" of a Socratic-style learning experience. We can witness the debates that occurred when Chinese medicine met the impressive technical skill of Western medicine at a vulnerable time in China's history. We can listen to this "inner circle" debate and then step into the continuing process of our medicine's development: How meaningful is this discussion? What is debated well? What remains to be asked? What does it mean for us today, foreigners practicing this form of Chinese medicine that was rapidly transformed during the last century, in part by our own culture's knowledge base, and then transplanted back into our soil, itself a terrain that is foreign to ancient Chinese philosophy? Where is the way forward to develop the inherent qualities of Chinese medicine, harmoniously with scientific knowledge and without losing its essence? This question is as topical and urgent now as it was a century ago.

This discussion is open to all practitioners who wish to learn together, to grow as practitioners by challenging their own certainties and then collectively making the most of this opportunity to deeply enhance the quality of our profession, regardless of affiliation to style or modality or school of thought.

Lois Nethery

How to use this book

The four chapters of this book consist of excerpts and articles related to each chapter's main topic. The majority of our source material is originally written in Chinese, for which we provide an English translation, while a small number of articles and excerpts included herein were already in English; we have only selected appropriate excerpts as applicable to this book. The beginning of each article references the source in English and Chinese, including specific page numbers. For materials from English sources, we preserved their original prose, despite the occasional flawed rationalizations and textual errors. We believe this will help the reader have a better contextual view of the state of affairs at the time of the writings.

Our English source material is limited to the following items:

1. *China and modern medicine: A study in medical missionary development* by Harold Balme in 1921.
2. Two articles from *The Caduceus Journal* in 1934 and 1937.
3. Five articles from *Chinese Medical Journal Foreign Language Publication* in 1955, 1960 and 1966.

In the above items, Chinese names and institutions do not include Chinese characters, unless included in the original text.

In our translations, personal names, institutions and books are listed in Pinyin Romanized letters and in Chinese; book titles, when applicable, may be accompanied by their English translation. For articles and publications appearing prior to 1949, we use long form Chinese (Fan Ti Zi 繁體字), and for later publications we use simplified Chinese (Jian Ti Zi 简体字). During the 1950s, the Chinese long script was modified to a simplified Chinese gradually; in the earlier part, fewer characters were modified but, as years went by, increasing numbers of characters became simplified. We have tried, as much as possible, to stay close to the source and so some articles contain a mixture of the two as it originally appeared.

For most articles, there is a section that follows after the title material for our own comments and, in some cases, there may be comment sections embedded in the body of the article. These comment sections are right-justified, appear in a contrasting font and commence with "Yaron:" These comments are strictly our own and are not part of the original article.

Chapter 1: Historical background prior to 1920

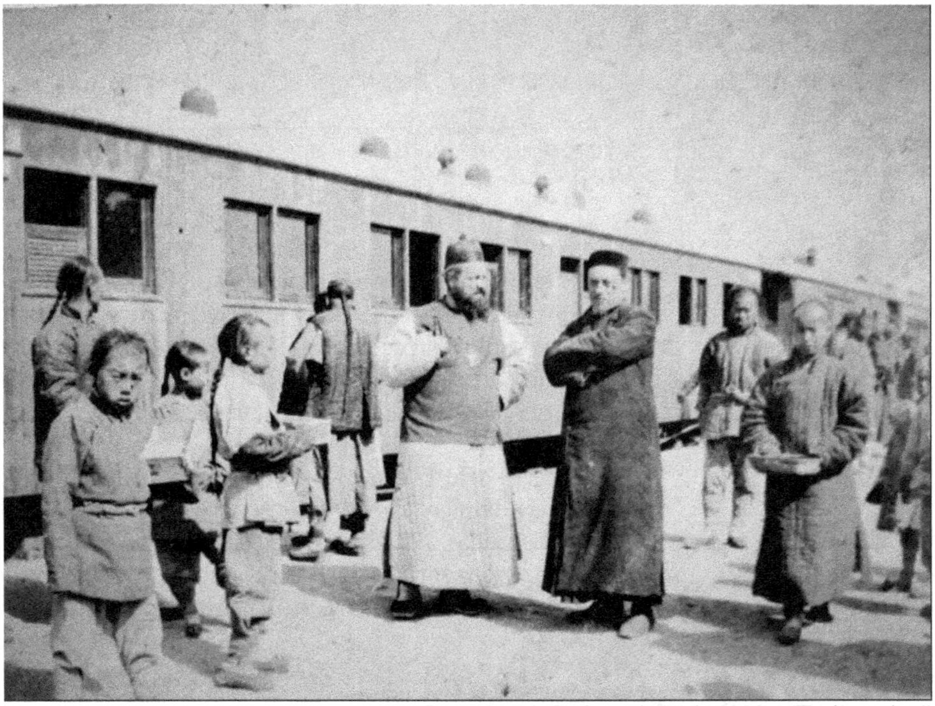

Photo by Mr P. Goux in early 1900s. "Train station"

"Anyone may be a doctor in China. There are no medical colleges, no examinations, and no diplomas. No license is required for practice. A man makes up his mind to practice medicine, and hangs out his sign. He buys a book or two, and begins to read. As soon as he can get a patient, he will diagnose his complaint, write a prescription, and accept the very small fee which is given to the beginner. After varying fortunes for a year or two, he makes a "marvelous cure," surprising no one, probably, so much as himself."[3]

[3] *China and modern medicine: A study in medical missionary development.* H. Balme, 1921.

China and modern medicine: A study in medical missionary development

1921 by Harold Balme F.R.C.S. (Eng.) D.P.H.

Dean of the School of Medicine, Shantung Christian University, Tsinan, China

WITH PREFACE BY Sir Donald MacAlister, K.C.B., M.D., President of the General Council of General Education and Registration of the United Kingdom, Principal and Vice-Chancellor of the University of Glasgow

LONDON, UNITED COUNCIL FOR MISSIONARY EDUCATION, EDINBURGH HOUSE, 2 EATON GATE, S.W. 1

Yaron: In line with the spirit of the entire book we present the "situation on the ground" through key figures living at that time.

This article is presented here to give a synopsis of the foreign missionary attitudes to the Chinese situation at the turn of the 20th century. Whereas factually it may be more or less correct and can give us a useful overview of the state of health care in China at that time, also bear in mind that the author is a Christian missionary and is likely to be biased by his particular agenda.

Following on from this excerpt, we contrast it with a historical synopsis written by Chen Bangxian in 1936, a Chinese medicine native historian, which illustrates how some Chinese may have viewed their own situation. This helps us achieve a more rounded view from people who were pro-modernization, both Western and Chinese.

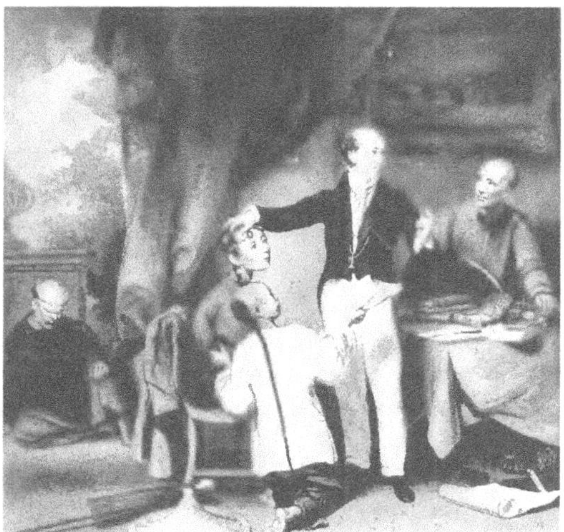

Thomas Richardson Colledge M.D., Founder of the first voluntary hospital established in China – The Ophthalmic Hospital, Macao. From the painting by G. Chinnery.

Pages 60 to 76

Chapter III: Methods of approach

> We cannot expect the Chinese to grasp with eagerness at our improvements; yet the cure of diseases, set down at once as fatal in their experience, must be likely to facilitate the introduction of our knowledge, and add most humanely to their comfort and civilization.
>
> *Sir Henry Halford, President of the College of Physicians, London, 1834.*

The introduction of western medicine to the various classes who compose the three hundred and sixty million inhabitants of China has followed two definite lines of approach.

In the first place, there have been those pioneer efforts which have been made since the days of Colledge and Parker, and still are made to-day, in order to bring the blessings of the art of healing to the service of the people throughout the length and breadth of the land.

Secondly, there are those new impacts which are being brought to bear upon different sections of the community through the medium of the out-patient dispensary and other agencies of every hospital. In any attempt to study this subject, therefore, both of these sides must be considered.

I

It is quite impossible to understand the work of the medical missionary pioneer in China, to appreciate his methods, to sympathize with his difficulties, or to estimate his success or failure, unless one first has a clear idea of the problems which have faced him, and their underlying causes.

1) *The Redemption of the Medical Reputation*—The first, and in some respects the most serious, of these problems arose from the attitude which the Chinese people, especially the educated classes, adopted towards medicine in general. This was due on the one hand to their tendency to associate sickness with the influence of evil spirits, and on the other hand to the low standard of medical science in China until quite recent times. A medical *profession* could not, by any stretch of imagination, be said to exist. Still less was there any recognized

standard of practice. The better educated of the old-fashioned practitioners had a certain general acquaintance with the action of drugs, and a rough and ready knowledge of the treatment of some conditions, yet on the other hand the most enlightened of them had never had the advantage of the most rudimentary study of the fundamental sciences—chemistry, biology, anatomy, physiology, etc. Thus it is clear how much justification there has been for the people's attitude, seeing that medicine was looked upon as very little more than a mixture of quackery, commercial exploitation, and superstition. Dr. O. L. Kilborn has well described the position:

> Anyone may be a doctor in China. There are no medical colleges, no examinations, and no diplomas. No license is required for practice. A man makes up his mind to practice medicine, and hangs out his sign. He buys a book or two, and begins to read. As soon as he can get a patient, he will diagnose his complaint, write a prescription, and accept the very small fee which is given to the beginner. After varying fortunes for a year or two, he makes a "marvelous cure," surprising no one, probably, so much as himself. Likely as not his cure was effected by the method by which pins saved a great many lives in the small boy's composition—"By people not swallowin' of 'em". The medicines which brought about the cure were entirely harmless; nature's methods were not interfered with; and a cure was effected quickly and well. Now the new doctor's fame goes up, his patients increase, and his fees also take a rise.[4]

It is one thing to introduce modern medicine in a country where medical science has already won its way, and the doctor's position is thoroughly assured; it is quite another thing to try to do so in a country where medicine is held in disrepute, and the physician looked down upon by the educated classes. Yet such were the difficulties which the pioneers of medical missions were called upon to overcome in every province of China. They had to prove, by the solid merit of their work, that modern medicine does rest upon a basis of exact science, at the same time as they were exhibiting, by life and precept, that great message of redemption—physical, moral, and spiritual—which they had come to proclaim.

[4] Heal the Sick, by O. L. Kilborne, p. 86 [*Note from Chinese Medicine Liberation authors: All footnotes from original source*]

2) *The Winning of Goodwill*—The second problem which faced the pioneer is one which happily we can now begin to speak of in the past tense. The traditional Chinese policy of isolation and exclusion, which expressed itself in suspicion, fear, and prejudice towards everything and everyone from the West, engendered a deep antipathy towards the mission hospital, just because it was foreign. No sooner was a hospital opened, particularly in the inland provinces, than the doctor's motives became at once the object of discussion and criticism, and in many cases the most extraordinary rumors were circulated as to the horrible practices which he was supposed to be indulging in secretly. There was a time, for example, in the province of Hunan, when an influential official, Chouhan by name, published a series of inflammatory pamphlets declaring that the missionary doctors took the eyes from infant children for medicinal purposes and were guilty of the most flagrant crimes in their operations upon women. And this was typical of the reports that were often spread abroad concerning the work of the hospitals.

   It must not be thought for a moment that the success which crowned Parker's efforts in Canton followed so inevitably or so rapidly in the more remote portions of the country, where the dreaded foreigner was less well known. In such places the pioneer had to proceed with great caution, carefully picking his cases, and avoiding, as far as was possible, all risk of failure. At the same time he sought, by every means in his power, to cultivate the friendship and win the confidence of the people around him, and especially of such patients as were bold enough to entrust themselves to his care. But there was always with him the serious thought that he carried in his hands the lives of his colleagues and the reputation of his profession, and that any false step might jeopardize the prospects not only of his own work but also of the whole mission for which he stood.

3) *The Overcoming of Limitations*—The third great difficulty arose from the lack of proper facilities for up-to-date medical work—no suitable premises to work in; no apparatus nor equipment; no nurses nor trained assistants, possibly not even an educated Chinese helper willing to be trained for such a work; not the least semblance of sanitation, nor of intelligent measures to prevent the spread of disease. The pioneer doctor had nothing but a limitless mass of human suffering and ignorance around him, a few instruments and drugs in his hand, an unshakable sense of vocation, and a dauntless faith in the sufficiency of God.

II

Such, then, were some of the grave problems which confronted the men who attempted to blaze the trail of medical missions in China. And it is to their patient and triumphant work that the remarkable change of attitude towards western medicine which has been seen in China during recent years must be ascribed.

To combat such difficulties was a problem of strategy. The following is a description, in a hitherto unpublished paper, of how Dr. William Wilson, of the China Inland Mission, set to work to win his way in the far inland province of Shensi. After referring to his unsuccessful efforts to secure a foothold in the provincial capital, where the literati instigated a riot and forced him to leave, Dr. Wilson writes:

> Commencing work in Hanchong, so far in the interior, where foreigners were little known, and foreign hospitals not at all, it seemed the wisest plan to concentrate at first all our energies on a vigorous, efficient, and attractive out-patient department, and, later on, as the confidence of the people was secured, to develop a surgical in-patient work—even then at first limiting ourselves to operative cases where a speedy and complete recovery could be anticipated, before undertaking more serious surgical cases.
>
> We were fortunate in obtaining very suitable premises, one part constituting our dwelling-house, and the other, with a long street frontage, furnishing us, when fitted up, with a large well-stocked dispensary and consulting-room, together with commodious waiting-room for men and women respectively. Here we were soon rewarded with the joy of receiving steadily increasing numbers of patients, suffering from all kinds of diseases, most of them similar to those met with at home, but in a far more aggravated condition, due to the deplorable consequences of native treatment. In a vast number of cases, such as skin diseases, ophthalmia, burns, ulcers, wounds, and all kinds of open sores, the utterly irrational methods of native treatment only perpetuate and aggravate the condition… Thousands of such cases present themselves to the medical missionary, and while not perhaps particularly interesting from a professional point of view, he may continually rejoice that he is afforded abundant opportunity of curing diseases, alleviating a vast amount of suf-

fering, and winning thereby the real affection and goodwill of his patients, to say nothing of the higher privilege still of daily carrying out Christ's twofold command to heal the sick and preach the gospel.

The Chinese doctor's ignorance of anatomy tells, of course, very seriously in cases of fracture of bones and dislocation of joints, and our treatment of a few such cases in our early days inspired a most encouraging confidence, resulting in many such cases coming to us, even from long distances. Cases of injury or disease necessitating amputation or the removal of tumors are, by his own confession, beyond the power of the native doctor; but coming to the hospital as a last hope, and there being operated upon under all the advantages due to chloroform and antiseptic treatment, the reputation gradually spread to great distances, so that it was not long before we were able to fit up accommodation and undertake in-patient surgical work.

Another important branch of the work was the curing of opium patients, who used, as a rule, to stay with us for a month. In the case of young men of sound constitution, we found the best results were gained by an immediate and entire withholding of opium in any form, and the treatment of symptoms as they arose. The deliverance from the opium crave was thus the more quickly effected, though, for the first few days, the physical distress was sometimes considerable. In older men, or men of weak constitution, or very heavy smokers, experience taught us that a less drastic method was preferable, and such would for two or three weeks be treated with medicine containing a steadily diminishing quantity of opium, till at the end of that period no opium was being taken. Many hundreds of these passed through our hands, and in nearly all instances were able to return home freed entirely from this terrible crave and the demoralizing effects of the opium habit; best of all, many proved by their after lives that they were not only delivered from the bondage of opium, but had entered into the liberty of the children of God.

> To make our medical work more widely known, and to inspire the people with confidence, we were glad to avail ourselves of the Chinese custom of accepting from grateful patients of the wealthier class the large handsome honorific tablets, on which the donor inscribes in letters of gold his name and official position, the history of his disease and finally, in very flowery language, his unbounded gratitude to the doctor who has so successfully undertaken his case. In a few years, more than ten of these, some as large as an average dining room table, had been presented, and adorned the street frontage of our hospital and the walls of the dispensary and waiting-room.
>
> The presentation of these tablets, as is customary in China, was always the occasion for a somewhat imposing ceremony. The grateful patient, accompanied by a dozen or more of his friends, marched through the streets in full official dress, accompanied by a band of musicians, and in the procession an honored place was assigned to the tablet, carried by bearers and festooned with scarlet silk.
>
> The formal presentation and speeches over, the tablet was hung in the place allotted to it, and the guests were invited to a feast, after which a general inspection of the hospital and any objects of interest usually occupied their attention for an hour or two; thus was afforded a fresh opportunity for friendly intercourse between the missionary community and these representatives of the literary and official class, which, especially in those days, was the most difficult class to reach. Such occasions naturally gave scope for conversation as to our real purpose in coming to their land, and on leaving, each guest was presented with portions of the Scriptures and other Christian books.

Concurrently with the opening of out-patient dispensary and hospital, as described by Dr Wilson, attempts were also made in many centers to extend the work of the medical mission over a wider area by means of itinerating tours. Important cities and market towns were thus visited on regular days, usually once a month or thereabouts, and on each visit patients were seen and evangelistic addresses given. This work, whilst not very satisfactory from the professional standpoint, certainly helped to familiarize the people of the district with the objects and work of the medical mission hospital, and probably encouraged some patients, who would not otherwise have done so, to take the journey to the medical mission station for purposes of in-patient treatment. From such humble beginnings many a branch of the Christian Church in China has sprung.

III

It is not only in the more remote parts of China that contacts are made with new sections of the community in the manner described above. Hardly a day passes in the out-patient clinic of any mission hospital but there are included, amongst those who come for help, numbers of men and women who have never before been brought into touch with western medicine, and who have not the slightest acquaintance with the teachings of Christ. They have come because of their physical need, which hitherto they have found no one able to relieve. But away back in their village or country town they have met another patient, possibly suffering from some affliction very similar to their own, who has told them of the relief that he has already obtained at this particular hospital; and this is what has led them to take the journey and make their way to the out-patient department.

Readers of missionary publications are sometimes so impressed with the progress that has been made at particular stations that they are apt to lose sight of the enormous mass of untouched population which forms the hinterland of each and all such centers. It is from this teeming hinterland that these patients come, and it is just this fact which invests the out-patient dispensary of every mission hospital with all the importance of a great Extension Department. It is here that first impressions are going to be formed—impressions which in many instances will never have the opportunity of being corrected or amplified by subsequent residence in the hospital wards, or by closer contact with those who profess to represent and serve the Greatest of all Physicians. It is here also that the patient will make up his mind, not merely about the western doctor and his methods of investigation and treatment, but also about the new truths which, as he learns, the hospital is intended to promulgate. It is no small matter for the doctor to stand up before men and women of this kind and to reflect that he and his assistants represent—if one dare to use the term—the only manifestation of the Great Father that some, at least, of these patients will ever meet. A discourteous reception; dry, perfunctory preaching; slipshod methods of diagnosis; impatient or hurried treatment—these things, which might under ordinary circumstances be easily excused on grounds of pressure, take on a new significance when it is remembered that these are the impressions which it will take longest of all to efface, and that they will effectually distort the image of the Christ which the doctor would fain have presented to the patient's view.

There is only one deduction that can be drawn from this: the out-patient work must be treated very seriously—far more seriously than is sometimes the case in hospitals to-day, where the doctor, overburdened as he often is with the pressure of the wards and of the countless other duties that fall to his lot, is apt to relegate his out-patient department to the care of a poorly-trained Chinese assistant and evangelist. Here in the West emphasis is being increasingly laid upon the importance of senior members of the leading hospitals taking an actual share in the treatment of out-patients; and the same is true in China. Even where a qualified doctor is single-handed it is a great question whether he would not, in the long run, be doing a bigger and better service to China by deliberately limiting himself to such numbers (in-patients and out-patients) as he could do real justice to. This does not mean that he should concentrate all his time and attention on a favored few, whose cases should be investigated with greatest minuteness; but it does mean that he should organize the work so as to safeguard the impression which is being made on the patients, and prevent the possibility of anyone who has been received in the out-patient department going away with the feeling that he has not been properly looked after, or his case not thoroughly investigated.

Nothing is more difficult than to curtail the number of patients, especially in a country where terrible suffering and disease abound on every side, but it must never be forgotten that, in any case, western doctors are not able to do more than touch the barest fringe of the work. It is often stated, for instance, that in some particular province or district there is only one fully qualified physician to half a million or a million people, as if forsooth he were able in some way to be of some service to such a number. The probability is that not one in every hundred ever come near him when they are sick, nor could he possibly attend them if they did.

There are four points in connection with the out-patient side of the work which are specially worthy of notice.

1) It is of the utmost importance that patients should always be regarded as guests, and be received with courtesy and kindness by the gate-keeper or registrar whom they first meet. He is the first representative of the hospital to come in contact with the new patient, and first impressions go a long way to determine the patient's attitude to the institution.

2) Any evangelistic service which is conducted for the patients should be of a character worthy of the great cause which is to be proclaimed, and calculated to emphasize the winsomeness and graciousness of the Message. It must never be forgotten that the patient has not come to the hospital for the sake of attending a religious service. He has come because he is sick, possibly he is in pain, and he wants to be helped. He will not as a rule object to listen to an evangelistic address while he is waiting for the hour at which the clinic is due to open; but if that address is to grip him it must be presented thoughtfully, earnestly, and with every possible consideration for the condition of the hearers. A very good plan that has been tried with success in at least one hospital in China is as follows: As the out-patients begin to gather the evangelist and his helpers, instead of keeping up a continuous preaching performance as is so often the case, mingle with the patients, and get into general conversation with them one by one. They find out where they have each come from, and what it is that has brought them to the hospital, at the same time explaining to them, in a simple way, the procedure that is to follow—how long it will be before the doctor comes; in what order they will be seen; where they will get their medicines; what they will have to do if they need to be admitted to the wards, etc. In these and similar ways they gain the confidence of the patients, and make them feel that they have their interests at heart.

About twenty minutes before the clinic is to open a bell is rung, and an announcement is then made that a short service will be held, at which all are asked to sit quietly, special stewards being appointed to show into their seats any fresh patients who may arrive during this time. The service opens with a brief introduction, in which the evangelist, or better still the doctor himself, explains simply why such a gathering is held. He tells them of the great Gift which the hospital tries to represent, and points them in simple language to the Father who cares for them all. Having made this introduction, and shown them how that Father may be approached by all who care to do so through the use of prayer, he asks them all to stand reverently in their places while he offers up an intercession on their behalf. Prayer concluded, an earnest address is given, usually on some incident in the life and teaching of Jesus Christ, and a strong appeal is made to all to study for themselves the truths of the gospel.

As the hour for the opening of medical work strikes, a second bell is rung, and at this signal the evangelist and his helpers leave the platform and mingle once more with the people. The early-comers, whose registration number will entitle them to be seen first, are directed to the proper door, while the evangelist sits with those who have some time to wait, explaining in more detail what has been said during the service, offering portions of the Scriptures or other books for sale, and attempting to draw them into conversation. In this way he soon learns to recognize those who are coming regularly for treatment, and in some cases is able to obtain an invitation to visit them in their own homes, there to follow up the impression that has been formed.

3) The investigation of the patients, prior to the adoption of any particular line of treatment, should be as careful and complete as possible. Superficial medical practice ill accords with a fervent religious service. If the work of a mission hospital out-patient department is to be properly done, both the religious and the professional sides should be treated as of the utmost importance, and neither should be sacrificed for the sake of the other. It would be better to give up the evangelistic service or the medical work altogether than to treat either so carelessly as to convey the impression that it was only of very secondary importance. To do real justice to the medical care of the out-patients, the enthusiastic work of the doctor himself is essential, and he needs to have a well-trained staff and adequate equipment. In a country like China, where parasitic and blood infections abound, the more modern hospitals are finding that they need not only well-fitted examination and dressing rooms in their out-patient departments, but that a small clinical laboratory in constant use is also an indispensable adjunct for thorough investigations. Fortunately the Chinese make excellent technicians, and it is not difficult to train them in laboratory methods.

4) The human side of the work is the supreme thing and must always be paramount. It may not be very easy for the doctor himself, in the rush of his work, to spend a large amount of time talking with individual patients, but his attitude towards them and the attitude of his helpers will count for everything. Here, for example, is a poor old man who has tramped fifty or a hundred miles in the hope of recovering his sight, because he has heard of someone else who was operated on for cataract with most successful result. But a glance is sufficient to show that his trouble, unfortunately, is due to a very different cause. His is a case of absolute glaucoma, for which nothing can possibly be done. It is a bitter disappointment for the old man, and very hard for him to

> understand; but it is going to make all the difference to him if the doctor spares a few moments to talk to him sympathetically about it, and then perhaps leads him to one of the nurses or other helpers, who will explain more fully why his case is incurable. And after all, it is these human impressions which are the most potential.

Some years ago a Chinese patient suffering from cataract consulted a friend of mine, and was successfully treated. Subsequently there came from his district a procession of seven blind men, walking one behind the other, each touching the shoulder of the one in front. They had tramped for many days across the mountains, in hope of a similar cure. When they reached the hospital it was immediately evident that no cure was possible in any of their cases. But they were received and treated as guests, and their confidence and friendship were won. For very many years one of those blind men was an untiring and successful evangelist, not only to the blind but to those who were more fortunate than he; this all resulted from his stay in that hospital. It certainly pays to treat the human factor as the most important of all.

Following is from same publication, pages 107–122

Chapter V: The new profession in China

> The greatest need of China is not, after all, for highly trained scientists, although they are essential; it is not, after all, for the greatest technical skill, although that is absolutely necessary if the great end is to be attained. But the great need of China is scientific knowledge and technical skill dominated by an idealistic loyalty to the highest and best things in human life; and that idealism that is most enduring, that can be most counted upon, that is least likely to fail, is an idealism based upon a deep and abiding religious conviction.
>
> *George E Vincent, president of the Rockefeller foundation, March 4, 1920.*

It was characteristic of men of such farsighted vision as Colledge and Parker that they saw, from the very commencement of their medical work in China, that the vast needs of the country could never be met except by the trained efforts of her own sons and daughters. And since China at that time had no medical College of her own whatever,[5] they at once realized that one of the chief contributions which medical missions must offer should be the direction of the training of the Chinese youths in Western medical science. Not only was this object included in the first statement of the medical missionary society, which as we have seen they founded in 1838, but already, in the preceding year, Parker had commenced to train three assistants in his hospital at Canton. Naturally enough such training consisted almost entirely of oral instruction of a practical character of very much the same lines in the old apprenticeship days in this country, for there were no Chinese medical textbooks that could be employed, nor any facilities for laboratory work. But the clinical teaching which Parker gave these men was so successful that one, Dr. Kwantao, subsequently obtained reputation as surgeon and occultist that was almost as widespread as that of his teacher. On one occasion he was sent to work by the Viceroy of Szechuan, nearly 2,000 miles away, upon whom he operated for cataract. He also performed various major surgical operations, one of which was the removing of a tumor which is said to have measured some three and a quarter feet in circumference—a performance which, in those days, must have made an enormous impression on the people, to say nothing of the patient!

The work of training Chinese assistants which Parker thus inaugurated was continued by various medical men who succeeded him, notably by Dr. John G Kerr of the American Presbyterian Mission, who, in a remarkable life of nearly 50 years of medical missionary service at Canton, not only helped to instruct some two hundred students but also made invaluable contributions to the building up of the new Chinese medical literature, which, as we have seen, Benjamin Hobson had been the first to undertake.[6] Kerr personally translated over 20 medical textbooks, compromising thirty-two volumes.

I

Thus was medical education commenced on a humble scale in China, and for the next 50 or 60 years similar classes for the students were organized in various parts of the country, in connection with different mission hospitals. Most of these students came from poor homes and were deficient in general education; but in spite of so many handicaps many of them became valuable workers and rendered great assistance in various hospital centers, both as physicians and evangelists.

[5] The so-called Imperial Medical College at Peking, established from the time of the Yuen Dynasty (A.D. 1280–1368), merely existed for the conferring of degrees on court physicians. No instruction was given, nor were examinations conducted.

[6] Vid. p.46.

Meantime the first steps were being taken towards the provision of a new supply of fully trained Chinese physicians, by the sending abroad of students whose knowledge of English was sufficient to enable them to pursue their medical studies in Europe or America. The first of these was Mr. Wang Fun, who was sent to Edinburgh through the generosity of some British merchants in Hong Kong, and who graduated there with distinction in 1855. He returned to China in 1857, in connection with the London Missionary Society, and Dr. Henderson wrote of him a few years later: "There is not a medical man now in China who has a better knowledge of his profession in all its branches than Dr. Wang Fun."[7]

Many years elapsed before Dr. Wang's example was followed, and indeed it is only in very recent times that a considerable number of Chinese have left their country to study medicine abroad. Most of these have gone to Japan, where, unfortunately, they have not as a rule attached themselves to the higher-grade Japanese medical schools, and thus have failed to secure the full benefits of modern medical science. There have, however, been some notable exception, especially amongst those students who have proceeded to Europe and America, the most conspicuous being Dr. Wu Lien-Teh, a graduate of Cambridge, now Director of the Plague Prevention Service of North Manchuria; Dr. S. P. Chen, also of Cambridge, who has charge both of the Central Hospital and of the Isolation Hospital, Peking; and Dr. F. C. Yen, of Yale, Dean of the Hunan-Yale Medical College at Changsha.

In this connection mention must be made of a brilliant little group of Chinese women students who have studied medicine in America. The first of these was Dr. Y. May King, an adopted daughter of Dr. McCartee of Ningpo, who graduated from the Women's Medical College of the New York Infirmary in 1885, took various post-graduate appointments, and finally returned to China to work in connection with the Reformed Church at Amoy. She was followed a few years later by Miss Hu King-eng, the daughter of a Foochow pastor, who subsequently returned to do splendid work in her native town.

In 1892 no little excitement was caused at the Medical School of the University of Michigan by the arrival of two Chinese girls to study medicine. They were protégés of Miss Howe of Kiu-kiang, the one Miss Mary Stone (Shih Mei-yu) and the other Miss Ida Kahn. They completed their course in 1896, and no more popular figures

[7] Memorials of James Henderson, M.D., p. 179.

took part in the graduation exercises of their year than those two dignified Chinese women in their native dress, of whom President Angell said: "Their future career will be watched with every expectation of eminent success." Their return to Kiu-kiang was made the occasion of an extraordinary popular ovation, the Chinese welcoming them with a huge demonstration in which some forty thousand firecrackers were let off! Dr. Mary Stone remained in Kiu-kiang, where in 1916 she treated no less than twenty-four thousand cases at the Danforth Memorial Hospital and where she developed excellent school for the training of Chinese midwives.[8] Dr. Ida Kahn responded to an invitation to open up medical work in another huge city, Nanchang, where by the successful treatment of the wife of an official she opened the gates to Protestant missionaries.

II

The year 1881 is one that should long be remembered in connection with the development of medical education in China, for it saw the opening of the first medical school established in the country on a modern basis.[9] Its inception was due to Kenneth Mackenzie, who, on hearing that several Chinese students who had been sent to America for collegiate education were being recalled by the Government, at once memorialized the Viceroy of Chihli, Li Hung Chang, petitioning that eight of them might be placed under his care "for the study of medicine and surgery, with a view to their being utilized eventually as medical officers by the Government." Li Hung Chang not only acceded to this request, but also placed suitable premises at Mackenzie's disposable at Tientsin and became responsible for the financial upkeep of the school, giving Mackenzie full freedom for missionary work amongst the students.

Three classes were admitted to the school during Mackenzie's lifetime, each taking a three-year course. All instruction was given in English, mostly by Dr. Mackenzie himself, who revived valuable assistance from Dr. Atterbury of Peking and from some of the British and American naval surgeons stationed at Tienstin. Nineteen men were graduated in all, and though Mackenzie wrote in 1887 that his hopes had not been entirely fulfilled, Dr. Fred Roberts was able to write in the following strain four years later:-

[8] Dr Mary Stone has recently removed to Shanghai, where she has established a large nursing home and private hospital.
[9] Medical Schools were established in China in the reign of Sheng Tsung (A.D. 1068), of the Sung Dynasty, and were still further developed in the Yuen and Ming dynasties. Subsequently, however, they fell into abeyance.

> You will be glad to know that the former labours of Dr. McKinsey, in connection with the government medical school under his charge, have been far from fruitless. Up to the time of his death it seemed to him almost like labour in vain, seeing that the graduates were not successful in obtaining appointments. It is very different now. In close proximity to our own hospital is an imposing building, the Viceroy's hospital, managed for the most part by three of McKinsey's former students, and with the prospect, if well conducted, of doing much good in the healing of the sick. In Port Arthur there is a naval and military hospital and dispensary which is much appreciated by the soldiers, and it also is worked by former students. Others again have been appointed to Wei Hai Wei, a naval station. Dr. Chang has been accepted many months ago for the post of house surgeon to the Alice Memorial Hospital (L.M.S.) Hong Kong; while last but not least, Dr. Mai has been for some time successfully treating the father of the Emperor in Peking.[10]

It is interesting to know that this medical school is still in existence, being now supported by the provincial government of Chihli, and known as the Peiyang Medical College, Tientsin.

In 1887 the Hong Kong College of medicine was opened, with Dr. Manson (now Sir Patrick Manson) as its first Dean. The London Missionary Society was closely connected with the college from its inception, the Society's hospitals being used for practical instruction, and their physicians assisting in the teaching work. It was in that college that Dr. Sun Yat Sen received his education, and formed that friendship with Dr. James Cantile (then professor of Anatomy and Surgery) that was to play so dramatic a part in his future career.

[10] John Kenneth Machenzie, by Mrs Bryson, p. 376.

***

Other small medical schools slowly came into existence, namely as a development of those classes for student-assistants which had been started in connection with various mission hospitals.[11] It was after the Boxer uprising of 1900, when the need for constructive and educative work on a broad basis was brought home to all friends of China, that the first attempt was made to establish a School of Medicine in Peking. This was the first medical college to be established in China by the combination of both British and American medical men, and through the cooperation of missionaries is Chinese representing different religious denominations. It was organized by Dr. Thomas, of the London Missionary Society, who was fortunately successful in securing the patronage and financial support of the dowager Empress and many of the leading Chinese officials, and he received invaluable assistance from such men as the late Sir Robert Heart, Sir Ernest Sasso and Douglas Gray. The college was recognized by the Chinese government from the outset, the Board of Education giving a special diploma to all graduates and making an annual grant for its support of the institution. A very able group of men was obtained as members of the teaching staff, many of whom, alas, passed away in early life. Such men were the late Dr. H. V. Wenham—a man of exceptional charm and brilliant gift, who had gone to China with a view to organizing such an institution himself, and with characteristic unselfishness threw himself into the Peking scheme—and Dr. J. G. Gibb, of St. Bartholomew's, Dr. J. M. Stenhouse, of London Hospital, who died of wounds received during the recent war, and Dr. Francis J Hall, an American physician—men to whom the cause of medical education in China owes a large debt of gratitude. This college in Peking had the distinction of conducting its medical teaching in Chinese, aided by text-books which a special committee had translated into that language.

It was not long before other centres followed Peking for the lead, and missionary medical colleges, both denominational and union, were opened all over the country, with commendable zeal but questionable wisdom. There was not ample room for them all, and many more in addition, if the needs of so vast a country were taken into consideration; but the suitable men who were available to staff such institutions, and of funds from which to supply the extensive buildings and equipment needed, were both so limited that there was no hope unless the number of these colleges was

[11] A series of successful classes of this nature had already been organized by Dr. H. W. Boone at Shanghai, Dr. Van Someren Taylor and Dr. Osgood at Foochow, Dr. Dunean Main and Hangchow, Dr. Christie at Moukden, Dr. Gillison at Hankow, and many others.

produced for any of them would be adequately manned and furnished. At the biennial conference of the China Medical Missionary Association in 1913 a resolution was passed urging that no further medical schools be established until the eight union colleges then in existence were made sufficient.[12] It soon became evident that even that number was far beyond the power of the missions to render effective.

In addition to the eight missionary medical colleges just referred to, all of which were confined to men students, three medical schools for women had also been established in China. In the South, Dr. Mary Fulton—one of the pioneer women physicians in the far east—laid in 1899 the foundation of what has become the Hackett Medical College, Canton. In central China another pioneer worker, Dr. Margaret H Polk, made a similar effort at Soochow; whilst in the north a Union Medical College for women was established in Peking. These three schools not only differ widely in their location, but also in the language employed for the instruction of the students, Cantonese being used at Canton, English at Soochow, and Mandarin at Peking.

Many valuable women workers have received their training in these institutions, but unfortunately the women's colleges, like the others, have been so starved for lack of workers and equipment as severely to cripple the efficiency of their medical instruction. Important steps are now on foot looking to the concentration of women's medical education in their one or two thoroughly efficient schools, and possibly to cooperation with one or other of the men's medical colleges. Such a plan, combined with a large expansion of staff and improved buildings and equipment, should ensure that the important work of training women medical students for the unique service that they can render to their suffering sisters in China will be placed on a satisfactory footing.

III

Meantime, however, important new factors began to appear on the scene. In the first place there came into existence a body of Chinese medical men who had received their training on modern lines, mostly in Europe and America, and who subsequently formed themselves into a National Medical Association of China.[13] The leader of this group, Dr. Wu Lien-teh, who is still known in England as Dr. G.

---

[12] These eight were situated at Moukden, Peking, Tsiman, Hankow, Chengtu, Nanking (with Hangchow), Foochow, and Canton.

[13] Vide Appendix IV.

L. Tuck—the name he adopted while at Cambridge—lost no time in memorializing the Government for the establishment of modern standards of medical education and outlined a suggested syllabus for the purpose. At the same time, various of the Chinese provincial governments began to show their keen interest in this work, not only by opening provincial medical colleges (as at Soochow, Hangchow, etc.), but also by cooperating in the development and support of some of the missionary medical colleges, notably that connected with the work of the Yale Mission at Changsha, and with the Moukden Medical College.

In the second place, other organizations interested in the progress of China began to take a share in the work of medical education. The University of Hongkong, which was established in 1907, incorporated the former College of Medicine. In a similar way were founded the Harvard Medical School at Shanghai; the German Medical Colleges at Shanghai and Tsingtao (both since closed); and the Japanese Medical College at Moukden. But none of these organizations made so large a contribution to the cause of medical education, nor has exerted so profound an influence in the setting of modern standards, as has been effected by the Rockefeller Foundation of New York. During 1914 and 1915 the Foundation dispatched two influential commissions to China, including some of the leading university and medical men of the United States, "to enquire into the condition of medical education, hospitals and public health." After making an extended tour through a large part of China, in which they visited practically all the medical colleges, and personally inspected some eighty-eight hospitals, they issued a careful report, entitled *Medicine in China,*[14] in which they made a series of recommendations to the Foundation, of which the following is a brief summary:-

1) That the Rockefeller Foundation should undertake medical work in China,
2) That the Foundation should, so far as possible, cooperate with existing missionary institutions "which have already done such good work in China."
3) That medical instruction in which the Foundation is concerned should be on the highest practicable standard.
4) That the English language should be the medium of instruction in those medical schools with which the Foundation should become connected.

[14] Published by the Rockefeller Foundation, 61 Broadway, New York.

5) That the Foundation should commence its activities in Peking and ___, if a suitable scheme could be formulated for association with the missionary medical colleges in those two centres: and that, in addition, some assistance should be given to the Canton Christian College and to the Yale Mission in their plans for medical education at Canton and Changsha respectively.

6) That assistance should be given to the development of a higher standard of professional efficiency in various hospitals, commencing with those situated in the fields tributary to the medical schools aided by the Foundation. This assistance should take the form of grants towards the support of increased medical and nursing staffs, business managers, etc., and the provision of laboratory equipment for the improved diagnostic measures.

7) That encouragement should be given to the training of nurses.

The recommendations of this Commission were adopted by the Foundation and a special organization erected for the purpose of putting them into effect: this has been designated the *China Medical Board* of the Rockefeller Foundation.

The First act of this new Board was to enter into arrangements with the London Missionary Society by which the Board acquired the whole property of the Union Medical College, Peking, vesting it in a new Board of Trustees, upon which the various missionary societies interested in the work in Peking, and the China Medical Board, are equally represented. An extensive property, formerly owned by one of the Chinese princes, was purchased, and here there has been erected what is no exaggeration to describe as the most beautiful of modern building in the whole of China, and one of the best-ordered and best-equipped medical schools and hospitals to be found anywhere in the world. An adaptation of Chinese architecture has made it possible to give to the buildings, in addition to the usefulness for which they were planned, beauty of design in harmony with the great architectural monuments in Peking, and pleasing both to the Chinese and to the westerners. A sum approaching two million pounds sterling has been expended on this school, and every effort has been made to ensure that each department should be staffed by expert medical men, and furnished with everything necessary for up-to-date scientific work.

The missionary societies are cooperating in the selection of teachers for the school, and a number of the men who have already received appointments have been drawn from the ranks of medical missionaries. That whole cost of upkeep of the institution, which is, of course, very considerable, is being borne by the Rockefeller Foundation, and there is no question that their action in thus founding a first-class medical school in the capital of China has done more to raise the whole prestige of modern medicine and of medical education than any other step hitherto taken in the country.

Following is from same publication, pages 127–133

V

The theory of medical training and practice described in this chapter is based upon an assumption which has frequently been called in question—that only the fully qualified doctor is good enough for China. Those who challenge this assumption argue that in face of such an un-relieved mass of suffering as the population of China presents, and in a land where indigenous medical methods are so crude, it would be better to aim at quantity rather than quality, and for the mission colleges to turn out hundreds of students with a superficial knowledge of how to treat common ailments or to administer practical first-aid, instead of a mere handful, year by year, of students highly trained and qualified after long and expensive years of study. Such an argument suggests that we are improvising a temporary Red Cross organization to deal with an acute situation which has suddenly developed and which will rapidly improve. If this were the case, there might be some justification for such an *ad hoc* policy. But that does not represent the state of the case at all. We are engaged in the tremendous task of assisting a great and ancient nation to work out a worthy system of medical education and practice. Amongst the leaders of that nation are already to be numbered an influential group of medical men and women who are fully conversant with the best science of the West, and who are eager to see similar standards adopted in their own country. One of them has already expressed himself publicly in the following words:

> However necessary modern medicine may be to this country, I would rather see fewer well qualified men and women with high ideals than a great many poorly-qualified practitioners with indifferent ambitions. For the one class makes for progress, whilst the other leads to stagnation, if not retrogression.[15]

---

[15] Dr Wu Lien-teh, President of the National Medical Association of China, speaking in Canton, January 25th, 1917.

In face of such an utterance as that, how could the representatives of missions possibly justify a policy which, in the West, would be stigmatized as nothing short of "flooding the country with quacks"?

It will no doubt be urged that partially trained men can do a great deal to relieve suffering, and that they can always keep in touch with an up-to-date and well-staffed hospital, to which they can send all their difficult cases. But the real fact is, as everybody knows, that the poorly-trained man is the last person in the world to admit that he has met a difficult case. He would lose face if he did so—or at least he thinks he would.

Furthermore one must remember that the analogy of India and Japan, where a double standard of qualified doctor and licensed medical assistant is frankly recognized, does not hold good in China, where there is no authority to control the activities of the partially trained Chinese doctor. If he is in practice by himself, there is therefore every likelihood of his professional standards gradually degenerating, thus bringing the mission which trained him into disrepute. It is considerations such as these which have led to the adoption by the China Medical Missionary Association of the highest scientific standards (comparable to the best hospital-schools of London, Edinburgh, or Baltimore) in those medical colleges whose diplomas they recognize. And this contribution to the life and ideals of the Chinese people represents an achievement of which the Association, and the Missions which called it into being, has every right to be proud. Not only has this policy been followed in the general medical curriculum, but the Council on Medical Education has also taken the progressive step of outlining a two-year course of pre-medical study in the laboratory sciences, to be taken by students previous to entering upon their five years' medical training. This requirement is now enforced at the leading medical schools, and not only ensures a sound scientific foundation in the pre-medical subjects (chemistry, physics, and biology), but also allows for a re-arrangement of the medical curriculum by which the final year can be wholly devoted to clinical and pathological investigations. This emphasis upon practical work in laboratory and ward is of special importance in China where centuries of memorizing, whilst they have produced a marvelous faculty of recollection, have also left an unhappy legacy of passive mental receptivity, to the discouragement of aggressive thought.

There is always a demand for the well-trained graduate. The Government, the railway companies, the national army and the progressive communities in the Treaty Ports vie with mission hospitals throughout the country for his services. And the demand will certainly increase faster than it can possibly be met. Thus there is becoming established in the mind of the Chinese people an appreciation of the trained and competent doctor with which neither quackery nor superstition will be able to compete. To meet this growing demand not only is there a need for an increasing number of fully-qualified Chinese physicians, but it is essential that all medical science should be available in the language of the people. The China Medical Missionary Association has been fully alive to this fact. Special Publication and Terminology Committees have been at work for many years, translating several of the leading medical text-books,[16] and preparing a full vocabulary of scientific terms. Dr P. B. Cousland, of the English Presbyterian Mission, has been set aside for the direction of this work, whilst in recent years a strong translation department has been organized in connection with the Tsinan Medical School, under the able leadership of Drs T. Gillison and P. L. McAll and their Chinese associates. At first this important work had to be carried on without any certain guarantee that the scientific terms so created would be recognized by the Chinese Government. That stage has now happily passed. Within recent years the Central Education Board and other official bodies have appointed their own representatives to act with the Terminology Committee, thus giving an official imprimatur to their decisions. All medical terms are now being revised and added to by this joint body, the Chinese Government defraying the cost of publishing them and the China Medical Board also assisting most generously in this essential work of translation and publication. It is impossible to conclude this chapter without referring to the encouraging attitude which the Chinese Government is beginning to adopt towards the development of medical education.

This was clearly shown by the great step which was taken by the Board of the Interior in November 1913 in giving permission for human dissection and post-mortem examinations to be practiced in medical schools, thus removing the last obstacle to the effective teaching of anatomy and physiology. More recently, at the Conference of the China Medical Missionary Association in 1920, the 133rd representative of the Board of Education gave an important address, in which he outlined the policy of the Board as including the provision of a modern medical college in each province, the opening of an institute for research, and the registration of

[16] Amongst those already translated, or shortly to be published, are Gray's Anatomy, Halliburton's Physiology, Cunningham's Practical Anatomy, Lewis and Stroh's Histology, Osler's Medicine, Rose and Carless's Surgery, Fuchs' Ophthalmology, Stengel's Pathology, Hiss and Zinsser's Bacteriology, Hare's Therapeutics, Hutchinson and Rainy's Clinical Methods, Holt's Diseases of Childhood, and many others.

medical practitioners. One provincial governor—the progressive Governor of Shansi—has already commenced to erect buildings for a future school of medicine, and is now sending government students to Peking and Tsinan in the hope that they may ultimately form members of the teaching staff of the Shansi Medical College. Other schools are gradually being opened by the central and provincial governments as funds permit, and there is every reason to expect that in course of time China will be covered by well-staffed and well-equipped institutions. It will probably take many years to reach that stage, and meanwhile medical men and women from Great Britain and from North America are counting it the highest privilege to be allowed to assist China in this tremendous task.

Following is from same publication, pages 156–170

Chapter VII: Research and public health

> To wrest from nature the secrets which have perplexed philosophers in all ages, to track to their sources the causes of disease, to correlate the vast stores of knowledge, that they may be quickly available for the prevention and cure of disease—these are our ambitions.
>
> SIR WILLIAM OSLER, *The Vocation of Medicine and Nursing*, 1919.

WHEREVER western medicine spread in China—pioneered, as we have seen, by the missionary doctor—the possibility of advancing medical science and benefiting human sufferers by patient research and careful investigation was always before the minds of its most progressive leaders. Although the medical missionary does not go abroad with the primary purpose of scientific discovery, his sphere of service includes within its orbit everything that will help to throw new light upon the incidence and causation of disease, and will mitigate or prevent the sufferings of the people. Thus it is that the prosecution of medical research and the promulgation of public health measures are matters of vital concern to the true success of the medical missionary enterprise.

That remarkable trio, Colledge, Parker, and Bridgman, were fully alive to this fact from the outset, and in the first official pronouncement of the objects of the Medical Missionary Society in China, issued in 1838, they referred to it in the following terms:

> Countries are not more characterized by the form and nature of the soil and its productions, than they are by the prevalence of certain maladies and a partial or complete exemption from others. The contemplation of disease as influenced by the position and height of a country, its inland or maritime location, and the general habits of the people, conducts the student to a most engaging range of medical philosophy, while it discloses many important lessons to assist him in the way of benefiting his fellow creatures. The advantages derivable from such a contemplation have been acknowledged at all periods, and in all quarters. To secure these advantages it is required that a book should be kept in all the institutions connected with this Society, into which an entry will be made of all important cases, with a notice, not only of the disease and the treatment pursued, but also of the province, habits, and other circumstances bearing upon the history of each individual...

A knowledge of the language will open another door of enquiry, namely in relation to the substances used in Chinese pharmacy and to their peculiar modes of preparation. As the reciprocations of health and sickness are various in different countries, so Providence has displayed a corresponding variety in the distribution of remedies. This correspondence between the prevailing disorders of any country and the remedies which the hand of nature has provided is often very striking, and will become more so as the subject is investigated. We may therefore look for a great many valuable additions to our dispensatories, while an extended acquaintance with disease under new modifications will help to enlarge and complete our system of nosology.

Long before the China Medical Missionary Association came into existence in 1886, men were beginning to contribute original papers to the pages of the scientific journals. As early as 1842 William Lockhart published a "Treatise on Chinese Midwifery" in the *Dublin Journal of Medical Science*, whilst ten years later Benjamin Hobson read before the China Branch of the Royal Asiatic Society an important paper on "Leprosy in China and the East."

I

There were many difficulties attending the pursuance of scientific research in China in those early days, chief amongst which was the superstitious fear which the Chinese cherished towards any interference with the cadaver, owing to their traditional attitude regarding the spirits of the departed. In spite of that fact, Parker performed his first post-mortem examination as long ago as 1849, whilst Dr. James Henderson, in his report for 1862, not only referred to a number of similar autopsies in the London Mission Hospital, during the preceding year, but even stated that he had been able to give to Chinese practitioners in that city a series of demonstrations of surgical operations performed upon the dead body.

A second disability arose from the conditions under which medical work had to be carried on at first, owing both to lack of adequate staff and equipment, and also to the need for avoiding anything that might offend the susceptibilities of the people. It may be confidently stated that the largest sacrifice which the medical missionary of former days had to face in undertaking work in the interior of China was the sacrifice of his scientific ambitions, and the lack of opportunity for professional consultation and cooperation. He found himself surrounded by a mass of fascinating problems to which he longed to devote time and thought, and by a wealth of clinical cases which he longed to investigate; but how to carry out this desire, and at the same time do justice to the great objective which had brought him to China, was indeed a matter of serious difficulty.

In most instances the doctor was the solitary administrator of a large and busy hospital, and in all probability the only medical adviser for a scattered community of missionaries and other European and American residents, in a vast district where communications were far from easy, and transport very slow. He had to carry the responsibility for the daily treatment of in-patients and out-patients, for the engaging and supervising of every member of the hospital staff, for the keeping of accounts, for the superintendence of the records of the institution, for the maintenance of the necessary stock of supplies, and for the conduct of all correspondence with home supporters. The organization and carrying out of the spiritual work of the hospital—possibly, also, of the total church or school—was upon his shoulders, and represented to him the most important work of his life. Often enough the superintendence of building operations in the hospital and elsewhere, to say nothing of innumerable clerical duties and committees, put in a claim for the remnant of his time and strength. How then, in face of such endless duties, was he ever to find the necessary leisure and energy for scientific pursuits?

It says much for the professional keenness of the medical force in China that, in spite of all these many difficulties, there have always been a number of physicians who have found means of maintaining the scientific side of their work, and the pages of the *China Medical Journal* during the last thirty-three years of its existence, as well as occasional articles in the *Journal of Tropical Medicine* and other medical periodicals, bear eloquent testimony to the valuable contributions which have been made in the past by such men and women.[17]

Recent years have witnessed a great advance along these lines. The biennial conferences of the China Medical Missionary Association, which at one time were largely devoted to the discussion of questions of general medical mission policy, are becoming increasingly valuable from the scientific aspect also. At the last conference[18] over one hundred original theses were sent in by members, with the result that simultaneous meetings of a technical character were held every afternoon throughout the conference. Four separate sections were formed, representing Anthropology, Medicine, Surgery, and Special Diseases. In each section important papers were read and helpful discussions took place. At the same conference an "Anatomical and Anthropological Society" was inaugurated, for the purpose of pursuing special investigation in that department.

Prior to that date, at a similar gathering of the Association, a special Research Committee had been appointed, with a view to stimulating scientific investigation and collecting reliable data. This Committee has issued a number of valuable reports from time to time, and has already made some important contributions to our knowledge of medical conditions in China, particularly in the department of helminthology. Two former members of that Committee, Dr. W. H. Jefferys of ___ and Dr. J. L. Maxwell (Jr.) of Formosa, prepared an excellent text-book on the diseases of China. It is full of most interesting information concerning the distribution of disease in the Far East, and was published in 1910 by a Philadelphia publisher.[19]

---

[17] *Vide* list in Appendix I, page 209.
[18] February 1920.
[19] *Disease of China*, by Jefferys and Maxwell.

II

The main investigation that has so far been carried out in China has followed three distinct paths—historical, physiological, and clinical—and it may be of interest to give some indication as to the lines upon which it has proceeded, or is proceeding today.

1. Historical Investigation

From earliest days the exponents of western medicine in China have recognized that amidst much that is unscientific and unreliable in Chinese medical lore there must assuredly be a great deal of correct and useful observation, particularly as regards the course of various diseases, and the action of such medicaments as are in general use amongst Chinese practitioners. Unfortunately, as was pointed out in the opening chapter, the absence of a professional spirit amongst the doctors, or of any conception of cooperation with regard to medical knowledge, has prevented the publication of such discoveries, so that the task of the historical investigator is a very difficult one. But there is every reason to believe that a fund of interesting information, and possibly also the knowledge of new remedies for some complaints, awaits the patient search of the scientific student who has time and skill for the unravelling of the secrets of Chinese therapeusis.

Of those who have made the chief contributions to our knowledge of Chinese medicine the most noteworthy are the American missionary, Dr. J. C. Thomson of Macao,[20] whose interesting writings have filled many pages of the *China Medical Journal*; Dr. James Henderson of ____, who crowded more useful activities into his brief five years of life in China than anyone before or since; and Dr. John Dudgeon, the first Englishman to hold the position of Professor of Medicine in a Chinese College.[21]

Dr. Henderson's paper on "The Medicine and Medical Practice of the Chinese," which was read before the North China Branch of the Royal Asiatic Society in 1864, and for which he was awarded the Fellowship of the Royal College of Surgeons, Edinburgh, is one of the most lucid contributions ever made to this subject.[22] Commencing with the beginnings of medical knowledge in all parts of the world, Henderson showed convincingly at what point China had missed the stream of progress, and gave a graphic description of anatomy and physiology as interpreted in Chinese

[20] Not to be confused with Dr. J. C. Thomson of Edinburgh, who worked for many years in Hongkong.
[21] This was the Tung Wen College, Peking, to which a scientific department was added in 1865, and of which Rev. W. A. P. Martin, L.L.D., became President in 1869.
[22] *Proceedings, North China Branch, Royal Asiatic Society*, 1864.

medical literature. His article also included an extensive list of Chinese medical works, commencing with the earliest treatises, ascribed to the teachings of Shen-Nung and Hwang-Ti many centuries before Christ, and concluding with the famous "Yu-tswan-e-tsung-kin-kien," published in ninety volumes in the year 1740.

Most of the books which Henderson mentions consist of dissertations by ancient physicians on every imaginable complaint and symptom; elaborate theories, mostly of a philosophical nature, as to their causation; and innumerable prescriptions for their relief. In addition to these, however, is the great Chinese Materia Medica (Pen-ts'ao-kang-muh), which was compiled by Li Shi-chen in the middle of the sixteenth century by command of the Emperor, and which contains some seventy volumes and eleven hundred illustrations. This interesting work, although over 300 years old, refers to a large number of drugs well known to practitioners of western medicine (such, for example, as sulphur, magnesia, calomel, aconite, etc.), and specially mentions one drug (probably hyoscyamus) as being of value as an analgesic for surgical operations.[23] The book also includes a vast number of substances which practitioners in the West have never learned to regard as of medical value. It classifies all drugs into the following varieties:

Water, fire and earth.
Minerals.
Vegetables (herbs, grains, culinary herbs, fruits and trees).
Animal (insects, scaly animals, shelly animals, birds, hairy animals, human secretions, etc.).

Dr. J. B. Neal of Shantung, now President of the Shantung Christian University, carried out a series of analyses in 1888 and the following years, with the aid of his assistants, and their results served to show which of the ordinary drugs procurable at the Chinese drug-shop were free from impurity, and what adulteration was present in those that were impure. A similar investigation, of great practical value, was made by Dr. W. Wilson and Dr. Douthwaite, who published methods for purifying and utilizing many of these drugs, thus effecting a large and most welcome saving in their hospital drug bills.

[23] Wa-T'o, the father of Chinese surgery, who lived in the third century A.D., is said to have performed a large number of major operations, including laparotomies, upon patients who had been previously drugged with Cannabis Indica. He is also credited with the use of a special powder, which he applied to his operation wounds to prevent them suppurating! Unfortunately, this courageous adventurer came to an untimely end, for on advising a military officer, who had consulted him about severe headaches, to submit to a trephining operation, the latter promptly had him executed for making a suggestion tantamount to an attempt on his life!

A very interesting and comprehensive list of Chinese medicines (including 1,575 varieties), prepared by Mr. F. A. Morgan, was published by the Imperial Maritime Customs in 1889, whilst in 1911 Dr. G. A. Stuart of Nanking brought out a valuable work entitled *Chinese Materia Medica: Vegetable Kingdom*, embodying the results of much careful research. The death of Dr. Stuart unfortunately prevented the completion of his investigations into the other volumes of the Chinese Pharmacopoeia. That great work has never yet been translated into English, although Mr. Daniel Hanbury and others have published very valuable notes upon it.[24] The subject of Chinese pharmacology thus remains practically virgin soil for the investigator, and a vast number of drugs referred to in Chinese medical books have never yet been identified or classified. Possibly some of the enterprising graduates of the newer medical schools in China will enter this fascinating field of research, and make discoveries which will lay the whole world under a debt of obligation to them.

2. Anatomical and Physiological Investigation

In addition to the efforts of the newly formed Anatomical and Anthropological Society in China, which has already published an interesting series of papers as a supplement to the *China Medical Journal*, one of the chief tasks to which the Research Committee of the China Medical Missionary Association has addressed itself has been the collecting of accurate data, as to the physical conditions of the average Chinese, in comparison with Europeans and Americans of equal age.

This investigation, carried out especially by Dr. Duncan Whyte of Swatow and Dr. Arthur Shoemaker of Peking, has already established definite standards as to height, weight, chest measurement, urinalysis, etc., which are essential to a correct appreciation of the effects of disease, or to any scientific determination of dosology for Chinese patients.[25]

Similar statistics are also being gathered with regard to various anatomical measurements, etc.

In addition to these investigations a most important branch of research work has recently been commenced in the study of the food-value of the chief articles of Chinese diet. Physiological text-books dealing with the subject of Dietetics are necessarily founded upon a study of those substances which go to make up the

---

[24] Vide *Pharmaceutical Journal and Transactions*, July, August 1860; May, July, October, November, December 1861; February 1862.

[25] Amongst these standards are the following:
Average height: Adult male in North China, 5 ft. 7 in., male in South China, 5 ft. 4 in., female in South China, 4 ft. 11 ½ in. Average weight of adult, 116 lbs. Chest measurement of adult, 28 in. to 31 in.

ordinary western diet, and, for that reason, are of but little value in a country where the staple food differs widely from western standards. Of what advantage is it to the physician in China to be told the number of calories in half a pound of beef-steak when his patient's chief meal consists of two large bowls of rice, a little fresh vegetable, and some bean-curd? It is plain that this whole subject of Dietetics needs to be studied afresh in every country, if scientific deductions are to be drawn from it for use in disease.

One of the first papers published on this topic was written in 1915 by Dr. J. B. Neal,[26] and consisted of a series of studies carried out by himself and his students in the physiological laboratory of the Tsinan Medical School. A further investigation, dealing specifically with the analysis and food-value of Chinese bean-curd, was made in the same laboratory by Dr. P. C. Kiang and Professor Adolph during 1919, whilst a similar research was conducted at the Peking Union Medical College by Professor Wilson and Miss Embrey. The results of these investigations were presented at the Medical Conference in 1920.[27] A start has thus been made, and the next few years will no doubt add fresh contributions to the knowledge of the subject, which will make it possible to deal scientifically with the vast range of digestive disorders which are met with amongst the Chinese.

3. Clinical and Pathological Investigation

But the chief investigations which have so far been carried out have been in the clinical field and, more recently, in the fields of pathology and bacteriology, and in this respect China naturally offers an unrivalled opportunity for research. Numerous conditions are met with in that country which are seldom found in the West, and those complaints which are common to all lands are seen in an aggravated and unusual form in China, owing to long years of neglect, or to irritation from sepsis and other causes.

Space does not avail, nor would it be appropriate, to give any detailed list of the conditions which are commonly seen in China, but it may be stated that practically every ailment recognized by western physicians is to be found in the Far East, and a good many others besides—although a few diseases, such as appendicitis, acute rheumatism and lobar pneumonia, appear to be distinctly more rare in certain parts

[26] *China Medical Journal*, 1916, p. 9.
[27] Vide *China Medical Journal*, 1920, pp. 268, 503.

of China than in Europe. Tuberculosis, in all its forms, is every bit as rampant in China as in Europe, and it is a strange fact that while the Chinese patient has developed an excellent immunity from certain microbic infections—for example, from typhus or infection from ordinary cocci—he appears to have an extremely poor resistance to the tubercle bacillus. Venereal disease is also universally met with, too often accompanied by sepsis, and characterized by deep ulceration and necrosis. Tumours of every size, shape, and age are to be seen anywhere daily, while dyspeptic troubles of every description, malignant disease, rectal complaints, and ophthalmic conditions are all extremely common.

Of the conditions which are less frequently seen in western countries than in China mention must specially be made of intestinal parasites, which formed the first subject of investigation conducted by the Research Committee of the China Medical Missionary Association. A large number of varieties of metazoal parasites are met with in China, particularly in the Yang-tse valley, and their distribution, symptomatology, etc., have been carefully worked out in recent years by medical missionaries in that area. In many cases this has meant considerable original research, particularly in regard to the recognition of metazoa, hitherto barely known in China (*e.g.* schistosomum japonicum, fasciolopsis buskii, etc.), and the result of this study has been of the greatest service in throwing light upon conditions not previously understood. These helminths are now shown to be responsible for a wide range of abdominal and blood diseases and obscure fevers, and in all the more up-to-date hospitals in China a routine faecal examination is conducted upon every patient admitted to the wards.

Malaria, kala-azar, beri-beri, elephantiasis, leprosy, and a host of other tropical diseases are also very common, particularly in central and southern China, whilst the dysenteries, the typhoid and para-typhoid groups, cholera and other diseases of the intestinal tract, are met with in almost every part of the country.

In addition to the great researches of Sir Patrick Manson, much valuable work has already been done by medical missionaries and others in investigating and describing some of these conditions. It is to the late Dr. O. T. Logan of Changteh, Hunan, and to Dr. F. W. Goddard of Shaoshing, that we owe much of our present knowledge of the distribution of intestinal parasites in China. It was Dr. S. Cochran, of Hwai Yuan, who first discovered that the Leishman-Donovan bodies of kala-azar were present in the lymph-nodes of patients affected with that disease. It was Dr. E. C. Peake of Tientsin who described the new blood parasite which appeared to be responsible for the condition of anaemia and dropsy from which many inhabitants of the flooded districts of Chihli suffered in 1918. It was Dr. Duncan Whyte of Swatow who drew attention to the prevalence of thrombo-angiitis obliterans amongst Chinese patients. And many others might similarly be named. Interesting statistics have also been published in many of the hospital reports as to the incidence of disease in different parts of the country. In this connection reference must specially be made to the valuable information regarding vesical calculus in China which has been collected at the Canton Hospital, where over three thousand operations for that complaint have now been performed.

But when all has been said, it must be confessed that up to the present time only the fringe of clinical research in China has been touched. A large variety of fevers and other complaints exist, the etiology of which is completely unknown, whilst innumerable other problems are awaiting investigation. With the better equipment which hospitals are now securing, particularly in the matter of laboratory apparatus, and with the larger staffs and the advent of keen Chinese graduates, this promising field of study can be attacked with new hope of success, and every year should see additional discovery to our general knowledge of Chinese medical conditions and their treatment.

Following is from same publication, pages 180–192

Chapter VIII: The outlook today

> Methinks I see in my mind a noble and puissant nation rousing herself like a strong man after sleep, and shaking her invincible locks; methinks I see her as an eagle, mewing her mighty youth, and kindling her undazzled eyes at the full mid-day beam.
>
> – *Milton,* Areopagitica.

Nearly a hundred years have passed since Thomas Colledge opened his first hospital in China. The time has come when we may ask ourselves what has been the harvest of these years.

Has modern medicine inspired a nobler conception than the practice of the old Chinese physician? Has it replaced conjecture and superstition with assured diagnosis and scientific truth? Is there promise of a high professional standard and a new ideal of service? Is there hope of advance and success in fighting the great battle for China's true health?

I

Before we attempt to estimate the effect which has been produced by the introduction of western medicine into China, we must first notice how pitiably under-staffed the medical forces have been and still are, and how insignificant is the total work which has so far been accomplished when calculated in purely quantitative terms. Let us examine the case critically, and see if there is not justification for this sweeping assertion.

At the present time the total number of fully qualified western-trained physicians practicing amongst the Chinese probably does not exceed 1500—men and women.[28] Now let us suppose that each physician can, on an average, give adequate medical attendance to 2,000 people. This is probably an exaggerated estimate, for in Great Britain, with one physician to every 1,100 of the population, and with all those additional safeguards to health which preventative medicine, sanitation, and welfare movements have built up, the profession is far from being over manned. But let us suppose that by energetic effects our 1,500 fully qualified physicians in China can do full justice to the physical needs of 2,000 people each—what, after all, does it amount to? It merely means that adequate medical care is provided for 3,000,000 people out of a population of approximately 860,000,000. In other words, there is no chance of the quackery of the unqualified being replaced by the competent medical treatment of fully trained physicians until the number of qualified doctors in China is one hundred and twenty times as many as it is today.

A similar figure can be arrived at by a different method of estimating. Statistics which have been compiled in connection with the operation of the National Insurance Act in Great Britain demonstrate that about sixty per cent of insured persons require medical attendance each year, and that the average number of medical visits (either at the doctor's surgery or at the patient's home) works out at about six per annum.[29] If such figures were applied to China it would mean that about 216,000,000 people would need to consult a physician each year, and that their total visits would amount to 1,296,000,000. But the total number of patients seen in all hospitals and dispensaries in China, or in the private consulting rooms of western trained Chinese physicians, probably does not exceed 1,800,000 per annum, whilst

[28] The number of western trained doctors in China is often quoted as 2,000, but that figure would include a large number of students who have received practical training in mission hospitals etc., but have never had the opportunity of taking the modern medical course, and who should not therefore be counted amongst the fully qualified practitioners.

[29] From information supplied by the Ministry of Health. If the number of medical visits annually be calculated on the total number of insured, and not on the 60 per cent who require medical attendance in any year, the average works out at 3.6 per annum.

the total number of visits which they pay is less than 5,000,000.[30] This means again that out of 120 sick persons who need competent medical help only one obtains it.

It may, of course, be argued that such a comparison loses sight of the fact that a large number of people in this country (especially those whose medical attendance is provided for by insurance) seek a doctor's advice for conditions which are quite trivial. On the other hand, in China there are a number of serious medical disorders which are not now seen in the West, thanks to the success of preventative medicine and sanitation. The incidence of disease is much greater there than it is in our own land, and, speaking generally, disease is apt to assume a much more serious form, and as a consequence the number of patients requiring medical help is very much larger. We are more than safe therefore in using these figures in comparison, and may assert that with all our medical missionaries and nurses from Europe and North America, and with our other western trained physicians, it is doubtful whether we are yet touching more than 0.8 per cent of China's patients. In other words, 992 out of every 1000 sick people in China still have no fully qualified medical help.

II

Whilst, however, it must be admitted, in face of such figures, that the practitioners of Western medicine are still too few in number to make any appreciable impression upon the total amount of sickness and suffering in China, there can be no question as to the far-reaching influence of their work, particularly among the progressive classes, and in the large cities and treaty ports.

In the first place, it is questionable whether there has been any other agency at work in China during this last century which has done so much to gain the confidence and goodwill of the people, and to dispel that miasma of fear and suspicion which beclouded all intercourse between East and West in former years.

It is startling to notice how great progress has been made in this direction. Only a few short years ago every political or social upheaval in China, every occasion of discontent and anxiety, was accomplished by an outburst of anti-foreign feeling, often culminating in riots and bloodshed. Did the heavens appear as brass and refuse to send the needed rain upon the parched crops? Then it was the foreigner whose presence was irritating the gods and producing the disaster. Did pestilence appear in

[30] Of these totals, the returns of mission hospitals show a little over 1,000,000 patients per annum, paying slightly less than 3,000,000 visits.

the district and carry out hundreds of children whose parents lived in daily defiance of the laws of hygiene? It was the western barbarian who had bewitched them and who, under the cloak of religion and charity, was poisoning the wells and hatching nefarious schemes for their undoing. Did bandits roam the countryside, and unpaid soldiers loot the helpless villagers? There would never be peace so long as these strangers were permitted to live amongst them. And so on.

But what a contrast today, when political revolution is invariably accomplished by proclamations holding the life and property of the foreigner inviolate; when the first act of the officials, at times of disorder, is to dispatch troops to reassure and protect their western guests; when good feeling and gratitude and appreciation are the commonly expressed sentiments of all classes towards the work of the foreign doctor. The hospitals' own work and influence have been the largest factor in bringing about the change. They have represented a new and tangible expression of brotherhood and sympathy which none could gainsay, even in times of misunderstanding and hostility. Thus they have won their way, not by the amount of suffering and sickness which they have relieved, but rather by the spirit which they have manifested.

In the second place, the mission hospital has been one of the most effective means of presenting and spreading Christianity in China. This it has done, not merely by dispelling misapprehension and producing a favorable atmosphere for the unprejudiced reception of the truth, but also by creating an ideal opportunity for the systematic teaching of the Christian message.

Many a patient who has entered a hospital ward with little or no interest beyond the immediate needs of his pain-racked body, has had his whole imagination fired by the story of the life of Jesus Christ that has been told him there; and many such have gone out of the hospital professed followers of Him, witnessing to His power in districts where formerly His name had never been heard.

Again, it may be confidently claimed that the practice of modern medicine, in the hands of men and women who have endeavored to make their medical work a true expression of Christ and His teaching, has had a profound effect upon the attitude which the Chinese have themselves come to adopt towards the indigent and needy. A new sense of responsibility is being manifested in China today, especially by the younger and better educated Chinese who have come under the influence of Christian teaching, and this expresses itself in an increasing effort to assist the poor and the suffering.

I well remember, on one occasion, being asked to address a large company of students in North China on the need for public health measures. I wanted to speak about community life and social service and such-like, but I found it most difficult to discover any adequate expression in the Chinese language with which to convey these ideas. That was less than ten years ago. To-day, one can hardly pick up any Chinese newspaper—one certainly cannot pick up a student publication—without being confronted with these new terms on almost every page. A new social conscience has awakened. We see it in the birth of the nursing profession. We see it in the "model city" of Nantungchow, with its modern banks and mills, its refuges for the aged and afflicted, its blind and deaf asylums, its orphanage and its schools. We see it in the model prisons, now a feature of several of the chief cities of China. We see it in the free dispensary which is maintained by the boys of Nan Kai School, that great educational establishment at Tientsin under the able leadership of Mr. Chang Po-ling. We see it in the Boys' Clubs; in the night schools; in the Y.M.C.A. work amongst the returned coolies from France: and in the special investigations into the economic conditions of various classes of workers. As we watch these innovations in ancient China, we realize that a new force of enormous potentiality is at work today, and that it is the Christian leaders who are pioneering the reforms.

Before the Revolution of 1911 the work of the Red Cross, and the humane treatment of the wounded in battle, were almost unknown in China. Today the Chinese Red Cross Society has its branches in every province, and its hospitals in numerous cities.

Another hopeful sign of the times is the way in which the Chinese people are extending financial support towards the hospitals and medical schools which have been organized in their country. Ever since the day when How Qua, the landlord of the building in which Parker had his first hospital, refused to accept any rent, the Chinese have repeatedly given proofs of their appreciation of such forms of medical charity, and of their willingness to share in the financial support of these institutions. Recent statistics have shown that over fifty per cent of the cost of upkeep of the mission hospitals in China today is borne by the Chinese themselves, and that no less than twenty-seven per cent of the hospitals are now entirely self-supporting, apart from the salaries of the foreign staff.[31]

Such financial assistance is not confined to private subscriptions and fees: for in many instances it is also derived from official sources. The most striking example of such co-

[31] *An enquiry into the Scientific Efficiency of Mission Hospitals in China*, pp. 33,37.

operation is the agreement entered into by the officials of the Hunan Government and the Yale Mission in China for the establishment of the Hunan-Yale Medical College and Hospital at Changsha. The Hunan Government has undertaken to provide no less than $50,000 per annum towards the institution, in addition to large sums towards the purchase of land and the erection of the initial buildings; and although constant revolution and military occupation have since impoverished the province to a pitiful extent, a most determined effort has been made to fulfil the compact.

Similar generosity has been shown in other cases. The officials and gentry in the city of Anking have for some years past contributed the sum of $8,000 per annum towards the support of the American (Protestant-Episcopal) Hospital in that centre, whilst within the last few months the provincial government of Shantung, at the insistence of the Civil Governor, has passed a bill approving of an annual appropriation of $5,000 from the provincial budget towards the support of the University Hospital at Tsinan.

But the most encouraging feature of all has been the action which the Chinese have taken in many cities in establishing and supporting hospitals and dispensaries of their own. The Central and Isolation Hospitals at Peking, erected and maintained by the Chinese, and now under the able superintendence of Dr. S. P. Chen (a graduate of Cambridge, and S. Thomas's Hospital, London), are excellent examples of first-class institutions which we may confidently expect to see multiplied all over China. In other cities also, Government Hospitals are now beginning to spring up. Many of these, it is interesting to note, have both "Eastern" and "Western" departments, patients being allowed to choose whether they will be treated by Chinese medicine or in accordance with western methods, in either case receiving medical treatment freely, or at very small cost.

These new Chinese hospitals are affording an excellent opportunity for co-operation on the part of medical missionaries and nurses, and in some of the larger cities local medical societies are now being organized for the purpose of providing a common ground on which the staffs of the Government and Mission Hospitals can meet for social intercourse and mutual consultation. At the same time applications are being received by the Nurses' Training Schools, which, as we have seen, are at present all connected with medical missions, for a supply of trained nurses for the new Government Hospitals.

It will thus be seen that while the quantitative side of the work which has so far been accomplished by the practitioners of Western medicine in China has been very insignificant, the qualitative side of the enterprise has been extraordinarily impressive and effectual. This at once brings us face to face with the significant fact that it is not the amount of work done by the medical missionary of today which is the most important factor in his success; it is the kind of work he is able to perform which means everything. He cannot hope to do more than touch the barest fringe of China's suffering and sickness. But where he does touch, he can see to it that his impress is true and vital, and that the tiny contribution which he is able to make is of such a quality as to reach to the very depths of China's physical and spiritual need, and to give her the very best that can be offered in the Name of Christ.

There was a time, not so many years ago, when the whole problem of world evangelization was worked out as a kind of mathematical problem, and many a fervid appeal that has been made on the basis of the number of foreign missionaries who would be required to evangelize the whole of China in a given time.

But we are learning more and more in these days that the saving of the world is not a question of mathematical formulae; it is problem of spiritual agriculture; not the physical presentation of a certain dogma to the people of a country by a host of foreign agents, but the sowing of spiritual seeds which have the capacity of indigenous growth and of limitless reproduction. It is the quality of the seeds we plant that matters most.

Some years ago a kindly-disposed American missionary in the province of Shantung was greatly distressed at the poor character of the peanuts, from the cultivation of which thousands of the Chinese in that province eked out a precarious existence. On the next furlough he spent a large amount of time consulting agricultural experts in his native country, and attempting to secure from them a better specimen of peanut for introduction into China. He had no means to set up every small farmer with nuts, but he could ensure that those which he introduced were the very finest that were grown in his own land. And today farmers all over that extensive province are under a deep obligation for his kindly thought and far-reaching effort.

Surely the same rule applies to the medical missionary enterprise. It is altogether beyond the power of missionary societies to cure all the ills of China, and probably God never intended that they should. In every country He is raising up people of the land to be His witness, and to do the great work of evangelizing and uplifting. But to us has been entrusted the inestimable privilege of setting some of these new forces into operation; or, to change the metaphor, of sketching an outline which other and abler hands will fill in. How infinitely important then that we sketch it aright, a worthy image of Him whom we would represent to His children who at present do not know Him.

Following is from same publication, pages 199–206

IV

It is not enough that these things should be understood in China. Their importance must be fully appreciated in Britain and in America also before ever they can become actualities out there. And that is why this book has been written. Four outstanding needs confront us:-

1) A deliberate far-sighted policy, which constantly takes stock of the whole medical missionary enterprise, must be maintained by the Boards at home as well as clamored for by the men in the field. Such a policy must ever look to the devolution of medical responsibility on to Chinese shoulders, the education of all classes in the means for fighting disease and ignorance, and the impressing of the whole Chinese Church with its duty and privilege in the care of the sick. It must keep careful watch upon the newer movements in China, readjusting itself continually to the requirements of a changing scene, and deliberately throwing on the scrap-heap such methods as no longer serve their end in the most effectual manner.

   This will often entail the sacrifice of individual or denominational interests for the sake of the larger good, but if, in the process, such sacrifice brings about the uniting of Christian forces, the increased efficiency and economy so secured will more than compensate for the loss. There is a failure somewhere in our Christian faith and practice—or at least in our missionary statesmanship—when two or more under-staffed mission hospitals exist separately in the same city, each unable to do thoroughly effective work. And such an example cannot but weaken our witness to the love of God and the unity of our faith, as well as proving a serious detriment to medical progress and efficiency.

   There are still some cities in China where such a state of things exists. But there are others in which the medical missionary efforts of different Societies have been united with striking success, as, for example, in the University

Hospital at Nanking, the Union Hospital at Huchowfu, etc. Where formerly there were three hospitals in Nanking, each belonging to a different mission, and each under-manned and ill-equipped, one excellent union institution is now in existence to which all these missions co-operate, and in the conduct of which each doctor is able to develop his own special department.

These great union medical schemes have a value that is far greater than the sum of the efficiency of the several units. They stand not only for a wealth of medical experience and knowledge, but for a united presentation of that which is the heart and the common ground of Christian truth.

2) A sustained attempt must be made to secure the services of trained Chinese physicians in all our hospitals and other branches of medical missionary work, and to accord them positions of full responsibility and trust. There is no student of the missionary enterprise who will not agree with this in theory, but so far as we have gone at present, it would be ridiculous to pretend that the policy of missions towards promoting the full development of Chinese leadership and initiative is carried out at the expense of the foreign missionary and his ideas. There are but few Mission Boards which are yet prepared to subsidize Chinese work without demanding control. Many missions have not even appointed a qualified Chinese doctor on their hospital staff, much less entrusted the lives of their representatives to his care—whilst in many other centers the Chinese doctor is regarded merely as the employee of the mission, or designated an "assistant" at best.

Chinese physicians or surgeons who have taken the full medical course in a modern medical school, and are elected to positions in our mission hospitals, must be given exactly the same status as their European or American confreres, and regarded as true colleagues and fellow-members of the great medical fraternity. The most efficient of them must be promoted to administrative posts, where their responsibility will be as great and as independent as the foreign members of the staff, and where they will be given equal opportunity to try out their ideas and make their own mistakes.

Where this is done, and where the hospital is so equipped as to offer them proper facilities for their medical work, there is every reason to hope that their services may be secured. Of 115 men who completed their medical training between the years 1906 and 1919 at the Union Medical College,

Hankow, the Medical Department of the University of Nanking, or at the Tsinan Medical College, no less than 110 have served for longer or shorter periods in mission hospitals, and the great majority are still doing so—and that in spite of the fact that only a comparatively small percentage of them were under any obligation to return to such work.

3) The work that still waits to be done in China urgently demands a large increase of medical men and women from the home countries. They are needed for pioneer work; for medical education; for public health developments; and, most of all, for the staffing of the existing hospitals, eighty per cent of which were only able to report the presence of a single missionary doctor each during the year 1919.

This kind of work calls pre-eminently for the Honors men and women of our medical schools. It requires a professional experience and keenness which are able to take full advantage of the enormous field of clinical research which China presents, and to make a thoughtful contribution towards the solution of some of her innumerable problems. But most of all it requires a depth of culture and refinement, and a solidarity of Christian character, which can regard with sympathy a point of view often far removed from its own, and can display humility and self-effacement even when circumstances are most trying.

If China did not also offer a sphere of useful service for the man of humble attainments, many of us would soon go home. But in the vastness of her need there is room for every well-qualified medical practitioner who is prepared to devote himself to the redemption of her people and the relief of her distress, and who is sufficiently young and elastic to adapt himself to an entirely new environment.

God give us men! A time like this demands
Strong minds, great hearts, true faith and
ready hands.

Surely it is high time that the professors of our home medical colleges should bear in mind the vast needs of Asia, and should constantly present the facts of the situation to their classes. Cannot we appeal to them to lay before their most promising students, year by year, the great adventure of science and of service to which the pathetic cry of the suffering millions of China is summoning men and women? And furthermore, is it unreasonable to ask that more direct lines of communication be established between the profession at home and its members in distant outposts? Why should not some of the leading physicians and surgeons of London and New York come and visit our hospitals in China—not as globe-trotters, but staying long enough to acquaint themselves with the conditions of medical life and practice out here—and give us the opportunity of sharing in their experience and skill? Better facilities should at the same time be provided in the laboratories and wards of the large hospitals of the West, so that medical men from China on furlough, or Chinese medical graduates proceeding to Europe or America for post-graduate study, should have full opportunity of being brought into touch with the latest methods of investigation and treatment, and of securing expert advice and assistance in attacking the unsolved medical problems of the Far East. [32]

4) This great and beneficent service for China can never be satisfactorily accomplished until Christian people in the homelands recapture the spirit of the men who founded and endowed our own great institutions of healing—such as Rahere and Thomas Guy and others like them—and are prepared to employ a similar munificence on behalf of the East. Numbers of our mission hospitals and medical schools here in China are suffering today from impaired efficiency and retarded progress on account of inadequate financial support. The furlough of the missionary doctor, which should be largely devoted to the replenishing of his professional and spiritual resources, is too often taken up with the effort to secure funds for the maintenance of beds and cots in his wards or the completion of his hospital buildings. This should no longer be, now that we have reached a day when the unity of the world and the brotherhood of its people are subjects which constantly occupy our thoughts and our conversation.

China is no longer an alien land. She has become our neighbor, our fellow-counsellor around the Table of Versailles, a member with us in the Council of the League of Nations. And if she suffers, we too must suffer with her.

If this battle for the redemption of China is worth our fighting, it is worth our sacrifice also. Such sacrifice has already been given by many humble followers of the Christ, who gladly lived upon small incomes voluntarily reduced, in order that China might share the richest blessings they possessed.

[32] The China Medical Board has already generously awarded a large number of fellowships to medical missionaries on furlough and Chinese medical graduates, to enable them to pursue post-graduate study in North America or Great Britain.

The healing of the world
Is in its nameless saints.
Each separate star is nothing;
A myriad scattered stars
Break up the night,
And make it beautiful.

And after all is not this the fundamental philosophy of the Christian life, that the seed should die in order that it might bring forth fruit? That was what the Cross of the Son of God meant. And after the Cross came the Resurrection.

Book excerpt end

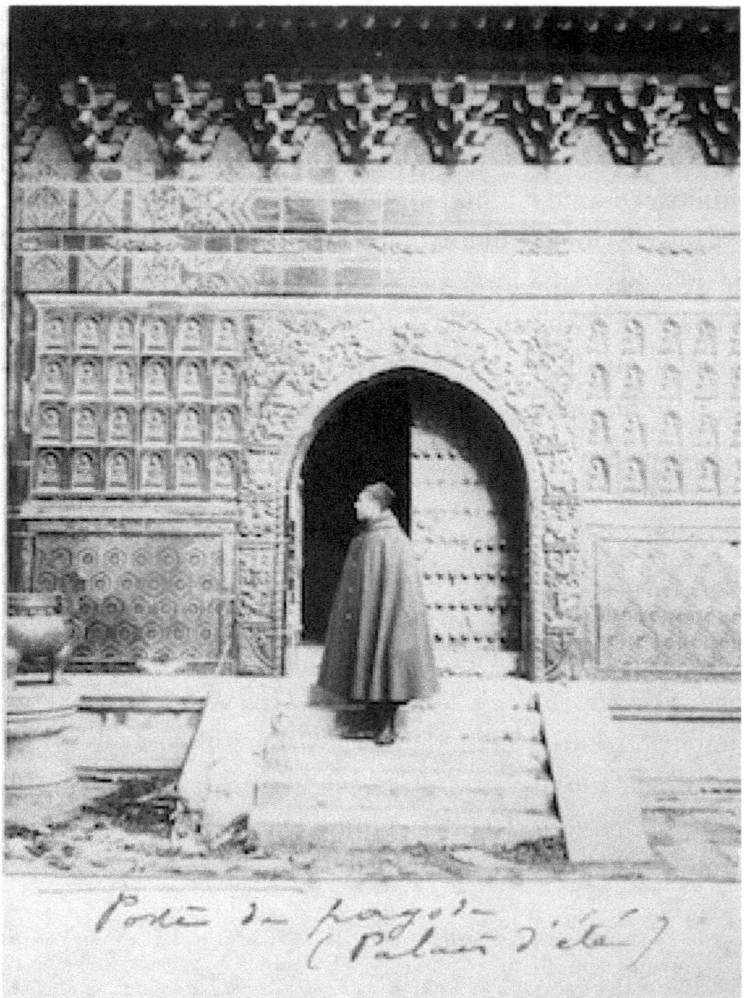

Photo by Mr P. Goux in early 1900s. "Door of Pagoda (Summer Palace)".

The medical history of China 中國醫學史

1936 by Chen Bangxian 陳邦賢

Source: *Part of the First Assortment of Chinese Cultural History Collection of Works*, Published by the Commercial Printing House, December 1st of the 25th year of the Republic (1936)
中國文化史叢書第一輯商務印書館出版
二十五年十二月一日

Chapter 3: Medicine in recent times 近世的醫學

Subchapter 2: The importation of Western medicine 西洋醫學的輸入

Pages 185–194

During medieval times, some foreign countries such as India, Persia and Arabia imported medicine into China, which was recorded in *Medicine in The Middle Ages Zhong Gu De Yi Xue* 中古的醫學. According to the written histories, medical art of the West gradually infiltrated into China prior to 1600. During the Tang Dynasty, Buddhism entered heavily into China, which then influenced the medicine as well. In the Yuan Dynasty, among the foreigners at official posts, there were some doctors; for example, Frank Isaiah[33] was an official dialectologist/ astronomer/ doctor who established a hospital in Beijing in 1272. As with other Christian religious followers, he founded many churches in Henan and also practiced medicine. During the end of the 13th century, some Roman Catholics came to China. A Franciscan, John of Montecorvino, came to Beijing in 1294, not only to do missionary work but also to practice medicine. After 1600, there were more and more Europeans coming to the East, displaying new medicine in China, such as Father Jean Torrenz (1575–1630), who came to China in 1621. He was specialized in philosophy and medicine, and his greatest work was to correct the calendar. He also had some dedication in medicine; his book *A Summary of the Human Body Ren Shen Gai Shuo* 人身概說 is the earliest book about anatomy imported into China. Father Michael Boym (1659) had been to China as well and made some contribution with a book about the pulse, tongue coating and simple explanation of herbs. Father Dominique Parrenin (1669–1741) had translated some medical books. Brother Bernard Rhodes (1645–1715) came to

[33] The Persian records show that in the thirteenth century the Great Kahn had Christian physicians attached to his court. "This .... is interesting for the Mongol history, which in one place says that Aisie (perhaps Isaiah) was a Fuh-Lin man (Frank) a linguist, astrologer and physician, actually asserts that he served Kyuk Khan and that subsequently in 1263 was chief physician and astrologer to Kub-lai; in 1273 he is once styled a Mussulman and his hospital at Peking was officially called the Broad Charity." (E. H. Parker's *China and Religion*, p. 181)

China to practice medicine in 1699; he had won the crowds' trust and cured imperial concubines and so was hired as the imperial physician. Brother Jean Joseph Casta arrived in Beijing in 1715 and had been hired to treat imperial concubines. His heart was set on curing the sick poor people; unfortunately because of that he contracted an infectious disease, was seriously ill and passed away in 1747. Other than that, people like Brother Etienne Roasset (1689–1758), Brother Emanuel de Mattos (1725–1764), Brother Louis Basin (1712–1774), Father Pierre Cibat (1727–1780) and Russian missionaries, not only did missionary work in China, but also provided medical help to many poor people.

In addition, there was some introduction to Western medicine in *Yixue Tiao* 醫學條 from *Xifang Yaoji* 西方要紀 by Giulio Alenio and *Hydraulic Machinery of the West Tai Xi Shui Jie Bing Fa* 泰西水結冰法, by Sabatino de Ursis. According to Huang Bolu's 黃伯祿 *Zheng Jiao Feng Bao* 正教奉褒 and Pierre-Marie-Alphonse Favier's *Mid Chapter* in *Yanjing Kaijiao Lüe* 燕京開教略:

> "Kangxi 康熙 Emperor[34] accidentally had malaria and was cured by missionaries Claude de Visdelou and Jean de Fontaney with Western medicine and quinine bark and they were rewarded."

During that time, Western medicine developed more in Macau. In the chapter *Foreigners in Macau Lüe Xia Juan Ao Fan Pian* 略下卷澳蕃篇 from the book *Brief History of Macau Ao Men Ji* 澳門記 by Yin Guanren 印光任 and Zhang Rulin 張汝霖:

> "In Macau there is Dr. Anthony who is famous for surgery."

And said,

> "There are different kinds of medicine distillates such as styrax, clove oil, sandalwood oil, bay oil, all in bottles."

Also said,

> "Several doctors practiced in a medical temple in eastern Macau; among all foreigners, widows, widowers, orphans, childless, or who has disease but no access to any treatment, they can go to the medical temple… there is a lunatic temple which insane foreigners inhabit. It was guarded by soldiers who have monthly salary."

[34] Lived 1654–1722 CE.

These paragraphs are about Western medicine imported into China in the late Ming and early Qing Dynasties. Therefore, we know that, at that time, the foreign intelligentsia didn't import Western medicine in a large volume, so much so that it did not attract the locals' attention. The history of Western doctors coming to China and the establishment of hospitals in China was recorded in Zhang Xinglang's 張星烺 *Ou Hua Dong Jian Shi* 歐化東漸史:

> "... in late Ming and early Qing Dynasties, there is no reliable record that the missionaries of Catholicism Society of Jesus were making many efforts on importing Western medicine. Western medicine got into China with Lutheran Protestants' entrance into China. The earliest was the vaccination of cowpox, which some say was brought by the Spanish in 1803 (the 8th year of Jia Qing 嘉慶). According to written history, Alexander Pearson from British East India Company brought the vaccination of cowpox into China in 1805. He had practiced medicine in Guangzhou and had written a book explaining the vaccination of cowpox; George Staunton not only translated this book into Chinese, but also taught the skill of the vaccination to Chinese apprentices. The most important one is Hequa 海官,[35] who became a famous doctor and administered cowpox vaccination to about a million people within thirty years. Hequa also passed on this skill to his son and founded a hospital to apply the vaccination. In 1820 the surgeons Livingston and Morrison, in the East India Company, founded a small hospital in Macau to cure poor local people with the help of Chinese apprentices. In 1827 the surgeon L. R. Colledge in the East India Company founded an ophthalmology hospital in Macau; he also founded a nursing home which contained forty-five people the next year and had admitted more than four thousand people. Other than the workers from the East India Company, Chinese businessmen also donated money to this first Western medical hospital in China. The next year, L. R. Colledge founded a small hospital in Guangzhou for both Chinese and foreigners with the help of two surgeons, J. A. Bradford and Cox. Colledge had an essay,

[35] In the text, both Chinese characters and Roman letters of the name are given. Hequa is a southern dialect.

Suggestion With Regard to Employing Medical Practitioners as Missionaries to China, which aroused common people's attention in the U.S.A. In 1834 Peter Parker, an American, established a hospital for only Chinese expatriates in Singapore. The next year, the hospital was moved to Guangzhou, specializing in ophthalmology. In 1838 Parker, Rev. E. C. Budzman and Colledge organized the Canton Medical Missionary Society. Parker was the fully authorized diplomat representing the U.S.A. in 1844, while afterwards, in 1857, he became an official ambassador and left China to return to the U.S. In 1879 he was the president of the China Medical Missionary Society in the U.S.A. and passed away in the U.S.A. in 1888. He was the first missionary who was also a surgeon in China. The second one is a British man William Lockhart, who arrived in Guangzhou in 1838 and became the president of the hospital founded by Parker the following year. Lockhart went to ___ in 1843 and founded Shandong Road Hospital in ___ international Settlement. He also founded a hospital in Beijing, which later became the foundation for Peking Union Medical College Hospital. In 1839, Benjamin Hobson, a British man, arrived in Guangzhou to be the president of Macau Hospital; later, he went to Hong Kong to be the president of London Missionary Society Hospital. In 1857, he went to ___ to be the president of Shandong Road Hospital. There were more and more surgeon-missionaries coming to China. More and more Western medical hospitals have been built. Although at the beginning of the medical establishment, many foolish people were against it, saying that foreigners were taking kids' hearts and eyes to compound drugs, as time went by, those surgeon-missionaries had proved that Western medicine was better than the old Chinese medicine and so it earned the locals' trust. Western medical hospitals had well-organized systems, while Chinese medical hospitals mostly had no organized system. Western medicine alleviated people's sufferings and saved people's lives and so Chinese people's prejudice against Christianity gradually subsided. The initial goal of the Medical Missionary Society was profound. The great

> achievement of every hospital was not only curing patients and decreasing deaths, but also training up many Chinese apprentices and translating Western medical books into Chinese to spread Western medical knowledge in China. Today, the Western hospitals founded by the missionary society are better than Chinese private and public hospitals in both quality and quantity. In addition, those provincial missionary society hospitals such as Swatow (Shantou 汕頭) English Presbyterian Mission Hospital 英國長老會的醫院, Fengtian Scottish United Presbyterian Mission Hospital 蘇格蘭聯合自由會醫院, Hangzhou England Kwang-Chi Hospital 杭州大英醫院, Hankou Renji Hospital 漢口英國醫院, Shanghai London Missionary Society Hospital (Renji Hospital) 上海倫敦傳教會醫院, Episcopal Church of the United States of America Hospital 美國聖公會醫院, Jinan Cheeloo Hospital 濟南齊魯醫院, Huaiyin Renji Hospital 淮陰仁濟醫院, Peking Union Medical College Hospital 北京協和醫院 etc., all have great capital and are large scale; they are famous nationwide and have saved many people's lives to lead the medical industry towards a Westernized direction…"

Even though this paragraph admires Westerners and loses too much of our own self-confidence, yet it is a correct historical text about the importation of Western medicine.

During Xianfeng 咸豐[36] and Tongzhi 同治[37] reigns in Qing Dynasty, there were many books explaining the medicine of the West; this bibliography was shown in Shulu's 述廬[38] *Tong Xue Shu Mu Kao* 通學書目考 and Liang Qichao's 梁啟超 *Western Studies Booklist Xi Xue Shu Mu Biao* 西學書目表. Among these, the more important is Ding Fubao's 丁福保 *Hygiene Questions and Answers Wei Sheng Xue Wen Da* 衛生學問答 Chapter 9:

> "As in Benjamin Hobson's *Five Western Medical Books Xi Yi Wu Zhong* 西醫五種, although the theory was old, it covered generally the whole corpus, such as internal medicine, surgical medicine and gynecology."

[36] 1850–1861 CE
[37] 1861–1875 CE
[38] Zou Lingyuan 鄒淩沅

Hobson was a Briton who, while living in Guangdong 廣東, authored many books, such as *Summary of Western Medicine Xi Yi Lun Lüe* 西醫論略, *Internal Medicine Modern Theory Nei Ke Xin Shuo* 內科新說, *Gynecology and Pediatrics Modern Theory Fu Ying Xin Shuo* 婦嬰新說 and *Entire Body Modern Treatise Quan Ti Xin Lun* 全體新論 etc. This was the starting point for the importation of Western medicine into China.

Also said,

> "Headlam's *Confucian Medicine Ru Men Yi Xue* 儒門醫學, John Glasgow Kerr's *Introduction to Inflammation Yan Zheng Lun Lüe* 炎症論略, Duncan Main's *Yi Fang Hui Bian* 醫方彙編, Yin Duanmu's 尹端模 *Bing Li Cuo Yao* 病理撮要 and *Yi Li Lüe Shu* 醫理略述 are all simplified, while John Glasgow Kerr's *Encyclopedia of Western Medicine Xi Yi Nei Ke Quan Shu* 西醫內科全書 and *Summary of Explanations for Western Drugs Xi Yao Lüe Shi* 西藥略釋, Hubo's 虎伯 *Nei Ke Li Fa* 內科理法 are detailed."

John Glasgow Kerr was from Ohio in the United States; he studied medicine in Jefferson Medical College in Philadelphia. In 1854, he came to Guangzhou and gave his opinions in the conference of China Presbyterian Missionary Society. He explained that Chinese medicine did not include dissection and anatomy, physiology, chemistry or physics and that the therapy was only herbs without surgical skills. Therefore, it would always result in death or disability if one encountered a serious disease. "The annual death toll in China," he said, was "much higher than that in Europe, and so we should save them," etc… He founded, in Canton, the Universal Love and Salvation (Pok-Tsai) Medical Center 博濟醫局 to practice medicine and dispense drugs. He established a medical school and sought students to teach his medical knowledge and skills. During his leisure time, he translated[39] *Hua Xue Chu Jie* 化學初階, *Ti Zhi Qiong Yuan* 體質窮源, *Ti Yong Shi Zhang* 體用十章, *Ge Zheng Quan Shu* 割症全書, *Yan Zheng Xin Lun* 炎症新論, *Guo Za Xin Fa* 裹紮新法, *Nei Ke Quan Shu* 內科全書, *Nei Ke Chan Wei* 內科闡微, *Xi Yao Lüe Shi* 西藥略釋, *Yan Ke Cuo Yao* 眼科撮要, *Fu Ke Jing Yun* 婦科精蘊, *Hua Liu Zhi Mi* 花柳指迷, *Pi Fu Xin Pian* 皮膚新篇, *Wei Sheng Yao Zhi* 衛生要旨, *Ying Han Bing Ming Biao* 英漢病名表 etc. In 1879, he added women's medical education. Canton (Pok-Tsai) medical center lasted for forty-five years; about 39,440 patients were admitted there, 48,918 patients had surgeries by him and 1,284 people had stones removed from their urinary system.

[39] Into Chinese.

Also said:

> "Furthermore, as for whole body there are *Quan Ti Chan Wei* 全體闡微, *Quan Ti Tong Kao* 全體通考, and *Ti Yong Shi Zhang* 體用十章. As for medicine, there are *Xi Yao Da Cheng* 西藥大成 and *Wan Guo Yao Fang* 萬國藥方. As for pediatrics, there are *Er Ke Cuo Yao* 兒科撮要 and *Er Ke Lun Lüe* 兒科論略. As for gynecology, there are *Fu Ke Jing Yun* 婦科精蘊, *Tai Chan Ju Yao* 胎產舉要 and *Chan Ke Tu Shuo* 產科圖說. As for Sexually Transmitted Diseases, there is *Hua Liu Zhi Mi* 花柳指迷. As for ophthalmology, there is *Yan Ke Zheng Zhi* 眼科證治. As for dermatology, there are *Pi Fu Xin Bian* 皮膚新編 and *Pi Fu Zheng Zhi* 皮膚證治. These are all absolutely reliable."

Afterwards, Zhao Yuanyi 趙元益[40] (Pen name Jinghan 靜涵), from Xinyang 新陽, translated *Confucian Medicine Ru Men Yi Xue* 儒門醫學, *Nei Ke Li Fa* 內科理法 and *Xi Yao Da Cheng* 西藥大成 and other books so that the influence of Western medicine became profound.

There were some Chinese people studying abroad for medicine, such as Huang Kuan 黃寬, who was the earliest one, as recorded in Yung Wing's[41] 容閎 *My Life in China and America Xi Xue Dong Jian Ji* 西學東漸記:

> "Huang Kuan studied medicine diligently at the University of Edinburgh for seven years and graduated at the third place, which earned an honor for all Chinese students. He went back to China in 1857, started practicing medicine and helped a lot of people. With his extensive medical knowledge and good skills, he thus became a good surgeon in the east of Cape of Good Hope. He continued staying in Canton and practiced medicine. As a result he earned more and more fame and wealth and was even more welcomed than other Western surgeons. He passed away in 1879; many Chinese and Westerners paid their last respects at his funeral, not only for his outstanding medical skills but also for his enthusiastic personality."

---

[40] Zhao Jinghan 趙靜涵（1840－1902 CE）
[41] Southern dialect name.

Dr. Huang Kuan (Huang Chuoqing 黃綽卿) was from Xiang-shan 香山 County in Guangdong 廣東. He had followed Brown, an American, to the United States and studied for four years there, graduating from a liberal arts college. Afterwards, he went to University of Edinburgh and was awarded a PhD and then he stayed in the United Kingdom for another two years. He went back to China in 1857 and stayed in Canton, and had been a surgeon in Hui Ai Hospital 惠愛醫館 and the president of Hong Kong National Hospital 香港國家醫院. He was specialized in anatomy and very admired by many Western medical scientists. John Glasgow Kerr had Kuan Huang's financial support when he was founding Canton (Pok-Tsai) Hospital 博濟醫局. At the first year of Tongzhi 同治[42] reign, Mr. Li Wenzhong 李文忠[43] had invited him to be the surgeon in the military affair center but he resigned after half a year. Mr. Ding Yusheng 丁雨生 regarded highly of him and was trying to persuade him to take that position again but he refused. See how aloof he was from politics and material pursuits.

This is about people who studied abroad for medicine on their own expense. There were other people studying abroad for medicine on public expense. The information about those students who studied abroad was recorded in the 32nd year of Guangxu 光緒 Reign[44] the 9th lunar month. In *Guan Xu Zheng Yao* (光緒政要) it says:

> "By the order of the emperor, today the academic department introduced the students who studied abroad for medicine to the monarch... Xie Tianbao 謝天保 was rewarded as a medical scholar...Xu Jingwen 徐景文 was rewarded as a medical scholar... Chen Zhonghu 陳仲虎 was rewarded as a medical bachelor... Cao Zhiyi 曹志沂 was rewarded as a medical bachelor... Li Yingmi 李應泌 was rewarded as a medical bachelor... Fu Ruqin 傅汝勤 was rewarded as a medical bachelor..."

Above is the general situation of the importation of Western medicine into China.

[42] 1861 CE

[43] Li Hongzhang 李鴻章 1823–1901 CE, politician, general and diplomat in late Qing.

[44] 1907 CE

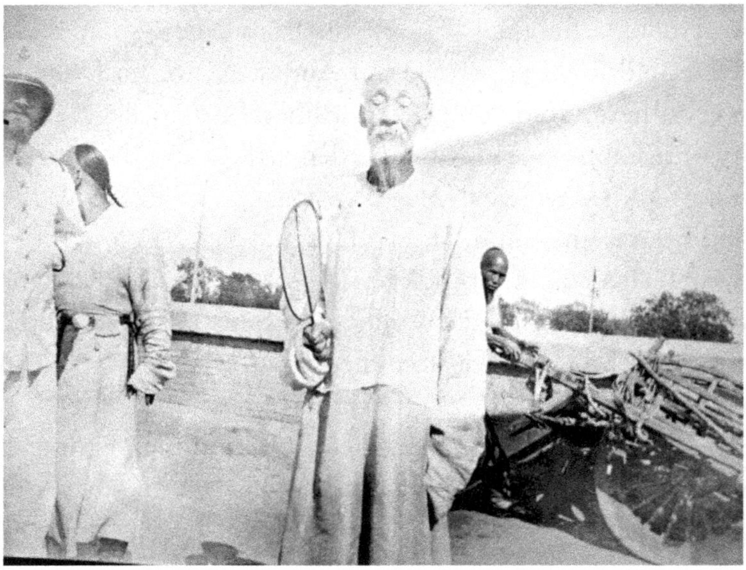

Photo by Mr P. Goux in early 1900s. "Mandarin from Li Hongzhang's entourage"

Following is from same publication, pages 222–231

Subchapter 5 : Medical Education in the Qing Dynasty 清代的醫事教育

Section 1: Westerners teaching Chinese medicine 外人教授華人醫學

Westerners teaching Chinese students in China started in 1835, when Peter Parker founded Canton Christian Hospital 廣州基督教醫院 and started training Chinese apprentices as assistants. This, one can say, was the first time that Chinese people studied Western kind of medicine.

In 1843 the British Dr. Hobson taught Chinese people Western medicine in Hong Kong Hospital 香港醫院 and translated English medical books into Chinese, such as *Quan Ti Xin Lun* 全體新論 (which was about dissection and physiology),[45] Xi Yi Lüe Lun 西醫略論 (specializes in surgical clinical experiments), *Fu Ying Qian Shuo* 婦嬰淺說 (nursing methods and pediatrics) and *Nei Ke Xin Shuo* 內科新說 (including internal clinical medicine and basic pharmacognosy) etc.

Shanghai Tongren Hospital 上海同仁醫院[46] was founded in 1881. Dr. Boone taught Chinese people medicine in this hospital. It became St. John's University Hospital afterwards 聖約翰大學醫學部.

[45] Comments in parenthesis are in the original text.
[46] St. Luke's Hospital.

In 1883 the Soochow Hospital 博習醫院 was founded in Suzhou 蘇州, which had an affiliated department to teach Chinese people Western medicine. The founders were Dr. Walter R. Laucbuih and William H Park. Dr. A. R. Parker taught chemistry and physics, Dr. Park taught internal medicine, clinical experience, pediatrics and drug compounding. Dr. Laucbuih taught anatomy, physiology and pharmacognosy.

Meanwhile in Hangzhou, Dr. Duncan Main founded Kwang-Chi Hospital 廣濟醫院 to teach Chinese people Western medicine.

In 1885 Mr. Sun Yat-Sen 孫中山 studied medicine at the Canton (Pok-Tsai) Medical school 廣東醫學校, founded by the Christian missionary John G. Kerr.

In 1887 Dr. Boone started training up nurses in Shanghai.

In 1888 Mr. Crews taught medicine in Beijing.

In 1892 Mr. Sun Yat-Sen was in the first graduating class of Hong Kong medical school 香港醫學校.

Hospitals founded by Westerners are as follows (in order of year of establishment):

Canton (Pok-Tsai) Hospital 博濟醫院 in Guangzhou 廣州
Hwa Mei Hospital 華美醫院 in Ningbo 寧波
Renji Hospital 仁濟醫院 in Shanghai 上海
Shantou English Presbyterian Hospital 汕頭基督醫院 in Shantou 汕頭
Kwang-Chi Hospital 聖公會廣濟醫院 in Hangzhou 杭州
Tsingchow Kwang Teh Hospital 基督廣德醫院 in Shandong Province Yidu County 山東益都
Dr. John Kenneth Mackenzie Memorial Hospital 馬大夫紀念醫院 in Tianjin 天津
Rankine Memorial Hospital 普濟醫院 in Yichang 宜昌
Wesleyan Mission Hodge Memorial Hospital 普愛醫院 in Hankou 漢口
Methodist Hospital 衛民博濟醫院 in Shangdong Province De Xian 德縣 County
Sheng King Charity Hospital 盛京施醫院 in Liaoning 遼寧
Yilisha Hospital 伊利沙醫院 in Liaoning 遼寧
Fuying Hospital 婦嬰醫院 in Tianjin outside South Gate (Qianmen) 天津南門外
Christian Women Hospital 基督教女醫院 in Fujian Province Xiapu County 福建霞浦縣
St. Luke's Hospital 同仁醫院 in Shanghai
Church Missionary Society Men's Hospital 福寧男醫院 in Fujian Province Xiapu County

C.M.S. Pakhoi General Hospital 北海普仁醫院 in Guangdong Province Beihai City 北海市

Shadyside Presbyterian Hospital 基督教醫院[47] in Shandong Province Wei County 山東濰縣

Church of Scotland Mission Hospital 基督教醫院 in Liaoyang 遼陽

Love and Mercy Hospital 仁慈醫院 in Huaiyin 淮陰

Soochow Hospital 博習醫院 in Suzhou Tiansizhuang 蘇州天賜莊

Hopkins Memorial Hospital 同仁醫院 in Peking 北平

Weerbosch Hospital 韋伯希醫院 in Xiamen 廈門

Renji Hospital 仁濟醫院 in Wuchang 武昌

Hospital of the Rhenish Mission 普濟醫院 in Guangdong Dongguan 廣東東莞

Tooker Memorial Hospital for Women and Children 婦孺醫院 in Suzhou 蘇州

Christian Gynecology Hospital 基督教婦科醫院 Jilin Province Chaoyang County 吉林朝陽

Renze Hospital 仁澤醫院 in Ningbo 寧波

American Presbyterian Mission Hospital 華美醫院 in Jinan 濟南

Drum Tower Hospital 鼓樓醫院 in Nanjing 南京

Hope & Wilhelmina Hospital 救世醫院 in Xiamen City Gulangyu Island 廈門鼓浪嶼

Chengtu Eye, Ear, Nose and Throat Hospital 眼耳喉專科醫院 in Chengdu 成都

Kiating Canadian Mission Hospital 仁濟男女醫院 in Jiading 嘉定

Fuyin Hospital 福陰醫院 in Jiangyin 江陰

Wiley Memorial Hospital 懷禮醫院 in Fujian Province Gutian County 福建古田

Women's Missionary Society Hospital for Women & Children 婦孺醫院 in Chengdu 成都

Bachman Hunter Hospital 德門醫院 in Jining 濟寧

These hospitals were mostly founded by missionary churches, the shortest one lasted 40 plus years, while the longest lasted for more than a hundred years. Most of the hospitals accepted numerous Chinese students. One can say that the initial stage of absorbing the new medicine in China was the missionary medicine.

Section 2: Medical schools founded by Westerners 外人設立的醫學校

In 1901 Hackett Medical College 夏葛醫學校 was founded in Guangdong.

In 1903 Peking Union Medical College 協和醫學校 was founded in Beijing, which was permitted by the Department of Education in 1906.

[47] Some of the English hospital names are not direct translation from the Chinese in this text, but rather the actual hospital names as they were at that time.

In 1904 Cheeloo Medical College 齊魯醫學校 was founded in Jinan.

In 1908 Erich Paulun, a German, founded a Tongji Hospital 同濟醫院 in Shanghai and the German Medical School was affiliated with the hospital 同濟德文醫學校.

The Church founded North China Union Medical College for Women 中國協和女子醫學專門學校 in Beijing.

In 1909 the Church founded He Gaituo Women Medical School 赫蓋脫女子醫學專門學校 in Guangzhou.[48]

In 1911 Tsingtao German Medical College 德國醫學校 was founded.

The medical schools founded by Westerners are attached below:

The College of Medicine of St John's University 聖約翰大學醫學部

C.M.S. Kwang Chi Medical School 廣濟醫學專門學校

Hockett Medical College 夏葛醫學校

Hankow Medical College 大同醫學校, which was combined with other schools to form Cheeloo University School of Medicine 齊魯大學醫科

National Tung-Chi University 同濟大學

The Medical Department of University of Nanking 金陵大學醫科, which was combined to form Cheeloo University School of Medicine 齊魯大學醫科

Peking Union Medical College 協和醫學校

West China Union University, College of Medicine 華西協和大學醫學校

Peking North China Union Medical College for Women 北京協和女子醫學校, which was combined to form Cheeloo University School of Medicine 齊魯大學醫科

Cheeloo University School of Medicine 齊魯大學醫科

He Gaituo Women Medical School 赫蓋脫女子醫學專門學校

Section 3: Medical schools founded by Chinese government 自辦的醫學校

In Beijing, the School of Combined Learning 北京同文館 established specifically a Science Department, which then, in 1865, properly started official research into the knowledge of medical science. Dr. Dudgeon was appointed as professor. This was the starting point for new medicine education in China.

---

[48] This women's school was originally founded in 1899 by an American Doctor Fu Mali, and initially was called Guangdong Women Medical Hall. The study curriculum was 7 years long and included preparatory course 2 years, bachelors 4 years, and practicum 1 year. It was divided into departments: internal medicine; surgery; gynecology; obstetrics; pediatrics; ear, nose and throat; and pharmacology. In 1920, the school had 49 women students.

In 1881 Viceroy's Hospital Medical School 醫學館 was founded in Tianjin 天津 and its first class graduated in 1885. This school was officially established and managed by the government and, in 1893, its name changed to Peiyang Medical College 北洋醫學校. Lin Lianhui 林聯輝 was appointed to be the principal, while the establishment of the school was the work of Li Hongzhang 李鴻章 in 1893.

The Medical College 醫學堂 was ordered to incorporate into the Imperial University of Peking 大學堂[49] on July 24th 1898 and the regulations were designed by Sun Jianai 孫家鼐.[50]

Zhang Baixi 張百熙 reported "Authorized School Regulations 學堂章程"[51] on July 12th 1902, which specified the special departments and subjects of the school, medicine being one of them. It also had "Affiliated Medical Practical Clinic Regulations 附設醫學實業館章程".

In November 1902, Yuan Shikai 袁世凱 founded Peiyang Military Medical College 北洋軍醫學堂 in Tianjin, which, in 1906, was incorporated into the Army Department Medical Bureau 陸軍部軍醫司 and renamed to Army Medical College 陸軍軍醫學堂.

In March 1903, the Imperial University of Peking 京師大學堂 established the Medical Clinic 醫學實業館 and recruited several dozen students. It taught Chinese and Western medicine and later became Peking Medical University 醫科大學.

On November 26th 1903, Zhang Zhidong 張之洞, Zhang Baixi 張百熙 and Rong Qing 榮慶 reported "Authorized School Regulations 學堂章程"[52] and "Constitution of the Imperial University of Peking 大學堂章程". The documents indicated that there were preparatory courses and undergraduate courses in the university. Undergraduate courses included medicine and needed three to fours years to complete, while preparatory courses needed three years. There were three categories in "Higher Educational Institution Regulations 高等學校章程", the third for preparing entry to Medical University 醫科大學 and needing three years to complete.

In February 1905, the Imperial University of Peking 京師大學堂 changed the Medical Practical Clinic 醫學實業館 to the Medical Clinic 醫學館. It also built a building in Hou Sun Garden 後孫公園 outside Qianmen 前門. On December 13th 1906, the Department of Education 學部 ordered to change the Medical Clinic into Peking

[49] Same as 京師大學堂

[50] 1827–1909, a senior Chinese official, appointed "Guanli Daxuetang Shiwu Dachen," or (education) minister for the Imperial University's affairs.

[51] Full document name is 欽定學堂章程

[52] Full document name is 秦定學堂章程

Specialized Medical Clinic 京師專門醫學堂 and taught separately Chinese and Western medicines.

In 1907 the Peking Medical Clinic 北京醫學館 ceased its activity.

In intercalary February of 1909, the Department of Education ordered Qu Yongqiu 屈永秋 to supervise the Imperial University of Peking 京師大學堂.

The Army Medical College 陸軍醫學堂 was founded in Guangdong.

In 1911 in Zhejiang Province the budget resolution for higher education was planned, estimated and was about to have been put into place "The 4th old facility, the higher medical specialized school 高等醫學專門學堂, is to be executed as planned", which showed that the government took high value in medical education.

Prior to Xinhai Revolution 辛亥革命,[53] in addition to the Army Medical College 陸軍醫學 there was also another government sponsored Navy Medical College 海軍醫學堂. It is a pity that there is not enough information about it.

Section 4: People who studied medicine abroad 留學外國學醫的

The first Chinese studying abroad in Europe, Huang Kuan, another name Chuoqing, was from Guangdong Province Xiangshan County, and came back to China in 1856. He was studying medicine in Edinburgh University in Scotland. After graduation, he researched pathology and anatomy and earned a medical PhD.

In 1906, among the students studying abroad on public expense, Xie Tianbao and Xu Jingwen were rewarded as medical scholars while Cao Zhiyi, Li Yingmi and Fu Ruqin were rewarded as medical bachelors by the monarch. From this we can see that the Qing Government already sent people to study medicine abroad during that time.

In 1907 the Department of Education and Chiba Medical College 千葉醫專校, in Japan, cooperated and established regulations of acceptance of Chinese students, and the fee was shared by every province. These are the historical materials about sending students to study medicine in Japan.

Excerpt end

[53] 1911 revolution that over threw the Qing government.

Medical book study

Source: Compilation of Discussions about Chinese Medical Education 中醫教育討論集

The following is an advertisement appearing at the very beginning of the book.

National Beiping Library
Library Supplement Publication
New Book Introduction

Author - Duo Ji Yuan Yin 多紀元胤 (Japanese: Taki Mototane)
25th year of the Republic of China September
Photocopied by Shanghai Chinese and Western Medicine Research Society
Special Compilation of Index for Book and Person Names

Four thick volumes of Jiangnan and History Book
Attached with new style book clips
Actual price 8 dollars
Registered mail fee 23 cents

In ancient times, medicine practitioners of our country were professionals to help others. As a tendency of last century, individual practitioners worked for their daily living. They learnt several books from private teachers and practiced here without pursuing further. The knowledge from collections of empirical prescriptions was never comparable to books from the three schools of Confucianism, Buddhism and Taoism. Starting from Liu Xiang 劉向 and his son Xin 歆 up to Ruan Xiao Xu 阮孝緒 of Liang Dynasty, Confucianism gradually developed without a question. Buddhism and Taoism also established their special publications respectively during the Six Dynasties and after the Song Dynasty to become different from the content of the classics. This did not only challenge Confucianism but sometimes overrode it as well. The medical skill or literary catalogue of knowledge was not previously developed. Yin Zhong Chun 殷仲春, of the Ming Dynasty, had a medical catalogue but it was just a simple piece of literature and was not regarded as valuable. Academically, there was useless and little knowledge in the study of medicine's origin or doctrine. That was the reason our Chinese Medicine was declining day by day.

Although the classics of our country were preserved through unrest and disorders of different dynasties, the scholars were unable to recover their former appearance, even with their entire lifetimes of effort, because of catastrophic fire damage. Medicine and Buddhism doctrines simultaneously spread to the east after the Sui and Tang Dynasties. Coincidentally, the national conditions of Japan thrived with little risk of military upheaval. Even when there were civil wars in Japan, they were not so cruelly disastrous as in our country. As a result, lost books from before the Song Dynasty in our country were still largely kept by Japan.

The book *Medical Study* contained 80 chapters that were largely not seen in our various medicine books stored throughout the dynasties. From a systematic perusal of the entire book, we can note a rough sketch of changes in our medicine's history over the centuries.

The author of this book, Mr. Duo Ji Yuan Yin 多紀元胤, was a Japanese supervisor of the Medical Institute in Japan's Wen Zheng years (Dao Guang of Qing Dynasty) and died at age 39. He wrote several books, including *Classic of Difficulties Syndrome Dredging Nan Jing Shu Zheng* 難經疏證, *Body Culture Ti Ya* 體雅, *Disease Culture Ji Ya* 疾雅, *Medicine Culture Yao Ya* 藥雅 and *Sickness Cases of Famous Doctors Ming Yi Gong An* 名醫公案. This famous scholar read extensively with comprehensive knowledge and published his writing during that period. He was the authority of Jiang Hu (Tokyo) medicine. He completed this book by continuing the will of his father Yuan Jian 元簡. According to the historical records of all dynasties, scholars distinguished medical books from all stored catalogues including poetry and terrain geography. They acted like Zhu Yi Zun 朱彝尊 to examine these classics. They put the book name first then the chapter numbers. They indicated whether the book existed, was lost or was never seen. Further, they recorded the preface and postscript of individual scholars with their resume but did not add any remarks. The books were considered as Medical Books, the scholars of the Tang and Song Dynasties followed the ancient method and compiled them under medical books. Moreover, the medical scholars of the Jin and Yuan Dynasties strived to establish their doctrines. That made the origin and history of Chinese medicine of the past thousand years as clear as glancing of fingers in one's palms. This is inevitably regarded as the most valuable classic in medical history. In the past, Yang Xing Wu 楊惺吾 visited Japan and always tried to copy the materials. However, subsequently the front matter was sadly lost. Mr Ye Gong Chuo 葉恭綽 also always invested much money to copy this book that was regarded as a treasure in the world. The book contained no carved plates but was copied into several editions and kept at home individually by the students of his school. After the passing away of Yuan Yin 元胤, his younger brother Yuan Jian 元堅 compiled the book with preface and directory added. Fan Xing Zhun 范行準, Song Da Ren 宋大仁, Zhou Ji 周濟 et.al. of the Chinese and Western Medicine Research Society advocated to print this book for the benefit of our people. This should not be only gratefully received by the medical field but should also not be ignored by the Chinese Cultural History department.

(Above copied from 152nd Edition, Library supplement of Da Gong Bao 大公報 Newspaper of October 15, 5th Year of the Republic of China (1916))

6 Tong Le Avenue, Lao Ba Zi Road, Shanghai

Article end

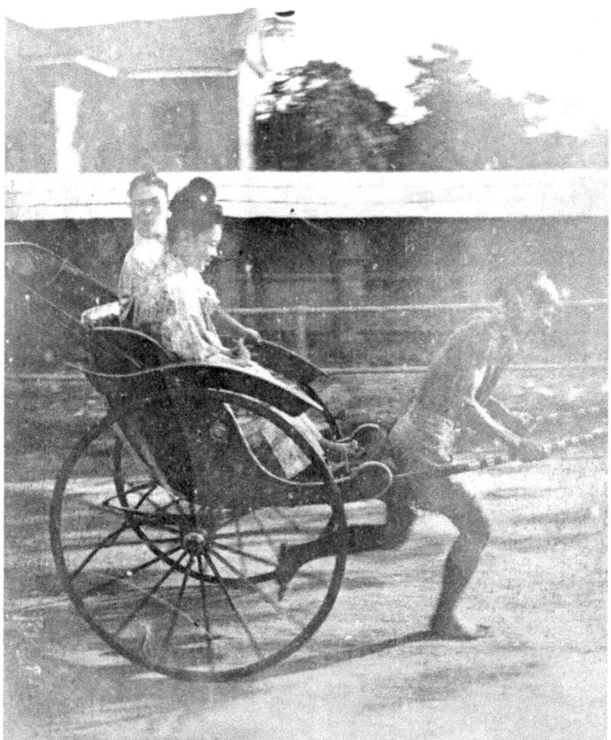

Photo by Mr P. Goux in early 1900s. Photo probably taken in Manchuria in or near Chien Hai Quouan

The main idea of source of acupuncture

1956 by Song Ruizhe 宋睿哲

Source: *The New Chinese Medicine Magazine* 新中醫藥 第七卷第八期, August 1956

Yaron: This article is not entirely dedicated to the pre-1920s time period; however, we can see the style in which early history narrative is pulled forward to the 1950s.

Pages 351–354

History of acupuncture

Partial article, point 5 until end

5. The decline of acupuncture

The decline of acupuncture can be attributed to two causes: one is that the doctors of later generations emphasized herbal decoction and underestimated the [beneficial] effect of acupuncture. Also doctors felt too embarrassed to have patients disrobe to have acupuncture. When they saw normal people doing scraping and bloodletting they looked down on these therapies. So acupuncture gradually declined. The other reason is that, since the lifting of the ban on maritime activities, European and American cultural influence has increased, so some people lean towards Western medicine rather than Chinese medicine and acupuncture is a main subject in Chinese medicine. In short, the decline of acupuncture can be blamed on a semi-feudal society and retroactive government. There are still some people regarding this precious national legacy as nothing but evil remnants.

6. The rebirth of acupuncture

Chairman Mao paid special attention to acupuncture in Yan-an 延安 in 1944. During that time, learning acupuncture was fashionable in doctors' groups. The devotion to acupuncture was tremendous during the Second Sino-Japanese War. Since our nation was established, due to the government's promotion, the development of acupuncture has changed a lot. As for the academic research about acupuncture, there was a symposium "acupuncture therapy" on March 7th, 1951 by Central Ministry of Health, also there was an acupuncture experiment institute, which is the current acupuncture research center in Academy of Chinese Medicine.

Acupuncture not only regains its glory, but also develops towards the scientific field and devotes more to people's health.

7. The general situation of our cultural legacy "acupuncture" in other countries

We Chinese are one of the earliest civilized races; Chinese medicine is also the earliest invented medicine, so it has influenced the development of medicine in other countries. Acupuncture especially is the most prominent kind amongst all forms of Chinese medicine to influence the world.

It has been fourteen hundred years since Chinese medicine entered Korea and its reliability is still the same. Acupuncture is even more popular in Korea than in China.

Chinese medicine entered Japan a mere twenty years later than into Korea. The research on Chinese medicine is very varied in Japan, and it's noticeable how important acupuncture is in their medical system, such as the article "Acupuncture Scholar Zhen Bo Shi 針博士" and "Acupuncture Student Zhen Sheng 針生" in "*Da Bao Ling* 大宝鈴". In 1465–1487 CE, Japanese ambassadors who had been to China said, "There were two famous doctors named Wasuke 和介氏 and Tamba 丹波氏 two hundred years ago. They specialized in curing abscess, carbuncle, whitlow, malignant boil, furunculosis, and scrofula etc., they did acupuncture and moxibustion on eight acupoints which had obvious effects." There are books transmitted from these two people now. It is a part of the Chinese acupuncture culture in Japan today. There are many people as well doing other research about acupuncture in the different departments.

Dr. Harada 原田 and Dr. Kashida 樫田 researched the effects of acupuncture treatment and published the experiments about its subcutaneous effect and the influence on blood, vessels, blood pressure, peristalsis, fatigue curve and skin tissue etc.

Dr. Ochi 越智 published *The effect of acupuncture on kidney mechanism, especially the influence on diuresis*.

Dr. Aochi 青地, Dr. Tokieda 時枝 and Dr. Hara 原 concluded research about acupuncture treatment: Acupuncture has influence on red blood cells, hemoglobin, white blood cells, blood serum, complement and immune process; moxibustion has influence on blood clotting time and blood sugar. They also published an article about the nature of moxibustion.

Dr. Hara has published research about the effect of moxibustion on skin, the healed inclination of tuberculosis on animals by moxibustion, and the effects of moxibustion on human beings.

There is other research about acupuncture shown as below:

Acupuncture has three effects as found: 1. stimulation; 2. inhibition; 3. induction. Okamoto's 岡本 "electrical air hypothesis". Okubo's 大久保 "mechanic stimulation hypothesis". Miura's 三浦 "transformation hypothesis". Other research such as insulating of the acupuncture stimulation, influence of acupuncture on blood and the reason for effectiveness of stopping bleeding by acupuncture.

There was much published scientific research about acupuncture since Meiji era, such as Dr. Miura's, Dr. Kimura's 木村 and Dr. Okubo's research.

Dr. Yoshimura 吉村 has research about acupuncture examination of some facial nerve disorder. Dr. Goto 後藤 found out that the reason acupuncture works is the reflexion of Heite sensation allergy band. Dr. Fuji 藤井 has scientific reports about pediatric dermatology, such as influence of acupuncture on the blood, the influence under the stimulation of sympathetic nerve and the influence on diameter of blood vessels.

There are so many books about the treatment, such as Sakamoto's 阪本 *Essence of Acupuncture Medicine*, Komai Kazuo's 駒井和夫 *Book of Moxibustion Therapy*, Okubo's *New Book of Acupuncture Treatment*, Sakai Matsuhari's *Kyuten New Therapy*, Uyama Kenji's 宇山健二 *Therapy for Palsy and Arthritis*, Yamazaki's 山崎 *Acupuncture Points Section Diagram*, Tamamori's *Acupuncture Essence*, Yasui's 安井 *Acupoints Compromise Volume*. Others are like higher level of acupuncture teaching materials, such as *Corrected Fourteen Meridians Acupoints* (by Yanagitani 柳谷), *The Basis of Therapy* (by Shirota 代田) etc., there are too many to name. Also there are so many acupuncture institutes, such as training schools. This is the general situation of acupuncture in East Asia.

Chinese medicine entered Western Europe in 17th century and, according to the investigation in Rome, it was passed by a Dutch surgeon, Wilhelm Ten Rhyne. According to Dr. Liu Yongchun's 刘永純 report, acupuncture entered Europe by a catholic missionary DuHalde, and had good reception. For example, a musician's father had mentioned in his book about acupuncture therapy in 1816, and a famous professor had published an experiment of effective acupuncture treatment in 1826.

The *Encyclopedia of Chinese Medicine*, published in 1863 in France, included not only Chinese medicine and veterinary medicine but also detailed acupuncture knowledge. Until now, almost every French doctor who studies acupuncture has this book.

In 1829 Dr. George Soulié de Morant came back to France from China and dedicated the acupuncture knowledge that he had been studying for thirty years to French medicine to provide the foundation of acupuncture in France. He had books published and the medicine he prescribed worked wonders, also he could clearly explain some difficult words and paragraphs in ancient Chinese books. His work *L'acuponcture Chinoise* combined *Zhenjiu Dacheng* 針灸大成 and his own clinical experience. Two books, *Acupoints* and *Instructions of Acupoints*, are published already; the *Diagnosis* and *Disease and Therapy* aren't finished yet. Other works include the French version of *Huangdi Neijing*, whose translator, Soulié de Morant, accomplished another book, *Chinese Acupuncture*, with another medical doctor. There are many compliments to Chinese acupuncture, such as, "Chinese acupuncture is very similar to electrical therapy but has better effects, it's very incredible which can't be explained by modern science" by a medical doctor Louis Jules Ernest Malinvaud. "Acupuncture's effects are amazing and much better than common treatments" by a professor of medicine. "[A]pplying acupuncture on acupoints with some stimulants can redistribute vigor and create a new balance to help the patient's recovery..." by a medical doctor Pouqueville.

A doctor Filliozat had said, "Europeans also know the method to treat rheumatism and waist pain is to have needles deeply into the muscles on the waist for ten minutes, which can be applied to any muscle pain, and it was from the experiment of acupuncture therapy."

Another doctor said, "among all the methods entering into body from skin [level] to adjust internal tissue to improve the body condition, none is as good as Chinese acupuncture treatment. Because it also has priceless value and glorious achievement..."

A doctor Laveran said, "The current reflexology nowadays is simply a part of Chinese acupuncture medicine." All these statements demonstrate the French admiration toward Chinese acupuncture.

As to the acupuncture institutions, there are two "acupuncture associations" in Paris. Each one has more than three hundred members. They arrange meetings twice a month for communication of experience that is recorded in the monthly magazine. There is also an "acupuncture workers association" which aims to guarantee the existence of the profession.

There is an "acupuncture international conference" once a year, organized by the association, as a platform for international communication of acupuncture experience.

There are "acupuncture courses" held by the association, facilitating academic knowledge, to make both theory and practice equally important. The courses are for two years to train acupuncture practitioners.

Today in Paris, five public hospitals have established "acupuncture therapy departments" and treated fifty to sixty people each session. It shows that Chinese acupuncture is reliable for foreign people. This is the general situation of acupuncture in France.

Medicine in Germany is always more advanced, and Germans researched Chinese acupuncture earlier as well. They translated *Illustrated Manual of Acupoints Bronze Figure* into German. Other acupuncture books were mostly translated from French to German, such as in *German Acupuncture Medical Association Magazine* Volume One pp50–56 was translated from French *Acupuncture Therapy*, but the names of the acupoints remained the original Chinese pronunciation. The number of each acupoint is according to the order of the direction on the fourteen meridians. This is the general situation of acupuncture in Germany.

In 1916 a British doctor wrote *Chinese Acupuncture Experiments* published in *Tropical Health Magazine*, gaining attention in the United Kingdom. Thereafter, many people started researching Chinese acupuncture.

In the United States, *Tulsa Sunday World Magazine* had an article about China on February 3rd, 1946, named *A Way Indicated by Ancient People*. In the content, it described acupuncture as "the five thousand-year-old medical experiment" and "earnestly curing diseases," and it also said "its development has the truth of the fifty centuries," and called this kind of treatment the "puncture turning method". It recorded that a Viennese surgeon had used acupuncture to cure malaria. It also recorded that "Dr. Ma Haitai, who was born in the United States, was the first one into China to learn Chinese medicine, and also encountered many people who were learning Chinese medicine… Dr. Ma and his partner had Chinese government help to found the 'Chinese and Western Medicine Doctors Research Association' in 1943, especially discussing the 'puncture turning therapy'… Their goal is to find the scientific proof." The original article was by John Luterzuch from the United States. From here, we can see that acupuncture had entered into the United States. Two doctors, Dula and Bock in Chicago University, have been researching Chinese acupuncture and they are the first to discover that acupuncture has special effect to relieve pain among current medicine, and also found the root from the view of neuroanatomy and gave it high compliment. After the Chinese medicine hospital in

San Francisco was established, it started the acupuncture department, and we can see through this how important acupuncture is.

Since the great physiologist, Ivan Pavlov, developed high-leveled neuropathology [research], it became a big turning point in medicine in the world. So Russian medicine is also the most scientific and advanced medicine in the whole world. In Pavlov's experiment, the situation of adjusting the imbalance of cerebral cortex by stimulating the sensor on the skin is identical to acupuncture clinical practice. Pavlov's theory inspired acupuncture research and, meanwhile, acupuncture treatment also provided Pavlov's theory important evidence. That's why in June 1952, the vice-president of the Russian medical science institution Huiwei Kenuowaluofu 惠維柯諾瓦洛夫 asked us to translate Zhu Lian's 朱璉 *New Acupuncture* into Russian. It shows that Russian medicine highly values Chinese cultural legacy—acupuncture—which works on the nervous system. So we can see that acupuncture is going to serve all people's health in the world.

Article excerpt end

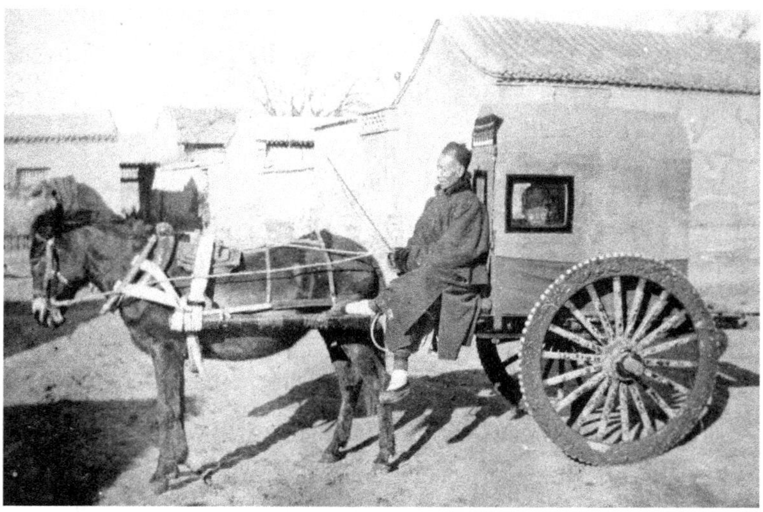

Photo by Mr P. Goux in early 1900s. Photo probably taken in Manchuria

Beginning our discussion with Mr. Taiyan's opinions about Chinese medicine and five elements theory

Oct 1956 by Zhang Cigong 章次公

Source: *The New Chinese Medicine Magazine* 新中醫藥第七卷第十期

Yaron: This article includes a long description of ancient history and is being used for a current debate about five elements theory, namely, should it be included in the new Chinese medicine curriculum or not?

This article may fit other chapters in this book—the formation of schools and curriculum as well as ideological influences. Therefore, as we progress in this book, especially the ideological influences chapter, you can return to this article for review.

Pages 437–438 and 446

Zhang Taiyan 章太炎, from Zhejiang Yuhang 餘杭, is a great master of Confucianism classic books and is also very good at medicine. So his opinions on medicine are definitely superb and difficult for us to approach. As to Chinese medicine, he denies downright the theory of five elements, as in his letter to Wu Jianzhai 吴檢齋 (Chengren 承仁) regarding the growth and decline of Chinese medicine:

> Some say Chinese medicine is philosophical medicine or [some] say that five elements theory is credible; the former is just a subterfuge and the latter is ridiculous. Yu's 禹 Dafu 大府 used "water, fire, metal, wood, earth and grain" showing its practical application within the population. The government official responsible for five elements said, Goumang 勾芒, Zhurong 祝融, Houtu 后土, Rushou 辱收, Xuanming 玄冥 (the gods of five elements), are like the government officials of the salt method, lightning Qi and river path; they exist because there is a demand and they pertain to everyday usage. In *The Great Plan Hongfan* 洪範 it describes characters of five elements but doesn't mention anything about generation and restriction Sheng Ke 生剋. You Zaijing's 尤在涇 *Yi Xue Du Shu Ji* 医学讀書記 put forth a discussion debating five elements theory. However, in order to defend the old school's theory, he trimmed his words a bit but

> his meaning was still obvious. There is no other sage of medicine comparable to Zhang Zhongjing 張仲景. Among his works, he mentions the theory of five elements only at the beginning of *Ping Mai* 平脈, *Bian Mai* 辨脈 and *Golden Chamber Jin Kui Yao Lüe* 金匱要略. Other than this, he rarely mentions it. Even if we don't talk about the theory of five elements, which part of Chinese medicine is harmed? Does the theory of five elements belong to philosophy? It's like 'Weichen 緯讖 school' in Han Dynasty which can fool people but can't be philosophy. Besides, there were already different opinions over the connection between five organs and five elements in the new version and old version of *Book of Documents Shang Shu* 尚書. Although Zheng Kangcheng 鄭康成 was following the new version, his comments to *Zhou Guan Ji Yi* 周官疾医 said, "Lung qi hot matches fire, heart qi less hot matches earth, liver qi cool matches metal, spleen qi warm matches wood, kidney qi cold matches water," which seems to follow the old version. From this we know that the distribution of the five elements was not consistent, just like the yellow and red celestial equators not conforming to the Jiu Dao 九道. In recent times the Jiu Dao is called the lunar orbit and it is not connected to the measurement of the astronomy… I had said about that the shape of the organs and blood vessels, in the past people couldn't understand them after they had dissected bodies roughly, so we should follow the standard of Western medicine. In the past, people saw the theory of five elements as symbols. Gradually, some ridiculous theory appeared; for example, the theory of generation and restriction is like people's five organs nourishing and restraining each other. Charlatans from later generations totally follow this ridiculous theory, without any experiments, and this tendency should be changed."

In Mr. Taiyang's point of view, except that the words about five elements in *Ping Mai* and *Bian Mai* were misunderstood as Zhang Zhongjing's words, the other contents of his opinions are very true and they fit science. We know that *Yi Jing* 易經 talked about Yin-Yang but not five elements. The theory of five elements didn't come into existence until the end of Warring States Period. Liu Shipei 刘師培 said:

> "*Yi Jing* started in Fu Xi 伏羲 period and finished during the time of King Wen of Zhou and Confucius. In Fu Xi period, there was not the theory of five elements yet. King Wen of Zhou and Confucius didn't follow five elements. So, in *Yi Jing*, there was not a word relating to five elements. In Western Han Dynasty, the people who were in the group of Jiao 焦 and Jing 京 said following *Yi Jing* caused unnatural disaster, so they mixed it with the theory of five elements, which already made it not the original version. Mr. Zheng 鄭 used metal, wood, water, and fire to explain the four symbols Si Xiang 四象 in his commentary of *Yi Jing*. Ma Rong 馬融 said that four seasons gave birth to five elements in his commentary. Confucians of the Song dynasty created the diagram of pre-heaven and post-heaven and said that the river picture and Luo diagram He Tu Luo Shu 河圖洛書 are based on five elements, which is totally wrong."

The theory of five elements was completely developed by Zou Yan 鄒衍 around the end of the Warring States Period. It was not a famous school before Zou Yan. So there was no direct commentary on five elements in Zhuangzi 莊子 and Han Feizi's 韓非子 books [and it was like this] until Xunzi 荀子 criticized Mencius' words and five elements in *Fei Shi Er Zi Pian* 非十二子篇. Some more contemporary people like Mr. Gu Jiegang 顧頡剛 pointed out Zou Yan's mistake and his words were credible. However, the theory of five elements had a lot of attention after Zou Yan became highly regarded by vassals Zhu Hou 諸侯, and we can see the influence on *Lüshi Chunqiu* 呂氏春秋. Since Han Dynasty, the influence of five elements on the academic cultural field was increasing; it even affected the medical field. The generation and restriction of five elements was not related to medicine originally; the focal connection might be Zou Yan.

The *History of Warring States Zhanguo Shi* 战國史 by Yang Kuan 楊寬 (published by Shanghai People's Publishing House in September 1955) included some comments on the representative of Yin-Yang School, Zou Yan, "…at this time Zou Yan used the restriction of five elements to establish the theory of the Cycle of Five Virtues Wu De Zhong Shi Shuo 五德終始說… Zou Yan saw that the Zhou dynasty kings were perishing and there would be another dynasty, so he built up this kind of theory. Although he used the restriction of five elements to explain the replacement of dynasties, it can't explain the motive force behind the restriction, so he had to attribute it to God's will. His theory of Cycle of Five Virtues was originally materialism, but it still fell to mysterious and religious superstition."

Mr. Yang 楊 said, "His theory of the Cycle of Five Virtues was from the original materialism," which is incorrect. Because the theory of the Cycle of Five Virtues was not the simple Five Origins Theory Wu Yuan Shuo 五元說 from *Hong Fan* 洪範 but, [rather], idealism which is based on imagination; of course it falls into mysterious and religious superstition. Wen Tingshi 文廷式, in *Chun Chang Zi Zhi Yu* 純常子枝語, said, "The theory of five elements emphasizes visual observation and daily usage, so it mentions wood instead of wind, earth instead of ground." Although it was still simple Five Origins Theory, it has become complicated. As to Zou Yan, he was the leader of the alchemists Fang Shi 方士 in the Kingdoms of Yan 燕 and Qi 齐 and so he certainly knew medicine; that is why Zou Yan was recorded as accomplishing the book *Zhong Dao Yan Ming Fang* 重道延命方[54] in *Book of Han—Liu Xiang Zhuan* 漢書刘向傳. Furthermore, he also established the theory of "Nine Provinces Jiu Zhou 九洲".[55] These above also affected *Neijing*. In Western Han Dynasty, some people like Dong Zhongshu 董仲舒 inherited Zou Yan's knowledge. Xia Cengyou 夏曾佑, in *The Combination of Confucianism and Alchemists Rujia Yu Fangshi de Rouhe Zhang* 儒家与方士的柔和章 from *Chinese Ancient History Zhong Guo Gu Dai Shi* 中國古代史, had said, "Ge Hong 葛洪 from Jin Dynasty 晋 had quoted Dong Zhongshu's book *Li Shaojun Jialu* 李少君家錄 in *Bao Pu Zi Lun Xian* 抱朴子論仙 as saying that:

> "Mr. Li 李君 had an immortality formula but he was too poor to buy the herbs so he became a government official to make money; finally he made it and became immortal.
>
> "This sounds unusual, but in *Chun Qiu Fanlu* 春秋繁露, all the methods for praying for rain or stopping rain are including witchcraft: gathering snakes, burying toads, burning male chickens or old pigs, getting dead people's burnt bones. Then Zhongshu's knowledge is actually combining "Wugu 巫蠱", "Yansheng 厭勝", "Shenxian 神仙" and "Fangshi 方士" all together. It is the combination of *Gongyang Chunqiu* 公羊春秋 and alchemists' Fangshi 方士 opinions. As to Yin-Yang of Dao in *Yi Jing* 易经, it is closer to alchemists Fangshi, and the title "Daoist

---

[54] In the article this book name was printed incorrectly as 重运延命方

[55] Used in ancient China to symbolically represent a division of islets in the Shang and Xia dynasties.

> Daoren 道人" originated from Jingfang's 京房 name (*Book of Han—Jing Fang Zhuan* 漢書京房傳). The school of etiquette, the grand ceremony of worship of heaven and earth, and people similar to Shengong 申公 and Gongyudai 公玉帶 are all Confucian scholars or alchemists Fangshi. Han Confucian scholars and alchemists Fangshi were divided."

Didn't Liu Shipei 刘師培 say, "Scholars who have dealt with classics combined five elements with medical treatment and they all have different theories about it. Because it mentions five elements in both *Lingshu* and *Suwen*, Confucian scholars thought the theory of five elements was the same as that referred to in *Hong Fan* 洪範, therefore the theory of five elements that those Confucian scholars passed down was combined with medical texts so much so that they even changed some original text in medical books to resemble explanation from Confucian classical books. That is how ancient medical books were based on Confucian classical books and were transmitted down." Lü Simian 呂思勉 said, "There are some texts of the theory of Yin-Yang and five elements mixed in *Suwen* because of alchemists' Fangshi philosophy being similar."

Above are the opinions of scholars from recent times over the relationship between five elements and medicine. We can see that the theory of Chinese medicine should get rid of the theory of five elements. Now I'll quote another two Chinese medicine doctors' explanations of the relationship between five elements and Chinese medicine—the conclusion is that five elements should be abandoned. First is Fu Xuechang 富雪厂, a famous Chinese medicine doctor from North China, and we know that he had researched *Huangdi Neijing* well. He thinks the [theory of] generation and restriction of five elements is a big obstacle in the development of Chinese medicine. He said:

> "The generation and restriction of five elements is truly the obstacle of Chinese medicine. I had researched the theory of five elements; it was from the end of Zhou Dynasty and became popular in Han Dynasty. During Tang and Song Dynasties, the Confucian scholars said *Neijing* was falsified in Han Dynasty, and half of my conclusion is based on this. *Lingshu*, *Suwen* and *Shennong Ben Cao Jing* did exist in the period of Huangdi Shennong.

There is Yin-Yang Qi in heaven and earth and people live within. Plus heredity from parents, family customs, people are definitely affected by dominant Qi. When the dominant Qi affects too much, disease happens. So ancient sages regulated Yin-Yang and recorded them as rules when they were working. That is why the theories of organs, nutrient and defense system, formula and herbs are all based on Yin-Yang instead of the theory of generation and restriction of five elements.

People from Han Dynasty had a superstition on five elements so they secretly added the theory of five elements in the explanation of ancient medical books and this is one disaster in the development of Chinese medicine. We can see that through Zhang Zhongjing treating disease without applying five elements but using six meridians. And when Wang Shuhe 王叔和 was collecting and organizing old medicine books, he didn't do it well enough to exclude the wrong theories, which is another disaster in the development of Chinese medicine. After Song Yuan Dynasties, the Chinese medicine doctors started talking about five elements without reading Hua Yuanhua's 華元化 anatomy book or doing any experiments; they pretended they were smart in front of fools, and this is also a disaster in the development of Chinese medicine.

I inherited medicine from my family when I was a teenager; I was researching pulse-taking methods and studying other doctors' experience for decades, finally got over the threshold of medicine and completed a book, which can explain the fine essence in ancient classical books, it can serve as reference book for later generations and cure the diseased medicine. There is no theory of five elements but rather only simple and important words. So if I give it to other scholars I'll tell them that this is Huang Nong Zhongjing's 黃農仲景[56] family tradition, and it is also my family tradition, so you should treasure it. (From North China National Medicine college—*Teaching notes on the four diagnostic methods secret of success Huabei Guoyi Xueyuan Sizhen Yaojue Jiangyi* 華北國医学院四診要訣講义.)

[56] Huang Di, Sheng Nong and Zhang Zhongjing

Then let's see the words from the famous deceased Chinese medicine doctor from South China, Ye Guhong 葉古紅:

> "The words of experience are gold fragments, while the theory of five elements is sand and stones. Now organizing the old knowledge is like picking out gold from a cover of sand. The generation and restriction of five elements is useless and we need to get rid of it. As to some myths such as leading heaven and in underground spring Sitian Zaiquan 司天在泉, it needs to be destroyed. The knowledge about the people's livelihood and the growth of human race shouldn't be affected by those myths."

He also said:

> "Among all the things in the universe that we don't know the truth [about] yet, none can be stronger due to the theory of generation and restriction of five elements. So, each day that we don't destroy the theory of five elements, is one more day it blocks all people's daily lives."

This is correct. Medicine is part of science, so why are we putting so much unnecessary decoration of idealism on it?

If we can't even figure out which school in the academic history the theory of Yin-Yang and five elements belongs to, or how it grew and developed, or how it connects to five transitions Wu Yun 五运, how can we stretch the relationship between five elements and medicine? That would be exactly as Mr. Taiyan 太炎 said, "That's ridiculous!"

In short, the theory of five elements has been changed by alchemists Fangshi so it is not the original one. It's not the simple materialism anymore but just another abstract name. Because it's a famous school in every dynasty, the doctors easily mixed it into medical books due to political reasons; then it became the main structure of the medical theories. One should be clear about the fact that the value of any given topic name is solely based on the principle behind it allowing it to develop. If an affair is not applicable to some principles or theories but we still force the use of them, then the conclusion will definitely be wrong. Chinese medicine has its own specialty and this is not deniable, but its advantage is not about the generation and restriction of five elements, which can't guide the clinical practice. Mr. Taiyan has said, "If we don't mention five elements, which part of Chinese medicine is harmed?"

For example, it's a fact that we use Dahuang 大黄 to remove congestion and Danggui 当歸 to alleviate pain in Chinese medicine; is it based on the generation and restriction of five elements or based on pattern differentiation by Zhang Zhongjing? Obviously, it has nothing to do with the theory of five elements, and the same goes for acupuncture and massage.

Article end

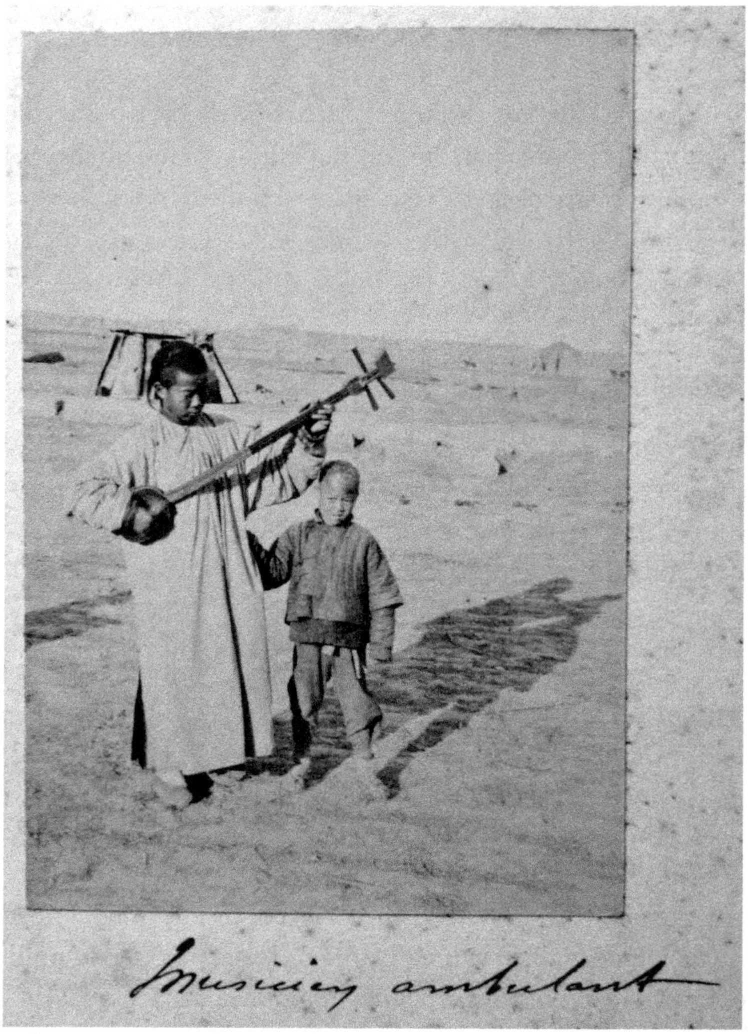

Photo by Mr P. Goux in early 1900s. "Traveling musician"

Discussing with Zhang Cigong 章次公 about Yin-Yang and the generation and restriction of five elements

Dec 1956 By Tang Yuqiu 唐玉虬

Source: *The New Chinese Medicine Magazine* 新中醫藥 第七卷第十二期

Pages 551–553

I just read the Zhang Cigong 章次公 article, "*Begin with Mr. Taiyan's Opinions about Chinese Medicine and Five Elements Theory*," the point of which is to get rid of the major obstacle of Chinese medicine: the theory of five elements. Mr. Cigong is a leader in the field of Chinese medicine today and won't have random words. There is definitely some reason, which silly I couldn't figure out, for him to encourage us to abandon the theory of five elements. I repeatedly read his essay for several days and finally got the point: that Mr. Cigong was misled by Zhang Taiyan 張太炎[57] and Liu Shipei 刘師培. Generally speaking, if famous people say something slightly wrong, it is easiest to mislead people. In addition, the people who were misled have difficulty to admit their misunderstandings. Xun Qing 荀卿[58] had said, "When one has sufficient arguments for his points or one's opinion has logic, then it's enough to fool the masses." In the past, Su Dongpo 苏东坡 had valued the Sheng Sanzi 聖散子[59] which thereafter, none-the-less, caused so many deaths. Therefore, scholars who speak words always treasure the statement: "Words abound under heaven yet there is not one error." Mr. Cigong was mislead by Taiyan and Shipei and I'm going to explain it. Taiyan and Shipei have said, "There is only natures of five elements in *Hong Fan* 洪範 but not the theory of generation and restriction. *Yi Jing* 易經 talks about Yin-Yang but not about five elements. King Wen of Zhou and Confucius didn't follow five elements." They also said, "You Zaijing's 尤在涇 *Yi Xue Du Shu Ji* 醫學讀書記 as if it was criticizing the theory of five elements, but in order to defend the old school's theory, he trimmed his words a bit." I'll list You Zaijing's Q&A about five elements first and then supplement an explanation.

In a rhetorical way, You Zaijing said, "*Yi Jing* talks about the Eight Trigrams Ba Gua 八卦 but didn't mention five elements. *Hongfan* talks about the nature of five

[57] The article writes Zhang Taiyan as 章太炎, which is a typo.

[58] The philosopher Xunzi 荀子

[59] Sheng Sanzi Fang 聖散子方 is a herbal formula name.

elements but doesn't mention the theory of generation and control Sheng Ke 生剋. Therefore we know that the theory of five elements was not from the sages but rather falsified by alchemists Shu Shi 術士 from Qin and Han Dynasties.

I [Zaijing 在涇 himself speaking] say, why don't you observe the River Map and Luo Card He Tu Luo Shu 河圖洛書? The numbers of He Tu: 1 and 6 at the bottom is water; 2 and 7 at the top is fire; 3 and 8 on the left is wood; 4 and 9 on the right is metal; 5 and 10 in the middle is earth. The numbers of Luo Shu: cap 9 shoe 1 these are the numbers generating water. To the right of[60] 1 there is 7, which is the completing[61] number of fire. To the right of 7 there is 9, which is the completing number of metal. To the right of 9 is 3, which is the completing number of wood.[62] 5 is in the middle and is the number of earth. So He Tu is going counter-clockwise, spinning leftwards, and with a generating order of the five elements, while Luo Shu is going clockwise, spinning rightwards, with a controlling order of the five elements.

It's very interesting that the control cycle is going clockwise and generation cycle is going counter-clockwise. Besides, He Tu is spinning leftwards and generating, while across it is controlling. Luo Shu is spinning rightwards and controlling, while across it is generating. This takes place because the life springing mechanism is hidden in the midst of decline, while generation Qi is always hidden in the prosperity.[63] Generation without control means it is only going forwards without backwards; the Qi will easily be exhausted. Control without generation means it is continuously declining without growing; the instrument will easily come to its end. Generation and control is the natural principle of Heaven and Earth, and we should know it without doubt. Besides, the control here means to restrain the excess and bring it back to normal—it does not mean to totally extinguish it. The control inhibits it from floating and surging and like this brings it back to the root. It is a sign of generation. Even though it is controlling, yet it's actually nurturing."

You Zaijing's opinion over the generation and control of five elements is very pointed. Zhang Taiyan was not convinced and he satirized Zaijing for trimming the words. Taiyan also criticized him for not answering the question at hand, namely,

[60] To the right means from the bottom going to the right to the top to the left in a counter clockwise direction. In Luo Shu 1 is at the bottom, 7 on the right, 9 at the top, while 3 on the left. Progressing from 1 to 7 to 9 to 3 are all called going to the right.

[61] Generating and completing numbers are from the River Map, where 1,2,3,4,5 are drawn as an inner circle and are claimed to be the generating numbers of the four directions plus center, while 6,7,8,9,10 are drawn as an outer circle and are said to be the completing numbers of same directions.

[62] 3 is the generating number of wood; however, in this article, we keep the mistake as being the completing number of wood.

[63] The dichotomy of this sentence seems to be wrong if we compare it to the prior sentence, but we have kept it as in the article.

why does *Yi Jing* only talk about the Eight Trigrams without five elements and *Hongfan* only talk about the nature of five elements without the theory of generation and control? Why does he only use He Tu and Luo Shu to supply an answer? Today I'm going to supplement his answer.

Yi Jing only talks about the Eight Trigrams because the Eight Trigrams already include five elements. There is no need to talk about five elements when the Eight Trigrams are mentioned. Haven't Taiyang and Shipei studied *Yi Jing* before? Qian 乾 and Kun 坤 are pure Yang and pure Yin, Qian is Father and Kun is Mother. One Father and one Mother give birth to three sons and three daughters. Zhen 震 is Eldest Son, Kan 坎 is Middle Son and Gen 艮 is Youngest Son, while Xun 巽 is Eldest Daughter, Li 離 is Middle Daughter and Dui 兌 is youngest Daughter. *Shuogua* 說卦[64] said, "Qian is metal," and "Kun is the ground," which is earth. It also said, "Xun is wood". The image commentary[65] *Xiang Ci* 象辞 of the Jing 井 hexagram said, "There's a water well on top of wood." The image commentary of Jian 漸 hexagram said, "There is wood growing on the mountains." *Shuogua* said, "Kan is water, Li is fire." The image commentary of Ji Ji 既濟 hexagram said, "Water is on top of fire crossing over." The image commentary of Wei Ji 未濟 hexagram said, "Fire on top of water is not crossing." It also said, "Gen is mountain," which is a solid formation of earth, and it also said "Dui is nourishing, Dui is autumn," which means it is also metal. It also said, "Zhen is thunder, Zhen is in the east," which means it is also wood.

These quotes above are talking about the Eight Trigrams and they are also talking about five elements. Therefore, if one talks about the Eight Trigrams and five elements together it will be a repeat. *Yi Jing* is the accomplishment of King Wen, Duke of Zhou and Confucius; how can one say that King Wen, Duke of Zhou and Confucius didn't follow five elements?

Now let's talk about *Hongfan* only talking about the nature of five elements without a theory of generation and control. In the *Book of Historical Records of the Zhou Dynasty Zhou Shu* 周書 in chapters *Great Plan Hongfan* 洪範 and *Counsels of Great Yu Yu Shu Da Yu Mo* 虞書大禹謨 both only talk about five elements without a theory of generation and control. The reason is that the five elements mentioned therein were the same as the

---

[64] Shuo Gua 說卦 is one of the ten wings to supplement the *Yi Jing*.

[65] Xiang Zhuan 象傳 is one of the ten wings to supplement the *Yi Jing*.

five materials Wu Cai 五材 in *Twenty-Seventh Year Zuozhuan Xiang* 左傳襄 (which is metal, wood, water, fire and earth). *Zuozhuan* said, "There are five materials in nature that people can use." *Hongfan* said, "Water nature is to moisten and flow downward," and this character can help people irrigate fields. "Fire nature is to flare up," and this character can help people burn things. "Wood nature is to bend and straighten," and this character can help people make their tools. "Metal nature is to transform," and this character can help people cast utensils. "Earth nature is to sow and reap," and this character can provide people with food.

This is the same as the five elements in *Liufu* 六府 in *Counsels of Great Yu Da Yu Mo* 大禹謨 which only uses the material in order to point out to people what to use. Therefore, it was unnecessary to mention the theory of generation and control. However, *Hongfan* talks about five elements as "1 is water, 2 is fire, 3 is wood, 4 is metal, 5 is earth." They are all generating numbers.[66] The five elements mentioned in *Counsels of Great Yu* were "water, fire, metal, wood and earth," which follows the order of control.

Although in *Hongfan* and *Counsels of Great Yu* there is no mention of five elements' generation and control, didn't it demonstrate to people the generation and control? When, in the past, people studied *Shang Han Lun*, they needed to focus on the word "Void" (Wu 無).[67] Today, the five elements in *Hongfan* and *Counsels of Great Yu* are implying the theory of generation and control even if it is not literally mentioned in both books. Mr. Taiyan is very smart, so why can't he think of this instead of simply listening to other people saying that *Hongfan* talks about material only without generation and control of five elements, and therefore he would not follow five elements.

My conclusion is that when *Yi Jing* talks about the Eight Trigrams, it also means the five elements, so there is no need to mention five elements again. King Wen and Confucius were following the theory of five elements, the five elements in *Great Counsels of Yu* and *Hongfan*. In these texts it was the same as in *Zuozhuan* for people's daily use so it didn't need to mention generation and control. Nonetheless, it still implied generation and control. Since creating the trigrams in antiquity, Fu Xi already hid within the Yin Yang and five elements theory of generation and control. Why would people think that Yin Yang and five elements came about first only with Zou Yan during the Warring States Period?

---

[66] Generating versus completing numbers as in the River Picture.

[67] The medical principle behind the *Shang Han Lun* is not explained in that text; the reader has to read between the lines in order to get at the principle.

Taiyan also said, "The connection between five organs and five elements was inconsistent in the old version and new version of *Book of Documents Shang Shu* 尚書, although Zheng Kangcheng 鄭康成 followed the new version but when explaining *Zhou Guang* 周官 and *Ji Yi* 疾医 he followed the old version. So we know that the distribution of five elements was not originally consistent." I'm going to give my opinions here. Ou Yang 歐陽, in the new version of *Book of Documents,* said, "Liver is wood. Heart is fire. Spleen is earth. Lung is metal. Kidney is water." The old version of *Book of Documents* says, "Spleen is wood. Lung is fire. Heart is earth. Liver is metal. Kidney is water." Xu Shen 許慎 said, "*In the Proceeding of Government in Different Months Yue Ling* 月令,[68] in spring we offer sacrifices to Spleen, in summer we offer sacrifices to Lung, in late summer we offer sacrifices to Heart, in autumn we offer sacrifices to Liver, in winter we offer sacrifices to Kidney. It is the same as in the old version of *Book of Documents*."

Zheng Kangcheng refuted it, saying, "*In the Proceeding of Government in Different Months Yue Ling* 月令, we offer sacrifices to the different positions of four seasons and the steps coming before and after each of the five organs. These shouldn't be the same as the Qi of five elements. Today, in the treatment method of disease, the Liver is wood, Heart is fire, Spleen is earth, Lung is metal, Kidney is water, and then patients can recover. Otherwise, the disease will get worse." As to what Zheng had said, when talking about five elements, it follows the new version of *Book of Documents*, which is different from Xu's words. However, Zheng's comments of *Yi Shi* 醫師 and *Ji Yi* 疾醫 articles in *Tian Guan* 天官 chapter of *Rites of Zhou Zhou Li* 周禮 still followed the old version of *Book of Documents*, but he himself explained that "This is based on *In the Proceeding of Government in Different Months Yue Ling* 月令, where the medical method regards Heart as south, Liver as east, Lung as west, Spleen as center, Kidney as north, and this is also based on five colors."

I totally understand Kangcheng's idea that the way to offer sacrifices was different from the way of medicine. Kangcheng originally didn't mean to destroy the theory of distribution of five organs based on five elements from the old version. To the contrary, he respected this theory a lot. The distribution of five organs based on five elements was, in our medicine, the same from past to present. Now Taiyan wants to destroy our medicine's theory by using Kangcheng's words; this is Taiyan's mistake. Besides, the reputation of the old version of *Book of Documents* is that it is mostly

[68] A chapter in the *Book of Rites*.

falsified, and yet, Taiyan used its words to destroy the theory of five elements, which makes me wonder of his intention.

Taiyan also said that the theory of five elements is actually from the "Chen Wei 讖緯 School"[69] in Han Dynasty, which can fool people but can't serve as a philosophy. This is also the mistake of Zhang Cigong that the five elements theory of generation and control had been made up by Zou Yan and became gradually mixed into the knowledge of medicine. Fu Xi looked above and observed heaven's phenomena, looked below and observed the earth's ways; looking close, he inspected his own body; looking far, he inspected all the other things, then he drew the Eight Trigrams and doubled them to become sixty-four hexagrams. Between heaven and earth, all the myriad things and all human affairs have this profound principle of 64 hexagrams. This is the way Fu Xi got the idea of the trigrams, and not by mere imagination departing from heaven and earth, the myriad things and human affairs.

Huangdi and Qibo researched the human body, five Zang and six Fu organs, twelve meridians and merged it with the five elements theory of generation and control. (Even though *Neijing* is said to have been compiled during the Warring States Period, most of the content was definitely Huangdi and Qibo's theory passing down by oral transmission and becoming written down in Warring States Period.) The principle is the waning and waxing principle of Yin-Yang from the *Yi Jing* and is closely connected to it like inhale and exhale. It is not an empty discussion about something foreign to the human body. Zou Yan's theory of the Cycle of Five Virtues and the Chen Wei sayings of the Han Dynasty are made up and absurd, so much so that, in the Sui Dynasty, "Chen Wei School" was banned, but the medical theory of Yin-Yang and five elements remained unharmed. This proves that the theory of Yin-Yang and five elements in the medical field was the ancient way of simple materialism and also the guiding principle for pattern differentiation. How can it be compared to "Chen Wei School" and regarded as silly? Probably only a silly person may think it's silly.

Taiyan also said, "In the past, people saw the theory of five elements as symbols. Gradually, some ridiculous theory appeared; for example, the theory of generation and control is like people's five organs nourishing and controlling each other. Charlatans from later generations totally follow the ridiculous theory without any experi-

---

[69] Chen and Wei is the combined name for early Han Shamans compiling mystical books and later Han Confucians annotating Confucian classics in a mystical way respectively. It represents the school that believes in spirits and Gods and not in logic and common sense.

ments and this phenomenon should be changed." Human being is alive, and machine isn't. When a machine loses a small piece then it can't work. But if a person has one organ taken, such as gallbladder, spleen, kidney, partial lung, liver or stomach, the person won't die right away but can live for a while. Isn't that showing the five organs nourishing each other? When one organ was cut off, other cooperating organs will help to work together and maintain the life for a while, and this is the experiment.

Assuming liver is excess and liver qi governs rising, if lung qi is too weak to control liver qi, then liver qi will keep rising and cause hypertension or cerebral hemorrhage. Then the lungs might get distended and cause cough and hemoptysis. Or the spleen and stomach might get congested and the desire for food decreases.[70] This is called "Over-control what you control, counter-control what you are not supposed to control." Can't the organs also harm each other?

Medicine emphasizes experiments very much. How can one get medicine without experiments? The five elements theory of generation and control come from experiments on people. It's not like the theoretical studies which has only literature research without any practical application, sitting in a room chatting empty talk. Even more so, if one doesn't understand yet the theory of nourishing and controlling between the five organs, from where can he talk about medicine at all? Now, probably because Mr. Taiyan hadn't seen any example in his lifetime that some people are still alive after they had their gallbladder removed, he couldn't figure out the nourishing and controlling relationships between five organs and so held his own viewpoint. However, the wrong theories of the past shouldn't be held again to enlarge the mistake.

Zhen, Kan, Gen, Xun, Li, Dui: these six Trigrams are from Qian and Kun Trigrams. Yet, the *Yi Jing* principle does not come about with only Qian and Kun. Metal, wood, water, fire, earth: these five elements were developed from Yin-Yang, yet the physiology and pathology of Chinese medicine cannot be deduced based only on Yin-Yang. There are five qi of weather: wind, cold, heat, dampness and dryness. There are five characteristics of herbs: cold, hot, warm, cool and even. There are five organs in human body: Heart, Liver, Spleen, Lung, and Kidney, which all can't be categorized with Yin-Yang alone. It only works if we categorize them to five elements.

There are grades in Yin-Yang. Let's take five characteristics of herbs as an example: hot is the most Yang, warm is less Yang than hot, cold is the most Yin, and cool is

[70] Lung metal is supposed to control Liver wood, but here the wood counter-controls the metal. Liver wood is supposed to control Spleen earth, but here the wood over controls the earth so it becomes weak.

less Yin than cold. Even-natured is in the middle, which is like a harmonizing factor for cold, hot, warm and cool. So we use warm herbs to treat cool disease, hot herbs to treat cold disease, cool herbs to treat warm disease, and cold herbs to treat hot disease, then the disease gets cured. Warm belongs to wood, hot belongs to fire, cool belongs to metal, and cold belongs to water. If we get rid of five elements then we should also abandon five characteristics of herbs, but then how do we treat disease? Five elements are developed from Yin-Yang, so to abandon five elements means to give up Yin-Yang as well, but then how can we differentiate the symptoms and treat the disease? The reason that warm belongs to wood is because trees are prosperous in spring and the spring breeze is warm so it belongs to wood and Liver responds to it. The reason that hot belongs to fire is because fire is vigorous in summer and in summer the weather is so hot so it belongs to fire and Heart responds to it. The reason that cool belongs to metal is because metal is vigorous in autumn and the weather is cool in autumn so it belongs to metal and Lung responds to it. The reason that cold belongs to water is because water is vigorous in winter and the weather in winter is cold so it belongs to water and Kidney responds to it. Earth is even, broad and thick, and it can bear the weight of things, so it is associated with Spleen which is in the middle and supplies things all around. This is how ancient people used five elements to categorize the four seasons and five organs.

Huang Kunzai 黃昆載 said, "Five elements generate each other through Qi and not through materials, otherwise they would not be generated." Ancient people explained five elements in *Book of Documents* as "Five kinds of qi flow Liu-Xing 流行 in the empty space, that's why we call it five elements Wu-Xing 五行." This also shows that we can't stubbornly talk about the five elements' generation and control being only in the living body. There were already correct explanations for five elements in terms of generation and control; for example, fire generates earth, earth generates metal, metal generates water, water generates wood, wood generates fire, and fire controls metal, metal controls wood, wood controls earth, earth controls water, water controls fire. We already talked much about this so I won't explain more on it.

Shi Shoutang 石寿堂, in *Yi Yuan* 医原, had said, "When one element is too much, it becomes harmful in both generation and control cycles." *Neijing* also said, "Excessiveness causes harm, restraining excessiveness brings back harmony and infinite vitality." This shows the five elements theory of generation and control is strongly connected to physiology and pathology.

The president of Chinese Academy of Sciences, comrade Guo Moruo 郭沫若, has said, "Yin-Yang and five elements is anti-superstitious and closer to science. It's a big progress that five elements were developed from Yin-Yang." A medical progressive has told me, "Yin-Yang and five elements is high-level science." Recently, the draft of Chinese medicine history from the Academy of Chinese Medicine said, "The theory of five elements is the 'ancient atomic theory' analyzing materials in universe into five fundamental elements." This exactly corresponds to the last two explanations.

Zhu Zi 朱子[71] said, "Heaven gives birth to the myriad things via Yin-Yang and five elements." One can see that in the universe there is Yin-Yang and five elements qi flowing all the time. All people and every single thing have pre-heaven Yin-Yang and five element Qi and all are affected by post-heaven Yin-Yang and five elements Qi. The earlier philosophers said, "Every single thing is a micro Taiji." Mencius said, "I can relate to every single thing," which has the same meaning. In *Zuo Zhuan* 左傳, Liu Kanggong 刘康公 said, "Man receives the center of heaven and earth and thus he has life."

Five elements originally have inclination, only humans have the completeness of non-inclination, while all other things[72] have their inclination. Therefore plants and minerals, as well as beasts, birds and fish from the animal kingdom, each of them receives one of the inclinations: cold, hot, warm and cool. Humans alone receive all of them so there is no inclination and therefore they are complete. That's why Mencius said, "I can relate to every single thing." Although things have their inclination, Yin-Yang and five element are included in all of them only in different amounts, therefore "every single thing is a micro Taiji." What, in antiquity, was called "Taiji" might be the same as the scientific term "atom" in the present.

Now we are heading into the era of science, so we should explore the most valuable in our native medicine, seek its true principle and develop it, then combine it with science. We can't refuse to research it in order to save some troubles or just because people used not to do it in the past. Otherwise, there will be no high achievement in the academic field. Scholars shouldn't be like this, especially the leading ones. Learning is an affair carried throughout generations; if we cannot resolve a problem in a certain era we should allow the generations to resolve it, instead of grabbing the son of heaven and making him order all the vassal princes, hoping to reach every-

[71] Zhu Xi 朱熹 of the Song dynasty.
[72] "Things" means every single thing in the world other than humans; animals, plants, minerals etc.

thing immediately. "Listen and follow most of the things other than the unknown ones, see and follow most of the things other than the uncertain ones." This is the real attitude of scholars.

I've read *Opinions on Chinese medicine and scientific evidence* (from *Xin Zhong Yi Xue the 7th scroll the 8th period* 新中医的七卷第八期) by a Russian internal medicine professor Vadim Gabrielevich Vogralik 華格拉立克, acknowledging that Russians have already studied our medicine thoroughly and meticulously. However, we, Chinese medicine doctors, like thick branches are still not willing to pay careful attention to the fine details, and once we encounter an obstacle, we are ready to give up on it. Since we don't put our hearts to it, we are really ashamed to face other developed countries.

What is this Russian internal medicine doctor's opinion over Yin-Yang and five elements in Chinese medicine? He said, "The theory of Yin-Yang and five elements is related to the inner organs and to the basic idea of medical treatment. These theories are time-verified with deep research, and include accurate and improved thinking and do totally match the principle of dialectic materialism." Others can have precise and correct vision to see Yin-Yang and five elements in our native medicine and yet Chinese medicine doctors, who should pass on our native medical knowledge, are going to roughly abandon five elements. Isn't it what Zhuge Kongming 諸葛孔明[73] said "undervalue ourselves and quote the wrong phrase will lose the meaning"?

The ancients said, "Only goodhearted people can accept others' words." I admire Mr. Cigong, but this time without first doing much research about five elements he devoted his crude opinion. Here I just provide my opinions from the meaningful words of the ancients, and if it's not disobedient, please grant instructions. Hope all of us in our homeland can get the correct knowledge and progress.

Article end

[73] Same as Zhuge Liang 諸葛亮, politician and militarist (181-234 CE)

Chapter 2: Founding of Chinese Medicine schools, education and teaching materials

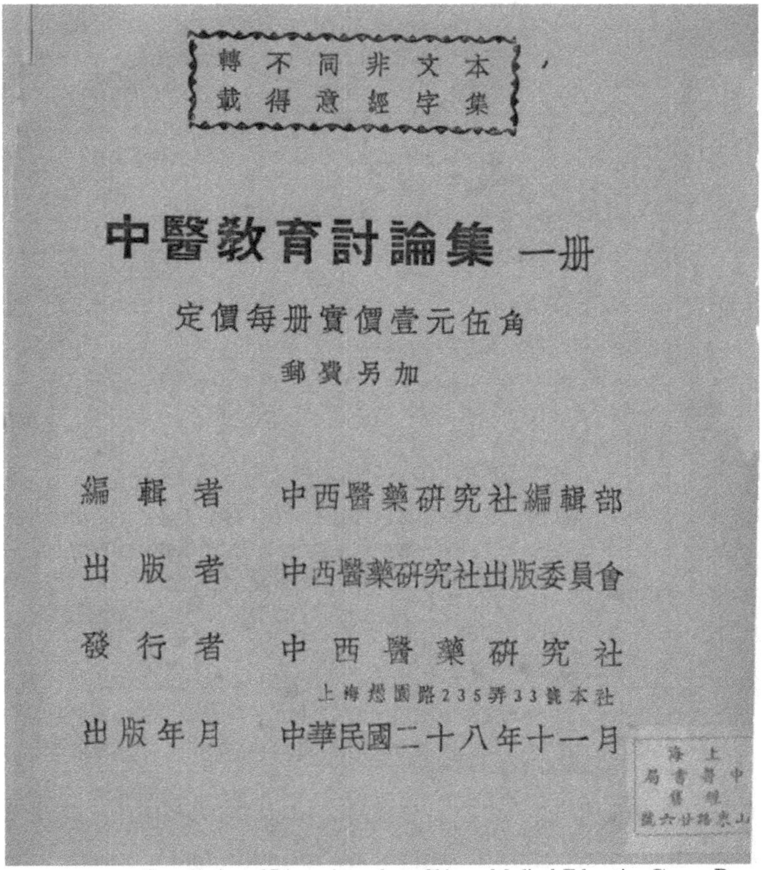
本集文字非經同意不得轉載

中醫教育討論集 一册

定價每册實價壹元伍角

郵費另加

編輯者 中西醫藥研究社編輯部

出版者 中西醫藥研究社出版委員會

發行者 中西醫藥研究社

上海愚園路235弄33號本社

出版年月 中華民國二十八年十一月

Compilation of Discussions about Chinese Medical Education Cover Page

"Zhang Taiyan 章太炎 once said, 'though calligraphy, chess and martial arts are not tested in schools, their level of competency can be tested easily. If students do not focus on their studies and merely treat their graduation certificate as a voucher to practice medicine, it is perhaps something inevitable for Western medicine to overtake us.'"[74]

---

[74] *On Chinese Medicine Education*, by Ye Jingqiu.

Preface of *Discussions about Chinese Medical Education*

Nov 1939 by Song Da Ren 宋大仁

Source: *Compilation of Discussions about Chinese Medical Education* 中醫教育討論集

Yaron: The following preface is a good overview of the situation for Chinese medicine in the first half of the 20th century. It describes the difficulties facing Chinese medicine, the confrontations and possible solutions. Note the nature of this compilation, the style of debate, as well as the chaos of the war.

This compilation is important because, first, it is close in time to the events themselves and second, the collection of articles selected may also express the message they hoped to convey.

We have translated most of the compilation but also bring other source materials from the same time period to compare other opinions. Keep in mind that the compilers here are in the modernizers' group of Chinese medicine. Therefore, articles supporting the old way of Chinese medicine are rather few. Even though there were many practitioners supporting the old ways, their political influence and their role in establishing the official Chinese medicine schools and Chinese medicine curriculum was very minor. Their voices faded away as the years went by.

This collection of articles, mainly representing the modernizers, is actually an accurate reflection of who called the shots at that time, of who decided what Chinese medicine should and will be like.

Chinese Medicine was remarkably developed in the Han and Tang Dynasties. However, skills were mainly taught by individuals in private. The Government did not set any criteria to regulate medical learning initially. In the Tang Dynasty, medical and acupuncture practitioners were taught and appointed through qualification examinations. After the Song and Yuan Dynasties, medical courses were established. Students, having passed the examinations, were appointed as Imperial Doctors or Medical Officers. The courses were established for public servants and not for the general population to learn the medicine. Towards the end of the Qing Dynasty, the Medical Practice Institute 醫學實業館 was established in Capital Teacher's University 京師大學. Some students were taught Chinese while others Western medicine. Later, the Institute was renamed as Capital Teacher's Professional Medical Institute 京師專門醫學館.

Meanwhile, Duan Fang 端方 governed the Two Rivers area. He deemed medical subjects relating to life and specially ordered all medicine practitioners in the province to attend examinations. Those attaining middle or higher levels were granted a license for practicing medicine. In Chinese and Western hospitals, he established Medicine Research Institutes. Licensed practitioners were appointed to teach in the Institutes.

This was the beginning of Chinese medicine education and practicing examination enforcement. Shortly afterwards, the Qing Dynasty was overturned and the Republic of China was newly established. Education Minister Mr. Wang Da Xie 汪大燮 deemed that Chinese medicine was not scientific. He strongly suggested abolishing Chinese medicine in medical courses and to focus on modern methods. Then Yu Bo Tao 余伯陶 and others organized the so-called Petition Group for Salvation of Medicine. They elected representatives to petition the State Council and Education Ministry 國務院教育部 in the hope to retain Chinese medicine. They established the Divine State Medicine School Shen Zhou Yi Xiao 神州醫校 in order to protest.

In the 4th year of the Republic of China (1915), the Shanghai Chinese Medicine Specialized School 上海中醫專門學校 was denied approval to be established. But in fact, the Chinese Medicine School had been already operating. All graduates were registered by individual local governments through examinations and were approved for operating a private practice.

Before the 17th year of the Republic of China (1928), there were very few Chinese Medicine Schools. Starting from the Central Health Meeting proposal to abolish the old medicine, the public was in panic. Not only were organization of nation-wide Medical Unions and election of representatives to file petitions underway, but also Chinese Medicine Schools were established one after another in all areas. Chinese Medicine Schools far outnumbered Modern Medicine Schools. Teaching content in particular became more varied than before.

All graduates, whether from academic societies, training institutes or teaching institutes, were granted certificates. There were Examination and Consultation Committees for setting Chinese Medicine Special Examinations in various local governments. Most committee members were professors or directors of respective schools so that candidates usually had no problems passing the examinations. All bills to abolish traditional medicine by the Central Government were invariably suspended and not enforced. Nevertheless, the status of the Chinese medicine profession and the academic system of Chinese medicine were still not well recognized just the same as before. There were no written documents to regulate or forbid as no one was concerned about it. Local governments, in fact, had acquiesced to the existence of Chinese medicine.

Starting from Tan Yan Kai 譚延闓, Hu Han Min 胡漢民 and others who initiated to organize the Central Bureau for Native Medicine Zhong Yang Guo Yi Guan 中央國醫館 and to apply the principle of scientific means for the management of Chinese medicine. It left a refreshing impression. All the institute's costs were subsidized by the Central Government. Capable personnel were gathered to collectively sort and arrange the old medicine's literature. Useful literature was retained for scientific studies. However, after ten years, the Bureau was burdened with costly expenditure without any achievement. There were some modern-minded participants in the Bureau, but they were unable to offer any contribution due to being a minority. The Officers in charge wished to abandon the existing obligation as an academic group, but instead changed the Bureau to an administration authority. They established branches and issued regulations for certain organizations. The knowledgeable personnel have complained about these organizations not existing to serve academic matters.

At the 5th National Committee Meeting in Nanjing, Feng Yu Xiang 馮玉祥 and others proposed bills for the equal status of Chinese and Western medicine, plus the establishment of Chinese medicine schools. The bills were passed and enforced by the Central Administration Committee. The lengthy suspended Chinese Medicine Regulation was issued by the National Government. The practitioners who graduated from Chinese Medicine School with certificates were listed as qualified personnel.

This then created the problems by which Chinese Medicine Schools were approved. Jiao Yi Tang 焦易堂 and others, totaling 53 personnel, proposed to the Education Ministry to prescriptively compile the Chinese Medicine Teaching Regulations and to add it into the education system, which will allow the establishment of Chinese medicine schools. Later, the Education Special Committee of the Central Political Congress examined the proposal and recommended the addition of special subjects to the Interim Subject Table of the Medical Professional School. The Health Ministry then purposely established the Chinese Medicine Council 中醫委員會 for the administration of Chinese medicine matters. The Chinese Medicine Education Regulation as a resolution in the 39th meeting of the Central Political Congress was: "The Education Ministry and Chinese Medicine Council of the Health Department jointly plan the interim subject table as issued by the National Government." Then the Chinese Medicine Council held several meetings with the Medical Education Council Secretary of the Education Ministry, but without result.

On the other hand, the Chinese Medicine Council announced they would collect relevant teaching materials. The Teaching Material Editing Committee of Chinese Medicine Schools was re-activated to organize it. However, the standard of how to gather materials was not agreed. The editing and preparing was confusing and inevitably stopped. Later the capital was moved to the West after the Incident of 13th August.[75] The popular topic of Chinese medicine education abruptly fell silent and no further information ensued for a long time.

In winter of last year, some personnel of the Chinese Medicine Council and Chinese Medicine Bureau developed the Chinese Medicine Education Society 中國醫藥教育社 in Chongqing. The council members drafted the interim regulation and table of subjects for Chinese Medicine Schools. The draft was submitted to the Commercial and Education Ministry via the Health Department for approval. After the consideration of the Commercial and Education Ministry, the Subject Table of Chinese Medicine Professional School was officially issued in May of this year and will be trialed from the 28th year (1939) without exception. After confusion for some 20 years, Chinese Medicine Education achieved legal status and came to its final proper place.

Although the interim subjects were announced, outlines of the teaching material were not yet issued. There were questions of how the textbooks were being compiled. Presently, Chinese Medicine schools in Shanghai each take its own initiative to hold meetings and employ professionals to compile the textbooks. The Chinese Medicine Education Society originally also had Organization of Teaching Materials Compilation Committee 教材編纂委員會 that is working on it. Nevertheless, no one knows how the result will be. According to past experience, it is hard to imagine optimal result, since most Chinese medicine practitioners would not agree to drop their own opinions for the art and instead follow sciences. In the past, as there was discriminating against Western science and a lack of uniform opinions, it was not surprising that no result was achieved.

We actually disagree to the establishment of independent Chinese Medicine Schools. If only for research purposes, we could simply establish Chinese medicine professional lectures in medical colleges or add medicine subjects in the University. There would be no other alternative means to develop principle without following scientific theories. As a matter of fact, there are sufficient, even excessive, Chinese medicine professionals to meet the nation-wide requirement. For example, in the area of

[75] August 13th to 22nd, 1937 is the first phase of the Shanghai battle of the second Sino-Japanese war, a time when China and Japan entered a de facto state of war.

Yangtze River and Zhejiang, the number of Chinese medicine professionals far exceeds the total number of modern doctors in the countryside many fold. In terms of equality, we should not request any further expansion in numbers. To our understanding, the number of Chinese medicine practitioners produced in recent years hasn't reduced but to the contrary has increased, despite having no legal status recognized by the Government. The mode of private teaching has not changed. If today the legal status of the Chinese Medicine School is recognized, there will be permanent confrontation between the modern and old medicines. It is questionable if this will be of any benefit for the improvement of Chinese medicine.

Under the current circumstances, let us not delay in offering supplementary education in Chinese Medicine, which will apply science though research into the experience of the old medicine for further improvement. We should not offer education for the production of new Chinese medicine professionals. Though Chinese education has been suspended for 20 years, we are not concerned about the threat against the loss of principle. In conserving the old medicine there is no need to rush. Presently, the authority pushes unnecessary urgency and also delays the urgent priority. This action is baffled. The unregistered Chinese Medicine Professional Schools have been operating and continue to be newly established. Though the Medicine Education Committee has been drafting the outline of teaching materials, there is no definite expected date of completion.

The officials of the Medicine Education Committee are purely scientific modern medical doctors. Even when Chinese medicine practitioners participate as members, they are not skillful in both the modern and old medicines and not experienced in clinical practice. The issue of rules and regulations will not meet the actual requirement.

Particularly, the specific teaching materials and textbooks were not completely arranged in the recent past. If compiled by teachers of individual schools, we envisage it will be that they will comprehensively understand the sciences or adequately follow the true principles or strictly hold the proper attitude. We criticized some gentlemen like Lu Yuan Lei 陸淵雷 and Tan Ci Zhong 譚次仲 because their suggestions, in communication and thinking, are not comprehensive. However we widely searched the whole country and are unable to find gentlemen like them to show some inclination to modern knowledge. Moreover, some scholars cannot accept their colleagues and falsely accuse them of surrendering to Western medicine. This makes us deeply hurt. Who will be our teachers in this vast territory? We cannot but be endlessly sad regarding the future of Chinese medicine education!

This book was set to be printed in the autumn of the 26th year of the Republic of China (1937), shortly before the Shanghai War broke out. Our medical society location was in the war area and, in panic, was moved to escape. Half of the stored books we were unable to take and they were burnt to ashes. Fortunately, this edition was preserved due to being printed and not yet bound at that moment. This edition was printed two years ago; the materials might be outdated but the current circumstances have not changed.

As teaching material standards are not yet confirmed today, this edition may still be valuable and important as a draft reference for the Medical Education Committee. We have resumed collecting and re-binding the set by including the full text of the latest announced subject table, the opinion of our society members and previously unrecorded relevant articles. As the original draft was printed earlier, publication will be delayed for several months if we go for a new compilation before printing. Therefore, we attach the earlier version in this set. Note that the compilation's format may not be orderly. In any case, the articles following the announcement of the subject table will naturally be collected for convenient examination. The compilation may not be complete nor without omission concerning the important articles of the discussion of Chinese medicine education of recent years. Nevertheless, we have here opportunity to hear the views of advocates and opponents. Readers who can view them calmly and dispassionately may be arbiters on the correctness of such views.

Regarding standards for establishing Chinese medical schools, if science is not skillfully applied for means of improvement, then there will be no benchmark for acceptance or rejection when arranging teaching materials. Moreover, there will be no hope to improve clinical practice. Even though foundational studies have already been incorporated into modern medicine, the theory and application still seem disconnected. This confers no benefit at all! This is why stubborn members take the view that the subject table is a distraction and not important!

We deeply hope that the Education Authority will consider our opinions to thoroughly compile all the individual teaching materials of Chinese medicine again. The eligible candidates for compilation should have Chinese medicine clinical experience as well as knowledge of modern medicine theories. The equipment for schools should also be of the same standard as Medical Professional Schools. Moreover, tutorials for practicing Chinese medicine practitioners, training of teachers, establishment of research organizations and outlawing of private teaching are all important objectives of today. The Authority should lay down the foundation by consulting with the Health Department and enforcing the respective decisions. Otherwise, wasteful debate over the subject table is only an impediment to promoting medicine's development.

We feel the risk and need to say it. We can't gauge the level of antipathy from the entire society. Some noted members might understand the situation. They should have insights regarding pros and cons and the determination to innovate. We hope we might be consulted as necessary.

Song Da Ren 宋大仁 at Zhongshan 中山 at Chinese and Western Medical Research Society 中西醫藥研究社. November of the 28th year of the Republic of China (1939)

Article end

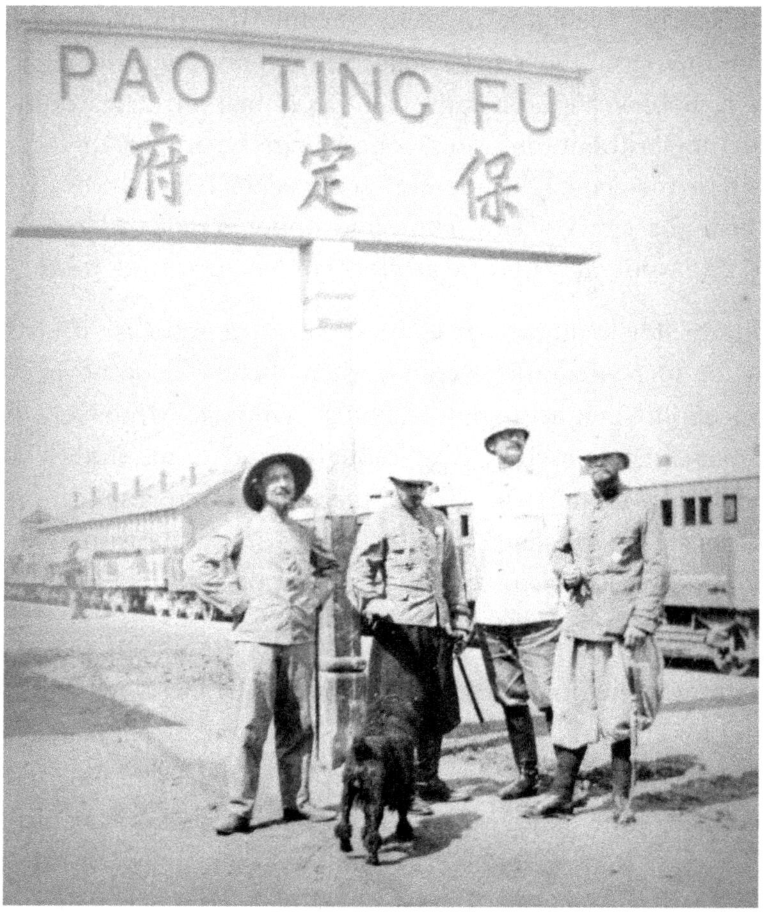

Photo by Mr P. Goux in early 1900s. "Train Station"

Chinese Medicine College curriculum schedules announced by Education Ministry

Republic of China May of the 28th year (1939)

Source: *Compilation of Discussions about Chinese Medical Education* 中醫教育討論集

Yaron: This was the first legal official curriculum of Chinese medicine education, comprising mostly Western medicine requirements. This comes at the end of decades of debates between Chinese medicine purists, reformers and opposers. At that time, it appears that the only legitimate way out was a curriculum dominated by modern science.

This legislation comes on the eve of a decade of war, first with Japan and then a civil war. Because of the wars, the curriculum was never implemented, at least not in any significant way. From the Communist takeover in 1949 (or "liberation" as they coin it) it resumes where it left off, Chinese medicine's status being reinstituted in their own way for their own benefit, as we shall see in Chapter 4 on ideological influences. Chapters 2 and 3 of this book are dedicated to the events and debates taking place up to this point in time, while Chapter 4 continues after the Communist "liberation". In a way, this official and legal curriculum is the junction, connecting the Nationalist and Communist eras.

How Chinese medicine was transformed up to this point and from this point onwards should be seen as a single process with different bends and twists. The events preceding and following this point in time are not entirely independent of each other. The Republicans used Chinese medicine for certain objectives and so did the Communists. There exists an overarching theme of "create a certain kind of Chinese medicine to fulfill an objective".

In order to create a Chinese medicine that fits the sought-after objective, a Chinese medicine selection process was instituted. People creating these new styles of Chinese medicine needed to select what could be included and excluded from the curriculum, who can be named a Chinese medicine practitioner and who not. In this book, we hope to discover the objectives creating the new styles of Chinese medicine and the selection process that took place.

Pages 1–6

The motion of establishing the Chinese medicine schools has been passed by the Central Political Committee 中央政治委員會. The Education Ministry 教部 acted under the order from Executive Yuan 行政院 to announce the temporary Chinese medicine schools' curriculum schedules and gave the order to the department of education in each province to supervise and report on application of curriculum schedules from their respective Chinese medicine schools. The better-quality schools are permitted to start operating as legitimate Chinese medicine schools. Below are the temporary Chinese medicine schools curriculum schedules.

Temporary Chinese medicine schools' curriculum schedule and allocation of teaching hours

i. Common subjects and basic science:
36 hours Central Idea of The Party
108 hours Chinese Literature
32 hours Biology
96 hours Practicum (128 hours in total)
68 hours Chemistry (including Analytical Chemistry and Organic Chemistry)
204 hours Practicum (272 hours in total)
36 hours Physics
108 hours Practicum (144 hours in total)
72 hours Chinese Medical History
Total 760 hours.

ii. Anatomy:
98 hours Anatomy, Histology, Embryology, Neuroanatomy
294 hours Practicum
Total 392 hours.

iii. Physiology and Pharmacology:
72 hours Physiology and Biochemistry
216 hours Practicum (388 hours in total)
98 hours Pharmacognosy, Chemical Pharmacology, Herbal Prescription
294 hours Practicum (392 hours in total)
Total 680 hours.

iv. Pathology:

72 hours Bacteriology, Parasitology
216 hours Practicum (288 hours in total)
72 hours Pathology
216 hours Practicum (288 hours in total)
Total 576 hours.

v. Diagnostics and Internal Medicine:

216 hours Physical Laboratory Diagnostics and Internal Medicine
128 hours Practicum
340 hours Clinical practice (684 hours in total)
64 hours Pediatrics
88 hours Clinical practice (152 hours in total)
48 hours Psychiatry and Neurology
48 hours Clinical practice (96 hours in total)
48 hours Dermatology and Sexually Transmitted Diseases (STD)
48 hours Clinical practice (96 hours in total)
Total 1028 hours.

vi. Surgery:

160 hours Surgery
300 hours Clinical practice (460 hours in total)
48 hours Ophthalmology and Ear Nose Throat (ENT)
64 hours Clinical practice (112 hours in total)
Total 572 hours.

vii. Obstetrics and Gynecology:

36 hours Gynecology
60 hours Clinical practice (96 hours in total)
16 hours Obstetrics
48 hours Clinical practice (64 hours in total)
Total 160 hours.

viii. Acupuncture and Massage:

32 hours Acupuncture
32 hours Clinical practice (64 hours in total)
16 hours Massage
16 hours Clinical practice (32 hours in total)
Total 96 hours.

ix. Other:

64 hours	Public Health
128 hours	Practicum (192 hours in total)
16 hours	Radiology
16 hours	Practicum (32 hours in total)
16 hours	General Forensic Science
16 hours	Practicum (32 hours in total)
96 hours	Wartime Rescue Training

(during period of outdoor hygiene study in summer and field maneuver time).
Time spent on Physical Education can be decided by each school.

Students need to pass every subject every academic year in order to graduate.

The lecture time of all the subjects above is 1640 hours in total, Practicum is 1932 hours in total, and clinical practice is 461 hours in total.

Some explanation follows:

1) All Chinese medical schools in the country will apply this curriculum schedule starting from the 28th year (1939).

2) The education committee of the Education Ministry will compile all outlines of teaching materials.

3) All the subject hours on the allocation sheets are flexible, according to the local situation of each school, while the flexibility amount should not exceed twenty percent, and changed allocation should be approved by the Education Ministry.

4) All the basic and clinical subjects should include preventive medicine and public health, in order to comply with the principle that prevention is as important as treatment.

5) "Chinese literature" should include sufficient Chinese medical terminology.

6) We should emphasize Chinese cultural education and further assist those students who fall behind in the area of Chinese culture.

7) We should add psychology in "Psychiatry and Neurology".

8) We should place an emphasis on the differentiation and refining of herbal medicine in this country while at the same time teaching pharmacology.

9) While teaching Obstetrics we should recruit Western medical surgical teachers to demonstrate with this modality.

10) We should place an emphasis on local miscellaneous and epidemic diseases in clinical practice.

11) Orthopedics should be assigned to the surgical department, and its content should include surgical skills.

12) Subjects such as foreign language, sociology, health statistics, treatment theory, hospital management law, medicine ethics and so on should be electives and share the remaining teaching hours. If we have remaining time, then include more clinical practice.

13) Students should do Internship in a major hospital after the four-year course.

14) The principles of the exam are as below:
a. There should be an exam after finishing a subject;
b. Apart from the exam above, there should be a pre-phase exam and post-phase exam. The content of the pre-phase exam includes all the basic subjects; the content of post-phase exam includes clinical subjects. The pre-phase exam will be held at the end of the 2nd or 3rd year. The post-phase exam is equal to the graduation exam;
c. There are 2 kinds of exam: written and oral exams.

Subject Hours Allocation per Academic Year

1st academic year:

36 hours Central Idea of The Party
108 hours Chinese Literature
128 hours Biology
272 hours Chemistry (including Analytical Chemistry and Organic Chemistry)
144 hours Physics
144 hours Physiology and Biochemistry
196 hours Anatomy, Histology, Embryology and Neuroanatomy
72 hours Chinese Medicine History
32 hours Wartime Rescue Training and Physical Education
(See as mentioned above).

Total for the first academic year is 1132 hours.

2nd academic year:

144 hours	Physiology and Biochemistry
196 hours	Anatomy, Histology, Embryology and Neuroanatomy
288 hours	Bacteriology and Parasitology
288 hours	Pathology
196 hours	Pharmacognosy, Chemical Pharmacology, Pharmacology and Herbal Prescription
32 hours	Wartime Rescue Training and Physical Education (See as mentioned above).

Total for the second academic year is 1144 hours.

3rd academic year:

196 hours	Pharmacognosy, Chemical Pharmacology, Pharmacology and Herbal Prescription
342 hours	Physical Laboratory Diagnostics and Internal Medicine
230 hours	Surgery
152 hours	Pediatrics
96 hours	Psychiatry and Neurology
96 hours	Dermatology and STD
32 hours	Radiology
32 hours	Wartime Rescue Training and Physical Education (See as mentioned above).

Total for the third academic year is 1176 hours.

4th academic year:

342 hours	Internal Medicine
230 hours	Surgery
96 hours	Gynecology
64 hours	Obstetrics
112 hours	Ophthalmology and ENT
64 hours	Acupuncture
32 hours	Massage
192 hours	Public Health
32 hours	General Forensic Science
	Physical Education (See as mentioned above).

Total for the fourth academic year is 1164 hours.

5th academic year—Internship:

4 months Internal Medicine (including Pediatrics, Psychiatry, Dermatology and Sexually Transmitted Diseases (STD))
4 months Surgery (including Urology, Orthopedics, Ophthalmology and Ear Nose Throat (ENT) etc.)
1 month Gynecology and Obstetrics
1 month Acupuncture and Massage
1 month Public Health
1 month Vacation
12 months in total.

Subject Hours Allocation per Week

1st academic year:

1 hour weekly in both semesters for Central Idea of The Party.
3 hours weekly in both semesters for Chinese.
2 hours of lecture, 6 hours weekly of Practicum in both semesters for Chemistry (including Analytic Chemistry and Organic Chemistry).
2 hours of lecture, 6 hours weekly of Practicum in the 1st semester for Biology.
1 hour of lecture, 3 hours weekly of Practicum in both semesters for Physics.
1 hour of lecture, 3 hours weekly of Practicum in both semesters for Physiology and Biochemistry (both together).
1 hour of lecture, 3 hours weekly of Practicum in the 1st semester and 2 hours of lecture, 6 hours weekly of Practicum in the 2nd semester for Anatomy, Histology, Embryology, Neuroanatomy (four together).
4 hours weekly in the 2nd semester for Chinese Medicine History.
1 hour weekly in both semesters for Wartime Rescue Training.
Physical Education (see above).

12 hours of lecture, 21 hours weekly of Practicum, total of 33 hours in the 1st semester.
15 hours of lecture, 18 hours weekly of Practicum, total of 33 hours in the 2nd semester.

2nd academic year:

2 hours of lecture, 6 hours weekly of Practicum in the 1st semester for Physiology and Biochemistry (both together).
1 hour of lecture, 3 hours weekly of Practicum in the 1st semester, and 2 hours of

lecture, 6 hours weekly of Practicum in the 2nd semester for Anatomy, Histology, Embryology, Neuroanatomy (four together).
2 hours of lecture, 6 hours weekly of Practicum in both semesters for Bacteriology, Parasitology (both together).
2 hours of lecture, 6 hours weekly of Practicum in both semesters for Pathology.
1 hour of lecture, 3 hours weekly of Practicum in the 1st semester, 2 hours of lecture, 6 hours of Practicum in the 2nd semester for Pharmacognosy, Chemical Pharmacology, Pharmacology, Herbal Prescription (four together).
1 hour weekly in both semesters for Wartime Rescue Training.
Physical Education (see above).

9 hours of lecture, 24 hours weekly of Practicum in both semesters, 33 hours weekly in total.

3rd academic year:

2 hours of lecture, 5 hours weekly of Practicum / clinical practice in the 1st semester, and 1 hour of lecture, 3 hours weekly of Practicum in the 2nd semester for Pharmacognosy, Chemical Pharmacology, Pharmacology, Herbal Prescription (four together).
3 hours of lecture, 6 hours weekly of Practicum in the 1st semester, and 3 hours of lecture, 7 hours weekly of Practicum in the 2nd semester for Physical Laboratory Diagnostics and Internal Medicine (both together).
2 hours of lecture, 4 hours weekly of Practicum in the 1st semester, and 3 hours of lecture, 5 hours weekly of Practicum in the 2nd semester for Surgery.
2 hours of lecture, 3 hours of Practicum weekly in both semesters for Pediatrics.
3 hours of lecture, 3 hours weekly of Practicum in the 1st semester for Psychiatry and Neurology.
3 hours of lecture, 3 hours weekly of Practicum in the 2nd semester for Dermatology and STD.
1 hour of lecture, 1 hour weekly of Practicum in the 1st semester for Radiology.
1 hour weekly in both semesters for Wartime Rescue Training.
Physical Education (see above).

In the 1st semester, 14 hours of lecture, 22 hours weekly of Practicum, 36 hours in total. In the 2nd semester, 13 hours of lecture, 21 hours weekly of Practicum, 34 hours in total.

4th academic year:

3 hours of lecture, 6 hours weekly of Practicum in the 1st semester, and 3 hours of lecture, 7 hours weekly of Practicum in the 2nd semester for Internal Medicine.
2 hours of lecture, 4 hours weekly of Practicum in the 1st semester, and 3 hours of lecture, 5 hours weekly of Practicum in the 2nd semester for Surgery.
1 hour of lecture, 2 hours weekly of Practicum in both semesters for Gynecology.
1 hour of lecture, 3 hours weekly of Practicum in the 1st semester for Obstetrics.
3 hours of lecture, 4 hours weekly of Practicum in the 1st semester for Ophthalmology and ENT.
2 hours of lecture, 2 hours weekly of Practicum in the 2nd semester for Acupuncture.
1 hour of lecture, 1 hour weekly of Practicum in the 2nd semester for Massage.
2 hours of lecture, 4 hours weekly of Practicum in both semesters for Public Health.
1 hour of lecture, 1 hour weekly of Practicum in the 1st semester for Forensic Science.
Physical Education (see above).

In the 1st semester, 12 hours of lecture, 23 hours weekly of Practicum, 35 hours in total. In the 2nd semester, 13 hours of lecture, 22 hours weekly of Practicum, 35 hours in total.

Note: Although there are technically 18 weeks in a semester, the school calendar only needs to follow the allocation of the teaching hours instead of covering the whole 18 weeks, which means if the teaching hours are sufficient by week 16, the school can finish teaching and hold the exam.

Article end

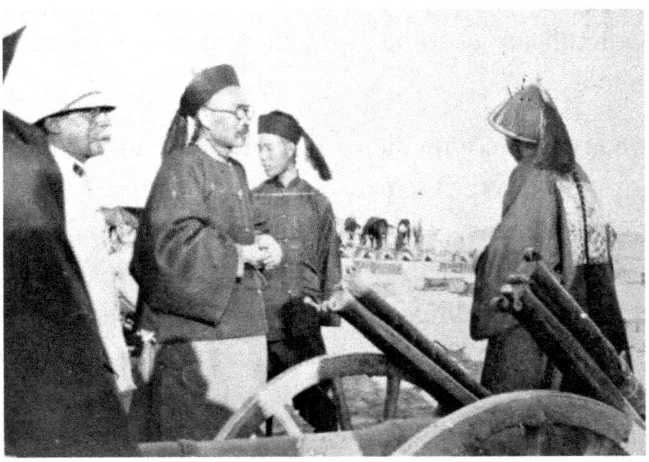

Photo by Mr P. Goux in early 1900s. "General Li, Colonel Guillet"

Advice to the Education Authority about problems that need solutions first within Chinese medicine education and a notice to the Society about enthusiastic Chinese medicine educators

By Xin Deng 新登 and Hong Guan Zhi 洪貫之

Source: *Compilation of Discussions about Chinese Medical Education* 中醫教育討論集

Yaron: Here is an example of the logic behind prohibiting independent Chinese medicine education. An idea suggesting that the proper place for Chinese medicine is within the broader modern medicine discipline, and even this because it is forced by necessity.

Pages 7–12

The Chinese medicine committee has been founded since the Chinese medicine regulations were announced, hence the inaugural Chinese medicine clinics or hospitals now have the same legal status as Western hospitals. There is also a specific Bureau to manage Chinese medicine. This shows the great progress of the administration of our Health Ministry, which is working to correct the attitude of neglect prevalent in the past. For this, not only do all Chinese medicine practitioners celebrate for reaching the goal they've been pursuing, but I too believe it should be like this and regard it as an advantage. Since Chinese medicine practice exists in our country today, it's reasonable to have a specific law to regulate medical behavior and that one of the necessary qualifications to be a practitioner is to hold a degree issued by a Chinese medicine school.

Now, there are miscellaneous Chinese medicine schools and considering that, in the past, they only needed to register in the Central Bureau for Native Medicine without approval from the Education Ministry, they all had different entrance qualification requirements, courses and years of study and, therefore, different Chinese medicine skill level for the students after they graduated. During that time the public expressed objection against this regulation and therefore the Health Ministry issued a definition saying: "A so-called Chinese Medicine School will mean a school that has been approved by the Education Ministry." Since then, Chinese Medicine Schools require approval by the Education Ministry before beginning operation. Now, Jiao Yi

Tang 焦易堂, among others, suggested a procedure for teaching Chinese medicine, which has since been approved by the 39th resolution of the Central Political Meeting: "The temporary Chinese medicine curriculum schedules are established by the Education Ministry and Chinese Medicine Committee according to the courses in medical college."

Isn't it gratifying that this issue finally achieved legal recognition after more than twenty years of debate? During the time that the Chinese Medicine Committee was planning together with the Education Ministry, and without having yet reached a conclusion, there came the July 7th incident in 1937 then following that was the Battle of Shanghai. The Government moved the capital to the west and the entire Chinese medicine education planned process had to be postponed. Subsequently, a new Chief was appointed to the Education Ministry. Some Chinese medicine personnel joined the Education Ministry and that helped accomplish the drafting of the Chinese Medicine Curriculum Schedule. Finally it was completed and announced in May of the same year. The Education Ministry then worked on drafting the standard for Chinese medicine teaching materials.

The main goal of a professional school is to develop people who have professional skills to work in a specific industry. In the motion that Feng Yu Xiang 馮玉祥 and others had submitted in the 5th National Congress, "to develop the academy, to benefit all people's lives," the development of professional people wasn't mentioned. Jiao Yi Tang 焦易堂, of the Central Political Meeting, suggested that "although the ordinance has been changed, as a way forward during the transition period, the procedure should not be changed again. According to the principle of equality, the foundation subjects and applied subjects mentioned in the original procedure are similar to the standard subjects in medical colleges, the only differences being *Wen Bing* 瘟病, acupuncture, massage, Chinese medicine orthopedics and so on, which can be named as special subjects." Jiao also said, "schools that develop medical practitioners should abide by the rules for colleges or higher institutions in regards to the length of schooling. They should only accept high school graduates as a standard entry requirement and should not set up new teaching procedures, just follow standard subjects in the medical college and add some special subjects."

He did not know both *Wen Bing* 瘟病 and *Shang Han* 傷寒 in Chinese medicine belong to the same category as seasonal infectious disease, thus how can they be named as special subjects without any exact definition? As for orthopedics, it belongs to the surgical department. These mistakes are all due to the lack of practical understanding of Chinese medicine.

The new curriculum schedule promulgated by the Education Ministry has been revised. However, the name of the school still remains Chinese Medicine Specialty School 中醫專科學校, according to the original content of the regulation. This is also because they are not exactly aware of the supply and demand between Chinese medicine and our society. Now, only learning something can never be regarded as a profession. Today, regarding the equality of the professions, the number of modern medicine practitioners in the entire country is less than ten thousand, yet there are many more Chinese medicine practitioners in Jiangsu 江蘇 and Zhejiang 浙江 area alone, more than modern medicine practitioners in the country as a whole. Despite this surplus, there are individuals who pass on the knowledge and skills privately, while the government still approves them to practice.

As for the issue of preserving the knowledge, there are many people who practice Chinese medicine and even if there were no Chinese Medical schools in the next twenty years, we would have no concern about this knowledge being extinguished, nor would we be concerned about the profession. If the regulation of modern medicine is too restrictive, with comparatively fewer limitations imposed on Chinese medicine schools, then modern medicine practitioners will be eliminated eventually. How can it be fair? This is definitely not the original goal of developing Chinese medicine academic knowledge!

But the professional ability of local Chinese medicine practitioners is rarely equivalent to qualifications according to Chinese medicine regulations. A few years ago, a certain Mr. Zhang 張 and Mr. Zhu 朱, in some Chinese medicine committee, who strove for equality between Western and Chinese medicine treatment, had criticized the government's prohibition that Chinese medicine practitioners cannot use anesthesia or modern medical instruments as violating the public ownership of academic knowledge. We are working hard to achieve some progress, but if Chinese medicine is to become a conventional treatment, then practitioners need to be able to use opium and morphine or, when a patient is diagnosed with infectious disease, the practitioners need to follow sterilization instructions for the patient. These were all incorporated into Chinese medicine regulations, so there should be no problem.

However, knowledge about Western medicine diagnosis of infectious diseases, prescription of anesthesia and instructions regarding the use of modern instruments is very lacking in Chinese medicine. Therefore the most pressing thing is to teach scientific knowledge to Chinese medicine practitioners. Because of this deficiency, we emphasize the development of Chinese medicine practitioners with a new modern curriculum schedule for Chinese medical schools, instead of establishing research institutions or using scientific theories to explain the old Chinese medicine texts, with which we can never solve the problem. Actually, we can add special courses or lectures to a modern medical college or Western medical university, and the lectures could be held by the people who are proficient in both Chinese and Western medicine, such as Weng Zhi Long 翁之龍 or Guo Ruo Ding 郭若定. If we set up separate schools, there will always be differences and therefore confrontation. Besides, the purpose of setting up separate schools is not the same as promoting research and therefore this is not a good strategy.

The first problem in establishing a Chinese medical school is the teachers and teaching materials; if we are unable to solve this then there will be more difficulties in the future. Today the general outline for teaching materials is still being drafted. Without knowing whether or not it's based on scientific theory and what the standard is until it's promulgated, then we can only consider it as reference and not enforce its application.

Compiling textbooks takes much time; surely it will be completed by teachers in each school. However, education of Chinese medicine should follow the national educational guideline and teaching materials should be composed according to Chinese medicine regulations, as well as be based on scientific principles, eliminating old mistakes and reassessing the value of Chinese medicine.

All basic subjects, such as anatomy, physiology, pharmacology, pathology, physical experiments, prescriptions and so on, should be no different from courses in Western medical colleges.

As for teachers and teaching materials, we can hire modern medicine professors to give lectures. Since the name of the school is "Chinese medicine", we should add Chinese medicine practical topics, which is rather difficult to establish. There are various applications for Chinese medicine terminology; if we wish to use these words with modern medical explanations, it will be then very difficult to diagnose and prescribe. No other word can substitute for "Yin-Yang" 陰陽 and "five phases" 五行.

As for disease patterns, there are Qi 氣, Blood, Wind, Phlegm, Coldness, Heat, Dampness and Fire, in pharmacology, there are five colors, five flavors, floating, sinking, ascending, and descending. These are very absurd and do not exist objectively. Therefore reasonable Chinese medicine practitioners are highly advised to abandon the old concepts, while preserving the practical experience. Diagnosis in Chinese medicine involves recognizing the symptoms but not the disease, and so there is no knowledge of pathogens.

As for treatment, it involves curing the symptoms instead of extinguishing the pathogens and it was recorded as formulas of herbs according to practical experience. But in the past, there was no diagnosis of disease and hence one patient could have had various diagnoses, while a wrong diagnosis would carry along wrong herb prescription, and so it is very difficult to rely on. Usually, most diseases in Chinese medicine are the not serious ones and this is why they can be cured based on symptoms and general observation. However, from scientific point of view this is not a proper way to treat disease. The so-called connection between the pathological change of the organs internally and the symptoms externally is not realistic. As a matter of fact, although the external symptoms are similar, the internal organs are not invaded by the same pathogen, so it is not effective if we only use one general relationship between symptoms and diagnosis. This is why, in recent years, Chinese medicine practitioners gradually gave up this idea and rather started emphasizing a disease diagnosis as well.

As for the names of Chinese medicine diseases, they are all different according to different books. Senior practitioners, such as the assistant director of the Central Bureau for Native Medicine Mr. Shi 施 and Lu Yuan Lei 陸淵雷 already noticed this problem early on, so they are working on changing old disease names to modern medicine disease names, which is admirable. However, some people are still striving to use the old names and descriptions of Chinese medicine diseases and their results are unexpectedly superficial. There is no value in using the old names; besides, it is not compatible with the new Chinese medicine regulations, which instructs that the Chinese medicine diagnostic textbook should record the modern names of the diseases. The old names have no benefit to the administration of health services. It is not indispensable to diagnose the old name of the disease, and it should follow the names of disease from modern medicine.

After changing the disease names, prescribing is still problematic. For example, it is said to be effective using Chinese medicine to cure dysentery, but without being sure whether it's bacillary dysentery or amoebic dysentery or even common intestinal infection, how can we prescribe for bacillary or amoebic dysentery or intestinal infection? Although it is generally effective, it still lacks thorough consideration and we do not know the effects of other formulas and herbs. Seriously speaking, if we are unable to figure out the chemical and pharmacological mode of action then it should not be used in practice. Nowadays, it is legal to establish a Chinese medicine school; the priority should be to research the application of herbs.

Regarding compilation of textbooks, one should follow the principle of literature research, organizing the contents by frequency of use, while at the same time comparing Western and Chinese medicine disease names, in order to reach a better efficacy. It is not impossible, but certainly needs many people's brainpower and a certain amount of time. It is even more difficult to find practitioners who are proficient in both Western and Chinese medicine to research the Chinese medicine literature. This is why I disapprove of establishing Chinese medicine schools first instead of working on developing teachers and teaching materials.

As for practical learning, if we start by learning modern medicine then we will become familiar with physical examination skills. As for prescribing Chinese herbs, if we continue to teach it according to accumulated experience kind of knowledge, then although we have separately learnt science, we will not be able to apply to our practice. This is ridiculous; there is no progress in such a medicine's development. Apart from that, there should be special topics in Chinese medicine colleges that are different from general medical colleges, such as Chinese medicine history, prescribing formulas, acupuncture and massage. Chinese medicine history is part of cultural history. Compared to other medicines' history books, it is simpler and contains errors and is therefore far from a true account of history. Thus far, there is no suitable Chinese medicine history book worth reading, and it cannot simply be supplemented by way of modern medicine history research.

As for prescribing formulas, this refers to the methodology of prescribing herbs, and should be included in the same subject grouping as Chinese herbs rather than being an independent subject. In any case, the methodology of prescribing Chinese medicine does not conform to scientific principle, and so how can we use that?

Regarding acupuncture and massage, although it is worth studying, there is no book illustrating it from a scientific point of view. Charlatan acupuncturists know nothing about it. Although recently some practitioners have been studying it, rarely can they use scientific theory to explain it, let alone improve it.

In short, it is not appropriate to decide on topics within the Chinese medicine school without scientifically researching them, despite benefits that Chinese medical practice may have. I hope our education authority, in the spirit of guarding Chinese medicine and preserving the national essence, will encourage medical colleges to have some Chinese medicine lectures and include scientific research. Meanwhile, educating current Chinese medicine practitioners about scientific knowledge is more meaningful than establishing Chinese Medicine Schools. This is what I sincerely hope; is anyone in power willing to take my opinion and apply it?

Lastly, the curriculum schedule mentions that after four years of study, the Chinese medicine student should practice in a good Chinese medicine hospital for one year. We have no idea if a "good" Chinese medicine hospital includes any modern medical scientific equipment or not. I will not comment on this, but there are some problems regarding the establishment of Chinese medicine hospitals; I will write another article discussing it.

Article end

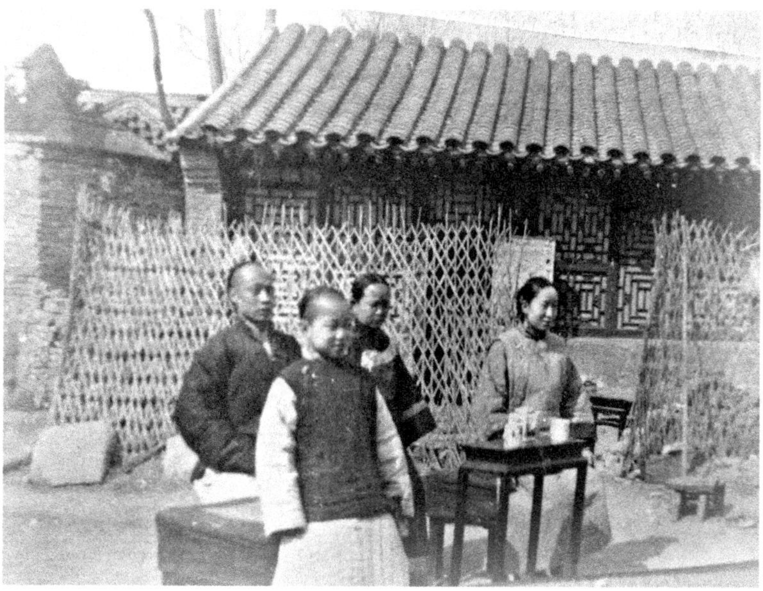

Photo by Mr P. Goux in early 1900s. "Chinese interior"

Medical historical novel 醫學演義

Published 1927

Source: *San San Medical Publication*, 3rd Vol. 22 Issue
三三醫報第三卷二十二期

Yaron: Some practitioners attempted to merge Chinese and Western theories. This style of "some proficiency in Western medicine and scientific theories and reformulating Chinese medicine theory as scientific" was a trend in the early decades of the 20th century, however, it was not the dominant trend. Decades later, during the Communist era of the 1950s and '60s, this style was "reinvigorated" and, to a certain degree, continues up to this day.

Introduction to physiology 生理說意

There are four main principles in physiology: anatomical physiology, chemical physiology, the entire body physiology and natural physiology. These four are different and here's my introduction.

Anatomical physiology includes systems and organs dissection so we know the function, it also includes the entire body dissection so we know the layers under the skin. For example, brain nerves travel around the entire body and govern sensation and motion. Spleen has sweet meat juice which digests food. However, man is the soul of the universe, so the organs and systems can't solely be named by their function. That's why this subject is called anatomical physiology, which means we understand the function of organs and systems through an anatomical procedure.

When we categorize chemical medicine by the origin substances, there are two main categories, metallic and non-metallic; we also have other elements inside our body, such as hydrogen, nitrogen, carbon, oxygen and ferric phosphate, ferric sulfate etc. These are all related to physiology. Iron travels in blood with oxygen and keeps the body warm. Phosphorus is produced in ministerial fire in Liver Yang and it's the origin of bone. Sodium travels in and out of a cell through its membrane. Protein works at the ion pumps and together with hemoglobin travels in blood. We get the physiological knowledge from chemical experiments so it's called chemical physiology.

Inside a human body, there's physiology of one Qi penetrating through the entire body. The classics say that heaven Qi descends and Qi flows through to the ground.

Earth Qi ascends and Qi flow rises into the sky. Mr. You 有氏 said that heaven Qi is Yang Qi while earth Qi is Yin Qi. Yin ascends then Yang descends, Yang descends then Yin ascends, these are natural cycles that flow just like an endless circle. From this point of view, a human being is similar to heaven, so Yin liquid in kidney ascends while Yang Qi of the heart descends, the interaction of these two things result in many interesting natural reactions, so we classify this kind of knowledge as the entire body physiology.

Taiji 太極 generates two polarities which generate four phenomena which generate eight trigrams and this is where the shape and function of five elements begin. Therefore Zhongjing 仲景 said, "Heaven distributes five elements to generate all creatures in nature. Human has five organs to work with these five elements, and then they start generation and restriction actions," which is a main part of ancient Chinese medicine. Recently, a few in the medical intelligentsia remarked that "everything in nature was attributed to five elements in the past, but now we should abandon five elements, because human is different from heaven and earth." They don't know that it is natural physiology to have five elements pairing with five organs.

However, the organ names, representing five elements, don't have the same meaning as physical organs in pathology and treatment. The effect of herbal formulas is largely based on five elements theory which is "physiology in nature". Although the names of five physical organs represent five elements, it is still too far-fetched to make the correlation. In my opinion, five elements theory is natural physiology, yet people don't know about this.

Chinese medicine followers think that anatomy is incredible while Western medicine followers think that entire body physiology is a guess. Chinese medicine followers regard analysis as "too many details" while Western medicine adherents regard five elements as a disadvantage. Both sides will only talk about their own theories. Sigh! How come doctors today have such narrow vision? Humbly, I introduced the general idea of physiology as advice for both sides.

The entire body physiology 全體生理

A human body is like a natural machine; there are external systems of skin, muscles, tendons, bones as well as internal systems of nerves, respiration, circulation, digestion, urinary, reproductive organs and metabolism. They all exist in one body and work together; just like small parts in a single machine, every part works together when the machine is operating. Man is divine amongst the myriad things. He has sensation and motion and he also can think and do work; while the central nervous system governs all these functions, there is one Qi that goes through and circulates in the entire body. This is my opinion about the entire body physiology.

Mr. Wang 汪氏 said that everything comes out from the heart and that five organs six viscera are all connected to the heart. Heart is the monarch amongst the officials. In heaven the sun is the main thing while in the human body heart is. This is why we regard the heart as the governor of human physiology. However, it's not true. According to anatomists, the function of the heart is to inject blood into body circulation. It is a chunk of muscle and not the governor of the entire body. Westerners say that brain is the governor of the entire body. The cerebrum dominates sensation, the cerebellum dominates motion, the pons dominates blood transportation, the medulla oblongata dominates respiration, twelve pairs of cranial nerve govern the sensation and motion of things and thirty one pairs of spinal nerves govern the entire body. Although the brain covers everything, just like the pivot in a machine, however, there is one thing that governs the brain and allows it to start its function.

There are many similar examples, the atmosphere covering the earth to nourish it and generate all creatures. It's also like a machine generated by steam, which then may start working. This is Formless governing Form and only Formless can generate Form. Formless is Qi transformation. Therefore Mr. Jiayan 嘉言 said that Qi accumulates in heaven while Form accumulates on earth, and then the human being is created. Only Qi can form a physical shape, therefore it is said that "when Qi gathers then shapes exist, Qi scatters then shapes disappear." Qi matters a lot to the existence of a physical shape. There are many kinds of Qi in the human body, such as nutrient Qi, defensive Qi, collateral Qi, breath Qi and viscera Qi and there is a difference between each of them. The main Qi that manages the nutrient, defense, collaterals, breath, viscera and the endless circulation is the big Qi in the chest. This big Qi is an example of the entire body physiology.

People's life and death depends on the origin Qi. The origin Qi is invisible and untouchable, it conceals inside Qi and blood and so it governs Qi and blood. "Yin-Yang open and close" exist in it and breath is generated from it. It keeps the body warm without fire and moistens the five organs without water. Life keeps going as long as this origin Qi hasn't run out. Therefore, the origin Qi is another example of the entire body physiology. Experts at preserving health call it ancestor Qi which means a vigorous Qi between heaven and earth. In *Suwen* 素問 *Sheng Qi Tong Tian Lun* 生氣通天論, it said "the Qi of the blue sky is clear and then the Will is proper, then Yang Qi can become solid if the will is followed." It also said that "following the natural rhythm allows one to connect the clear spirit."

These are all examples of Formless being in charge of the entire body physiology. When Qi mechanism declines then the circulation stops, Qi transformation disconnects from the body and seven kinds of body fluid become dead materials. People who don't know this still try to use physical flesh and blood products to supplement the body. However, they don't know that the Qi dominates the entire body physiology and that it is dying, and so the physical body still dies. Why bother to take physical flesh and blood products? Therefore, we treat the Qi before we treat the body, Qi governs the body. And we treat spirit before we treat Qi because spirit is the origin source of Qi. In pre-heaven the body is generated by Qi, in post-heaven spirit leads this Qi. Shen 神 is spirit. Therefore we should maintain philosophical concepts while studying physiology.

Simple explanation of Western medicine and Chinese medicine 西藥略釋與中藥

John Glasgow Kerr translated the book *Manual of Materia Medica* and it has been popular for quite a while. It has four volumes and the first article is talking about the characteristics and function of each drug and how to take it. It was classified by the characteristics and there are categories of laxative, emetic, tonifying, astringent, rising up, harmonizing, exterior dispelling etc. Each one explains clearly the origin, characteristics and effects of the drug. Gradually this book has become the bible of medical students.

However, there are so many mistakes in this book. For example, it says that Talc Hua Shi 滑石 is a combination of magnesium and oxygen and that it can neutralize the stomach acid when it's too much. It criticizes the *Chinese Materia Medica Zhong Guo Ben Cao* 中國本草 for exaggerating claims that Talc cures stone stranguria, jaundice, beriberi and edema. The acid in abdomen is accumulation of damp heat in stomach from a Chinese medical point of view, and damp heat toxin may go down to bladder and transform to stone stranguria. Western medicine treats acid reflux or sand stone stranguria mostly with salty drugs, Talc is one of them, which is slippery and make the patient prone to diarrhea. Talc is heavy and going downwards, so it's the main herb to treat damp heat syndrome. Jaundice, edema and beriberi are damp heat syndromes, how could John Glasgow Kerr say that Talc can't treat these symptoms? It's very clear that they want to abandon Chinese medicine. Other descriptions in his book are similar to this one; we don't have to review them one by one.

Red Halloysite Chi Shi Zhi 赤石脂 has been shown in the past to have many functions, but today people say that it only contains some minerals and has no other medicinal function so it shouldn't be taken as medicine. According to *Well's Principles of Chemistry*, the mineral in Halloysite combined with carbon becomes calcareous, combining with silicon and oxygen becomes several kinds of stone. So stones which are slippery as wax all have this combination and that's why it has another name: soap stone. The mineral in Halloysite is potassium according to *Manual of Materia Medica*. However, according to *Well's Principles of Chemistry*, Halloysite is not the combination of potassium, carbon and oxygen. One can see that John Glasgow Kerr was so confident in his claims because he knew that Chinese medicine practitioners know nothing about chemistry.

Here is another example: nacre, dragon bone, oyster shell, sea-ear shell, stalactite, actinolite, mica, amber, fluorite and other stone kinds of herbs all have different functions, which were clearly recorded in *Compendium of Materia Medica*; today people claim that they all have aluminum, carbon and oxygen and the function is similar to fire powders which can only neutralize acid. They say that there is no other function related to physiology. This claim was easily agreed to by Western chemists.

However, in chemistry, the most interesting part is usually the impurity and not the main part. The main part usually is the chemical structure while impurity matters more when referring to a substance function. Mr. Hengqu 横渠 had said that one is birth and two is formation, which fits chemistry very well. Chemistry means to divide and transform in order to research the original material, combine and transform in order to increase impurity. Therefore *Yi Jing* 周易 said that one Yin one Yang is called Dao. We can't decide the function only by one aspect of the original material. For example, the original material of diamond and pencil is carbon—can we regard both of them as coal?

Therefore elements like oxygen, hydrogen, nitrogen, carbon and other kinds totally change to something else when there's only one little difference in the chemical structure. It's not wise to use the wrong knowledge to attack Chinese medicine. A combination of two different things can have totally different characteristics from the original ones, so a poison combined with another poison might turn into a nontoxic thing; the combination of two nontoxic things might become a poison.

In *Manual of Materia Medica* there are mostly made-up paragraphs. However, many people in our country are tricked by this book and they can't tell right from wrong. Even the authors of *Chemically Experimented New Materia Medica Hua Xue Shi Yan Xin Ben Cao* 化學實驗新本草 and *Family Materia Medica Jia Ting Ben Cao* 家庭本草 and other books extract words from *Manual of Materia Medica* and regard those as rules to follow. Recently anything new is in fashion in our country; people only follow Westerners' lead and abandon our own traditional knowledge as garbage. This happens in the medical field, which is not the only one but the worst one.

Today, the Department of Education promulgates the curriculum of medical schools, which does not include a single Chinese medical book. People now regard the subject of microorganism and pathology as advanced knowledge. Alas, the textbooks they're using are translated books of poor quality and yet they still attack Chinese medicine. I advise everyone to distinguish true from false while studying medical books. Don't be fooled!

Article end

Shanghai Chinese Medicine College Formed

1927 by Zhang Zanchen 張贊臣

Source: *San San Medical Publication*, (Advertisement extracted from newspaper), 3rd Vol. 31 Issue. 三三醫報第三卷三十一期

Mr. Xie Liheng 謝利恆, the former principal of Shanghai Chinese Medicine Specialized School 上海中醫專門學校, has written *Chinese Medical College Dictionary*, which has three million words, and claimed fame around the world. Lately he established Shanghai Chinese Medicine College 上海中醫學院 on no. 379 of North Zhejiang Road, which lies west of Shanghai-Nanjing Railway Station. Mr. Xie's Chinese medical theory is very concise, subtle and profound, while the new theories are difficult to develop without thorough research. Yet, as for the country's teaching system, there are only few proper measures to apply and so he established this college. The system copies Dalton Plan, which pays attention to every professor to pass down Chinese medicine knowledge and also to the development of superior Chinese medicine practitioners. Four major subjects are taught: internal medicine, surgery, gynecology and pediatrics. Courses start with physiology, pathology, pharmacology and diagnostics individually. They also include ancient experts' words and clinical experience, combine the two together to understand the entire concept in detail and then accomplish a big achievement.

Article end

Proposal for Establishing Zhejiang's Chinese Medicine Professional School

Jun 1925

Source: *Compilation of Discussions about Chinese Medical Education* 中醫教育討論集

Yaron: In the face of modern medicine becoming ever more dominant, critical to the Chinese medicine survival struggle was the inclusion of Chinese medicine education in the official public school system. This kind of recognition by the Department of Education would officially validate Chinese medicine as a subject worth studying.

In debates on Chinese medicine theories and their validity, during that time modern science often held the upper hand, especially in the urban population and in the eyes of the ruling party.

A call to include Chinese medicine in the public school system was viewed by many supporters of Chinese medicine as a way out—a way to maintain Chinese medicine through government recognition. This, likewise, was fiercely opposed by Western medicine advocates, as we shall see in the following documents.

The idea of accepting Chinese medicine schools into the public education system will be picked up again and implemented by the Communist government in the 1950s. This is yet another TCM thread that began early on in the 20th century and was picked up forcefully during the Communist era.

Pages 372–374

The prosperity of academics depends on the prosperity of schools. The prosperity of schools depends on the support of the government. Chinese medicine history begins with *Shen Nong* 神農, *Ling Shu* 靈樞, *Su Wen* 素問 and various other classics on Materia Medica, all of them relatively important to Chinese medicine. There are many famous persons in each generation commentating on the above classics. It is important to develop Chinese medicine in order to save lives. Since our country has established the school system, there is no school focusing exclusively on Chinese medicine, nor are there any regulations for Chinese medicine courses. This is not ideal for Chinese medicine's development.

Therefore, I list the following reasons to support Chinese medicine's inclusion in the school system.

Huang Di 黃帝 and Qi Bo 岐伯, as the monarch and prime minister, were concerned with illness in the population and taught medicine in the court. The book *Zhou Li* 周礼 recommends creating the occupation of "doctor". Song Shenzong 宋神宗 imitated *Zhou Li* 周礼, selecting students and teaching them the six subjects.[76]

The above examples reflect that governments and education departments in past dynasties were dedicated to advocating for Chinese medicine and taking care of the lives of the people. All countries around the world today are proud of their unique academic achievements and make efforts to be at the top of the academic world. But our country appears to be following the reverse strategy, which is devoted to developing Western medicine and excluding Chinese medicine from the school system. This is really not the way to respect people's lives and develop traditional culture.

Someone may say that Chinese medicine is not so efficacious, but which other art than Chinese medicine has saved people's lives for thousands of years? This is the first reason to include Chinese medicine schools in the official school system. Our country covers a vast territory, with abundant resources and a large population; the climate varies in the mountain compared to the plains and dampness or dryness is different in the east versus west, south and north. Furthermore, individuals differ in their constitutions. Doctors throughout the dynasties did their best to research deeply. Chinese medicine is quite effective; no other medicine system compares because they don't adapt the therapeutics to the abovementioned characteristics. There are many intelligent students in Chinese medicine who research deeply the medical works of past dynasties and develop Chinese medicine as a systematic science.

---

[76] The six arts of the Zhou 周 dynasty: Rites 禮; Music 樂; Archery 射; Charioteering 禦; Calligraphy 書; Mathematics 數

The second reason to include Chinese Medicine Schools in the official school system is to propagate Chinese medicine so that it may heal the world and its people. Several schools and hospitals of Chinese medicine have been established in Hankou 汉口, Shanxi 山西, Jiangsu 江苏, Guangdong 广东, Zhejiang 浙江 and so on, but the Ministry of Education hasn't approved the subject of Chinese medicine; thus, these schools have no official regulation.

The students of these schools cannot earn a medical degree, which limits their future career development. These schools cannot receive political and financial support from the state, only receiving private donations, so their development faces many difficulties. All of these are greatly related with people's lives but, unfortunately, the state takes them as unimportant issues, even abandoning Chinese medicine. This is the third reason to include Chinese medicine schools in the official school system.

Japan is similar to China in terms of culture and race; it has strictly prohibited Chinese medicine and promoted Western medicine since the Meiji Restoration. Taiwan is occupied by Japan and also promotes Western medicine. But there are many Japanese and Taiwanese who study Chinese medicine in our schools. I ask them about their reasons and they say Western medicine is less effective than Chinese medicine due to the differences in climate, local conditions, customs and individual constitutions. Thus, people have more faith in Chinese medicine. Because Chinese medicine is banned there, they travel thousands of miles to study Chinese medicine here. Accordingly, we can see that Chinese medicine is still believed by the society, even though it is banned by all these governments. The Chinese government abandons Chinese medicine, and excludes Chinese medicine schools from the official school system, which is contrary to society's opinion on this matter. This is the fourth reason to include Chinese medicine schools in the official school system.

Our country is very poor; patriotic citizens buy domestic goods in order to prevent a huge trade deficit. But in recent decades, the importation of Western medicine increased due to the development of Western medicine schools. Western medicine is divided into branches according to the different countries like Japanese medicine, German medicine or English-American medicine. They sell medicines from their own countries, thus shops selling Western medicines can be seen everywhere. It shows not only that people are paying more attention to health, but also that Western medicine sells very well. People are advocating the breaking off of economic trade relations with foreign countries after the May 30th incident,[77] but they continue

[77] May Thirtieth Incident, (1925), in China, a nationwide series of strikes and demonstrations precipitated by the killing of 13 labour demonstrators by British police in Shanghai. This was the largest anti-foreign demonstration China had yet experienced,

to buy Western medicine because there aren't any domestic alternatives. It is embarrassing that medical drugs are all provided by foreign countries. If the Chinese medicine schools could be inserted in the official school system, similar to those of Western medicine, then our country needn't spend so much money purchasing Western medicine products. This is the fifth reason to include Chinese medicine schools in the official school system. It is quite necessary to include Chinese medicine in the official school system based on the above five reasons, based on history and on today's situation.

I propose to the meeting the following methods for organizing a referendum, and then refer it to the Ministry of Education.

Methods:

- Chinese medicine schools should be included in the official school system and as a part of higher education.
- The curriculum standards for Chinese medicine should be developed by the National Education Association and Chinese medicine specialists, and published by the Ministry of Education.
- Each province should establish a public school of Chinese medicine.
- Each provincial medicine school should equate Chinese medicine majors to the same level of importance as those of Western medicine.
- Private schools of Chinese medicine should be approved by the Ministry of Education.
- Private schools of Chinese medicine should be supported by government financial aid.
- The staff, students and graduates of both public and private schools of Chinese medicine should enjoy the same treatment as all the other schools.

June, 14th year (1925)

Remarks by the editor: This proposal was presented in a conference held by the Chinese Education Improvement Society 中華教育改進社大會.

Article end

---

and it encompassed people of all classes from all parts of the country. The Chinese Communist Party greatly benefited by the anti-imperialist sentiment prevalent in the movement, and party membership swelled from several hundred to more than 20,000. http://www.britannica.com/EBchecked/topic/370754/May-Thirtieth-Incident

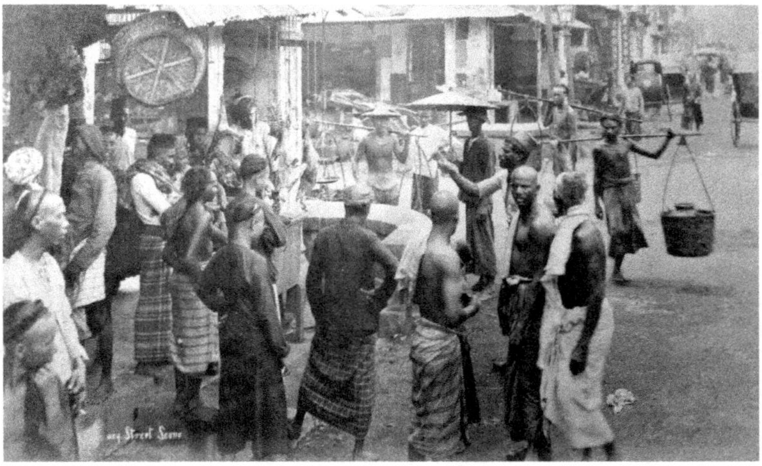

Photo by Mr P. Goux in early 1900s. "Street Scene".

Refuting the proposal for including old medicine schools in the official school system

By Yu Yunxiu 余雲岫

Source: *Compilation of Discussions about Chinese Medical Education* 中醫教育討論集

Yaron: Here Yu Yunxiu argues against including Chinese medicine schools in the official school system. Later on we have an entire section dedicated to "the great debates" where more of Yu's arguments can be seen.

Pages 374–379

I read reports of the meeting held by the Chinese Education Improvement Organization; including a Proposal submitted by the Chinese Medicine Association of Jiangsu Province 江蘇. It argues for the inclusion of Chinese medicine schools in the official school system and the Proposal provides eight reasons which are quite shallow. Originally, I thought the Proposal was inadequate, but some may hear such notions and think they are true. That Proposal was like a single spark that can start a prairie fire; it is really worrying. Now I have to refute it and inform our countrymen, in order to prevent the future crisis of the education and in the hope that all insightful scholars can debate against it.

The first reason mentioned by that Proposal is based on history, involving Shen Nong 神農, Huang Di 黃帝, Qi Bo 岐伯, Lei Gong 雷公, Bian Que 扁鵲, Zhong Jing 仲景 and Four Famous Doctors[78] in the Jin 金 and Yuan 元 dynasties. It says that these sages made all effort to develop Chinese medicine and therefore it should not be abolished.

If all professions with historical foundations were to be added to the official school system, then Yin-Yang 陰陽, divination and witchcraft should also establish schools and be included in the official school system. After Shen Yu 神禹 created the nine principles for good governance, the study of forecasting the harvest through climate changes, and predicting when good or bad luck eventually may arise, these subjects became very popular. In the Spring and Autumn Period (770–476 B.C.), Bi Zao 裨竈 and Zi Shen 梓慎 were the top astrologers. Si Maqian 司馬遷 wrote a biography for diviners, Ban Gu 班固 wrote a record called *Five Phases Wu Xing Zhi* 五行志, and discussed the study of Yin Yang and divination. This means there are many more historical records about Yin Yang and divination than records about Chinese medicine. Pao Xi 庖犧 drew the Eight Diagrams, Zhou Wenwang 周文王 developed lines in the Eight Diagrams, Confucius wrote Shiyi 十翼; the study of nine great masters and five divinatory signs were recorded in Han Dynasty's book Hong Fan 洪範 and the eight famous turtles were discussed in Gui Ce 龜策. There were many discussions on divination in the book *Zuo Shi Nei Wai Zhuan* 左氏內外傳. A diviner was higher than a doctor in the official rankings of the Zhou Dynasty. Therefore, in ancient times, divination was more important than medicine. Witchcraft and medicine belonged to the same profession. Shi Ben 世本 recorded that in the period when Wu Peng 巫彭 was a doctor, Jin Teng 金縢 said that Zhou Wuwang 周武王 was ill and Zhou Gong 周公 prayed to the ghost and god. Lun Yu 論語 recorded that when Kong Zi 孔子 was ill, Zi Lu 子路 prayed to the ghosts and gods. Zuo Zhuan 左傳 recorded that when Qi Jinggong 齊景公 was ill, Liang Qiuju 梁邱據 suggested executing Zhu Gu 祝固 and Shi Yin 史嚚 (being responsible for witchcraft ritual), with no mentioning of medicine. The *Nei Jing* 內經 also recorded that "Witchcraft ritual could treat diseases in ancient times". So doctors didn't exist in ancient times, only witch doctors. Zuo Shi 左氏 also said "It is acceptable not to use medicine when serving the emperor". It was really not common to use medicine to treat diseases in

[78] Liu Wan Su, heat theory 刘完素的火热说; Zhang Cong Zheng, purging theory 张从正的攻邪说; Li Dong Yuan, Spleen and Stomach theory 李东垣的脾胃说; Zhu Zhen Heng, tonify Yin theory 朱震亨的养阴说.

ancient times. It thus can be seen that, if setting up schools according to history, schools of divination should be established as a first priority. Medicine schools should only be established up after the schools of divination. That Proposal reveals the ignorance of the history of our own country, and considers Chinese medicine as the epitome of Chinese culture, while denouncing divination and astrology as an extravagance. That Proposal is superficial, not reflecting deep research of our historical roots. And the quoted books of Shen Nong 神農 and Huang Di 黃帝 aren't really classics. There were many Shen Nong 神農 books recorded in *Han Shu Yi Wen Zhi* 漢書藝文志 but none was on the materia medica. Lu Jia 陸賈 said in his book *Xin Yu* 新語 that "Shen Nong thought meats were not enough to support all people, so he tried to find alternative foods, he tasted hundreds of herbs with different flavors, and finally taught people to eat whole grains." In a quotation from *Zhong Jing Bu* 中經簿, Zhou Guan Ji Yi 周官疾醫 said, "There was a book named *Zi Yi Ben Cao Jing* 子儀本草經 with one volume." And then it quoted Liu Xiang 劉向: "Bian Que 扁鵲 asked Zi Yi 子儀 to take the pulse when treating Zhao Taizi's 趙太子 disease." Thus, the *Materia Medica* was not written by Shen Nong 神農, but by Zi Yi 子儀, who was a disciple of Bian Que 扁鵲 in the Six Kingdoms period. As for the *Internal Classic Nei Jing* 內經, it was also not a book written by Huang Di 黃帝. Kong Zi 孔子[79] compiled the *Shang Shu* 尚書; he selected articles in the periods from Yao Shun 堯舜 to the Spring and Autumn. Tai Shigong 太史公[80] stated, "Hundreds of scholars said Huang Di's 黃帝 works were not refined and elegant, therefore Chinese nobility was not willing to discuss them." Since Huang Di's 黃帝 books were considered vulgar and nonclassical during the periods of Kong Zi 孔子 and Shigong 史公, scholars and bureaucrats were ashamed of talking about them. *Nan Jing* 難經, in which the diagnostic method of Cunkou 寸口 pulse was created, was really a nonsensical and misleading book; it should be condemned as having been a negative influence throughout the ages.

Bian Que Zhuan 扁鵲傳, in *Shi Ji* 史記, recorded, "There was a person that had the ability of seeing through people, thus he was able to treat patients by seeing the disorders of internal organs, and he named it as pulse diagnosis" and pointed out that "The person who created pulse diagnosis was Bian Que 扁鵲." Bian Que 扁鵲 took pulses depending on the ability of seeing through people, and so it was quite

[79] Confucius.

[80] An official position in ancient time, here referring to Si Maqian 司馬遷.

foolish of later generations to respect and follow his pulse diagnosis without having such special ability. The book of Zhang Zhongjing 張仲景 was somewhat methodized, but it created the theory of six channels absurdly and in a disorderly way, which was the bone of contention of later generations. *Qian Jin* 千金 and *Wai Tai* 外臺, the compilations of formulas, were also collections of ancient practical experience which is rarely ever mentioned, but they could be valuable research materials for later generations. Influenced by the emptiness and superficiality of Song-Confucianism, the works of the four famous doctors from Jin and Yuan dynasties were unclear and absurd, though their academic opinions appeared assertive and coherent. *Internal Classic Nei Jing* 內經 was the theoretical foundation of that Proposal, but was far inferior to *Qian Jin* 千金 and *Wai Tai* 外臺, which listed the symptoms and relevant formulas to get the truth. So most of the examples thought to be valuable and provided by that Proposal are actually absurd and totally unfounded.

The second reason suggested in that Proposal argues, based on theories and experiments, that it is not effective to treat local diseases using foreign medicines. The theories of ancient medicine are no more than Yin Yang, five elements, six Qi, and twelve channels. Yin Yang, five elements, six Qi are the classifications developed by the ancients through observing natural phenomena. They are quite simple and not comparable to the understanding of natural phenomena by scholars nowadays. If we still insist on these ancient theories, it's just like we've abandoned civilization and regressed back into animal forms. If we try to prove the existence of the twelve channels anatomically, we will know it is a complete fallacy; refer to my work *Ling Su Shang Dui* 靈素商兌 for further details. Therefore, the theories of ancient medicine are naïve and absurd. Regarding experimentation, actually it is not related to Chinese medicine. Da Huang 大黃 is able to eliminate accumulations and Dang Gui 當歸 can relieve pain. All these are facts instinctively known by people, such as grains for relieving hunger, water for relieving thirst, which are related to experience and not experimentation. An experiment analyzes intricate natural phenomena by precise scientific method to explain the facts that are instinctively known by people and discovered by experience. It makes hard things simple, complicated to plain, hidden to visible, in order to avoid misunderstanding. It checks the truth repeatedly and carefully. What the Chinese doctors do follow is facts instinctively known by ancient people and their experiences. They don't know the natural phenomena clearly, and so how then can they know the truth of Nature and treat patients based on that? The treatise on *Abolishing the Medicine Fei Yi Lun* 廢醫論 by Yu Quyuan 俞曲園 states, "If cured by medicine, then also could be cured without medicine. If not cured without medicine, then also could not be cured by medicine." It is superficial to judge the therapy by the effect. The argument that, "the effect of Chinese medicine is quick and good" in that Proposal, is dominated by greedy egotism. It is really not an experiment.

Saying "medicine from foreign countries" is nonsense may deceive lay persons. Medicine for diseases is exactly like beans and grains for surviving. I never heard of people bringing local foods when they go abroad, nor foreigners who travel in China bringing their own foods. Europe, the United States and our country are all within the same planet, which belongs to the solar system, rather than being a different world. The laws of nature govern everything in the world, and being a part of this world, human beings are no exception. So when talking about bone and muscle, people can't avoid mentioning mechanics. When talking about the eye, people can't avoid mentioning optics. When talking about ears, people can't avoid mentioning acoustics. When talking about movement, people can't avoid mentioning kinesiology. When talking about the body's material, people can't avoid mentioning chemistry. When talking about cell growth, dissimilation and assimilation, metabolism and species breeding, people can't avoid mentioning biology. All in all, there is no difference between the East and the West. For diseases caused by the excess or insufficiency of substances in the body, if there is a kind of material that may correct it, and doesn't harm the body, then this material can be used as a drug for the treatment of such disease. There is also no difference between East and West about this. For example, sodium carbonate is used for hyperchlorhydria in Western medicine. The Chinese don't have hyperchlorhydria. Otherwise, Chinese people would also use sodium carbonate for hyperchlorhydria. As another example, saline is used for dehydration caused by cholera. The Chinese don't suffer from cholera, or rather suffer from cholera but without dehydration. Otherwise, Chinese people would also use saline for dehydration caused by cholera.

The so-called "foreign drugs and native diseases," "inefficacy due to physical differences between the East and West," and "wearing down due to the consumption of strong and powerful drugs," in that Proposal, are all malicious slanders that lack a reasonable foundation. I have found that there are Tibetan saffron and American ginseng in the formulas prescribed by Chinese medicine doctors; how can they explain this?

Article four in that Proposal suggests that "Western medicine originated in Rome," which is totally wrong. It actually originated in Greece, with Hippocrates being honored as the father of Western medicine. These facts were recorded in reliable historical records. The suggestion of medicine originating from Rome is completely wrong. More than that, Western medicine has changed a great deal since its founding in Greece. Over the past century, science and technology have achieved great advances, while the medicine has enjoyed great progress. The situation is completely at odds with the old sayings against Western medicine. The Proposal suggests that "Western medicine imitated the *Nei Jing* 內經; it spread across the world and became popular." This is really the opinion of a person who doesn't understand developments in the world.

The Proposal suggests that "the wisdom of Chinese medicine is no less than Western medicine." It is narrow-minded to compare the two medicines. We should know that the development of an academic subject relies on the mutual communication and assistance of the broader academic environment. The development of Western medicine relies on the progress of the natural sciences. Its basic theories are never contrary to natural law, thus it can develop with the sciences and gain popularity the world over. Meanwhile, Chinese medicine is only an old belief system based on Yin-Yang and Five Phases. Its fundamentals are not compatible with contemporary knowledge of the natural sciences. Even there if there was no competition from Western medicine, still it's not possible for Chinese medicine to become a systematized theory. Chinese medicine doesn't try to thoroughly improve itself; conversely, it is addicted to competing with Western medicine, which is so puzzling.

The fifth reason of the Proposal suggests that Chinese medicine communicate with Western medicine. There was already an article discussing in detail the inadequacy of that issue; it is wrong to suggest communication between them.

Modern medicine is a science. It firstly researches human birth, the body structure, its relationship with chemistry and physics and its positioning in nature. Then it researches the root of diseases, their causes and progression, with the newest and most sophisticated methods. Finally, the therapeutic method is selected, such as various supplements.

Therefore, treatment is the final step in contemporary Western medicine. Ancient Chinese medicine was just the opposite over its long history; it considered the treatment first off. This is probably because prehistoric humans didn't know what exactly a disease was, but paid great attention to finding a way to treat diseases they suffered from. For example, treating hunger with food, treating fatigue with rest, treating heat with ice, treating cold with fire, treating perceptual disturbance and movement disorders with exercise; all were instinctive treatments similar to those of primitive animals. However, the prosperity of Chinese medicine was based on this.

With increasing human wisdom and the development of philosophy, people tried to explain all natural phenomena by fantasy theories such as Four Substances, Five Elements and Eight Diagrams. Chinese medicine, unfortunately, could not be immune to these fantasy theories which tried to explain physiology and pathology by the combination of these theories, life experience and knowledge of anatomy. *Huang Di Nei Jing* 黃帝內經, the Indian *Guang Ming Zui Sheng Wang Jing* 光明最勝王經 and the Greek Four Humors of Hippocrates were all products of that time. There was some possibility of communication between Chinese medicine and Western medicine at that time because the basis of both was similar to each other and there were means of communication. But nowadays, with the development of science, Western medicine has become a completely new medicine. Meanwhile, Chinese medicine stands still and refuses to progress. Therefore, there is a wide gap between Chinese medicine and Western medicine. Furthermore, there is no such thing as Chinese or Western medicine, only old or new medicine. New and old medicines, with completely different theories, cannot communicate with each other now. For them to attempt communicating is just like reducing the intelligence and wisdom of evolved white and yellow people to maintain the same level of knowledge as that of the savages from Southern Africa or Taiwan. It is really backwards to do so.

The Proposal takes effective metal and stone as foreign drugs, while taking medicinal liquids and balms as our own medical materials. This is really neither consistent nor justified; these changeable opinions may collapse without being refuted. It is really immature to say "huge trade deficit" in the Proposal. If medicinal liquids and balms are our own medical materials, why can't we produce drugs? Nowadays, people would like to buy locally-produced cigarettes, towels and so on, but none of them originates from our country. People are always motivated by profit. So if Western medicine is widely used in the future, there will be more and more manufacturers of Western medicine. It is really not necessary to worry about that. We will even export drugs to foreign countries then. Chinese medicine doesn't try to make progress, but rather it stands still. It was acceptable during the period of isolation decades ago, but it is really not a sustainable solution nowadays.

So that Proposal confuses right and wrong, goes against generally acknowledged truth; it is not civilized, but savage. It violates laws of evolution and nature, going against academic development and the worldwide trend. It mocks scholars and foreign countries, which is really not a trivial matter. But the Chinese Medicine Association of Jiangsu Province published the Proposal brazenly, the Chinese Education Improvement Society passed it unexpectedly; it really is silly behavior, how can we not worry about the future of education? As for "people doing good deeds," I, more than anyone, want to. In our land, there are many wise gentlemen and as science develops so rapidly, this Proposal is unacceptable today. I think my refutation is a little bit unnecessary. But I cannot help but refute it due to my concerns. If this Proposal were to disappear from the academic world, even though ignorant of many things, I would be happy.

Article end

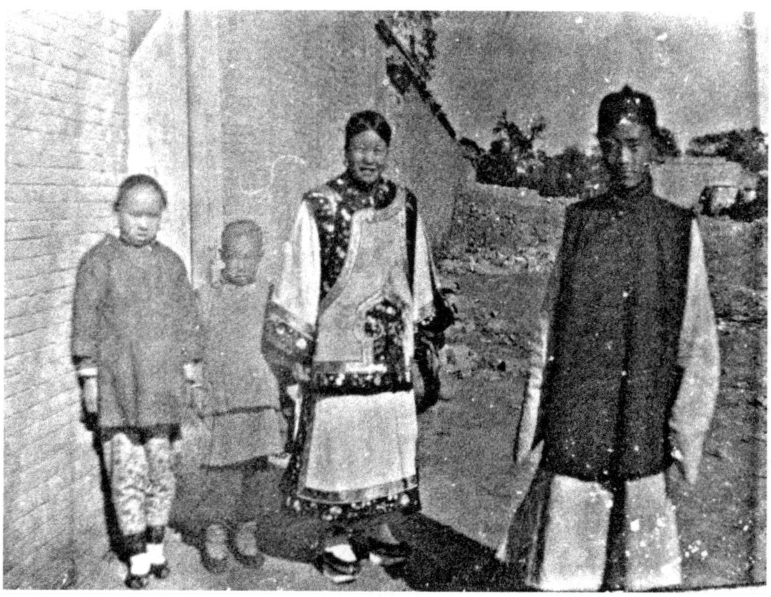

Photo by Mr P. Goux in early 1900s. "Chinese family".

Denouncement of Yu Yunxiu's refutation of the medical school system proposal

By Qin Bowei 秦伯未

Source: *Compilation of Discussions about Chinese Medical Education* 中醫教育討論集

Yaron: Qin Bowei is one of the important figures during the Republic and the early years of Communist rule. There are several articles from him throughout the book.

Pages 379–381

On October the 13th, *Shi Bao* 時報 published *Refuting the Proposal for Including Chinese Medicine Schools*[81] *in the Official School System* written by Yu Yunxiu. Ten days later, this article was republished in *Shen Bao* 申報. Chinese medicine will not disappear due to that text and people will not mistrust Chinese medicine because of its content. However, it may mislead lay persons, so I have to refute it.

That article mainly attacked the Chinese medical theories of Yin Yang, Five Phases and twelve Channels. Yin Yang is a concept of relativity, describing opposite and interactive actions. Take the Yin Yang of Qi as an example: Yin Qi governs the static and tends to be interior, while Yang Qi governs the dynamic and tends to be exterior. Yang originates from Yin; Yin originates from Yang. Only when Yin and Yang are in harmony, can essence-spirit be normal. If Yin and Yang separate from each other, essence-spirit will be exhausted. It is just like electricity with the division between positive and negative. Five Phases is a concept representing change. For example, earth generating metal in the *Nei Jing* 內經 is related to Spleen Qi transporting essence to the Lung. Fire restricting metal in the *Nei Jing* 內經 is related to heat accumulating in the Lung and causing lung weakness. When it says that Qian 乾 trigram means "heaven" but it does not specifically use the word "heaven" Tian 天, this means heaven is the principle and Qian is the practical aspect of it. Regarding the twelve channels, the *Nei Jing* 內經 already described their circulation in detail; it is able to be argued and proved, for example, by headaches. Occipital headache is attributed to the Foot-Taiyang, which can be cured by Herba Ephedrae Ma Huang 麻黃 and Ramulus Cinnamomi Gui Zhi 桂枝. Frontal headache is attributed to the Foot-Yangming, which can be cured by Radix Puerariae Ge Gen 葛根 and Radix

[81] Note: The original title is "Old Medicine Schools 舊醫學校" here changed to "Chinese Medicine Schools 中醫學校".

Angelicae Formosanae Bai Zhi 白芷. Headache on both sides is attributed to the Foot-Shaoyang, which can be cured by Radix Bupleuri Chinensis Chai Hu 柴胡 and Radix Scutellariae Baicalensis Huang Qin 黃芩. All these examples of headache can prove the theory of Twelve Channels. And acupuncture must use needling along the channels, otherwise it may cause fainting—how to explain this? So the theory of the Twelve Channels cannot be abolished and Yin Yang and Five Phases are also able to be justified. People may sneer at using a fixed formula to treat changeable diseases; it is a digression to discuss generation and restriction cycles if one is restricted to Five Phases stubbornly.

Western medicine is good at treating organic diseases, while Chinese medicine is good at regulating functional disorders. For example, hematuria is caused by the rupture of the vessel or bladder dysfunction according to Western medicine, thus repairing the vessel or performing a bladder operation is the way to treat hematuria. Chinese medicine considers hematuria as being caused by either hyperactivity of ministerial fire activating blood or deficiency of middle Qi failing to control blood, so it treats hematuria by clearing fire or tonifying Qi. So Chinese medicine is characterized by the concept of holism, while Western medicine is adept at reductionism. There are some disadvantages of ["allopathic"] reductionism; for example, in the past, Jia Lun 迦倫 always used warming methods to treat heat diseases, but nowadays Western medicine always uses cooling methods to treat heat diseases according to the thermometer reading. Western medicine ignores specific situations; for example, there are some heat diseases that must be treated by warming methods, some heat diseases that cannot be treated by cooling methods and other heat diseases where neither external warming nor cooling methods are effective. Chinese Medicine has Gui Zhi Tang 桂枝湯 to release the exterior heat, Bai Hu Tang 白虎湯 to clear internal heat and Zhen Wu Tang 真武湯 to clear deficiency-heat caused by floating Yang.

Even more surprising, Chinese medicine divides exterior heat into sweating and non-sweating types, and internal heat into excess and deficiency types. So I dare to say that Chinese medicine is irreplaceable due to its detailed descriptions of pathology and flexible formulas. That article tried to put Chinese medicine down by quoting Yu Qu Yuan's 俞曲園 opinion of abolishing Chinese medicine. In my opinion, medicine is only able to cure diseases, but it is not able to bring the dead back to life. Everyone will experience the life process from birth, maturity and aging to the final stage of life, which is a law of nature. Furthermore, the words of Yu Qu Yuan 俞曲園 originated from the words of *Han Shu Yi Wen Zhi* 漢書藝文志, which means people will not have to call the doctor nor go to the hospital whenever they get sick, just use the body's self-healing abilities. The body's self-healing ability is just the same as the immunity in Western medicine.

Western medicine was popular when Qu Yuan 曲園 was alive; why didn't he suggest abolishing Western medicine? Wow! He [Yu Yunxiu] studied medicine in Japan. I cite here the medical treatise of the Japanese Fu Hai Tuo Lun 夫海脫倫, stating "my art is being far from perfect, I urgently consult all kinds of medical treatments, examining them and deciding if they are appropriate or not. There is no knowledge or experience which is perverse to medicine, and that's it!"

Article end

Debates regarding the inclusion of Chinese medicine in the official school system

Feb 1926 by Xu Xiangchen 徐相宸

Source: *Compilation of Discussions about Chinese Medical Education* 中醫教育討論集

Yaron: An emotional nationalistic plea: allow Chinese medicine to survive because it is ours. This, in a way, will be used again by the Communists in the 1950s.

Pages 381–382

Dear Beijing Ministry of Education,

Our country is in danger because of social injustice and political unrest. If there is academic injustice, the situation will be even more confusing; can people survive in our country? Chinese people benefit from Chinese medicine, but intentionally belittle it. Are all sick persons sick because of Chinese medicine? If Chinese medicine does cause such disease, it should be made obsolete. It's better to keep both Chinese medicine and Western medicine and make them compete against each other, thus promoting the development of medicine. It's not proper to say that Chinese medicine is completely wrong and Western medicine is always right. This should be proven by facts, rather than arguing on a theoretical level. There was no need for Sun Yat-Sen 孫中山 to have an operation but doctors of Western medicine performed it. He got worse, and then turned to Chinese medicine doctors, all of whom refused to treat him because they thought the disease was incurable. I also thought it was not curable after reading the newspaper; the diagnosis was quite clear. Why do some still say that Chinese medicine is inferior to Western medicine? The Ministry of Education rebuked Chinese medicine for not meeting academic standards. Is it scientific principles or the principles of Chinese cultural studies? If it means scientific principles, Chinese medicine is not a product of science, so it shouldn't be restricted by science. If it means the principles of Chinese cultural studies, Chinese medicine belongs to Chinese cultural studies, and is related to Chinese history, Confucian classics and Chinese literature. If all Chinese cultural studies don't meet academic principles, should all of them be abolished? Do all issues of current government and politics fit scientific principles? Of course they don't. There is no excuse for that, even though the country is in an era of transition. If unscientific politics can be acceptable, why not Chinese cultural studies? I suggest organizing Chinese cultural studies with scientific methods, and to develop science guided by the spirit of Chinese cultural studies. I am sure all scholars will adopt this approach in the future. Obstructing the development of Chinese cultural studies, while promoting the science of foreign countries, the Ministry of Education is implementing suicidal policies of our culture. All Chinese have to take that seriously.

February, 15th year (1926)

Article end

The issue of including Chinese medicine schools in the official school system

Mar 1926 By Wang Yiren 王一仁

Source: *Compilation of Discussions about Chinese Medical Education* 中醫教育討論集

Page 382

People with prejudiced views cannot discuss the issue of public interest, and people with superficial opinions cannot see the essence of things. The issue of including Chinese medicine schools in the official school system, which hasn't yet been implemented, is up against stiff opposition from Western medicine groups. Isn't that biased and superficial? If so, how is it that they are qualified both to discuss the public interest and see the essence of things? Recently, three Western medicine groups publicly denounced Chinese medicine by quoting the preface of *Nei Jing* 內經 and *Shang Han Lun* 傷寒論. But *Nei Jing* 內經 and *Shang Han Lun* 傷寒論 are the most important classics of Chinese Medicine, far transcending later medical books. Thus, it is quite insane to denounce Chinese medicine by quoting the preface of those works. These groups think that the abuse of Chinese medicine practice should be held responsible for all medical malpractice. The abuse of Western medicine has killed many patients, which is rather shocking and so Western medicine should also be abolished.

In a word, Chinese medicine is effective. The theories and accumulated experience of Chinese medicine can save lives and the public has faith in it. It's only a matter of time before Chinese medicine is included in the official school system. I am pleased that many persons of great insight have refuted the Western medicine doctors' opinions.

March, 15th year (1926)

Article end

A letter arguing strongly for the inclusion of Chinese Medicine Schools in the official school system

May 1936 by Shi Yiren 時逸人

Source: *Compilation of Discussions about Chinese Medical Education* 中醫教育討論集

Pages 382–383

Dear Beijing Ministry of Education,

The whole country has been shocked since the Ministry of Education excluded Chinese medicine from the official school system. Chinese medicine, the world's oldest medicine, contains the most profound theories. Throughout history, Chinese medicine has made great achievements due to wise monarchs, reputable prime ministers advocating it and talented scholars endeavoring for four thousand seven hundred years. However, in recent years, a few people have attacked Chinese medicine—those who were self-interested and lacking respect for human life. Syndrome differentiation in Chinese medicine is worthy of research, it is more effective than the simple treatments of Western medicine. Justice and truth will prevail. I trust the Ministry of Education will take Chinese medicine seriously and rethink over the abolition of Chinese medicine. If Chinese medicine is worthy of preservation then it should also be included in the official school system. Western medicine proponents, who are prejudiced against Chinese medicine, may mislead lay persons.

The Ministry of Education should recognize and uncover the selfish behaviors of Western medicine proponents. Despite a number of shortcomings, such as slight differences in academic opinion across the various ages and regions, Chinese medicine has made great progress due to continuous effort. What is the intention of completely abolishing Chinese medicine? Our scholars should be responsible for promoting the academic development of Chinese medicine, while the Ministry of Education should be responsible for providing political support to save Chinese medicine. Therefore I strongly suggest including Chinese medicine in the official school system.

May, 25th year (1936)

Article end

On Chinese medicine education

By Ye Jingqiu 葉勁秋

Source: *Compilation of Discussions about Chinese Medical Education* 中醫教育討論集

Pages 461–464

The Republic of China rose after the last emperor of the Qing dynasty abdicated. The political system has changed a lot since then. Nevertheless, our traditional medicine has fallen into disrepute since the introduction of "new medicine". On January 1914, a representative of the Medical Association of Beijing had a meeting with Wang Daxie 汪大燮, the secretary of Education, to discuss the matter regarding the registration of the association. Here is the response from Wang: "I have already decided to abrogate the use of Chinese medicine as well as Chinese materia medica. I can hardly accept your application."

Subsequently, Yu Dexun 余德壎 and some others had gathered Chinese medicine doctors from all over the country to set up a group concerned with Chinese medicine and sent representatives to the State Council and various ministries to petition for preserving Chinese medicine. The Ministry of Education gave the following reply: "We appreciate your concerted effort in studying and preserving Chinese medicine. Nonetheless, in view of globalization and the advancement in technology, all scientific subjects should adopt the most up-to-date theories. Hence, the curriculum of specialized medical school has incorporated all kinds of science subjects such as anatomy and laboratory class. There is no way to begin without this basic scientific knowledge."

This regulation was adopted and promulgated by the Ministry in the Extraordinary General Meeting and after detailed discussions with medical experts and consultants. We hope that the development of medical science in our country will be able to meet the global trend. Only after that can we move on to issues and policies on public health. This is not discriminating against any kind of medicine. One should be more calculative before pleading for a specialized Chinese medicine school.

In 1915, Shanghai Chinese Medicine School filed the application for a second time. This time, the Ministry of Internal Affairs responded, "This Chinese medicine school is not considered part of our academic system and no Chinese medicine subjects are listed in the regulations." For those fighting for equality between Chinese and Western medicine doctors, the crux of the matter became that Chinese medicine schools were being isolated from the entire academic system. Thus, commissar Li Zonghuang 李宗黃 and 37 other commissars proposed to match the status of Chinese and Western medicine doctors in the Third Plenary Session. In addition, 53 commissars, including Jiao Yitang 焦易堂, also proposed the integration of Chinese medicine education into the official school system so that Chinese medicine schools can be established under legal regulations. These two bills have passed the censorship and now sent to the Central Political Committee for discussion and possible solutions. Those who are concerned with the development of Chinese medicine should not remain silent anymore and grab this chance to express their opinions.

When the Ministry of Education was having a meeting in Shanxi, Yang Baicheng 楊百城, Zhao Yikong 趙意空, Ran Jianhong 冉劍虹 and others intended to invite the department 公决咨部 and discuss the matter—reintegrating Chinese medicine into the official school system. Their arguments are summarized as follows: "The education system only includes Western medicine but not Chinese medicine. As such, there is no curriculum for those Chinese medicine schools to follow and no rewards for them to participate. It is nothing but a limitation of academic development through legal means. This policy is slowly strangling our own traditional culture. There is no other way for Chinese medicine to thrive without establishing its own schools and, in order to establish these schools, it is imperative to include them into the education system."

Before the promulgation of the Chinese medicine regulations 中醫條例, according to research by Suzhou Native Medicine School 蘇州國醫學校, there were thirty nine Chinese medicine schools, Colleges and research institutes 中醫學校學院研究院; this number now rose to more than a hundred and ten (see *Suzhou Native Medicine Journal* 蘇州國醫雜誌), all along without a promise of any reward. It is even more unreasonable to say that the education bureau is killing our own culture for excluding Chinese medicine in the curriculum.

In July 1919, Zhang Jilao 張季老 expressed his opinion on the lacking Chinese medicine curriculum to military governor of Shanxi Yan 閻: "Due to the inadequacy of teaching materials and teachers, the rift between the two systems of medical education is widening. It also poses difficulties in communication between them. I propose that we include physiology and chemistry as well as Chinese materia medica into the curriculum of Chinese and Western medicines respectively in a bid to unite students and also promote communications between them." Yan 閻 replied: "I, too, share the same aspiration. Yet I have made no progress in recent months, facing the obstacles exactly as how you have described in your letter. Alas, only those who have come through the obstacles know the underlying difficulties."

The major concern for any Chinese medicine school is the insufficiency of teaching materials. Even a talented person as Mr. Jizhi 季直, all he wanted is to foster communication between students. Both Zhang 張 and Yan 閻 care deeply about Chinese medicine. Their efforts are truly remarkable. However, Western medicine continues to flourish in Nantong 南通 and Taiyuan 太原, while Chinese medicine there has withered. In the summer of 1930, a committee, which is responsible for designing Chinese medicine teaching materials, was established in Shanghai for a short period of time. Guangdong 廣東 and Henan 河南 provinces alike had sent representatives to the meetings. Article VII of the aforementioned committee states that: "the aims of the committee shall be 1. To decide on the criteria for the selection of academic theories; 2. To decide on the writing style of the textbooks; 3. To decide on the curriculum; 4. To standardize the content and proportion of each subject; and 5. To prepare a demonstration for each subject."

Article IX states that: "the committee shall hold the second meeting this year during annual leave for one week." The first meeting was ended without any conclusions, not to mention the second. The Central Bureau for Native Medicine is an academic organization that gathers Chinese medicine talent from all over the country. With our capable members and the $5000 subsidy from the government per month, there should be no doubt that the institution will prosper. At the beginning, there are still discussions regarding the standardization of curriculum. Yet after all these years, all that we have come up with is a draft bill on the standardization of disease names.

Two years ago, the Central Bureau for Native Medicine had drafted the 3223rd order: "the diversity of school curricula between medical schools in different provinces has become a major obstacle to the training of professionals and the promotion of Chinese medicine. In view of this, we have designated new names to these institutions according to their functions. Those that aim to teach shall be called Native Medicine Schools while those that aim to do research shall be called Native Medicine Research Institutes. In addition, a drafted constitution with 21 articles shall be sent to the council and made public after passing the council meeting."

Nevertheless, the council made a surprising decision not long after. The 3550th order states that "the 8th annual council meeting of the 2nd council has come to the consensus that the bill is inapplicable and shall be abolished with immediate effect." The capriciousness of the council has made us feel disoriented. Now that commissars like Jiao have written to the Ministry of Education to urge them to come up with a standard curriculum for Chinese medicine education, they suggest that the curriculum should include foundation courses such as anatomy and physiology, public health, pathology, diagnosis, pharmacology, prescription methodology and medical history as well as practical courses including internal medicine, surgery medicine, gynaecology, paediatrics, science of seasonal febrile disease, infectious disease, otorhinolaryngology, acupuncture, Tui Na, orthopaedics and traumatology, sexual medicine and forensic medicine. They have included basic sciences like anatomy, physiology and public health, but why have they missed microbiology and immunology?

Just as *Nan Jing* 難經, a classic written by Qin Yueren 秦越人, has mentioned, "there are five types of exogenous febrile: seasonal febrile, 熱病…" Replacing exogenous febrile with seasonal febrile is something unheard of and I am not sure why they have made that decision. Zhang Taiyan 章太炎 once said, "though calligraphy, chess and martial arts are not tested in schools, their level of competency can be tested easily. If students do not focus on their studies and merely treat their graduation certificate as a voucher to practice medicine, it is perhaps something inevitable for Western medicine to overtake us." We should all be well aware and alerted for something like that to happen.

(From the foreword of *The Problem of Chinese Medicine in China* 中國醫藥問題) Pan Gongbo 潘公播 has stated, "I did not deny the efficacy of Chinese medicine. Instead, I believe that it is a valuable legacy from our ancestors. However, if we do nothing to change the status quo, Chinese medicine will inevitably be eliminated. On the other hand, if we standardize the curriculum and set up Chinese medical schools, we can control both the quantity and quality of the knowledge transferred. However, doing this alone is not enough to invigorate Chinese medicine once again. We have to bear in mind that the most effective way of protecting this legacy of ours is to organize it in a scientific way."

(From the editorial of *Shi Shi Xin Bao* 時事新報 of 20th February, 1937) Education and our country's constitutional development are so closely related that one wrong move would actually affect the whole game. We must revise thoroughly the nature of Chinese medicine. As for Chinese medicine education, we should first develop a comprehensive system of Chinese medicine or else it would be very difficult to recruit teachers, prepare teaching materials and examine academic theories. It will only cause distress if we merely focus on the end without considering the means. These are only some of my personal opinions but I sincerely hope that the authority can consider them seriously.

(Retrieved from Mingrijiaoyu 明日教育 of Dagongbao 大公报 in Tianjin 天津)

Article end

Proposal on the development of Chinese medicine

Nov 1925 by Wang Yiren 王一仁

Source: *Compilation of Discussions about Chinese Medical Education* 中醫教育討論集

Pages 383–384

A name is the reflection of a reality. A name without reality is meaningless. It is reasonable and appropriate to request that the Ministry of Education include Chinese medicine in the official school system, in order to promote the development of Chinese medicine. Some Western medicine groups and individuals adamantly oppose the Proposal, with the purpose of monopolizing medicine. They completely ignore Chinese medicine wisdom and the robustness of its experiments.

This article refutes that of Yu Yunxiu 余雲岫, which is prejudiced against the "Old" medicine. My friend Qin Bowei 秦伯未 has already indignantly refuted it based on truth, declaring Chinese medicine to be legitimate. Chinese medicine is spiritual and not materialistic, advocating experiments but not empty words. In the past ten years, Chinese medicine schools have been gradually built around the country. All want to rescue Chinese medicine from abolition. Therefore I petition the Ministry of Education to include Chinese medicine in the official school system. If Chinese government policy will not turn a blind eye then it should be quick to accept Chinese medicine in the official school system. The opposition from Western medicine is usually based on governmental policy; therefore, the Ministry of Education should support Chinese medicine swiftly.

I am a Chinese medicine doctor and I wholeheartedly welcome and endorse the proposals supporting Chinese medicine. Now, it is unavoidable that this will be derided and criticized by Western medicine proponents. Fortunately, Western medicine practitioners do exactly as I do. So to be completely fair is beyond my reach.

November, 14th year (1925)

Article end

On the recent news of including Chinese medicine in the official school system

Jan 1928 by Hu Ding'an 胡定安

Source: *Compilation of Discussions about Chinese Medical Education* 中醫教育討論集

Pages 384–385

I heard that a certain person called Wang 王, a Chinese Medicine doctor, recently wrote a book called *Chinese Medicine Problems*. This book, with thirty thousand more words, attempts to justify the inclusion of Chinese medicine in the official school system, which may mislead lay persons. For the purpose of including Chinese medicine in the official school system, the author is going to present the book to Mr. Hu Shizhi 胡適之[82] and hope that he, in turn, will transfer the book to Mr. Cai Zimin 蔡子民,[83] the president of the Administration of Universities. I became concerned when I heard this news. I have heard speeches by Mr. Hu 胡 and Mr. Cai 蔡 in China and Europe. These two gentlemen often travel overseas, so both of them have wide knowledge and modern thinking. I certainly don't believe that Mr. Hu 胡 will accept Wang's 王 request just because they are hometown friends. I also don't believe that Mr. Cai 蔡 will go against public opinion just because of a recommendation from Mr. Hu 胡. Even if Mr. Hu 胡 is willing to help Wang 王, and Mr. Cai 蔡 also accepts the request, there is no need for concern, because public opinion will decide which is right and which is wrong.

Western medicine, along scientific grounds, can argue against the Proposal to include Chinese medicine in the official school system. I believe Western medicine will achieve the final victory. I expose this to warn Western medicine practitioners. If the Proposal is beginning to revitalize, we will do our best to counterattack. Now let's wait for what will happen next.

New Medicine and Society, January, 17th year (1928)

Article end

[82] Hu Shih 胡适 (1891–1962) was a Chinese philosopher, essayist and diplomat. He was influential in the May Fourth Movement, one of the leaders of China's New Culture Movement, was a president of Peking University, and in 1939 was nominated for a Nobel Prize in literature. Source: Wiki.

[83] Cai Yuanpei 蔡元培 (1868–1940) was a Chinese educator, president of Peking University, and founder of the Academia Sinica. He was known for his critical evaluation of Chinese culture and synthesis of Chinese and Western thinking, including anarchism. At Peking University he assembled influential figures in the New Culture and May Fourth Movements. In 1928–1929 was the president of the Control Yuan branch of government. Source: Wiki.

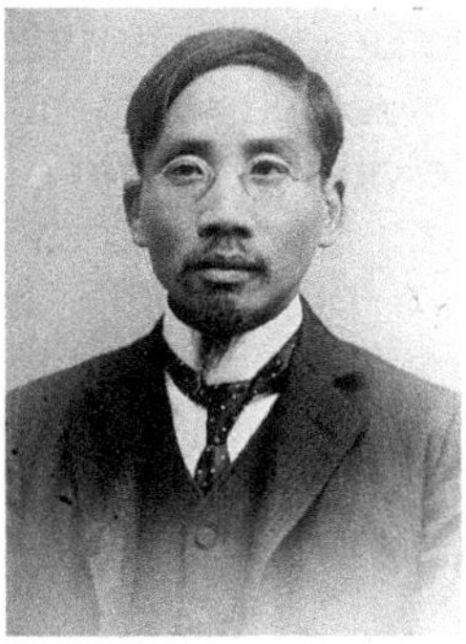

Cai Yuanpei[84]

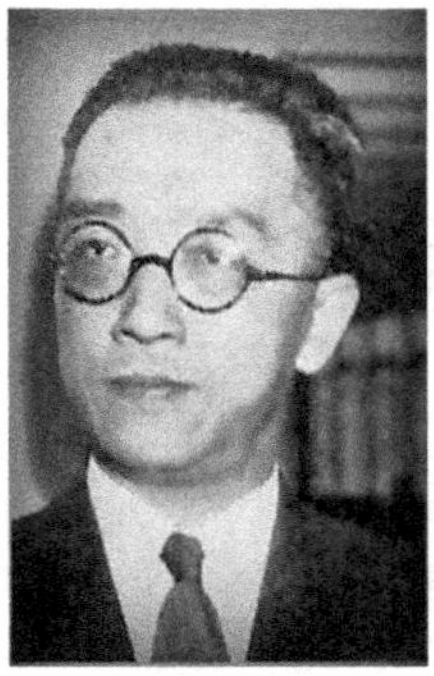

Hu Shi[85]

An open letter to the Provincial Education Committee

By Yu Yunxiu 余雲岫

Source: *Compilation of Discussions about Chinese Medical Education* 中醫教育討論集

Yaron: In the 20th century's early decades, there were Western medicine proponents antagonizing Chinese medicine yet being highly versed in classical Chinese literature. Such a person was Yu Yunxiu; educated on both sides, he was able to argue painfully against Chinese medicine.

His kind of argument, presented in the following letter, is priceless for us wanting to research and advance Chinese medicine in the 21st century. Yu's threatening narrative, that Chinese medicine theories are erroneous but herbs are valuable, influenced the early Chinese medicine "scientification"[86] attempts in a grand way. His arguments were often detailed and based in the ancient classics, refuting the ancient theories while validating modern science.

During the Communist era, such blunt attacks against anything Chinese and in support of the West would be abolished. We should realize that any "debate" during the Communist years was not really a debate between two sides, but a rather artificially-forced, one-sided doctrine.

[84] http://en.wikipedia.org/wiki/Cai_Yuanpei

[85] http://en.wikipedia.org/wiki/Hu_Shih

[86] Used throughout the book, this term refers to the attempts to make Chinese medicine more science-like or to conform to the norms of modern science.

> Therefore, it is beneficial for us to go back to the 1920s and '30s "free market" debates, especially by such versed practitioners as Yu Yunxiu. If we can contemplate and solve the problems he posed to Chinese medicine at that time, then we may be able to redefine Chinese medicine in the 21st century.
>
> Pages 385–390

As the representative of the Medical Association of the Republic of China, Chinese Medical Association, and Shanghai College of Physicians

Dear members of the Provincial Committee of Education,

Education has made significant progress since the founding of the Republic of China. In the past ten years, it hasn't been swayed by backwards proposals such as the restoration of imperial examinations, eight-part essay Ba Gu Wen 八股文 and so on. Though this has been a strong trend in the world, we cannot forget the efforts of those gentlemen who behave firmly and with determination. The Chinese Education Improvement Society Jiao Yu Gai Jin She 教育改進社 held a meeting in Shanxi Province 山西, passing the Proposal regarding the school system that was submitted by the Chinese Medicine Association of Jiangsu Province Jiang Su Quan Sheng Zhong Yi Lian He Hui 江蘇全省中醫聯合會, as reported in the press. That Proposal is ignorant of academic evolution, goes against the general trend, violates natural law, disrupts educational objectives and is very shallow and absurd. Those Chinese medicine practitioners don't pay attention to improving society; why are they confused and unable to distinguish right from wrong? My colleagues were still puzzled after much consideration; we figured it was a random mistake they had made, and that it wouldn't be carried out. Before long, the National Education Association Quan Guo Jiao Yu Lian He Hui 全國教育聯合會 accepted proposals from Hubei Province 湖北 and Zhejiang Province 浙江.

Those Chinese medicine practitioners continue to make mistakes. I am going to expose their ignorance; please observe impartially.

The Proposal pointed out that "Chinese medicine has been developed for thousands of years, and it is the single most important reason why China has the largest population in the world." It is a gross exaggeration, attempting to deceive lay persons; why are there so many scholars believing and accepting this? *Yi Jing Bian Qi Lun* 移精變氣論 in *Su Wen* 素問 states, "Today's doctors treat internal diseases with toxic herbs, external diseases with stone needles, some may be cured, while some may not." *Tang Ye Lao Li Lun* 湯液醪醴論 says, "Why can't people these days cure themselves by taking rice wine? Because nowadays, people have to use toxic herbs to treat internal diseases, and stone needles and moxibustion to treat external diseases." So we know that in the period of Huangdi 黃帝, doctors treated patients only with toxic herbs or stone needles, with unknown effects. *Yi Jing Bian Qi Lun* 移精變氣論 also says, "Nowadays, treatment is no longer like before. Nowadays, there are many quack doctors using gentle needling to treat external diseases and decoctions to treat internal diseases, which may lead to the failure of recovery or even the onset of a new disease." It indicates that prevention is better than cure. If disease has occurred, cure is not reliable and may be harmful. So the doctors in the period of Huangdi 黃帝 were not able to cure diseases and may have caused harm to the patients. In the Chun Qiu 春秋 Spring and Autumn Period, witch doctors were appointed to treat diseases who rarely used medicine. Xu Shizi 許士子 was accused of murdering the emperor, because he suggested that the emperor should take herbs. *Han Shu Yi Wen Zhi* 漢書藝文志, written by Ban Gu 班固, although including medical classics and prescriptions, also quoted a proverb, "Doing nothing for diseases is better than being treated by a doctor," as a warning. It shows that doctors in the Han Dynasty were quite immature, with most of them being punished for their mistakes and common people mistrusting them. In the preface of the *Shang Han Lun* 傷寒論, Zhang Zhongjing 張仲景 says, "If a mediocre doctor is entrusted with the treatment without restriction, the patient will be in mortal danger". He also states, "Nowadays, doctors have no desire to research the Ancient medical books Jing Zhi 經旨 to extend their knowledge. They only inherit from their own ancestors medical skills which are quite outdated. They devote themselves solely to the inquiry, and prescribe formulas after a very short inquiry. They usually take pulses hastily and incompletely; for example, ignoring Chi Pulse while taking Can Pulse, ignoring feet while examining hands, ignoring comprehensive analysis of Ren Ying 人迎, Can Kou 寸口 and Fu Yang 趺陽, ignoring the examination of Ming Tang 明堂 and Que Ting 闕庭." Therefore, we can know that doctors in the end of the Han 漢 Dynasty killed many more people than they saved. Based on the opinion of the Proposal, we can deduce that the size of our population would be larger without doctors. In the preface of *Mai Jing* 脈經, Wang Shuhe 王叔和 says, "Those medical books are remote from basic medical principles, and fundamentally impractical. They may lead a minor illness to a serious condition, and dash the hope of recovery from illness." Therefore, doctors in the Jin 晉 Dynasty were not competent to cure patients. Huang Fumi 皇甫謐 says, in *Shi Quan* 釋勸, "Huang Di 黃帝 created institutions based on the nine universal rules, Qi Bo 岐伯 removed intestines through an abdominal incision, Bian Que 扁鵲 saved patients from death in the Guo Kingdom 虢國, Wen Zhi 文摯 sacrificed his life in order to cure the King of Qi

齊王, Yi He 醫和 showed his medical skill during the period between the Jin Kingdom 晉國 and Qin Dynasty 秦代, Cang Gong 倉公 discovered medical secrets in the Han Dynasty 漢朝, Hua Tuo 華佗 preserved the essence of medicine with unique insights and Zhang Zhongjing 張仲景 created many marvellous prescriptions. It is to be regretted that there are no such talents nowadays, so I make an appeal to the emperor to support medicine." Shi'an 士安 (Huang Fumi 皇甫謐) started to study medicine after suffering from wind arthralgia syndrome, which was most probably because there were no reliable doctors. He said in the preface of *Jia Yi Jing* 甲乙經 that "people who ignore medicine are completely worthless". He didn't believe in the doctors of that time, so he researched medicine. We can know that doctors at that time were quite mediocre. Tao Yinju 陶隱居 (Tao Hongjing 陶弘景) wrote, in the preface of *Bai Yi Fang* 百一方, "It is quite easy to find herbalists in the centre of a city, but it becomes a little bit difficult in the suburbs and the situation in remote villages is more severe. Current medical books are usually voluminous, thus they are not practical in saving lives." It shows that the medicine is of limited value in treating diseases. In the preface to *Qian Jin Fang* 千金方, Sun Zhenren 孫真人 (Sun Simiao 孫思邈) wrote: "Though famous doctors have occasionally appeared since the Jin Dynasty 晉代 and Song Dynasty 宋代, most of them were only able to cure half of their patients." Even the famous doctors were unable to cure half of their patients, so we can easily imagine the situation of other doctors. How can we believe that Chinese medicine had saved a lot of people? Moreover, Sun Simiao 孫思邈 says, "Many quacks deceive the public in the name of medicine, so all people are ashamed to talk about medicine." Thus we know that there were many quacks in the Tang Dynasty 唐代; scholars and officials despised medicine, which was considered to be unnecessary. Can we say that the health of people relied heavily on quacks in that time? In *Lun Zhen Hou* 論診候, Sun Simiao 孫思邈 writes, "Alas, almost half of the patients lost their lives because of improper treatments." The doctors of the Tang Dynasty 唐代 were not competent to protect the health of people. Lin Yi 林億 revised the *Mai Jing* 脈經 in the Song Dynasty 宋朝. In a report to the emperor he wrote, "Since the establishment of the Eastern Jin Dynasty 東晉, the country had been divided into north and south and been thrown into turmoil. Actually, there were still many medical books being published, but most of them inherited incorrect theories, which misled the development of medicine." So reliable medicine disappeared since the Eastern Jin Dynasty 東晉. Honestly, I don't know what exactly the "medicine" in that Proposal refers to. In the middle of the Song Dynasty 宋朝, Gao Yangsheng's *Mai Jue* 高陽生脈訣 was quite popular, as evidenced by the preface of Chen Kongshuo's *Mai Jing* 陳孔碩脈經. Now we all know the ridiculousness of the *Mai Jue*

脈訣, but the health of the people of the Song Dynasty 宋朝 relied on it. In the preface to *Zheng He Sheng Ji Zong Lu* 政和聖濟總錄, the emperor wrote, "I regret that there are many problems in our country, such as low moral principles, improper social customs, long-term patients and absurd quacks". He then wrote, "Treating excess with tonifying, deficiency with reducing, such cursory and irresponsible behaviour causes half of the patients to die." Thus we learn the tricks of treatment played by the doctors of the Song Dynasty 宋朝. In the preface of the *San Yin Fang* 三因方, Chen Wuze 陳無擇 says, "Medical books compiled in the Jin Dynasty 晉代 and Han Dynasty 漢代 were completely impractical, complicated and farfetched. The revisions of classics were defective, and without clear principle. The common medical books had no basic principles, but had plausible theories, which were applied indiscriminately by quacks." So we are well aware of the facts of the medical situation in the Song Dynasty 宋朝. In the preface to the *Bao Ming Ji* 保命集, Liu Hejian 劉河間 writes, "Nowadays, doctors follow the ancestors' theories, and continue to use outdated prescriptions. They are ashamed of asking questions and not willing to learn new ideas. They rebuke good theories as inferior. Most of the patients are hurt after being treated by them, or even die." In the *Zhen Zhu Nang* 珍珠囊, Li Dongyuan 李東垣 says, "Later scholars only follow theories created by their ancestors and never try to develop new knowledge." Thus we can know the situation of medicine in the Jin Dynasty 金代 and Yuan Dynasty 元代. As for the words of Li Dongyuan 李東垣 cited above, these days doctors follow the ancient medicine from Shen Nong, and they cause many common people to die innocently. In the preface of the *Zheng Zhi Zhun Sheng* 證治準繩, Wang Nianxi 王念西 (Wang Kentang 王肯堂) noted that "There are five departments and seven situations.[87] But nowadays doctors don't follow these, it is quite a fortune to survive after being treated by them." Zhang Huang 章潢 wrote in *Tu Shu Bian* 圖書編: "All famous doctors in historical records were fortuitous." Yu Jiayan 俞嘉言 wrote, in *Yu Yi Cao* 寓意草, "There are many people learning medicine, but the medicine is still on the wane. Doctors only focus on the herbs, but ignore the diseases, which leads many patients to die innocently. Most people think it is caused by natural causes." Gu Tinglin 顧亭林 writes, in *Ri Zhi Lu* 日知錄, "Ancient quacks killed patients, nowadays quacks don't kill patients, but they are unable to cure patients. Patients become gradually worse and finally die. The doctors who don't kill patients will be regarded as virtuous." Shen Gui Yu 沈歸愚 writes, in *Ye Xiangyan*

[87] From *San Yin Ji Yi Bing Zheng Fang Lun* 三因極一病証方論 by Chen Yan 陳言 1174CE: 凡學醫，必識五科七事。五科者，脈病証治，及其所因；七事者，所因複分為三。故因脈以識病，因病以辨証，隨証以施治，則能事畢矣。For all who study medicine they must know the five departments and seven situations. Five departments are pulse, disease, syndrome, treatment and their cause. The seven situations result from the further division of the cause into three. Therefore because of pulse one knows the disease, because of disease one differentiates the syndrome, because the differentiation of syndromes that one can reach at the treatment. Like this the affair is complete.

Zhuan 葉香嚴傳, "Nowadays, doctors appear ignorant; they prescribe many unnecessary herbs." In *Shen Ji Chu Yan* 慎疾芻言, Xu Huixi 徐洄溪 quoted, "Nowadays, doctors don't learn from medical classics, they treat patients inconsiderately and they cause large numbers of needless deaths." In the preface of the *Ben Cao Bai Zhong* 本草百種, Xu Huixi 徐洄溪 writes, "During the Tang Dynasty 唐朝, doctors were unaware of the properties of herbs and preferred to use their own prescriptions. During the Song Dynasty 宋朝 and Yuan Dynasty 元朝, there were more herbs but most of them were not deeply researched. Doctors used herbs arbitrarily and mistakenly. Although used improperly, however, herbs or prescriptions occasionally may have been effective." In the preface of the *Yi Xue Yuan Liu Lun* 醫學源流論, Xu Huixi 徐洄溪 writes, "Since the Tang Dynasty 唐朝 and Song Dynasty 宋朝, few intellectual persons have dedicated themselves to the development of the medicine. What's more, the occupation of doctor has been regarded as a dishonorable one and the excellent medical theories have been lost. I worry that there will be no effective medicine from now on." In the preface of the *Lan Tai Gui Fan* 蘭臺軌範, Xu Huixi 徐洄溪 writes, "During the Song Dynasty 宋朝, there was nothing but Yin, Yang, Qi, Blood, cold, heat, reinforcing and reducing. All of these were superficial and sweeping. Doctors didn't know the basic herbs and prescriptions for a specific disease. Some doctors classified the disease and discussed the pathogenic factors first, then discussed the treatment. But such discussions were disorderly, the herbs and prescriptions were superficial and made up. Nowadays, however, doctors treat all diseases by several fixed prescriptions and herbs, ignoring the syndrome differentiation. They don't have academic opinions, and prescribe thoughtlessly, so they may easily harm patients." Huang Yuqiu 黃玉楸 writes, "Many laypersons work in the field of medicine and they cause numerous patients to die needlessly. It is really a serious situation. People die from medical malpractice, not wars. Natural disasters don't strike year after year, but malpractice occurs frequently, so the issue of malpractice is more concerning." Lu Jiuzhi 陸九芝 wrote, in the *Shi Bu Zhai Wen* 世補齋文, "The *Study of Cold Damage Shang Han* 傷寒 has been lost since Ye Tianshi 葉天士 and the *Study of Warm Heat Wen Re* 溫熱 has been also lost since Ye Tianshi 葉天士. The *Wen Re Jing Wei* 溫熱經緯, which was written by Wang Mengying 王孟英, listed the contents from Zhang Zhongjing 張仲景 and Ye Tianshi 葉天士, but it didn't include clinical considerations. When can such situations stop?" Lu Jiuzhi 陸九芝 in criticizing *Lin Zheng Zhi Nan* 臨證指南, says, "I didn't know why so many patients died after being treated by doctors of warm diseases. I only understood the reason after reading this book, which was a prepared response to the anticipated criticisms. It's because the more people die, the more doctors will gain fame." Based on the above quotations, we can know the situation of medicine in the Qing Dynasty 清代. In summary, doctors have tended to emphasize the ancient while ignoring the modern since the time of the *Nei Jing* 內經. Qi Bo 岐伯 and Huang Di 黃帝 admired the ancients, Bian Que 扁鵲 and Zhongjing 仲景 admired Qi Bo 岐伯 and Huang Di 黃帝, Wang Shuhe 王叔和 and Sun Zhenren 孫真人 admired Bian Que 扁鵲 and Zhongjing 仲景, being handed down from generation to generation. But in the times of these doctors, they mourned the ineffective medicines and the murderous quacks. People had lived in a society full of murderous quacks since the period of Huang Di 黃帝. However, there were some doctors who, differing from quacks, wrote books and developed theories in order to awaken people to the dangers related with medicine. Unfortunately, however, these doctors were quite rare; they were not able to bear the responsibility for protecting the health of all the people. It is really foolish to believe that the behavior of these ancient doctors was not similar to contemporary quacks. It is really not proper to provide these ancient doctors as arguments of the Proposal and advocate it publicly.

In order to prove that the ancient medicine should not be abolished, the Proposal also quoted the words of Chang Wei Zao Cheng 長尾藻城, a Japanese scholar. I want all scholars to know that ancient medicine should be researched, especially by scientific methods. I have published two articles on the research of ancient medicine; one was in *Xue Yi Za Zhi* 學藝雜誌, titled *The First Step of the Scientific Research of Domestic Drugs*, another one was published in *Tong De Medicine Magazine* 同德醫藥學雜誌, titled *The Discussion of the Research of Domestic Drugs*. I don't want to copy these two articles because they are long. In summary, the theories of ancient medicine are completely worthless topics to be researched. On the other hand, the herbs that have been in use for thousands of years are worthy of being researched.

Honestly, we don't oppose the research of ancient medicine; to the contrary, we thoroughly approve such research. But I suggest that if they want to promote the development of ancient medicine, they need to completely abandon useless theories and begin researching the efficacy of the herbs themselves. If they don't learn from historical experience, the research will be without benefit. If they don't use the newest scientific methods, the research will be superficial and lacking substance. The Herbal Research Institute should have equipment and qualified personnel with knowledge of advanced chemistry and advanced physics and the attainments of physiology and pharmacology. Without enough equipment and qualified personnel, the research will be without benefit or unreliable. There are no qualified personnel in the area of ancient medicine and they are quite rare in modern medicine. The viewpoint given by the Proposal, which suggests that research can achieve success by gathering clever students and collecting all the medical books compiled in different dynasties, is completely wrong. In order to promote the development of ancient medicine and the research of herbs, I suggest the following: 1) giving financial support to found research institutions; 2) searching for qualified personnel to conduct the research with a generous salary; 3) inviting some veteran doctors as consultants; and 4) collecting secret prescriptions from across the whole country as supplemental material for research. In this way, such achievements will be accepted by the entire world and the position in the academic hierarchy of the world will be improved. But the Proposal advocates founding Chinese medicine schools, setting the Chinese medicine course and organizing Chinese medicine books of all ages. These methods are diametrically opposed to the purpose.

At first, I wasn't concerned about all those fallacies, because I figured they were made accidentally by those scholars. But now I am worried that they may endanger education and disrupt national affairs. So I have to express my opinion frankly. And I admire their original intentions of promoting the development of Chinese medicine. I believe the truth will prevail.

Article end

A Letter to President Cai 蔡 of Ministry of Education

1928 by the Shen Zhou Medical and Pharmaceutical Associations[88] Shen Zhou Yi Yao Zong Hui 神州醫藥總會

Source: *Compilation of Discussions about Chinese Medical Education* 中醫教育討論集

Yaron: In the face of stern and persistent attacks by Western medicine and modern science advocates who refuted any Chinese medicine value, Chinese medicine practitioners often resorted to nationalistic claims for their defense, such as in the following article. It became a defense tactic to associate the imperialist rule and aggression against China with Western science and medicine, a hand well played later on by the Communists in their "anti-Rightist" campaigns.

[88] Established in 1912

In both instances, defending Chinese medicine in such a way was not useful. At that time it served a purpose: keeping Chinese medicine from extinction, at least legally. However, it harmed Chinese medicine by preventing the engagement with fundamental arguments that could naturally sift through right and wrong theories. In other words, if science proponents claimed Chinese medicine theories as false, then Chinese medicine proponents needed to counter-claim and validate those theories or, at least, those that were amenable to validation. The nationalistic anti-imperialist argument was a mere excuse, used and manipulated to avoid answering tough questions.

Today we need to rethink these tough questions—Chinese medicine does not belong to China anymore so the nationalistic argument has no significance whatever, just a lingering sentiment. The tough questions remain, while the old answers have faded away. Today, Western medicine proponents simply dismiss Chinese medicine as evidence-less alternative medicine and they don't need to investigate Chinese medicine for this claim. In the 1920s in China, however, Chinese medicine was the popular medicine. It needed thorough and deep confrontation by the modernists. Now, we can use these arguments against Chinese medicine to rediscover its true value, doing away with the nationalistic excuse.

Pages 390–392

We apply for permission to include Chinese medicine into the official school system, in order to promote the development of Chinese medicine. Medicine should be valued by its ability to preserve the lives of the people. Our medicine, which was initiated in the period of Qi Bo 岐伯 and Huang Di 黃帝, already has four thousand years' history. It is quite perfect and remarkable, having been created and improved upon in successive generations. It protects a population of more than 400 million, the largest in the world. So it should be advocated according to its great historical contribution.

The opposition always complains that Chinese medicine doesn't have uniform theories. They don't realize that its advanced theories are not amenable to being unified. Moreover, the non-uniformity will stimulate interest in research and promote scholarly thought. Apart from Chinese medicine, other advanced subjects such as politics, philosophy, economics and so on are not uniform. The classics, such as *Shang Han Lun* 傷寒論 and *Jin Gui Yao Lüe* 金匱要略, are systematic. And there are countless fine theories of different schools which can be taken as references. This is the second reason for including Chinese medicine into the official school system.

Detractors claim that the theory of six Qi in Chinese medicine is not provable and is inferior to germ theory. They also describe Yin Yang and Five Phases as absurd and superstitious theories. Diseases are caused by germs but these authors don't realize that germs are only able to invade the body if they are preceded by disorders of six Qi. So the treatments according to the theory of six Qi are able to cure diseases by killing germs. The theories of Yin Yang and Five Phases try to express abstract concepts in a convenient way. For example, Yin and Yang are just like the positive and negative in algebra. Metal representing Lung or Wood representing Liver are just like A for a known number and X for an unknown number. So these theories are quite different from those of astrologers. The theories of Chinese medicine are perfect and complete. This is the third reason for including Chinese medicine into the official school system.

Some people say Chinese medicine is similar to philosophy and far from an exact science. Though science is universal, there are still many problems that cannot be solved by scientific methods. And the treatments of Chinese medicine also have fixed approaches, for example, treating internal wind with pungent-cool herbs and some sweet-bitter herbs as assistants. This shows that Chinese medicine not only has clear rules, but also has the spirit of scientific formulas. This is the fourth reason for including Chinese medicine into the official school system.

In recent times, Chinese people have become biased towards Western things because of cultural imperialism. There is a risk that Chinese medicine gradually will be replaced by Western medicine. There are countless drugs and medical devices that could be imported from foreign countries. In that case, foreign goods will increase daily while domestic goods will decrease. Those excellent herbs will be abolished, and the unemployment of related personnel will be unavoidable. This is the fifth reason for including Chinese medicine into the official school system.

The purpose of the National Revolution is to struggle for the liberation of China from all unfair treaties. The imperialist powers have hostile tendencies and any of them can blockade our ports when there is a conflict. If we abandon Chinese medicine and become partial to Western medicine, our health system will undoubtedly be in danger. In order to avoid this risk, we have to advocate that the government support our own medicine. This is the sixth reason for including Chinese medicine into the official school system.

The military government is gradually being replaced by constitutional government. The present policies on education are not favorable for the development of Chinese medicine. If there are no specific schools or subjects, Chinese medicine will eventually disappear. So I submit this letter to the Ministry of Education, and hope the National Education Conference will approve the Proposal to include Chinese medicine in the official school system. In addition, the government should support the establishment of Chinese medicine schools and reorganize our own intrinsic culture. We can absorb appropriately the advantages of Western medicine and develop Chinese medicine as the true "new medicine". In that case, Chinese medicine will benefit all people. I sincerely submit this letter to Mr. Cai 蔡, director of Higher Education Ministry of the Republic's government.

May, the 17th year of the republic (1928)

Article end

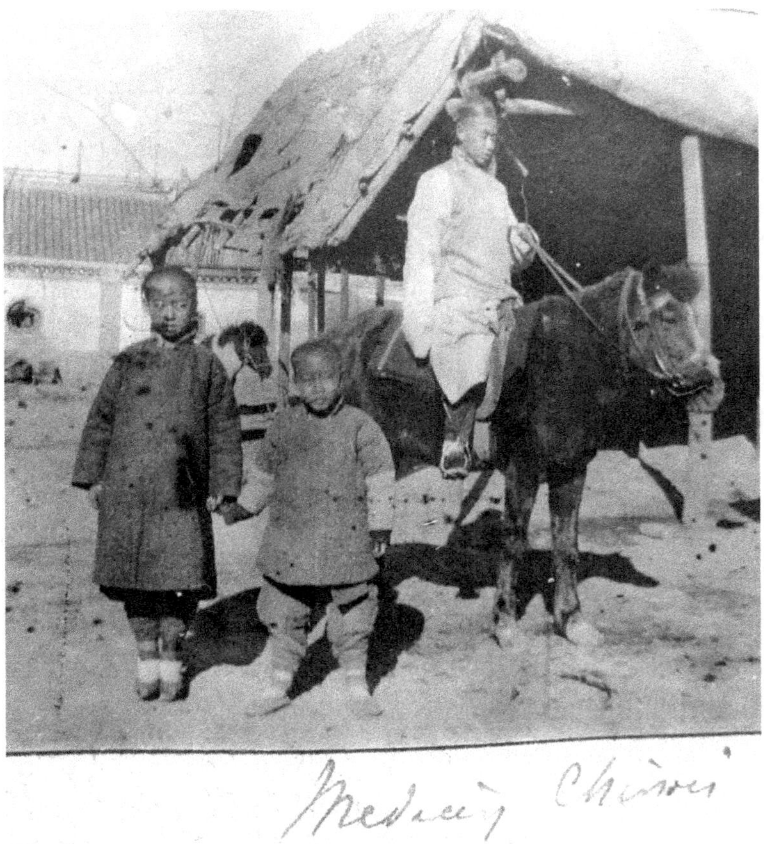

Photo by Mr P. Goux in early 1900s. "Chinese doctor".

Discussing the inclusion of Chinese medicine in the official school system

July 1928 by Wang Qizhang 汪企張

Source: *Compilation of Discussions about Chinese Medical Education* 中醫教育討論集

Yaron: Arguments against Chinese medicine in the 1920s and '30s were indeed harsh because most Chinese medicine practitioners at that time had very little education—a sort of medical profession that was mostly illiterate. Educated Chinese medicine practitioners were a minority within the profession.

The situation is, of course, very different today where the majority of Chinese medicine practitioners are highly educated. In this respect, some arguments in the following documents are no longer valid. Yet the core arguments for refuting Chinese medicine still remain and need to be countered now by contemporary educated practitioners.

Let's also keep in mind point number 9 in this document: history's third era being the scientific era of Chinese medicine. This perspective on Chinese medicine materialized in the Communist era.

Pages 392–415

Several years ago, during the warlord era, some educational activists set up an organization called The Chinese Education Improvement Society Zhong Hua Jiao Yu Gai Jin She 中華教育改進社, in order to advocate reform of the official school system. They lobbied wherever possible and tried to gain a monopolizing power in the education arena. Because of their efforts, the Proposal of including Chinese medicine in the official school system was unexpectedly accepted. Doctors of the Old Medicine were greatly cheered by the admission. But it was due to simple luck and was a temporary success, so this may only deceive them as well as laypersons. Matters that run contrary to scientific evolution can't persist. I said that our Chinese medicine was quite good in ancient times, but it was completely misrepresented by contemporary Chinese doctors. That's why Chinese medicine these days is neither fish nor fowl. Such proposals were not sufficient to preserve and develop Chinese medicine; to the contrary, they may cause its decline. Now that we arrived at the period of the Republic of China, the earlier premier had advocated the idea of saving the nation through science, which was warranted by the situation. This created a situation where all officials within the authorities have a scientific background.

All National Education Conference delegates have a global perspective and the aspiration to improve education. I am fortunate to be one of them and I am confident that I am well aware of world trends and the situation of domestic education. I have an obligation to make suggestions or offer proposals that are unbiased and fair. I have no intention to create power struggles with Chinese medicine or create unemployment for Chinese medicine doctors. A certain article was published in several newspapers, noting the responses of Chinese medicine after being denounced by Western medicine proponents. A branch of the Chinese Merchants Union, called the Chinese Herbal Materials Association, spoke in favor of Chinese medicine. I am really puzzled by that. Chinese Herbal Materials Association is a merchant organization, so why is it interfering in academic affairs? The proposals of reorganizing and improving the old medicine in the National Education Conference are not intended to destroy the livelihood of the people related to Chinese medicine. These proposals may promote the development of Chinese medicine. The Chinese Medicine Association also published an article with the title of "*Chinese Medicine Circles Should Discern the Situation*," which advocated that Chinese medicine should be included in the official school system. This article intended to unite Chinese medicine circles in order to gain benefit. Originally, I had proposed to preserve Chinese medicine via reorganization but, unexpectedly, my behavior aroused their suspicions. So I would like to talk about the methods of preserving Chinese medicine and discuss whether or not it is reasonable to include Chinese medicine in the official school system.

Firstly, the essence of our culture refers to the most important features of Chinese culture; in a broad sense, we can define all those traits that differ from those of other countries as quintessence. Should all such traits be preserved or only those that are valuable? If we preserve all, it means we close our doors to the rest of the world. If we preserve the valuable ones, we have to think carefully about which should be preserved. The things to be preserved should also be reliable for other countries. So we should have our aims, standards and basis. The doctors of Old Medicine believe their own medicine is excellent, while the doctors of modern medicine consider Chinese medicine to be always wrong. These opinions are based on each position and it's difficult to reconcile them. But there is not a perfect thing in the world; we need to be tolerant with different points of view and avoid extremes. Some doctors of the Old Medicine said that all people in history relied on Chinese medicine to survive. This was really an extreme view, which was not suitable to present to the public. Population growth is not only due to medicine. There are many factors that influenced the population; I am not going to discuss further here. So I oppose the preservation of all traits of Chinese culture. I hope the Chinese medicine doctors don't misunderstand what I have discussed about the essence of Chinese culture.

Secondly, in both the new and the old medicine circles, people only affirm their own theories and methods and they cannot merge each other's theories. This is because the old medicine is closely related to philosophy, while new medicine is closely related to science. Western medicine was also unscientific before the fourteenth century. Our medicine has many different kinds of theories and methods, which are quite complicated and may be confusing and so the current situation of Chinese medicine is quite similar to the situation of Western medicine in the fourteenth century. Western counties hadn't completely abandoned their own old medicine. Moreover, our new medicine also adopts many theories of old medicine, which have been proven via experimentation. In other words, new medicine conducts experiments by scientific methods, which is quite different from old medicine being based on subjective perception. Though science and non-science appear to be mutually incompatible, non-science gradually may become science with time. If we are aware of the history of Western countries, we can clearly see that. In order to preserve and develop the old medicine, I suggest the doctors of old medicine not be conservative, but rather be innovative and open-minded. Now we are in the twentieth century and it is quite inappropriate to be confined by the traits of the fourteenth century.

Thirdly, doctors of the old medicine always boast about how excellent and meritorious their medicine is. They believe the old medicine will develop well and that it is not necessary for them to argue with its opponents. These views sound attractive. Besides medicine, there are many other subjects with a long history, such as astronomy, geography, agriculture, military strategy and tactics and so on. It is not appropriate to set an independent school system for old medicine based on the *Ling Shu* 靈樞, *Su Wen* 素問, *Jin Gui* 金匱, *Jin Jian* 金鑒, *Nan Jing* 難經, *Ben Cao* 本草, *Shang Han Lun* 傷寒論 and so on. There are also many famous ancient books in other subjects, so should we also set an independent school system for them? I am able to list lots of such books for different subjects; for example, on law, we have *Guan Zi* 管子, *Zheng Xi Zi* 鄭析子,

Han Fei Zi 韓非子, *Yi Yu Ji* 疑獄集, *Zhe Yu Gui Jian* 折獄龜鑒, *Tang Yin Bi Shi* 棠陰比事, *Xing Tong Fu* 刑統賦, *Xing Fa Xu Lüe* 刑法敘略, *Xi Yuan Lu* 洗冤錄, *Wu Yuan Lu* 無冤錄, *Zheng Xing Lei Yao* 政刑類要, *Xiang Xing Yao Lan* 祥刑要覽, *Fa Jia Ai Ji* 法家哀集, *Da Qing Lü Li* 大清律例, *She Yu Zhi Yan* 折獄卮言, etc. On agriculture, there are *Qi Min Yao Shu* 齊民要術, *Nong Sang Ji Yao* 農桑輯要, *Nong Sang Yi Shi Cuo Yao* 農桑衣食撮要, *Nong Shu* 農書, *Jiu Huang Ben Cao* 救荒本草, *Nong Zheng Quan Shu* 農政全書, *Ye Cai Bo Lu* 野菜博錄, *Shou Shi Tong Kao* 授時通考, *Lai Si Jing* 來耜經, *Geng Zhi Tu Shi* 耕織圖詩, *Jing Shi Min Shi Lu* 經世民事錄, *Ye Cai Shi* 野菜識, *Nong Shuo* 農說, *Nong Pu* 農譜 and *Bin Feng Guang Yi* 豳風廣義. On astronomy, such as *Zhou Bi Suan Jing* 周髀算經, *Xin Yi Xiang Fa Yao* 新儀象法要, *Liu Jing Tian Wen Bian* 六經天文編, *Ge Xiang Xin Shu* 革象新書, *Sui Shi Guang Ji* 歲時廣記 in Song Dynasty, *Qi Zheng Tui Bu* 七政推步, *Sheng Shou Wan Nian Li* 聖壽萬年曆, *Gu Jin Lü Li* 古今律歷, *Si Shi Yi Ji* 四時宜忌, *Si Shi Qi Hou Ji Jie* 四時氣候集解, *Yue Ling Tong Kao* 月令通考, *Yue Ling Guang Yi* 月令廣義, *Jie Xuan Ji* 節宣輯, *Yang Yu Yue Ling* 養馀月令, *Ri She Lun* 日涉論, *Guang Yue Ling* 廣月令 in Ming Dynasty, *Gu Jin Lei Zhuan Sui Shi Bu* 古今類傳歲時部, *Jie Xu Tong Feng Lu* 節序同風錄, *Shi Ling Hui Ji* 時令彙記, *Yu Ri Shi Wen* 餘日事文, etc. On geography, such as *San Fu Huang Tu* 三輔黃圖 in the Five Dynasties, *Yuan He Jun Xian Zhi* 元和郡縣志 in Tang Dynasty, *Tai Ping Huan Yu Ji* 太平寰宇記, *Yuan Feng Jiu Yu Zhi* 元豐九域志, *Fang Yu Sheng Lan* 方輿勝覽 in Song Dynasty, *Ming Yi Tong Zhi* 明一統志 in Ming Dynasty, *Da Qing Yi Tong Zhi* 大清一統志 in Qing Dynasty, etc. And there are numerous historical records on prefectures and counties. Discussing international territories, there are texts such as *Fo Guo Ji* 佛國記, *Da Tang Xi Yu Ji* 大唐西域記, *Gao Li Tu Jing* 高麗圖經, *Zhu Fang Zhi* 諸蕃志, *Xi Ying Yan Xiao* 溪熒巖笑, *Zhen La Feng Tu Ji* 真臘風土記, *Dao Yi Zhi Lüe* 島夷志略, *Hai Yu* 海語, *Dong Xi Yang Kao* 東西洋考, *Zhi Fang Wai Ji* 職方外紀, *Chi Ya* 赤雅, *Chao Xian Zhi* 朝鮮志, *Yi Yu Lu* 異域錄, *Hai Guo Wen Jian Lu* 海國聞見錄, *Huang Qing Zhi Gong Tu* 皇清職貢圖, etc. On military, *Wo Qi Ji* 握奇濟 by Feng Huo 風后, *Liu Tao* 六韜 by Tai Gong 太公, *Sun Zi* 孫子 by Sun Wu 孫武, *Wu Zi* 吳子 by Wu Qi 吳起, *Si Ma Fa* 司馬法 by Sima Rangju 司馬穰苴, *Wei Liao Zi* 尉繚子 by Wei Liao 蔚繚, *San Lüe* 三略 and *Su Shu* 素書 by Huang Shigong 黃石公, *Tai Bai Yin Jing* 太白陰經 by Li Quan 李筌, *Wu Jing Zong Yao* 武經總要 by Zeng Gongliang 曾公亮 and *Ding Du* 丁度, *Hu Ling Jing* 虎鈴經 by Xu Dong 許洞, *He Bo Shi Bei Lun* 何博士備論 by He Qufei 何去非, *Shou Cheng Lu* 守城錄 by Chen Gui 陳規, *Wu Bian* 武編 by Tang Shunzhi 唐順之, *Chen Ji* 陳紀 by He Liangchen 何良臣, *Jiang Nan Jing Lüe* 江南經略 by Zheng Ruo Ceng 鄭若曾, *Lian Bing Shi Ji* 練兵實紀, *Ji Yao Xin Shu* 紀要新書, *Li Rong Yao Nü* 蒞戎要女 and *Wu Bei Xin Shu* 武備新書 by Qi Jiguang 戚繼光, *Jiang Jian Lun Duan* 將鑒論斷 by Dai Shaowang 戴少望, *Jiang Nan Shi Jian* 江南十鑑 by

Li Shun Chen 李舜臣, *Ba Zhen He Bian Tu Shuo* 八陣合變圖說 by Long Zheng 龍正, *Yu Zhe Bing Zhi* 雨浙兵制 by Hou Duanguo 侯斷國, *Bei Wo Ji* 備倭記 by Bu Datong 卜大同, *Jiang Jiang Ji* 將將紀 by Li Cai 李材, *Ling Xi Shui Lu Bing Ji* 嶺西水陸兵紀 by Sheng Wannian 盛萬年, *Zuo Shi Bing Lüe* 左氏兵略 by Chen Yu Mo 陳禹謨, *Lei Ji Lian Chu Zhu Shu* 類輯練出諸書 by Dong Chengzhao 董承詔, *Huo Qi Tu* 火器圖 by Gu Bin 顧斌, *Bing Ji Lei Zuan* 兵機類纂 by Zhang Pangyi 張龐翼, *Zuo Shi Bing Fa Ce Yao* 左氏兵法測要 by Song Zhengbi 宋徵壁, *Wu Bei Zhi Lüe* 武備志略 by Fu Yu 傅禹, *Li Dai Che Zhan Xu Lüe* 歷代車戰敘略 by Zhang Tai Jiao 張泰交, *Lian Yue Huo Qi Zhen Ji* 練閱火器陣紀 by Xue Xi 薛熙, etc. So we have many well-developed subjects with many rare books which could be used as textbooks. So we could set new schools for these subjects and include them in the official school system. Furthermore, we were always at peace because of the legal system. We have astronomy to correct time, geography to draw the map, agriculture to maintain life, military tactics to fight the enemy. For example, with the help of *Bei Wo Ji* 備倭記 by Bu Datong 卜大同, the Japanese army were not able to land at Qingdao and cause the Jinan Massacre. In that case, we are so powerful, and it is not necessary to set modern science schools, read foreign books, wear foreign clothes and speak foreign languages.

The doctors of ancient medicine usually learn from masters or teach themselves. These have been known as good means for medical education for thousands of years, so why do current Chinese medicine doctors want to imitate the Western school system and establish modern schools, publish textbooks and set up hospitals? Though there were schools in ancient times, such as the imperial college and academy, there were no schools of medicine, divination or astrology. Is setting up a Chinese medicine school an innovative way or old-fashioned way? We can know that the positions of these Chinese medicine doctors are not stable. Moreover, even if we set up some schools of Chinese medicine, publish textbooks and set up Chinese medicine hospitals, it is possible that most of the Chinese medicine doctors will still follow the old-fashioned theories, having no desire to improve Chinese medicine. It will remain in an unscientific and backward state.

There are two main problems for Chinese medicine according to the convention of the world school system and national educational policy. The first problem is that it is not permitted to separate one subject into two. For example, engineering is a subject, as well as agriculture and medicine. So there is no reason for medicine to be divided into Western and Chinese. We are now in the 20th century. Scientific Western medicine is the main trend in the world; it is not going to be replaced by ancient Chinese medicine. So, in order to survive, Chinese medicine has to be included in the Western medicine subject.

The second problem is that medicine is a subject of higher education. According to current education policy, people who want to receive higher education should have successfully completed the courses of primary and secondary school. Some Chinese medicine schools name themselves as college, a type of higher education. But as far as I know, some Chinese medicine students are only 13 or 14 years old and they haven't completed the courses of primary school and secondary school. These Chinese medicine schools don't follow the national education policies, so they are neither qualified nor reasonable to be included in the official school system. The new medicine doctors have to study six years in primary school, as well as the secondary school, and five years in medical college or seven years in medical university. It is not possible to shorten the length of schooling. But ancient medicine doctors usually start to treat patients after studying for three to five years. Could it be said that they are much cleverer than the new medicine doctors? Actually, it is highly irresponsible to train doctors like that. If we don't make reforms in education, it will never be possible for Chinese medicine to be included in the official school system and it will be definitely eliminated by its competition with Western medicine.

Two days ago, I met a friend, who is a Chinese medicine doctor, and discussed with him about this topic. He thinks that it is unnecessary to spend 12 years in primary and secondary school. It seems that education in the primary and secondary school is not directly helpful to the medical profession. But basic education is indispensable for modern professionals. The current ancient medicine doctors usually don't know the importance of basic education, that's why they are not able to realize the truth. In a word, I do hope Chinese medicine doctors can make complete reform to promote the development of Chinese medicine.

Fourthly, medicine is not a science for treating illness; *Chun Qiu Zuo Zhuan* 春秋左傳 noted, "the best doctors are able to solve problems of the country, while average doctors treat diseases of the body". The lower doctors are the ones who only focus on earning money. Contemporary doctors of the old medicine seem to devote their attention entirely to the treatment of illness. They don't understand the current situation, which has changed a lot.

Firstly, there is a strong trend towards international medical cooperation between countries; no country's medicine can perform well without consideration of other countries' medicine.

Secondly, medicine has become one of the most important political issues.

Thirdly, there are many new discoveries in the field of medicine, but it is not highly developed. Therefore, the objective is to prevent illness, because it is too late to treat after the onset of illness. We should be ashamed of the belated response to the importance of prevention. It is completely wrong that doctors only have a responsibility to treat illness.

Nowadays, China is no longer a powerful country; conversely, it is a backward country in international terms. We have to do our best to save our country from crisis and eliminate poverty and weakness. There are two reasons for China lagging badly behind the rest of the world. One is the belief that our country is still powerful and important in the world. The other one is the nationalist worldview. We are now people of the 20th century. People of a developed and free country cannot be secretive and closed-minded, nor will a country benefit from its citizens being closed-minded.

Let me give an example, people are allowed to migrate freely since the end of the maritime trade ban. Consequently, every year there are many international medical meetings to discuss the prevention of infectious disease and international cooperation. Our country used to ignore the prevention of infectious diseases and international cooperation. Nowadays, foreigners can easily reside in our country; what's more, they establish colonies in China and set up their own hospitals based on their medicine, because they dislike the poor hygiene of the Chinese people. But the Chinese who want to migrate to foreign countries have to undergo medical examinations and some people are kept in quarantine for several days. Every summer and autumn, when infectious diseases become common, not only are Chinese immigrants required to undergo medical examinations, but also their personal belongings are required to be disinfected. Chinese people are often despised by these countries. So we have to make every effort to improve ourselves and eliminate habits of poor hygiene. Then we can even point out their shortcomings.

It is necessary for us to join the international medical organizations, provide political and financial support to them and cooperate with other countries. It is really not appropriate that the doctors of the old medicine preach the prosperity of our country and the virtues of Chinese medicine.

Besides the treatment of illness, there are many other tasks for doctors; some are related to domestic affairs while others are related to international affairs. For example, issuing death certificates, testing vaccines and drugs, reporting of infectious diseases and stillbirths, forensic evidence, autopsy, food and water inspection, sanitation, the prevention and research of infectious diseases, school health, family health and so on. All these tasks are closely related to science. We can do nothing without the help of science. But doctors of the old medicine may have two different approaches. Firstly, they may be completely against performing these medical tasks, based on four thousand years of history. Secondly, they may undertake these tasks, but refuse to completely change their minds. I think neither approach can achieve success. I hope the wise doctors of the old medicine no longer stick to old ways and no longer advocate Chinese medicine in establishing an independent school system.

Fifthly, nowadays, science is changing quickly. Accordingly, medical books are continually revised. But ancient Chinese medicine, on the contrary, persists in believing its ancient books written thousands of years ago. In my opinion, ancient Chinese medicine tends to be more conservative and narrow, and the new medicine tends to be more innovative and liberal. Consequently, it is quite difficult to communicate with each other. For example, it is really stupid for a country person to jeer at high buildings and large mansions in the city. If Chinese medicine doctors refuse to change their mind and way of behaving, I am afraid that Chinese medicine will never make any progress. How could it jeer at Western medicine? The doctors of the old medicine usually don't trust, accept nor admire science; to the contrary, they oppose and slander science. But sometimes, they say that Chinese medicine has the implication of scientific spirit. If Chinese medicine can take action to develop such scientific spirit, it will gradually turn from unscientific to scientific, and make it possible to preserve itself.

Sixthly, those who have ever read ancient books know that medicine was identified with witchcraft. *Lun Yu* 論語 said a person could not be a good shaman without perseverance. *Guan Zi* 管子 said that the emperor liked divination and that he appointed shamans. *Zhan Guo Ce* 戰國策 noted that shamans were good at divination, but were not able to eliminate their own disasters, while the doctor was good at treating illness, but didn't know how to play a musical instrument. *Lü Shi Chun Qiu* 呂

氏春秋 recorded that shamans thoroughly understood death and life, and cured critical illness. *Shi Ji Xiao Wu Ben Ji* 史記孝武本紀 recorded that the emperor fell ill in Ding Lake 鼎湖, all shamans and doctors were called to be there. *Huai Nan Zi* 淮南子 recorded that both the doctors with needle-stones and shamans with sacrifices could cure bedridden patients. *Shuo Yuan* 說苑 said the emperor would ask the shamans to help patients when epidemic diseases were sweeping the country. *Lun Heng* 論衡 said the doctor was responsible for illness, and the shaman was responsible for avoiding disaster. There are many books that mentioned the role of shaman and doctor simultaneously. Ancient famous doctors such as Bian Que 扁鵲 were considered shamans at that time. Today, when people compliment an excellent doctor it is as if Bian Que 扁鵲 was reborn. So actually, it is not a compliment, it is contempt. After the Han Dynasty 漢代, some scholars wrote medical books which discussed herbs, not completely relying on witchcraft and incantations. So the position of doctor was higher than previously. The four occupations were scholar, farmer, artisan and merchant; therefore, a doctor was still not an important role in society. The theories of Five Phases and Six Qi, Yin and Yang, and generation and restriction, actually, still have traces of witchcraft and incantation.

I have to declare that I don't disdain the ancient Chinese medicine, and I hope that they will not misunderstand my words. The role and position of Chinese medicine in history was truly low. Nowadays, the situation has greatly changed and the intelligence of people has continually evolved. Scientific medicine from foreign countries is not only included in the higher education system, but also plays an important role in the international, political and military affairs. It is quite different from the old Chinese medicine. In order to improve the role and position of Chinese medicine, it should meet the need of contemporary people and follow the world trend. It should also endeavour to remove the traces of witchcraft and incantations. Basing itself on ancient books and methods, even if Chinese medicine happens to be included in the official school system, it won't be able to compete with scientific medicine. I have to advise the doctors of old Chinese medicine earnestly to change their stubborn ways.

Seventhly, the proposal of regaining economic rights is a way to awaken citizens of our country. But it doesn't mean to boycott foreign goods in a negative fashion. Due to the development of human intelligence and culture, we must learn from other countries' strong points and offset our weaknesses. In a highly competitive world, it is not appropriate to close one's doors to the rest of the world. So importation of some necessary goods from other countries is inevitable.

There are two solutions. Firstly, for the necessities that we are not able to produce or imitate, it's better to find a substitute; otherwise, we have to use the foreign goods. For example, because of its cool nature and tonifying action, the doctors of old medicine like to use American ginseng. The annual import quantity and cost of American ginseng are far more than those of imported drugs used by new medicine doctors. The doctors of old medicine always advocate the regaining of economic rights, so why they don't find a substitute for American ginseng? Why they don't plant American ginseng? Actually, it is not suitable to plant American ginseng in China, because the climate and soil are quite different, which may cause difference in its efficacy. It is just like copper, iron, cotton and rice, which should have specific regions of production. Nowadays, international goods trade is inevitable. According to what we know, the ancient medicine doctors use many foreign drugs. For example, Gao Li 高麗,[89] which belonged to China, now is occupied by another country. Isn't Gao Li Shen 高麗參 a product from our enemy? Therefore, we have to be flexible and never give up eating for fear of choking. It is no use talking without taking any action.

Secondly, for the common ordinary things, for which we have enough raw materials, it's better for us to be self-sufficient. For example, cement and bricks, used for buildings, originated in foreign countries. Chinese people didn't boycott them; on the contrary, they liked to use them. Through effort, today most of them are produced by domestic factories. The situation of clothing is the same. Actually, these are the correct ways to regain economic rights. We can even export these goods to foreign countries and promote the development of our industry and commerce. Japan was a quite poor country 50 years ago, but the Japanese knew how to regain their economic rights; they worked very hard, and now Japan is not only able to support itself, but also able to export goods to other countries. Honestly, Japan plays an important role in world industry and commerce.

The ancient medicine doctors rebuked overseas students for being flunkies and salesmen of foreign goods. Frankly, I don't agree with their opinions. I think those overseas students will form an elite that has the power to regain the economic rights. The doctors of the old medicine can do nothing but helplessly wait for death if our country is in conflict with foreigners. This is because they never try to find solutions

[89] Gao Li 高麗 and Gao Li Shen 高麗參 are Korea and Korean ginseng, respectively.

for the situation, believing that everything will be alright if they avoid buying goods exported from foreign countries. It is really terrible to be controlled by other countries. For example, the doctors of the old medicine have published many newspapers and magazines, such as *Yi Jie Chun Qiu* 醫界春秋, *Wei Sheng Bao* 衛生報, *Kang Jian Bao* 康健報 and so on, but there is no papermaking factory in China. If China is in a conflict with other countries, all our newspapers and magazines have to be stopped. Many doctors of the old medicine live in the foreign concessions of Shanghai 上海, where many materials are controlled by foreigners. But they don't refuse to use these materials. In order to regain our economic rights, we have to be more proactive. It is really not appropriate to apply old methods from thousands of years ago without any improvement. Considering the situation of China, the world and the century we are in, there is no other entity that can rescue China except science.

Eighthly, doctors of the old medicine united herbal workers to complain about their livelihood by publishing advertisements in the newspapers. Occupations should meet the development of society. No one would like to continue with a needless occupation. For example, now we use guns as weapons, rarely using bows and arrows. Did all workers relating to bows and arrows starve to death? Now we use paper, pen and ink for writing, rarely using paint and bamboo slip. Did all workers related to paint and bamboo slip starve to death? Now we use stereotype zincography and chalcography for printing, rarely using block printing. Did all workers related to block printing starve to death? The doctors of the old medicine are always conservative, so by definition they oppose new scientific ideas. Inexplicably, they wear factory-made clothes, not homespun. There are many persons employed making homespun clothes, but they are not likely to hold meetings for protecting their old livelihood, and we haven't seen many of them starve to death. The doctors of the old medicine used to make home visit by sedan chair; why do they prefer to use cars nowadays? The bearers are not likely to hold meetings for protecting their old livelihood and we haven't seen many of them starve to death. The doctors of the old medicine used oil lamps for light; unexpectedly, they now turn to electric light. In that case, should the oil lamp workers hold meetings to protest their livelihood? Rice was usually pounded in a mortar manually, but now it is done by the rice mill; should those manual workers hold meetings to protest their livelihood? I just provide the above examples, which are quite common in daily life. We can find more of such situations in our life, if we observe carefully and deeply.

These changes are the result of scientific development. If the ancient medicine doctors think such changes are not good, why do they use modern products? I don't think that the new government will ignore the potential problem of unemployment.

Actually, the proposals of the doctors of the old medicine aim to attack the new medicine. As the natives of Shanghai 上海, we all know there was a famous hand-made sock shop called Hong Mao Chang 宏茂昌 in Bao Shan Street 寶善街. I still remember buying many socks from it when we were young. With the influx of machine-made socks from foreign countries, business became worse and worse. Did all workers of this shop starve to death? No. The boss of this shop was flexible; he began producing and selling machine-made socks. On the one hand, he called on people to boycott foreign socks but on the other hand, he tried his best to develop his machine-made sock business. Now he has two sock factories, one in Bao Shan Street 寶善街 and the other one in Beijing Road 北京路. Their business became better and better. This is a really good example of how to regain economic rights. If the boss of the sock shop followed the old medicine way of doing things, refusing to change his mind, would there have been any chance for his business?

However, there are still some doctors of the old medicine who want to make some changes. For example, there was a good doctor of the old medicine who wanted his successive generations to study new medicine, rather than carrying on the old medicine. And several years ago, there was a Chinese medicine factory in Nan Jing Road 南京路 and Zhong Hua Road 中華路. But unfortunately, due to lack of scientific knowledge and global view, it finally went bankrupt. However, I admire such attempts. It is not possible to transform Chinese herbs into new-style liquid, powder, and pill without enough capital and deep research. In order to succeed in the pharmaceutical industry, scientific knowledge and global view are quite necessary. We know that foreign pharmaceutical companies usually spend millions of dollars and several decades researching one herb. Finally, I would like to warn the doctors of the old medicine with an old saying "Those who suit their actions to the times are wise".

Ninthly, as discussed above, China had some subjects similar to modern scientific subjects. Chinese subjects rely on imagination, whereas modern scientific subjects rely on evidence. With the development of material progress in recent years, many more things can be proven by science. For example, with the development of acoustics, we are able to produce gramophones and hearing-aids. With the development of optics, we are able to produce many appliances. With electricity, we have lighting, heating and powered machines. Now, we have telegraph and telephone to communicate with each other. We have cable picture transmission system to send pictures to faraway places. Airplane and submarine are used in current wars.

With scientific development, medicine has gradually changed from suppositional to evidence-based since the 14th century. Medical knowledge of twenty years ago is no longer applicable to the present. Science failed to develop well in ancient China, due to the worship of ancient classics and the old obstructionist policies of the emperors. The people were fettered by old conventions; no one desired to innovate. All this also influenced the field of medicine, which still follows old thoughts and refuses to reform.

I will give some examples to discuss whether Chinese medicine is suitable to be formed as an independent subject in the 20th century. Firstly, what the ancient medicine doctors relied on are some ancient classics. These classics are literary and philosophical, and value textual research. The words are obscure, while the medical theories seem profound. The doctors who have never studied *Ling Shu* 靈樞, *Su Wen* 素問, and *Nan Jing* 難經 are like water without a source, and a tree without roots. Actually such thoughts are not suitable at the present time, when human intelligence has made great progress. According to historical experience, we have to compare different academic tendencies, and choose the best suitable ones. It is not suitable to be fettered by only one theory or theories of a specific time. We can divide medicine into three periods. The first is the philosophical period. By studying medical books from Chinese medicine in the Han Dynasty 漢代, ancient Greek medicine and ancient Roman medicine, we can see the knowledge level and academic tendency of the people that lived in this period. The second is the farfetched analogy period. Herbs and formulas have been more and more important in Chinese medicine since the Han Dynasty 漢代. Due to the limits of the times, doctors were fettered by theories from the ancient classics. They had to use these theories to explain the usage of herbs. Therefore, the herbs are genuine but the theories are false. However, there was a rudimentary empiricism which could develop as a means for scientific research. Due to space limitations, I am not going to discuss the comparable situations in foreign countries.

But it was quite similar to nowadays Chinese medicine. I am afraid the ancient medicine doctors may oppose my opinion. I am going to analyze some famous books on Chinese medicine, in order to display the trend of the different times and the level of human intelligence. For example, *Ling Shu* 靈樞, *Su Wen* 素問, *Nan Jing* 難經, *Jia Yi Jing* 甲乙經, etc., all are books written before Han Dynasty. They are not called medical books 醫籍, but Classics Jing 經, which is similar to the category of philosophical books, such as Lao Zi 老子, *Dao De Jing* 道德經, *Fo Jing* 佛經, and *Nan Hua Jing* 南華經 and so on. They are based on speculation and analogy. Only the *Jia Yi Jing* 甲乙經[90] is somewhat related to medical practice; however, it is considered as a book written in the Sui Dynasty 隋朝, according to the *Qun Jing Gu Fang Lun* 羣經古方論 by Lü Fu 呂復. Also, the *Sui Shu Jing Ji Zhi* 隋書經籍志 notes that the *Jia Yi Jing* 甲乙經 has ten volumes but the author is unknown. Therefore, this book is not credible.

Furthermore, we don't believe that acupuncture could develop so well before the Han Dynasty 漢朝. If these books weren't expounded by the doctors after the Han Dynasty 漢代, they may be still classified as classic works of literature, which are not able to guide the treatment of diseases. In the Han Dynasty 漢代, Zhang Zhongjing 張仲景 wrote the *Jin Gui Yao Lüe* 金匱要略. It is full of mystery and quite difficult to understand. So it is considered as a classic 經典 by later doctors, and also called *Jin Gui Yu Han Jing* 金匱玉函經. However, with the progress of human intelligence, the medicine from the Han Dynasty 漢代 changed gradually from theoretical to practical, and doctors paid more attention to formulas and less to theory. But the theories used to explain the formulas were still greatly related to philosophy. This is an example of the "farfetched analogy period". Most doctors in that time had known that the formulas were more important than the theories in the treatment of diseases.

There were many books on formulas in that period, such as *Zhou Hou Bei Ji Fang* 肘後備急方 by Ge Hong 葛洪 in the Jin Dynasty 晋朝, *Qian Jin Fang* 千金方 by Sun Simiao 孫思邈 in the Tang Dynasty 唐朝, *Bo Ji Fang* 博濟方 by Wang Gun 王袞 in the Song Dynasty 宋朝, *Su Shen Liang Fang* 蘇沈良方 by Shen Kuo 沈括 and *Su Shi* 蘇軾, *Lü She Bei Yao Fang* 旅舍備要方 by Dong Ji 董汲, *Quan Sheng Zhi Mi Fang* 全生指迷方 by Wang Kuang 王貺, *Lei Zheng Pu Ji Ben Shi Fang* 類證普濟本事方 by Xu Shuwei 許叔微, *Tai Ping Hui Min He Ji Ju Fang* 太平惠民和劑局方, *Wei Sheng Shi Quan Fang* 衛生十全方 and *Qi Ji Fang* 齊疾方 by Xia De 夏德, *Fu Ren Da Quan Liang Fang* 婦人大全良方 by Chen Ziming 陳自明, *Ji Yan Bei Ju Fang* 集驗背疽方 by Li Xun 李迅, *Ji Sheng Fang* 濟生方 by Yan Yonghe 嚴用和, *Chan Bao Zhu Fang* 產寶諸方, *Ji Jiu Xian Fang* 急救仙方, *Xiao Er Wei Sheng Zong Wei Lun Fang* 小兒衛生總微論方, *Fu Xin Shi Yong Fang* 傅信適用方, *Chan Yu Bao Qing Fang* 產育寶慶方 and so on. In the Jin and Yuan dynasties 金源時代, there were fewer formulas books, for example *Xuan Ming Lun Fang* 宣明論方 and *Shang Han Zhi Ge Fang* 傷寒直格方 by Liu Wansu 劉完素 in the Jin Dynasty 金朝, *Rui Zhu Tang Jing Yan Fang* 瑞竹堂經驗方 by Sha Tu Mu Su 沙圖穆蘇 in the Yuan Dynasty 元朝, *Ru*

90 *Systematic Classic of Acupuncture and Moxibustion (Zhen Jiu Jia Yi Jing)*

Yi Fang 如宜方 by Ai Yuan Ying 艾元英, *Shi Yi De Xiao Fang* 世醫得效方 by Wei Yilin 危亦林 and so on. In the Ming Dynasty 明朝, there were much fewer formulas books, for example *Pu Ji Fang* 普濟方 by Zhou Dingwang Su 周定王橚, *Yi Fang Xuan Yao* 醫方選要 by Zhou Wencai 周文采, *Xiu Zhen Xiao Er Fang* 袖珍小兒方 by Xu Yongxuan 徐用宣, *Wan Min Jia Chao Ji Shi Liang Fang* 萬民家鈔濟世良方 by Wan Biao 萬表, *She Sheng Zhong Miao Fang* 攝生眾妙方 and *Ji Jiu Liang Fang* 急救良方 by Zhang Shiche 張時徹, *Bi Shui Ji Yan Fang* 避水集驗方 by Dong Bing 董炳, *Lu Fu Mi Fang* 魯府秘方 by Liu Yingtai 劉應泰, *Ling Mi Shi Ba Fang* 靈秘十八方 and so on. Most of the formulas in these books were not original.

In the Qing Dynasty 清朝, books of formulas were quite rare, examples being *Shang Han Lun Fang* 傷寒論方 by Xu Dachun 徐大椿, *Cheng Fang Qie Yong* 成方切用 by Wu Yiluo 吳儀洛 and so on.

In our opinion, the period with an even greater number of formula books will be developed in the third period, which is called the scientific period.

Surprisingly, Chinese medicine reverted to its old ways from the Jin and Yuan dynasties 金元, when doctors preferred to research ancient theories and discuss theoretical issues. In the Song Dynasty 宋朝, the situation was even more extreme, with the trend of reverting to the first period. The schools of thought on Confucianism originated in the Song Dynasty 宋朝 and the schools of thought on medicine originated in the Jin and Yuan dynasties 金元. Usually, schools of thought can promote academic progress. But the medical schools of thought in Jin and Yuan dynasties 金元 were empty, with little or no regard for practical problems. Examples include the argument between Liu Hejian 劉河間 and Zhang Yuansu 張元素, Zhu Danxi's 朱丹溪 critique of *Xuan He Ju Fang* 宣和局方 and so on. They slandered each other, confusing right and wrong. Therefore, it is quite difficult for Chinese medicine to regain the academic caliber of the times prior to the Jin and Yuan dynasties 金元; how dare they wish to include it in the official school system?

We have to be practical and innovative, especially for serious medicine. It is not productive to argue about empty theories. The third period is the scientific period. The new medicine originated after the 14th century, when doctors started to focus on the material world. Actually, medicine should be more practical. As a living being, the human body consists of substances that actually exist. People will be healthy if these substances maintain normality, and become ill or die if they become abnormal.

As we all know, the structure of living things is more complicated than non-living things, especially in the case of human beings. People have worked hard to unlock the secrets of the body for centuries, but we still only know a little about the body. So it is a long-term effort, we have to gradually improve medical knowledge.

Unfortunately, Chinese medicine has stagnated or even regressed to the stage it was during the Jin and Yuan dynasties 金元. There are many reasons for this, the most important being the shackle of feudalism. The Ming 明 emperor Zhu Yuanzhang 朱元璋 decreed that all talented personnel in the country worked in the Imperial Court. Naturally, it hindered the academic progress. With the change of governmental structure and the importation of foreign ideas, people became more and more open-minded. However, it is not possible for all people to change their minds completely in a short period. As we all know, China is a backward country now; naturally, therefore, Chinese medicine is also backward. But Chinese medicine doctors are still arrogant and anti-foreign. They are patriotic, but their behavior is foolish. I have spoken with some Chinese medicine doctors recently, which helped me to understand more about them:

Doctor	Thoughts	Age	Level of Ancient Literature	Level of Ancient Medicine	Purposes
1	conservative	over 40	high	high	doctrine, enrich
2	conservative	unspecified	high	average	enrich
3	conservative	unspecified	average	high	livelihood
4	conservative	under 50	low	average	enrich
5	indefinite	under 30	low	high	livelihood
6	indefinite	under 40	average	average	enrich
7	indefinite	under 35	high	high	livelihood
8	indefinite	over 40	low	average	livelihood

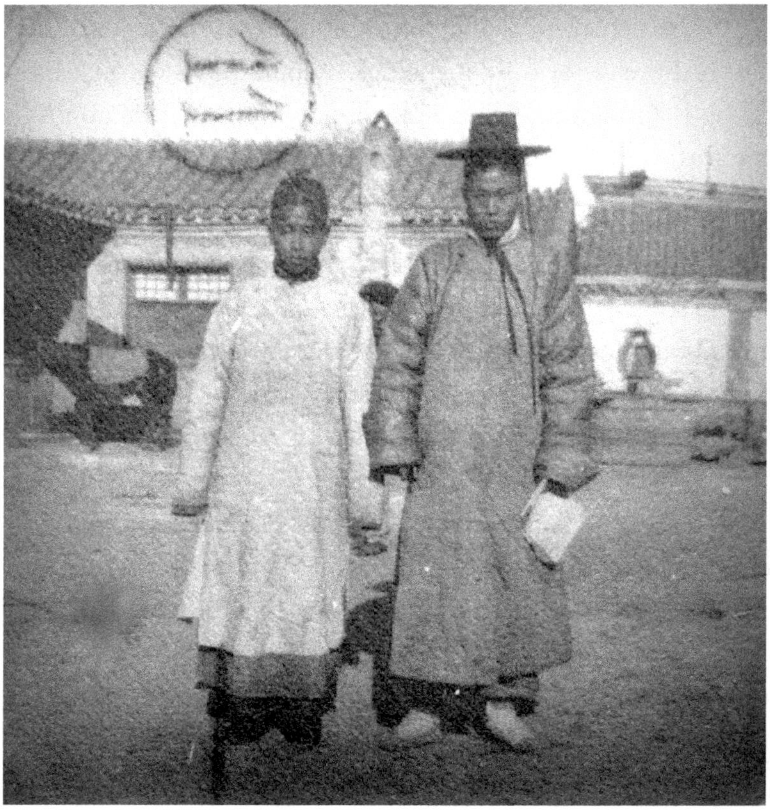

Photo by Mr P. Goux in early 1900s. "Chinese doctor with Korean interpreter"

The 3rd, 5th, 7th and 8th kinds of doctors earn their livelihood by practicing Chinese medicine. Some of them are not conservative, so it is possible to change their minds. Some of them have a low level of ancient literature, so they have fewer ideological shackles and don't have the ability to argue theoretical issues both orally and written. If the government can provide them with other means of livelihood, these doctors may move towards the right way.

The 1st kind of doctors, who are old and greatly influenced by ancient culture, usually read lots of medical classics. They know nothing about scientific subjects from foreign countries. They believe that the *Ling Shu* 靈樞 and *Su Wen* 素問 are the ultimate books created by great men, enabling doctors to cure all diseases. Besides money, they also worked for doctrine. Thus, it is not possible to persuade them to change their minds.

The 2nd, 4th, 6th kinds of doctors, who have no other means of earning a living except being a doctor, usually work only for money, so they deceive patients with quite average medical skills.

The 2nd kind of doctors with a high level of ancient literature knowledge, are the most dangerous of all because they can mislead common people with beautiful words. They are the core members who loudly call the public to support and preserve the essence of Chinese culture and the inclusion of Chinese medicine in the official school system.

The 1st kind is quite similar to the 7th kind of doctor. However, one works for money and ideals, the other for livelihood. Because the purposes are different, we cannot treat them the same. I met a doctor of the old Chinese medicine and I deeply admired his words. He said there were no methods to change the minds of elder doctors, but the government could help the young doctors to study the new medicine and keep the young students away from Chinese medicine. These words are like an alarm clock ringing at midnight.

Tenthly, I am quite tired these days because I had to treat too many patients due to the hot weather. But I still prefer to discuss with the doctors of old medicine about their medicine. What I say may not be totally right, but I think it will be helpful to them. As per what I have said before, according to the national education policies, Chinese medicine is not suitable to become an independent school system. Furthermore, it is not appropriate for the old and modern medicine to exist simultaneously. They have to be in the same medical education system with the same educational purpose. Everything should be unified in a unified country. It is not reasonable to separate Chinese medicine from the national medical school system.

It is a completely wrong way to include Chinese medicine in the official school system. It is only reasonable and possible to set some courses related to Chinese medicine in the proposal to the Ministry of Higher Education. If the doctors of the old Chinese medicine don't agree with my opinion, they can try to remove the new medicine from the official school system, as per the Proposal they sent to the Ministry of Higher Education, only keeping the useful aspects of the new medicine. But this is a really backwards step for the development of medicine, which wouldn't be supported by the majority of people. Besides, it is not possible to develop both the ancient and new medicine simultaneously. Honestly, I hope the doctors of the old medicine can cease such futile efforts. Here I analyze the doctors of old Chinese medicine with psychological methods:

	Clinic Business	Their Children's Job	Reason	Psychology	Other Factor
1	good	CM doctor	safeguard the heritage	carry forward the family tradition	believe CM will have a bright prospect
2	good	CM doctor	enrich	pride with the current success	want to transmit success from one generation to another
3	good	other job	disillusioned with CM	not confident about CM	too late for himself to change job
4	good	CM doctor or other jobs	no specific reason	only want a job	several children have chosen different jobs
5	bad	CM doctor	stubborn character	poor but happy	unwilling to give up family tradition
6	bad	CM doctor	have no alternative	disillusioned with CM	inability to provide better job opportunity
7	bad	other job	current trend	disillusioned with CM	contrite to be a CM doctor
8	bad	other job	social environment	open-minded	without intervention

We know that it is common for the children of doctors of old medicine to take other jobs, including becoming new medicine doctors. But it is quite rare for the children of new medicine doctors to be employed in Chinese medicine. This is a good example for the current trend. The doctors of old medicine, who agree with or support their children to change jobs, may not become completely disillusioned with Chinese medicine. However, at least they are not so confident about Chinese medicine. The 4th and 8th doctors have a casual attitude towards their children's job. The 3rd and 7th doctors are completely disillusioned with Chinese medicine. The 1st and 5th doctors are stubborn, they don't want to give up family tradition. The 6th doctor is unable to provide a better job opportunity for his children. The 2nd doctor just works for money. It is not strange that a mediocre doctor would like his children to do other jobs. But it is difficult to understand that the children of the successful doctors give up the family tradition and take other jobs. There must be some hidden reasons. In my opinion, only the 5th doctor truly loves Chinese medicine; he is happy, though he is poor. For the others, Chinese medicine is just a means of earning money in order to live. Therefore, we know that the proposals presented by ancient Chinese medicine doctors are not aimed for preserving the essence of Chinese culture, but their own livelihood. Their attempts and behaviours, such as rescuing old Chinese medicine, trying to include Chinese medicine in the official school system, defaming new medicine, opposing science and so on, are actually motivated by the magic power of money. If the government can change their source of livelihood, none of them will fight for old Chinese medicine. I will stop writing now, and if possible, I will discuss more about the proper procedures for dealing with the problem of Chinese medicine this autumn.

July, the 17th year of the republic (1928)

Article end

The opinions in Chinese medicine circles about compilation of standard teaching materials

Source: *Compilation of Discussions about Chinese Medical Education* 中醫教育討論集

Yaron: This illustrates the early beginnings of making Chinese medicine a uniform standard. This clearly was a response to the modernizers' claims that Chinese medicine is not only unscientific but also lacks a standard—each graduate reaches a different knowledge level and most only reach a low level of education.

Worth noting is the fact that while Chinese medicine faced legal extinction on a national scale, this gave birth to many small associations which later united under one umbrella or central federation. Under a centralized organization, there was power to decide what is and what will become of Chinese medicine on a large scale. Often, this power fell in the hands of a small group of people, for better or for worse.

Chinese medicine schools curriculum: my opinion

Pages 434–440 (partial article)

1. The rules of the Editing Committee for Standard Teaching Materials of the National Federation of Associations of Chinese Medicine.

Article 1 The aim of setting up the textbook Editing Committee is to encourage the forward movement of the Chinese Medicine profession, through standardizing textbooks and teaching contents.

Article 2 This Editing Committee will be nominated by all Chinese Medicine Schools and formed by one to three committee members.

Article 3 The central federation would assign three professionals as the principals of this committee.

Article 4 The central federation would hire seven education professionals, five Internal medicine experts, five pharmacologist experts, and each three experts in other different disciplines such as surgery, traumatology, etc and two medical students studying abroad, all serving as consultants.

Article 5 The Editing Committee will be assisted by the central federation in collecting different textbooks and receiving the feedback from old teachers and doctors.

Article 6 The Editing Committee will hold the first meeting in the coming summer vacation, lasting for 2 weeks, expenses of which will be paid by the central federation. It is permissible to extend this period if there is more to discuss.

Article 7 The agenda of the first meeting is as follows:

Determine the standard for theory.

Finalize the format of textbooks, and teaching materials.

Revise the study schedule.

Mark the ratio of each topic to the entire study curriculum.

Make samples for each course / subject.

Article 8 The Editing Committee will finalize the nomination of authors for each course before the end of the first meeting. The editing work should be completed within half a year.

Article 9 The Editing Committee will hold the second meeting at the end of the year and the catering expenses will be paid by the central federation.

Article 10 The aim of the second meeting is listed as follows:

Review all the submitted textbooks proposals.

Complete the remaining tasks not dealt with in the first meeting.

Article 11 The copyrights of each textbook belong to the central federation, while the editors receive 30% of the copyright fee.

Article 12 This regulation is passed by the administrative committee of the central federation and is being enforced.

2. My opinion of Chinese medicine schools curriculum

By Zhu Song 朱松[91]

Yaron: Here we see the urgent need to create a modern curriculum for Chinese medicine, the majority of which in the first two years is dedicated to modern medicine, while the last two years allows specialization in Chinese medicine.

Chinese medicine was to become a department within the bigger modern medicine. Even in its specialization phase it took the shape and format of modern medicine—teaching medicine by departments. This trend continues into the Communist-era TCM schools.

The Principle:

a. Chinese Medicine Schools should be considered specialty schools.

   Reason: Medicine is a specialty topic within the sciences, Chinese medicine is likewise, therefore Chinese medicine schools should be considered specialty schools.

b. Graduation should be limited to four years.

   Reason: The essence of specialty schools is to teach practical knowledge. Universities, on the other hand, emphasize theoretical studies, therefore in all countries specialty schools graduate after four years, which is one year shorter than universities.

c. Divide the four years course into two terms. The first term will teach the student how to prepare himself and improve his general knowledge, while the second term will make him a specialist.

   Reason: The first step in acquiring more knowledge is to equip students with more tools for further learning. Therefore, basic Chinese language, basic foreign language and basic scientific methods should be taught prior to further studies. Regarding studying, instructions on learning methods could be provided to students. Students should use pre-defined vocabularies, and give special attention to self-studying. In terms of accomplishing the objective of applica-

[91] This article was compiled by different authors. Zhu Song is the author of point 2.

tion, there should be enough freedom given in their learning, but it is necessary to ensure that students can apply scientific methods. The reason for having the above is to let them have a better opportunity for setting up research.

When dividing labor tasks in a society, there must be specialization. The students will gain professional success through assistance in the early phase of education, by teaching basic knowledge and scientific methods. For example, schools should adopt foreign-style tutorials and grading systems in order to provide more opportunities for students to have more academic contact with each other. (The above aims were also suggested by the Professor Dong Ren Jian 董任堅 as a scholar at National Chi Nan University 國立暨南大學.)

The above principles should be applied while establishing the four-year syllabus, including subjects taught and their contributing ratios.

First Academic Year

Focus on developing basic knowledge as essential tools for further learning.

- National Party platform- The President's honorary guidance
- Chinese Language
- Foreign Language
- World Culture and History
- Introduction to Philosophy
- Physics and Chemistry
- Biology
- Anatomy
- Physiology
- Military Studies

Second Academic Year

Focus on preparing for professional studies.

- National Party's Teachings
- Anatomy
- Physiology
- Bacteriology
- Biochemistry

- Chinese Medicine History
- Introduction to Surgery
- Introduction to Internal Medicine
- Chinese Pharmaceutical Studies
- Military Studies

Third Academic Year

Focus on professional study of medicine. (Same ratio of theoretical studies to internship.)

- Internal Medicine
- Surgery
- Formulas
- Gynecology
- Pediatrics
- Qi Transformations
- Public Hygiene
- Internship in Hospital

Fourth Academic Year

Focus on internship and advanced studies for future occupation.

- Diagnosis
- Treatment
- Medical Traumatology and Orthopaedics
- Laryngology
- Ophthalmology
- Acupuncture
- Tui Na
- Medical Ethics
- Internship in Hospital

3. Proposal on teaching materials' style and format

By Lu Zong Qiang 盧宗強

Yaron: Different opinions prevailed throughout Chinese medicine history and this was a major obstacle for creating a standardized and unified system. The following approach aims to remedy this situation.

Guangdong Guanghan Chinese Medicine Specialty School 廣東光漢中醫專門學校 representative Lu Zong Qiang 盧宗強.

Style and format need to be established for teaching materials such as textbooks, using principles for compiling and editing. It is like holding the wheel in a ship to decide its direction or walking by following the compass direction. There are two possible methods for editing textbooks: one method is to collect different opinions from all the related books and list them out, while the second method is to integrate several opinions and explain them in a new form.

With the former method, there are two unhelpful habits seen with past authors that might impair a book's content. Firstly, some scholars insisted on their own theories but refused to accept new thinking, while others believed that some random books were master works and they followed their silly theories. Secondly, using this method of collecting and listing different opinions this amounted to a huge collection. Without a specific goal for learning, it does not benefit the reader. It is also possible that some recorded opinions were contrary to one another, for instance Miu Zhongchun 繆仲醇 followers who don't investigate excess and deficiency; or Zhang Jingyue 張景岳 having prejudice about particular herbs without even making a diagnosis. Therefore, it seems that this first method of editing should not be used, due to its various adverse outcomes.

However, for the latter method there are different problems too. The first problem is that there is too much information that is difficult to integrate. This can result in omission of opinions from various scholars or difficulty deciding the degree of contribution from each scholar's opinions. The knowledge and meaning to be integrated might not be clear enough at the moment or might require more proof, which is the second problem. Apart from the above, integration of different opinions or knowledge can cause trouble due to failing to reference specific scholars or doctors. Also, without a united system in terms of different opinions, it might easily confuse the reader. Thus, from the above comments, it seems that neither is the second method very feasible.

Therefore, the correct method of completing the editing progress is suggested as follows: all related books should be referenced to integrate specific knowledge and comprehensiveness should be ensured. The referencing of each book mentioned or adopted should be clearly included. So as to prevent the above problems, a preface or a conclusion should be written from the opinions listed, or integration made, aiming to clarify the main idea or subject that it represents.

To sum up, students could learn the essentials, while also being able to drill down in specific points or theories, while the teaching staff should not be selfish in their teaching from the book. This can be further discussed and requires agreement from all concerned. Thank you.

4. Proposal on textbook style and format

By Bao Shisheng 包識生

Yaron: This is a somewhat unsuccessful attempt to preserve old theories while adding a modern structure of anatomy and physiology. This kind of physical explanation using ancient ideas—for example, how breasts form from Li Trigram and male genitalia from Kan Trigram—was most certainly the weakest point Chinese medicine could not hold onto in its struggle against modern medicine. More often than not, it was used by Chinese medicine antagonists as proof of old medicine's backwardness.

Today, Chinese medicine still struggles for recognition and a divide within the Chinese medicine community still exists—one group proposes a scientific narrative, while the other a philosophical one.

It is my honor that our society has gathered different professionals to discuss the style and format of teaching materials. It is not easy to prevent arguments among members towards a conclusion, though we should provide our opinions with more proof, in academic fashion, and be calmer facing the discussion. It would be a great joke in society if we kept discussion in this wrong way coming up with wrong conclusions, thereby weakening our reputation. Therefore, I first made my own four viewpoints, as follows:

1. Teaching materials should be strictly based on traditional Chinese medicine concepts. It should not be catering to the modern direction of science.
2. Teaching materials should be recognized by all doctors in the field of Chinese medicine.
3. Teaching materials should be produced according to science, to prevent vague expressions that may confuse readers.
4. Teaching materials should be suitable for all people to study with real positive effects in learning.

Chinese medicine theory

1. Anatomy

"Xian Tian Ba Gua 先天八卦 The Pre heaven Eight Trigrams" is the model of the Nine orifices of the body

Qian ☰and Kun ☷ are the parent trigrams of The Primordial Eight Trigrams. Fuxi 伏羲 observed and dissected the human body in order to develop the trigrams.

Kun, in fact, was formed by two eyes, two nose openings and two ears, which are the six clear apertures located on the human face. Qian was formed by one mouth and two openings below for elimination, called the three muddy apertures of the human body. Kun should be above, while Qian should be below. "Therefore, the point below the nose and above the mouth is the border dividing the two types of apertures and is called Ren Zhong 人中 the human center."

Not only do humans share the same characteristics, cattle do as well. It is the reason why the Pre-heaven Eight Trigrams can include all phenomena in the world. The nine apertures of the human body are the most important means enabling a human's ongoing life, which is well proven in Chinese medicine. It is also the reason why Chinese medicine is based on the Pre-heaven Eight Trigrams. If this life-enabling rule is abandoned, then most concepts could no longer be understood! It will become a great depression and sadness!

2. Physiology

"The Acquired Eight Trigrams" is the symbol of physiology

Its formation is due to the interchange of the Eight Trigrams converting Qian to Li ☲ and Kun to Kan ☵. Kan represents male and Li represents female. These two trigrams determine the physiological development of each gender.

The sex characteristics maturely developed in a male, including the sex organ, are due to the characteristic of Kan. Kan belongs to water which tends to flow down, going to the lower region of the body and triggering the formation there. While for females, breast development is due to Li, belonging to fire. Fire tends to go upwards and burn, triggering the formation of the breasts. The above is the natural rule of The Acquired Eight Trigrams.

Male belongs to Yang 陽, therefore the growth is based on Qi 氣. The lungs are affected and form a laryngeal prominence causing sound change. For female who belongs to Yin 陰 Blood Xue 血 is dominant, the liver helps the growth in terms of widening the pelvis during the reproductive years.

It can be observed that the physiological secretions of humans also symbolize the trigrams. Males produce semen, which is white in color and represents Kan's water of the same color. Menstruation in female is red, matching Li's fire in color. Thus, males frequently present with weakness of Qi and females with lack of Blood.

5. Theory adoption standard

Memorial Week and National Party Report.....According to National Party's rule
Sanmin 三民主義 Doctrine ....According to premier Sun 孫總理 text
Modern Translation of *Suwen* 素問 ....*The Inner Canon of Huangdi* 黃帝內經
Modern Translation of *Lingshu* 靈樞 ....As above
Anatomy ....*The Inner Canon of Huangdi* 黃帝內經

Referring to Western Medicine

Physiology	As above
Pathology in *Treatise on Cold Injuries* *Shang Han Lun* 傷寒論	Original text of Zhang Zhongjing 張仲景
Golden Chamber Miscellaneous Diseases *Jingui Za Bing Xue* 金櫃雜病學	As above
Epidemiology of Febrile Diseases 溫病病理學	Ye Tianshi 葉天士, Wu Jutong 吳鞠通
Pharmacology	*Divine Farmer's Materia Medica* *Shen Nong Ben Cao* 神農本草
Medical History in China	Chen Xiuyuan 陳修園
Processing of medicinals	*Leigong PaoZhi* 雷公炮製
Formulas	Zhang Zhongjing 張仲景 and Formula rhymes
Gynecology	[Blank]
Nanjing 難經 Study	[Blank]
Diagnosis	[Blank]
Tooth, Ear, Throat, Nose studies	[Blank]
Mental Treatment	[Blank]
Pediatrics	[Blank]
Surgery	*Wai Ke Jin Jian* 外科金鑒
Ophthalmology	*Yan Ke Da Quan* 眼科大全
Sphygmology	[Blank]
Forensic Science	[Blank]
Emergency Medicine	[Blank]
Acupuncture	*Zhen Jiu Da Cheng* 針灸大成
Clinical Internship	Instructed by teachers
Sexually Transmitted Diseases	[Blank]
Medical Traumatology and Orthopaedics	[Blank]
Internship and Practicum	Instruction by the teachers

6. The decision by the syllabus-creating committee of the National Native Medicine Council QuanGuo YiYao Zonghui Bian Zhi Xue Cheng Wei Yuan Hui 全國醫藥總會編製學程委員會

1) Chinese Medicine Schools should be recognized as specialty schools in the higher education system. Graduation should be set for five years.

2) After graduation, students are allowed to continue their learning in a research institute.

3) The study syllabus is as follows:

First Year

National Party's Guidance
Chinese Language, Foreign Language
History of Medicine
Pharmaceutical Studies
Biology
Anatomy
Physiology
Military Studies
Medical Chemistry
Basic Medical Knowledge
Public Hygiene

Second Year

Anatomy
Physiology
Military Studies
National Party's Guidance
Chinese Language, Foreign Language
Medical Chemistry
Pharmaceutical Studies
Pathology
Internal Medicine
Bacteriology

Third Year

Pathology
Pharmaceutical Studies
Internal Medicine
Surgery
Chinese Language
Formulas

Fourth Year

Diagnosis
Internal Medicine
Gynecology
Surgery
Pediatrics
Internship in Clinic

Fifth Year

Electives
Clinical Internship

Article end

The Central Bureau of Native Medicine Regulations and Guidelines 中央國醫館訓令

Source: *Compilation of Discussions about Chinese Medical Education* 中醫教育討論集

Yaron: The following is an initial attempt to centralize power into the hands of the Central Bureau of Native Medicine. There are 21 regulations in this draft aiming to create a unified Chinese medicine school system.

This measure was quickly abandoned, as we shall see in the article's last paragraph. A genuine standardization of Chinese medicine schools will have to wait until the Communist era some two decades later. We can see, however, that standardization attempts for a Chinese medicine unified school system began here in the 1930s.

Pages 440–445

To all,

This document is delivery of official instruction No. 3323

Upon inspection of several Chinese medicine institutes and clinics, there is a common phenomenon found in the study programs, and that is a lack of unity in the programs and existing differences between institutes. It certainly adversely affects students' learning and degrades our prospects of training more professionals. Therefore, a united standard for study programs should be strictly applied and complied with. Firstly, the different institutes should be named according to their purpose in Chinese medicine education. Institutes aiming to provide traditional medicine techniques and knowledge should be named as Native Medicine Professional Schools Guo Yi Zhuan Ke Xue She 國醫專科學社. Schools specializing in the research and advanced study of native medicine should be named as Research Institutes of Native Medicine Guo Yi Yan Jiu Suo 國醫研究所.

We are preparing to draft an outline with 21 standard rules and send it to the central meeting for approval. Thereafter, it will be promulgated to the entire country and all institutes must comply with the recommendations.

In addition to this letter, ten copies of the complete outline will be sent to the different institutes for reference, as well as single copies delivered to doctors to enable them to comply with this.

Sent to:
Shanghai Native Medicine Union 上海市國醫公會
Shanghai Native Medicine Academic Union 上海市國醫學會
ZhongHua Native Medicine Academic Union 中華國醫學會
Shenzhou Native Medicine Academic Union 神州國醫學會
China's Medical Institute 中國醫學院
Chinese Medicine Institute 中醫學院

Attached: The proposed temporary outline of a standard for Native Medicine Professional Schools and Research Institutes of Native Medicine to be carried out

On the 15th day of the 5th month of the 24th year (1935) was passed by the third central meeting of the Second Session of the whole chamber of members.

Regulation 1.

Native Medicine Professional Schools aim to provide traditional medicine techniques and knowledge; Research Institutes of Native Medicine specialize in the research and advanced study of traditional medicine.

Regulation 2.

Native Medicine Professional Schools and Research Institutes of Native Medicine should be established by either the members of the association or private organizations, according to the particular situation.

Regulation 3.

Alterations or any modifications of Native Medicine Professional Schools and Research Institutes of Native Medicine should be approved by the Central Bureau for Native Medicine Zhongyang GuoYiGuan 中央國醫館.

Regulation 4.

Enrolment requirements for Native Medicine Professional Schools and Research Institutes of Native Medicine should be as follows:

A. Students enrolling in Native Medicine Professional Schools should complete high school education from a school certified by the national education bureau or equivalent level of learning. Passing grade should be attained in a test offered by the Native Medicine Professional Schools in order to fulfill the requirements.

B. Students in Research Institutes of Native Medicine should have a license to practice medicine or have adequate research into the native medicine.

Regulation 5.

Native Medicine Professional Schools and Research Institutes of Native Medicine should collaborate with each other.

Regulation 6.

The duration of study in Native Medicine Professional Schools and Research Institute of Native Medicine should be as follows:

A. Students in Native Medicine Professional Schools should complete a four-year program plus one to two years of internship.

B. Students in Research Institutes of Native Medicine should complete the program in two to three years.

Regulation 7.

When establishing a Native Medicine Professional School or a Research Institute of Native Medicine, the founders should firstly assemble a board of directors and then compose regulations, providing them to the Central Bureau of Native Medicine Zhongyang GuoYiGuan 中央國醫館 for approval and a trial period of operation.

Regulation 8.

To receive a permanent approval, Native Medicine Professional Schools and Research Institutes of Native Medicine should fulfill the following requirements after one year's trial operation:

A. The operation fee should be supported by confirmed capital and assets.

B. Basic facilities should be provided, such as: library, sport grounds and campus land, as well as laboratories.

C. Detailed information about each teaching staff should be sent to the Central Bureau of Native Medicine for final approval and confirmation.

Regulation 9.

Native Medicine Professional Schools and Research Institutes of Native Medicine must provide a campus map with detailed explanations to the Central Bureau of Native Medicine for approval and inspection, which includes:

A. Official name of the Professional School or Research Institute.

B. Study programs categorized.

C. Address of the school or Institute and condition of school grounds and dormitories.

D. Source of capital and balance sheet recording income and expenditures.

E. School Regulations, Study Syllabus and arrangements of each study program.

F. List of contents of textbooks and index of books (separated and listed by departments).

G. List of books stored in the library and statistical index by category.

H. Contents of all the equipment and specimens used in laboratory, as well as list of medical tools used for treatment.

I. Résumés of all teaching staff.

J. Complete list of all students.

Regulation 10.

Native Medicine Professional Schools and Research Institutes of Native Medicine should hand their proposals and required documents, prepared by themselves or their board of directors, to the local branch of Central Bureau of Native Medicine and later to the Central Bureau of Native Medicine for backup. There should be detailed inspection by the local branch Central Bureau of Native Medicine, which will then provide comments for improvement.

Regulation 11.

Proposals for Native Medicine Professional Schools and Research Institutes of Native Medicine should be approved once the school condition satisfies the inspectors dispatched by the Central Bureau of Native Medicine.

Regulation 12.

Programs taught in Native Medicine Professional Schools should be decided by each school's agenda and arranged across several academic years. However, National Party's Guidance, Chinese Language and Physical Education are compulsory for every student.

A. Foundation Courses
   1. Anatomy and Physiology
   2. Hygiene
   3. Pathology
   4. Diagnosis
   5. Pharmaceutical Studies
   6. Formulas
   7. History of Medicine

B. Applied Courses
   1. Internal Medicine
   2. Surgery
   3. Gynecology (with Obstetrics)
   4. Pediatrics (with Measles Science)
   5. Ophthalmology
   6. Laryngology
   7. Odontology
   8. Acupuncture
   9. Massage Science
   10. Orthopedics
   11. Science of Sexually Transmitted Diseases
   12. Forensic Science

The programs listed above may be selected by Research Institutes of Native Medicine as part of their curriculum. However, an institute should write a note to inform the Central Bureau of Native Medicine.

Regulation 13.

A president should be elected by the board of directors in Research Institutes of Native Medicine and Native Medicine Professional Schools. The elected candidate should be nominated by the local branch Central Bureau of Native Medicine, which will notify the central Bureau of Native Medicine.

The president of the institute or school should be responsible for hiring an academic dean and operations director.

Regulation 14.

The teaching staff hired by the president of the institute or school should have experience in teaching their specific subjects or have prominent research reputation.

Regulation 15.

There should be regular official meetings held in the institute or school, organized by the dean or director.

Regulation 16.

The purpose of the official meeting is as follows:

1. Creation of a budget plan.
2. Arrangements and plans of study programs.
3. Approval of regulations in the institute or school.
4. Academic tests and examinations.
5. Discipline of students.
6. Facilities, equipment and matters for improvement.
7. Other important issues.

Regulation 17.

The graduation examination in the institutes or schools should be held under the monitoring of the supervisor sent by the Central Bureau of Native Medicine. The graduation certificate should be approved by the supervisor.

Regulation 18.

Native Medicine Professional Schools and Research Institutes of Native Medicine, if they are found to be in inferior condition or poor academic operations, should correct their mistakes according to the Central Bureau of Native Medicine comments of improvements. Schools and Institutes may be expelled from the registered list of Schools and Institutes of the Central Bureau of Native Medicine.

Regulation 19.

Native medical schools or institutes set up within the past year should register and hand the required documents to Central Bureau of Native Medicine according to Regulation 7. For schools set up more than one year ago, the trial operation steps may be ignored though the requirement to register still holds according to Regulations 8 through 10.

Regulation 20.

This standard outline, if found to be with mistakes or incomplete, could be reviewed by the Central Bureau of Native Medicine and discussed by the board of directors regarding any specific issues.

Regulation 21.

This standard outline should be enforced after approval by the central meeting of board of directors of Central Bureau of Native Medicine.

According to official instruction No. 3550, on the 21st of this month, the eighth central meeting of second session of board of directors decided that "*The proposed temporary standards outlining the Native Medicine Professional Schools and Research Institutes of Native Medicine to be carried out* should not be applied anymore. It is to issue that this outline is abolished." (The rest of instruction No. 3550 is omitted)[92]

Article end

[92] In this compilation of documents, the compilers first introduce instruction #3323 from the second meeting of the board, and then it introduces a later instruction #3550 from the eighth meeting of the board cancelling the earlier instruction. Instruction #3550 only includes the first paragraph of the instruction.

Problems regarding teaching materials in native medicine schools

By Qin Bowei 秦伯未

Source: *Compilation of Discussions about Chinese Medical Education* 中醫教育討論集

Yaron: A divided Chinese medicine on the eve of legal extinction was the worst option. Noted voices like Qin Bowei urged everyone to unite, a unity that is only possible when disagreements stop. The old style of contending schools had to stop in order for Chinese medicine to survive.

Pages 445–446

The objective for establishing Schools of Native Medicine is to cultivate talent. Our hope to further develop Chinese medicine lies with these schools' graduates. Therefore, for us establishing schools, the responsibility is great. Without doubt the fate of Native medicine relies on this.

There is a long-lasting problem hindering the development of Chinese Medicine: the mismatch of various theories. For example, the various schools developed during Jin 金 and Yuan 元 dynasties, the disparity between cold injury Shang Han 傷寒 and warm disease Wen Bing 溫病 has greatly confused students, with some even losing their faith in Chinese medicine. Nowadays, schools have been established as centers in which education in Chinese medicine is provided. Therefore, in terms of theoretical study, theories should be fixed and aligned to a united framework.

It is not hard to see that there are three trends within Chinese medicine schools: the conservative, the modern-minded and the compromising. The conservative schools object the modern elements, while the modern-minded abandons the classics and the worst is the compromising one without thorough views of either modern or old. One cannot disguise the fact that they cannot walk in the same pace. Now, that the Department of Education does not pass proposals regarding our schools seems harsh; some say it is unfair but actually the responsibility is borne by us for lacking a unified, systematic education system.

Unfortunately, despite the fact that last year there was an Editing Committee of Chinese Medicine Teaching Materials 教材編輯委員會 organized by the National

Chinese Medicine Association Quan Guo Yi Yao Hui 全國醫藥會, for lack of time and human resources, developing comprehensive and updated teaching materials was halted. Now the Bureau of Native Medicine Zhongyang GuoYi Guan 中央國醫館 has formed. Its most pressing issue should be creating standard teaching materials for the schools. Otherwise, the different schools will never cease their fights, leading to a weakened unity, from which the only possible outcome is lack of cooperation spirit.

Article end

Chinese Medicine Bylaws 中醫條例 literacy record summary

Source: *Compilation of Discussions about Chinese Medical Education* 中醫教育討論集

Yaron: These bylaws were officially passed in 1936 and authorized by the third acting president of the Republic, Lin Sen 林森. Lin was respected for his benevolent actions and behavior, yet was a political puppet of the prior president Jiang Jieshi 蔣介石 who was able to maintain power behind the scenes. The following year, 1937, saw the war with Japan and the entire government and Lin Sen moved to the new capital in Chongqing.

These bylaws never had a chance to materialize, at least not until the Communist era.

Pages 446–454

1. Chinese Medicine Bylaws original text

National Government Instruction—No.126—January 22nd of the 25th year (1936)
Applies to all subordinate government institutions.

This is to announce that the *Chinese Medicine Bylaws* have been established and begun being enforced unless with other specific instructions issued. Attached please find the *Chinese Medicine Bylaws* text to distribute to all subordinate bodies for reference.

Please see the attached.

President - Lin Sen 林森
Legislative Yuan Principal - Sun Ke 孫科

Chinese Medicine Practitioner Bylaws

January 22nd of the 25th year (1936)—Announced by National Government

Regulation 1

Up until the examination authority 考試院 establishes an official Chinese medicine examination, a person aged 25 or above could start their Chinese medicine practice after obtaining approval documents from the Interior Ministry and having fulfilled one of the following requirements:

1. Persons who obtained a passing grade in past examinations organized by the province or city government, or holding an equivalent certificate.
2. Persons given the official medical practitioner license by the province or city government.
3. Persons who graduated and obtained a certificate from an official Chinese Medicine School.
4. Persons who previously worked as a Chinese medicine practitioner for at least five years.

The standards for measuring the above requirements are set up by the Interior Ministry.

Regulation 2

All current Chinese medicine practitioners may temporarily provide their medical services until getting approval from the Interior Ministry.

Regulation 3

Practitioners who are approved by the Interior Ministry need to register with local authorities and present their certification.

Regulation 4

Practitioners are prohibited from treating, writing any prescription or writing diagnosis note for patients without personally seeing the patient. Also, death certificates and stillborn certificates may not be issued without personally inspecting the dead person. The format and clauses of death certificates and stillborn certificates is determined by the Interior Ministry.

Regulation 5

Chinese medicine practitioners should utilize sterilization methods and immediately and truthfully report to related local departments if patients present with epidemic diseases.

Regulation 6

Chinese medicine practitioners should bear legal responsibility to help the government Public Security Bureau and Courts in dealing with any issues related to social security, preventing epidemics and judgments.

Regulation 7

Regulations 4, 6, 7, 10, 11, 13, 15, 17 on Western Medicine Bylaws **西醫條例** should also be applied to Chinese medicine practitioners.[93]

Regulation 8

People who become disqualified from practicing medicine and who still perform unauthorized treatments will be penalized. Penalty is any amount less than one hundred dollars and should be paid to local government department.

Regulation 9

Any practitioner shall pay penalty with amount less than fifty dollars if he or she is found to not comply with any single listed regulation, unless punishments or sanctions have already been applied. If that person commits any criminal offense, he or she must be tried in court.

Regulation 10

The listed regulations are in force as at the date of announcement.

---

[93] See extract of this document, below.

Attached: (Extract) "Western Medicine Bylaws"

Regulation 4

It should be reported to the local department if the clinic started, closed, re-opened or relocated by the doctor or his/ her affiliated persons. Death of the doctor should be also reported to the department.

Regulation 6

The doctor should keep records with complete notes including patient's name, age, gender, occupation, disease name, medical record (history) and treatment applied. It should be stored for each patient for at least three years.

Regulation 7

A written prescription should record the following:

1. Own name, address should be included and then stamp, sign on it; and
2. Patient name, age, drug name, usage and dose with the complete date (day, month, and year).

Regulation 10

Doctors should report in less than 48 hours to the local Security Bureau upon discovery of any possible murder situation when examining dead bodies.

Regulation 11

Doctors are responsible for writing death certificates or diagnosis notes for the investigation; however refusal to do so is accepted with reasonable reasons.

Regulation 13

Doctors should not use any intoxicating drugs consisting of opium or morphine unless prescribed and needed for treatment.

Regulation 15

The local department has the right to stop medical services provided by, or the occupation of, doctors if the doctor exhibits any behavioral problems or mental impairment.

Regulation 17

Those doctors who were prohibited from providing medical service should surrender their own registered certificate to the local department for recording the reason and period on the certificate's back. Once recorded, the certificate may be retained by the doctor.

2. *Chinese Medicine Bylaws* Announcement: My heartfelt impressions

Jiao Yitang 焦易堂

> Yaron: Here we see another plea to standardize and make Chinese medicine uniform. We should keep in mind that this time period was harsh on Chinese medicine. Chinese medicine had been on the defensive for decades, struggling for recognition and, indeed, for its survival. At this point, achieving official and legal recognition was a major win for Chinese medicine, far surpassing any losses arising out of compromise.

The *Chinese Medicine Bylaws* legislation was announced on 22nd January, Year 25 (1936). It finally fulfills the initial step of my dream. Since it is related to our future and has great impact on our people, I have strong feelings for this law and wanted here to express them to all the people of China.

1. The motivation and influence behind composing the bylaws

Nowadays, people are becoming passionate about modern science and so, in the current situation, they largely neglect the development of Chinese medicine. The Government even did not establish a specific department to take charge of Chinese medicine until the formation of the Bureau for Native Medicine ZhongYang GuoYiGuan 中央國醫館. We, practitioners of Chinese medicine, recognized that this emergency required us to have theoretical revision, educational improvements, screening for practitioners and a unified syllabus for the entire system. Rules are required for making and implementing the above modifications in order to move a step forwards.

Therefore, the enduring *Western Medicine Bylaws* were referenced for setting up the new legislation. Since the situation for the practice of Chinese medicine today does not conform to the law and does not have equal recognition, we came up with a written proposal, *Chinese Medicine Bylaws*, and submitted it to the government's Central Political Council 中央政治會議. I knew that this would fulfill the public wishes as well as the wish of all Chinese medicine practitioners.

2. Steps towards announcement of the legislation

Since the Proposal has been raised, it has been weighed by the Central Political Council and each regulation was approved by the administrative department and, finally, delivered to the highest administrative ministry. However, problems were raised again in the ministry and the announcement has been postponed. Fortunately, supporters were still present in the ministry; Mr. Jiang 蔣, as vice-president, with a precious heart promoting our valuable culture, stated that the Central Political Council decided to put *Chinese Medicine Practitioner Bylaws* in effect in order to depart from the past and create a new century of the future for this profession!

3. Effects of the announcement of the new legislation

There are various effects of the announcement of the new legislation. Generally speaking, they can be classified into two perspectives. One is in the aspect of education, while the other is in terms of administration. For example, in *Regulation 1*, "Persons who graduated and obtained a certificate from a Chinese Medicine School could start their operation upon completion of an inquiry by the Interior Ministry".

All along, Chinese medicine was excluded from mainstream education system, but in fact there are many schools in different cities, created by local demand, that teach this subject and train professionals. It is impossible for a government agency to stop this trend. However, going unsupervised, Chinese medicine development can no longer be overlooked or else it may develop in an unfavorable way. It is not to say that there are no good quality schools but, rather, that there are too few such schools compared to those with lower admission standards and inferior quality teaching. Nevertheless, since the announcement of this new law we hope for improvement, especially having a prospect of entering into the mainstream educational system in the future to train more professionals. Complying with these rules will further encourage Chinese medicine education to make a move toward a systematic learning experience, which will contribute more to society in the future.

According to *Regulation 2*, "All current Chinese medicine practitioners may temporarily provide their medical services until getting approval from the Interior Ministry." In the past, there was no fixed department responsible for management of Chinese medicine and neither did the Health Bureau pay attention to Chinese medicine, causing an unfair public opinion. By enforcing the above legislation, registered Chinese medicine practitioners could still temporarily provide their services. However, in the past, standards and regulations governing registered practitioners varied in different locations, thus this particular rule should be modified. In order to maintain consistency, in the future there should not be any local examinations or registration by local agencies but, rather, all should be administered by the Interior Ministry. Then, qualifications and registration will become adequate and uniform, which will enhance the reputation of Chinese medicine practitioners via proper administration.

The above improvements, applied in these two ways—educational and administrative—I believe will remove obstacles from future development of Chinese medicine.

4. Related Chinese medicine sector people should be aware of the bylaws announced

According to *Regulation 6*,[94] "Chinese medicine practitioners should utilize sterilization methods and immediately and truthfully report to related local departments if patients present with epidemic diseases." We know that Chinese medicine practitioners are always accused of ignorance regarding sterilization methods by Western medicine doctors. Thus, from now on, under the new regulations, Chinese medicine practitioners should pay more attention to sterilization methods, since we all bear joint responsibility in any case involving sterilization malpractice.

We should be clear that *Regulation 7* includes several Regulations: "Regulations 4, 6, 7, 10, 11, 13, 15, 17 and certain Western Medicine Bylaws should also be applied to Chinese medicine practitioners." We should be aware of *Regulations 6* and *7* in particular of the Western Medicine Bylaws. *Regulation 6* of Western Medicine Bylaws states that "A doctor should keep records with complete notes, including patient's name, age, gender, occupation, disease name, medical record (history), and treatment applied. It should be stored for each patient at least for three years." *Regulation 7* states that "The written prescription should record the following:

[94] According to prior text this should be Regulation 5, however, we kept the mistake as is.

1. Own name, address should be included and then stamp, sign on it; and
2. Patient name, age, drug name, usage and dose with the complete date (day, month, and year)."

Regarding the two regulations above, disease name, drug name and its usage and dose are closely related to the academic field of modern medicine. Therefore, to prevent an unfortunate situation in which many contemporary Chinese medicine practitioners substitute Chinese medicine disease names with Western medicine disease names without a through consideration, the department should co-operate as soon as possible with the Bureau for Native Medicine and standardize rules, concerning the above problem, in order to eliminate confusion. Drug names and usage can cause confusion as well, especially names of herbs in Chinese medicine. In order to prevent confusion, we should standardize them as soon as possible.

Frankly speaking, the political and legal status of Chinese medicine has passed through turbulent times and now welcomes this courageous period of its development. As members of this profession, we should both reflect on the achievements already attained and work harder together for the development of Chinese medicine. We can do more than just this law enforcement and announcement. Therefore, please keep our motivation to investigate Chinese medicine as well as open our minds and accept new elements; this is our only way to develop Chinese medicine into a great and better one.

February 8th of the 25th year (1936) written in *Nan Jing Xin Min Bao* 《新民报》(南京)

Section end

3. The development process of *Chinese Medicine Bylaws* legislation: Feelings shared with colleagues

1936 by Zhou Liuting 周柳亭

Yaron: Chinese medicine becoming a mainstream medicine with its own clinics and recognized schools is an aspiration still alive in the minds of many today. In comparison, the reality for everyday Chinese medicine practitioners in the 1920s and '30s was much different from the situation today. Today, at least in the West, Chinese medicine is seen as "alternative"; despite gradually increasing acceptance by the population, its legal status, as a general rule, is on the fringe of mainstream medicine. It is not widely practiced in hospitals and not recognized or reimbursed by health insurance, especially herbal medicine.

In the 1920s in China, however, the situation was very different. Not too long prior, Chinese medicine was mainstream medicine but now the tides had turned and Chinese medicine was on the sudden brink of legal extinction. The difference was stark: from being "The" medicine, to being gone and done away with. Huge variability and differing opinions within Chinese medicine became unimportant. It was similar to when the Nationalists and Communists forgot their differences (at least momentarily) and fought as comrades in the Sino-Japanese war. Chinese medicine in those times became unified with one goal: survival.

Today, as we reflect back on that time, the compromises that had been made in the name of this unity can be questioned. Some of us may see these compromises as advancement while others as regression. Regardless of our general viewpoint, and since the situation today is different, it is prudent for us to reflect upon it again.

The story begins on December 15th of the 22nd year (1933); the 75 attending committees Zhu Hezhong 朱和中, Lu Zhiyi 呂志伊 and so on, in the third session of Legislative Yuan 43rd meeting, discussed and passed the proposed *Chinese Medicine Bylaws* put forth by the Legal Committee. However, it has been three years of waiting since the approval of these bylaws by all Chinese-medicine-related personnel. We all once believed that the announcement of this legislation and its enforcement would not stand a chance. The fabulous news, unbelievably, came by the end of the Fifth National Congress of Chinese Nationalist Party 中國國民黨第五次全國代表大會.

The supporters of Chinese medicine were all surprised after hearing this news. After that, the Bureau for Native Medicine cabled this news to all local branches to share the unbelievable crazy happiness and fixed a celebration for 8th February. It also fixed a commemorative anniversary on January 22nd of every year. The status of Chinese medicine was now recognized officially under protection of the law. Thus, here, I want to share my happiness and feeling with three main points, as follows:

1. The development of the legislation was largely linked to the establishment of the Bureau for Native Medicine ZhongYang GuoYiGuan 中央國醫館.

The establishment of Bureau for Native Medicine was proposed by members of the Central Council 中委 President Tan Yankai 譚延闓, Hu Hanmin 胡漢民, Chen Zhaoying 陳肇英, Zhu Peide 朱培德, Shao Yuanchong 邵元沖, Chen Lifu 陳立夫, Jiao Yitang 焦易堂 on May 7th, Year 19 (1930). In the 26th meeting of The Central Executive Committee Political Meeting 中央執行委員會政治會議, the Proposal and the organizational structure outline was sent to the central government, applying for Bureau for Native Medicine formation. It has been five years since its establishment and local branches of Bureau for Native Medicine have developed in different provinces and cities such as Jiangsu, Zhejiang, Beijing, Hunan, Hubei, Guangdong, Gaungxi, Henan, Fujian, Sichuan and Shanghai. There were even branches developed in foreign countries and cities, for example in San Francisco, the Philippines and North Borneo. The maintenance of these local branches and the development of Chinese medicine in these difficult times could not be attained without the work of Bureau for Native Medicine.

2. The announcement of *Chinese Medicine Bylaws* was promoted by the committees, Shiying 石瑛 and Jiao Yitang 焦易堂.

Mr. Jiao 焦, the president of Bureau for Native Medicine at that time, was fighting for Chinese medicine development alongside his work in the Bureau. I remember when he sighed, "It is my responsibility to fight for an official legal status as the leader of all Chinese medicine practitioners, but I have not yet succeeded!" Unlike Chinese medicine, *Western Medicine Bylaws* had been passed and announced in Year 19 (1930). At that time, a proposal for *Chinese Medicine Bylaws*, which included ten general principles and six chapters of rules, was completed. Mr. Jiao 焦, being the former president of the Legal Committee of the Legislative Yuan, joined 29 central committees such as Shiying 石瑛, Ye Chucang 葉楚傖, Zhangji 張繼, Chen Guofu 陳

果夫, Shao Lizi 邵力子, Dai Chuanxian 戴傳賢, Juzheng 居正, Chen Lifu 陳立夫 and others to put forth that proposal in the meeting. Several committees in Legislative Yuan, like Shiying 石瑛, were keen to protect Chinese medicine and proposed that the Bureau for Native Medicine should be responsible for the management of Chinese medicine, and that by doing this it will protect and benefit the public health. Fortunately, the law was discussed and finally passed in the 43rd meeting, assisted by Mr. Jiao's 焦 appeal to the members.

3. The final announcement of the legislation came from the proposal made in the Fifth National Congress of Chinese Nationalist Party last winter.

The *Chinese Medicine Bylaws* proposal was initially not announced due to some hindrance even after being passed in the Legislative Yuan. I was feeling frustrated and helpless until the opening of the Fifth National Congress last November. There were 26 central committee members including Feng Yuxiang 馮玉祥, Wu Jingheng 吳敬恒, Ma Chaojun 馬超俊, He Chengjun 何成濬, Lu Zhonglin 鹿鐘麟, Zhang Fakui 張發奎, Bai Wenwei 柏文蔚, Luosang Jianzan 羅桑堅贊 and 33 provincial representatives including Zeng Shushi 曾叔實, Te Suo'er 特索爾 and 23 representatives from the party branch in U.S.A., Mexico and so on including Huang Shejing 黃社經, Zhen Xiangquan 甄香泉. They proposed that Chinese medicine should share the same status and enjoy equality with Western medicine. Three statements made by them are as follows:

1. The *Chinese Medicine Bylaws*, now passed, should be immediately announced and enforced.

2. The Government should add "Chinese Medicine" into the list of recognized medical institutes and departments.

3. The Government should allow the establishment of Chinese medicine educational institutes and schools.

The Proposal was given to the Central Executive Committee to handle. In less than two months, under the directing of President Jiang 蔣, the Proposal was successfully accepted. On 22nd January, the law was finally announced and enforced. We were very happy that the fight for fairness and same status as Western medicine had finally succeeded and that Chinese medicine was protected by law for ever more.

Concluding the above three viewpoints, the announcement of the legislation "Chinese Medicine Practitioner Bylaws" was the joint effort of those supporting committee members and President Jiang 蔣. We should thank Mr. Jiang who was aiming to protect the local culture and benefit the general public by allowing the passing and enforcement of this legislation. I still remember that in Year 18 (1929) some members, such as Yu Yan 余岩,[95] suggested abolishing Chinese medicine in the Central Health Committee Meeting. It rattled the nerves of all practitioners, whether local or foreign and, as a result, a grand congress was held in Shanghai to discuss and oppose this issue by the entire Chinese medicine community. Likewise, Mr. Jiang, in accord with the hopes of the general public, opposed the abolition attempt. It is hard to imagine what would follow if Chinese medicine was abolished due to these malevolent suggestions and without the protection and help of Mr. Jiang. We should wholeheartedly thank Mr. Jiang again for his help in promoting Chinese medicine onto a wonderful stage. There is no doubt that Mr. Jiang should be forever remembered as key in this critical historical development of Chinese medicine.

Nonetheless, we should not settle with the current situation. It is our responsibility to complete the improvement and construction of a more comprehensive system—do you all agree? Being a member of Bureau for Native Medicine, my responsibility is to communicate with all people in this field. I have a few opinions to share as follows:

1. The aim of forming different associations or organizations is not to attack different ideas suggested by others. Therefore, we should be united and discuss and research together toward advancing and improving our knowledge.

2. The new legislation has been announced and put into effect. This should be the time for me to represent my organization, Bureau for Native Medicine, in requesting to standardize the names of different Chinese medicine institutes, societies and learning venues. Previously, local regulations required use of different names but now they should be cancelled and the national legislation should take effect. All institutions should be named "schools" to prevent any confusion and potential legal issues.

3. The Medical Advancement Organization YiYao GaiJin Hui 醫藥改進會 was originally established to correct mistakes in Chinese medicine and improve knowledge; however, some members in different provinces had fought with each

[95] Another name of Yu Yunxiu 余雲岫.

other. Please stop the fighting, and work for the common goal of improving different aspects of Chinese Medicine.

I hope that all my dear colleagues can work with a common goal of protecting and developing Chinese Medicine according to Mr. Jiang's 蔣 help and teaching! Furthermore, all members of the Bureau for Native Medicine should be more passionate and responsible in our work following the leadership of Mr. Jiao 焦. For example, the "Chinese Medicine Licensing Exam" has been proposed to the Examination Authority to be listed as one of the occupation exams. It is now awaiting passage and enforcement in the Legislative Yuan. Also, Prescription Standards Committee 處方鑒定委員會 has been established recently and has begun providing advice services on legal cases involving prescription issues. The academic curriculum outline was drafted and a proposal for unifying disease names was completed as well. The Editing Committee for Teaching Materials is now working on teaching materials textbooks for Chinese Medicine Schools in the entire country. Capital Native Medicine Hospital 首都國醫院 has already been established. The obstacles preventing enrollment of higher classes students into Chinese Medicine Schools was removed but, as colleagues, we should not forget the teachings of Mr. Jiang and, united, work harder to develop Chinese medicine into a more favorable profession!

(February 8th of the 25th year (1936) *Nanjing China Daily* 中國日報 - 南京)

Written by Zhou Liuting 周柳亭 in Bureau for Native Medicine (ZhongYang GuoYiGuan 中央國醫館) on February 8th, Year 25.

Article end

Full text of Proposal to the Education Ministry to draw up *Regulations for Chinese Medicine Education* 中醫教育規程 by Jiao Yitang 焦易堂 and others

Source: *Compilation of Discussions about Chinese Medical Education* 中醫教育討論集

Pages 454–455

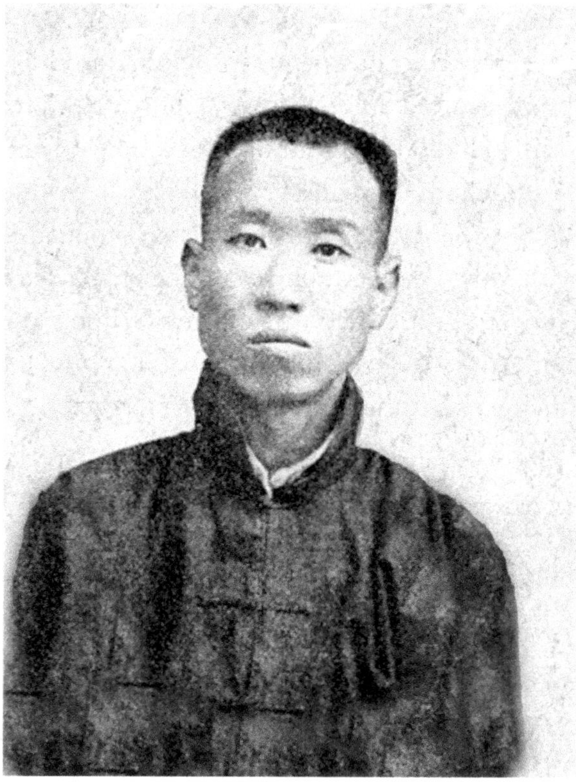

Jiao Yitang 焦易堂

(Objective): Following suggestion of promoting fairness between Chinese and Western medicine, made by committee members including Feng Yuxiang 馮玉祥 in the Fifth National Congress of Chinese Nationalist Party in January of the 24th year (1935), both the Proposal of setting up Chinese Medicine Schools and the fairness suggestions were passed to the Central Political Committee 中央政治委員會 for future discussion.

The *Chinese Medicine Bylaws* legislation was announced on January of the 25th year (1936). In *Regulation 1*, it states that registration requirements include obtaining a graduation certificate from a Chinese Medicine School. It certainly recognizes the importance of setting up Chinese Medicine Schools.

However, it has been a few years since that legislation announcement and the Education Ministry still does not include *Regulations for Chinese Medicine Education* as a part of the official school system. This makes it very difficult for Chinese Medicine Schools to develop and deal with their needed work. I don't think that the situation is going on the right track in matching the decision made in the Fifth National Congress of Chinese Nationalist Party. Therefore, I hereby request that the Education Ministry will include *Regulations for Chinese Medicine Education* in the official school system as soon as possible. This will remove the hindrance in establishing legal schools teaching Chinese medicine to train more professionals.

(Methods): Subjects in the curriculum, other then National Party's Guidance, Chinese Language and Physical Education, should be taught according to the following list:

A. Foundation Subjects:

1. Anatomy and Physiology
2. Hygienic Studies
3. Pathology
4. Diagnosis
5. Pharmaceutical Studies
6. Formulas
7. History of Chinese Medicine

B. Applied Subjects:

1. Internal Medicine
2. Surgery
3. Gynecology
4. Pediatrics
5. Febrile Disease Studies
6. Epidemic Diseases Studies
7. Ophthalmology
8. Laryngology

9. Dental Studies
10. Acupuncture
11. Massage Sciences
12. Medical Traumatology and Orthopaedics
13. Sexually Transmitted Diseases
14. Forensic Science

According to the subjects listed above, the Regulations Outline can be implemented after the agreement of, and discussion by, the Education Ministry together with the Chinese Medicine Committee in Department of Health 衛生處中醫委員會 and the Organizational Committee of Scholars in Chinese Medicine.

Proposed by: Jiao Yitang 焦易堂, Yang Jie 楊杰, Liang Hancao 梁寒操, Zhang Ji 張繼, Zou Lu 鄒魯, Feng Yuxiang 馮玉祥, Li Zonghuang 李宗黃, Fang Juehui 方覺慧, Shi Minting 石敏亭, Lu Zhonglin 鹿鐘麟, Ye Chucang 葉楚傖, Jiang Zuobin 蔣作賓, Xiao Jishan 蕭吉珊, Hong Ludong 洪陸東, Tan Zhen 覃振, Gu Zhengtou 谷正倫, Wang Yongbin 王用賓, Mao Zuquan 茅祖權, Zhou Bomin 周伯敏, He Jian 何鍵, Lu Dangping 魯蕩平, Peng Guojun 彭國鈞, Hu Wencan 胡文燦, Zhang Zhiben 張知本, Li Fulin 李福林, Miao Peicheng 苗培成, Luo Yiqun 羅翼群, Wang Fale 王法勤.

Jiang Bocheng 蔣伯誠, Liu Zhi 劉峙, Pan Gongzhan 潘公展, Ding Chaowu 丁超五, Wu Zhongxin 吳忠信, Li Wenfan 李文範, Yang Hu 楊虎, Yu Youren 于右任, Zhang Fang 張鈁, Kong Xiangxi 孔祥熙, Cheng Tiangu 程天固, Fu Bingchang 傅秉常, Xu Chongzhi 徐崇智, Mai Huanzhang 麥煥章, Huang Xuchu 黃旭初, Shang Zhen 商震.

Liu Jianxu 劉建緒, Xu Kan 徐堪, Fu Rulin 傅汝霖, Wu Jingheng 吳敬恒, Li Yuying 李煜瀛, Zeng Yangfu 曾養甫, Sun Lianzhong 孫連仲, Chen Diaoyuan 陳調元, Xue Dubi 薛篤弼.

Inspection Comments: Requesting to pass this draft to the Central Political Committee for further handling. Decision, after discussion it has been passed along.

Article end

Full text of an investigation report by a specialized education committee into Chinese Medicine Schools Proposal

Source: *Compilation of Discussions about Chinese Medical Education* 中醫教育討論集

Yaron: The Education Ministry did not want a separate Chinese medicine school system or two different kinds of medicine. Legislation for establishing Chinese medicine schools and giving them legal status was a transitional phase. Chinese medicine was to merge and become a branch of, or a department within, modern medicine. It was a compromise on the government's part not to abolish Chinese medicine abruptly and cause uproar in the population. Instead it would gradually allow it to become smaller within the big picture of modern medicine.

Establishing Chinese medicine schools that teach mainly Western medicine curriculum was a part of this plan; after all, modern educated doctors were in great demand in this vast country. Training Chinese medicine doctors to become more and more modern was part of the solution for modern healthcare shortages. The Communists, later on, with exactly the same objective in mind, continued this trend without interruption.

Pages 455–456

The full text of the investigation into Chinese Medicine Schools' Proposal, written by a Specialized Education Committee in the Central Political Committee is recorded as follows:

This is an investigation report done upon request, mainly about the proposal of 53 committee members including Jiao Yitang, suggesting to include "Regulations for Chinese Medicine Education" as a part of the official academic system in order to allow establishment of legal Chinese Medicine Schools.

Our meeting took place from 6th to 10th of March to discuss the above issue. All members agreed that the development of Chinese medicine is very much related to the general public, even though it is still not being included in our legal and educational system.

Chinese Medicine Schools are very different from other occupational schools. They require students to have higher educational knowledge and higher code of conduct. Therefore, it takes time to set up a comprehensive guide for Chinese Medicine Schools and their curriculum.

There should not be medicine classified into Chinese or Western, which is our final goal. The two existing laws for Western medicine and Chinese medicine are just temporary for the transition period.

It is easily seen that the subjects in Western Medical Schools are similar to the subjects mentioned in the proposal for Chinese Medicine Schools except for Acupuncture, Massage Studies, Medical Traumatology and Orthopedics. These subjects may be listed as "Special Subjects" and the offering of these subjects should be reported to the Education Ministry.

Report Conclusion is as follows:

1) Medical schools should be included in tertiary education and managed by its related regulations. They can only enroll students who have completed high school.
2) There should not be separate Education Regulations for Chinese Medicine Schools but, rather, one should reference those for Western Medical Schools. Offering of "Special Subjects" including Acupuncture, Massage, Medical Traumatology and Orthopedics should be reported to the Education Ministry for approval.
3) Native medicinal substances should be studied and analyzed at an institute appointed by the Education Ministry.

Article end

Medical science training should be actively promoted 醫學應積極提倡科學訓練

By Chen Zhiqian 陳志潛

Source: *Compilation of Discussions about Chinese Medical Education* 中醫教育討論集

Yaron: There were many opponents of Chinese medicine within government ranks. Their ultimate solution to the healthcare situation was to create one State or National Medicine and there was only one way to do it: train youngsters to become more educated in Western medicine.

For comparison purposes, when we look at the early Communist years, the propaganda claim then was that Western medicine needed to learn from Chinese medicine. Yet when we look at the curriculum actually taught in schools in the Communist years, it was just as before—youngsters needed to learn more Western medicine and science. On the surface it seemed different but in essence it was the same.

In fact, this style of educating Chinese medicine practitioners through a curriculum saturated with modern biomedicine began during the Republic and has continued up to today.

Pages 458–461

In the 3rd plenary session, Jiao Yitang 焦易堂 and various committees suggested to urge the Education Ministry to explicitly formulate regulations for Chinese medicine education and implement them into the official education system. Li Zonghuang 李宗黃 and other committees requested to carry out the original bill with an amendment in the fifth plenary session that Chinese and Western medicine will have equal status. Today, our country is in a difficult situation, with many things waiting to be done. Bills of this kind are of no importance and they shouldn't be proposed. However, if we consider the problems of medicine itself, there are a few points I would like Committee Jiao 焦, Li 李 and other committees to consider.

Nowadays, China is using Western engineering techniques to build houses that celebrities love to live in and highways and railroads that connect the world. I have never heard that we should preserve the skills of the carpenter and bricklayer to withstand modern engineering techniques. The people also hope that the Government would use the organization and equipment of foreign navies, but I have never heard people advocate keeping traditional training and weapons to enhance national defense. The only exception is using science as a basis for the development of medicine. It has raised intense reaction among the public and a great debate between Chinese medicine practitioners and Western medicine doctors. This is really funny!

The motives of committee Jiao, Li and other committees include:

1) Many patients cannot be cured by Western medicine but achieve good results after switching to Chinese medicine. Thus, both Chinese and Western medicine should be kept.

People who hold this view should understand that the strength of Western medicine lies in using scientific observation and experiments to examine the relationship between physiological changes and not just consider its methods of curing disease. It would be excellent if those in the field of Chinese medicine could accept science and understand scientific methods, fully applying scientific observation and experiments to examine the content and theories of Chinese medicine. However, most of Chinese medicine practitioners don't understand scientific methods and content. It is impossible to rely on Chinese medicine practitioners to examine their own theories. If there were some who were familiar enough with fundamentals of Western medicine and they did examine Chinese medicine, then the result would be Western medicine investigating Chinese medicine, but not Chinese medicine investigating itself.

Moreover, without a scientific enquiry, we cannot prove whether something is effective or not effective. Of course, individual cases should be considered. However, personal subjective experience would never be considered scholarship according to natural sciences and scientific method—there would never be universal evidence. If Chinese medicine practitioners and those who adore Chinese medicine still cling to individual cases as a proof and neglect the usage of modern scientific methods, I have nothing more to say. Chinese medicine will never become universally accepted scholarship. In the places of origin of modern medicine (Europe and the United States), many people still believe in folk remedies. However, until these folk remedies have been sorted out by scientific methodology, they can never be determined as effective or not effective. Those who are ignorant and incompetent shall never understand this point.

2) In recent years, executives in the Ministry of Health have received training from Western medicine, but did not learn Chinese medicine.

That those who learned Western medicine may not examine Chinese medicine theories is a loss for the Chinese scholars nowadays. No doubt, there should be scientific professionals in each Chinese medicine school, using scientific methods to sort out the essence of thousands of years of national culture. However, this kind of work would be extremely complicated and involved. Under today's situation, where both personnel and funds are limited, investigating Chinese medicine with Western technology cannot be done. It is not that people don't want to do it or that it shouldn't be done. When this kind of investigation is practically unavailable, then the truth cannot be found. It is best that Chinese medicine courses will be put aside, leaving Western medicine, with scientific proof, to be the basis of teaching. This is the reason why modern doctors do not understand Chinese medicine. Executives in the Ministry of Health didn't learn anything about Chinese medicine, not because they don't want to learn rather because those who run Chinese medicine schools simply don't know how to train these executives with Chinese medicine, and this fact has not been realized. Moreover, health administration includes vital statistics, communicable disease control, sanitation work and so on. These strategies are not found in Chinese medicine. If Chinese medicine were used to manage the health administration, wouldn't it be a joke?

3) Promoting Western medicine hinders the interest of businessmen to sell native pills, powders, extracts and pellets. The problem of livelihood became the center of debate between Chinese medicine and Western medicine.

Industry in China is lagging behind and production is low. Within the natural sciences field, there is extensive use of exotic products. This seems to have disadvantaged the country's economy. Selling Western produced drugs negatively affects the country's economy and it is a disadvantage. There are two ways to relieve this situation. First, encourage local production. Second, continue to use necessary foreign exotic products if needed. When people do not use weapons from Western countries, they could never copy from these weapons to produce their own weapons. This is also the case with Western medicine. If we want to produce our own Western drugs, we must borrow from the foreign exotic products to open our own market. This kind of initial loss cannot be avoided!

For those old pills, powders, extracts and pellets, if they are proved to be effective then they will not only sell in this country, but they may even sell to foreign countries. If some of them is proved ineffective, then these need to be eliminated. For sure, these ineffective medicines will not survive simply because of the suggestions of central committee. We need to bear in mind, people who are informed these days actually do not oppose the selling of pills, powders, extracts and pellets, rather they only suspect the efficacy behind these medicines. The Central Committee should encourage this kind of suspicion, in order to encourage others to use applied science in investigating Chinese medicine. Should we give up the foundation of the country's academic achievement, for the sake of the livelihood of only a small group of people? This is short-sighted. This kind of method to preserve native pills, powders, extracts and pellets is only helping eliminating themselves.

Apart from these, there are some conflicts between officials, making things difficult for each other. Furthermore, there are some personal problems that could not be investigated. I just hope that committee Jiao, Li and other committees would propose the following:

1) Stop naming Chinese medicine and Western medicine separately—they should collectively be called "State Medicine (Guo Yi 國醫)".

2) The Ministry of Health should set up a State medical research center, joining all of the well-known Chinese medicine practitioners and doctors to do medical research.

3) Be prepared to include research results into the medical curriculum.

In one country, there are two kinds of schools providing different basic trainings for one scholarship and career, this is a big joke. What's more, people (executives of health departments) with two disparate abilities are being treated the same, this is also ridiculous! If the Ministry of Education uses scientific training as the basis of medicine, whether the schools are called Chinese medicine schools or medical schools, the result eventually would become the same. Youngsters, who originally are supposed to learn Chinese medicine, would be directed onto the path of learning Western medicine, which will then shape how our "National Medicine" looks like.

From *Amongst the People* Bi-weekly periodical, 3rd Series 21st issue 民間半月刊三卷廿一期

Article end

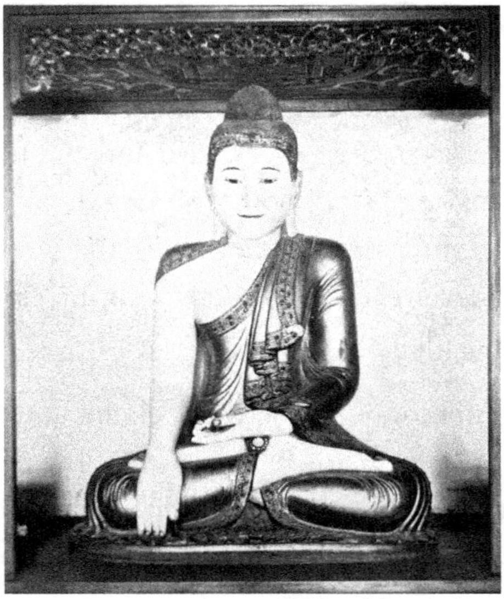

Photo by Mr P. Goux in early 1900s. "Buddha in the Rotunda".

After Chinese medicine education is included in the education system

By Jin Risheng 今日生

Source: *Compilation of Discussions about Chinese Medical Education* 中醫教育討論集

Yaron: A visionary voice echoes in the valley, "Used in this way, those young Chinese medicine practitioners, who learn in these Chinese medicine schools under the education system, are the pioneers destroying the Chinese medicine theory and speeding up the collapse of Chinese medicine. The collapse of Chinese medicine will become an inevitable trend and an inevitable fact. Brewing tea in a wine pot makes others upset; hardly will anyone take advice like this."

In my opinion, the following article is worth singling out as exceptional because, in those turmoil-filled times, when the "rescue Chinese medicine" banner was flying at an all-time high, the author maintains and points to other possible undesired outcomes. He seems less inclined to run along with an emotional herd. As we are still looking for a better and more proper Chinese medicine, his words ever more echo today.

Pages 473–478

We are living in an unusual era. Revolutionary consciousness is strong and the people began to join forces. Under these circumstances, two forces have formed. One is led by elders, another by youngsters, and both seeming to confront one another. Elders are discontent with the youngsters as they think the youngsters are too young and lack life experience. Youngsters feel discontent with the elders as they think the elders are too old and muddleheaded.

It goes without saying that there is a generation gap between elders and youngsters and it is impossible to bridge the gap between them. In times when the country is at peace with no wars, religion, state and cultural relics are prioritized and different kinds of pressure and brainwashing are used to occupy the thoughts of activists. When we were under abnormal oppression, the generation gap was less noticeable than it is now. However, not all trends could be oppressed and restrained artificially. No matter how much effort is made to suppress a trend, it is sometime futile.

This phenomenon can be observed in many historical examples. Zhang Taiyan 章太炎 stated one of these examples saying, "In the past when Buddhism expanded into China, those who practiced Taoism attacked and blamed Buddhism. Admittedly, Buddhism could not escape these attacks." The effects of oppression by political means can only temporarily last for a short period of time. It is unavoidable that the effects of oppression will die out eventually. If a certain kind of campaign is used as a tool for a political movement, this may be a temporary solution. However, under the influence of the law, this may affect the society as a whole. Recently, many people have discussed the problem of reading Chinese classics. Their main idea is that advocates who support and respect Confucius actually do not understand the teachings of Confucius. These commentators have certainly hit the point. I think the advocates who promote Chinese medicine are not that foolish and witless. Jiao Yitang 焦易堂, the director of Central Bureau for Native Medicine 中央國醫館, stated clearly, "let us see the young Chinese medicine practitioners aged 20 or even 30. Although they are learning Chinese medicine, they are giving up the metaphysical theories of Chinese medicine or at least they have doubts toward these principles. This is because Chinese medicine is experimentalist and does not emphasize theories." Mr. Jiao understands very well that, "Chinese medicine is experimentalist and does not emphasize theories," and his ultimate goal is to build a capital state hospital.

Mr. Jiao voiced his opinions during the 3rd plenary session. He urged the Ministry of Education to explicitly formulate regulations for Chinese medicine education and implement them into the official education system. Many people have doubts and feel puzzled, not knowing what future Chinese medicine practitioners will be like under the training and teaching of this so-called scientific course. There should be a clear definition for Chinese medicine, so as to make it easier for discussion. Ju Hu's 巨虎 article, *Who May be called a Chinese Medicine Doctor* published in Jing Bao 晶報[96] can be used for reference. The article is below:

> Chen Lifu 陳立夫 has said, *"Medicine is an important cultural aspect within the entire fabric of a nation." It's true; so many Chinese medicine doctors are now less indifferent than they were before. I think that before discussing the problems of Chinese medicine, in order to avoid pointless arguments and to have a focus, there should be a clear definition for the term "Chinese medicine". Then it will be easier to discover the truth. What is actually meant by the term "Chinese medicine"? Chinese medicine could be defined through its approach and spirit. Regarding its approach, Chinese medicine practitioners' assessments are based on perceptions and individual experience. They assume the patient is having a certain kind of disease, according to the pain felt by the patient mentally and physically. The Chinese medicine practitioner will then choose a so-called prescription from the books, applying the prescription based on his daily observation and subjective intuition. In most cases, the prescription contains twelve to thirteen kinds of plants and sometimes it contains animals, minerals or artificially-processed materials. In recent discussions with those who are prominent in the Chinese medicine profession, it was agreed by all that Chinese medicine internal medicine can be represented by cooked decoctions. Apart from decoction, there is acupuncture, moxibustion, massage and surgery for sores and ulcers.*
>
> *It should become here a separate discussion, however the number of people engaging it is extremely small: the spirit of Chinese medicine. Everyone focuses on collective observation. They are only looking for manifestation and seldom seeking the cause. Their entire mindset is set on being conservative and so confronting a disease they always have a definite diagnosis. However, when they engage the disease they seem helpless; they ask other brilliant ones*

[96] A small commercial gazette published in Shanghai in the 1920s.

to remedy it for them. Or only after they use a method and see if there is efficacy they determine the diagnosis and cause of the disease.

They make "X causes Y" their tool, yet apart from papers, ink, pen and ink stone, Chinese medicine practitioners do not have any tools. However, there are those Chinese medicine practitioners who do not write a prescription if they don't know the cause. They investigate the many facets of the root cause, they see the outer symptoms and they grasp what is inside.

It seems that whether Chinese medicine will vanish or not has become the center of the problem but I do have doubts. After Chinese medicine has vanished, does it mean that we cannot eat Da Huang coptis chinensis when we have constipation? If Chinese medicine doesn't vanish, does it mean Chinese medicine practitioners will never use microscope and X-rays? I am telling the truth in the above article. I welcome criticisms if I have missed out anything in the article."

If Chinese medicine is incorporated into the education system, the issue of teachers will become a problem. If we find Western medicine doctors to teach, what would it be like? Chinese medicine and Western medicine are rivals; Western medicine doctors only aspire to eliminate Chinese medicine. If we find Chinese medicine practitioners to teach just like before, dividing the curriculum into foundation and applied subjects, keeping the teaching model the same as in the past, teaching *Neijing* 內經, *Nanjing* 難經, *Shanghan* 傷寒 and *Wenbing* 溫病, then this is the best way just keeping it as it is. True gold doesn't fear fire; the power of Chinese medicine can be reflected by the following idiom "one dose and the doctor knows, two doses and the disease is cured." Chinese medicine has its own unique spirit. Why is it a must to include Chinese medicine education into the general education system? In order to have Chinese medicine education included into the official education system it will have to adapt to its environment. Chinese medicine has to become self-deprecating to cater and accommodate for the new trend. In this way, isn't it so that those who fight for including Chinese medicine education into the mainstream curriculum actually become the wrong-doers of the Chinese medicine profession? This is because Chinese Medicine Schools, which are included in the education system, are going to teach physiology and anatomy which are also taught in Western medicine schools. For example, teaching students that the liver is not on the left side and that modern anatomy cannot find a trace of twelve meridians Jing Mai 經脈. It is expected that Chinese medicine physiology, such as "sour flavor generates Liver, and Liver generates tendon," will not be included in the Chinese medicine textbooks under the official education system. However, after students graduate from these schools, how will they cure armpit pain that is, in Chinese medicine, a kind of disease related to the liver? Where will the basis for the theory come from? If pain medication injection is used instead of a decoction, then the way of Western medicine curing diseases is used. What is the point of having then these Chinese Medicine Schools? According to Mr. Jiao 焦, "let us see the young Chinese medicine practitioners of ages 20 or even 30. Although they are learning Chinese medicine, they are giving up the metaphysical theories of Chinese medicine or, at least, they doubt these principles." Used in this way, those young Chinese medicine practitioners, who are learning in these Chinese Medicine Schools under the education system, are the pioneers destroying the Chinese medicine theory, speeding up the collapse of Chinese medicine. The collapse of Chinese medicine will become an inevitable trend and an inevitable fact. Brewing tea in a wine pot makes others upset. Hardly will anyone take advice like this. One summer, I was confused after reading an article by Yu Yunxiu 余雲岫 that criticized the Chinese medicine concept of postpartum blood stasis. It happened that a friend, whose surname is Chen 陳, has asked me to cure his wife's postpartum abdominal pain. Of course, I did not dare use any herbs that remove blood stasis. Instead, I used herbs that calm hyperactive Liver and regulate the flow of Qi 氣. In the end, I failed miserably in curing her disease. Mr. Chen 陳 then found a better Chinese medicine practitioner through his old friends. The Chinese medicine practitioner used Ligusticum wallichii Chuan Xiong 川芎, Angelica sinensis Dang Gui 當歸 and Paeonia lactiflora Bai Shao 芍藥, and cured her disease. At that time, I hated Mr. Yu 余 as his argument had confused me. However, the truth is that I don't understand the theories of Chinese medicine and I think too simplistically. Do Ligusticum wallichii Chuan Xiong 川芎, Angelica sinensis Dang Gui 當歸 and Paeonia lactiflora Bai Shao 芍藥 really enhance blood circulation and remove blood stasis? Four-ingredient decoction Si Wu Tang 四物湯[97] is a famous decoction for curing gynecological diseases. It is a clear guideline and a precious experience left by our ancestors. I shouldn't blame others. Neglecting past experience is like leading yourself onto a wrong track, which certainly will have you face failure.

[97] A formula including the above 3 herbs.

Mr. Yu's 余 viewpoint is based on physiology of Western medicine. Now I casually applied his viewpoint to Chinese medicine, which is fundamentally different from Western medicine. How could I not face failure? In Shanghai 上海, there is a Chinese Medicine School proud of its teaching philosophy to abolish the old sayings and introduce new theories. This kind of school really confuses the "Chinese medicine youngster practitioners" as Mr. Jiao 焦 said. However, at the same time, the Chinese medicine community commented that although a certain school was teaching the new theories thoroughly and systematically, diseases naturally were not getting a cure. The feedback from the Chinese medicine community is true and they are not simply slandering the school. There are students who have graduated from this school and themselves are worried about not knowing how to cure disease. They then consult a certain Chinese medicine practitioner. This Chinese medicine practitioner is really great. Not only is he helping them cure their patients, he is also willing to teach those graduates, who don't have much clinical experience or a clue in curing disease. He tells the graduates to let go of all the things they have learned in school, focusing on three Chinese medicine classics including *Yixue Sanzi Jing* 醫學三字經 by Chen Xiuyuan 陳修園, *Shibing Lun* 時病論 by Lei Shaoyi 雷少逸 and *Tangtou Gejue* 湯頭歌訣 by Wang Ang 汪昂. These young Chinese medicine practitioners follow what he says and it really works, just like a panacea. This Chinese medicine practitioner is not familiar with the merged theories of Chinese and Western medicine; however, his experience is the reason for his success. Experience always works.

Jiao Yitang 焦易堂 said in the article, *A Letter to the Country's Medical Community* 敬告醫學界同人書 from the third issue of the *National Medicine Reporter Guoyi Gongbao* 國醫公報, "Chinese medicine uses various types of diagnostic methods: observation; hearing and smelling; asking; and touching, but only the five senses are used. Scientific inventions like thermometer, stethoscope, X-ray, electrical therapy machine, optical treatment machine and other diagnostic machinery should be used to improve the weaknesses and enhance the efficacy of Chinese medicine diagnostic methods. Usage of these scientific inventions is the reason why Western medicine could diagnose disease accurately and is effective in curing disease. Most of these machines are invented by scientists, not doctors, but if Western doctors can use these machines then why Chinese medicine practitioners can not do the same?" If, like Mr. Jiao suggests, in the future there is no difference between Chinese and Western medicines, then why is there a need to have Chinese Medicine Schools separately from Western Medicine Schools? Since we give it a name, "Chinese Medicine School", all of its behaviors and standards certainly cannot be the same as those of Western medicine

Schools. Otherwise, this would be like the behaviors of those elders and youngsters [mentioned above], which is ignorance. By promoting the idea of Mr. Jiao 焦 and other similar ideas, even though the original intent is to maintain the unique spirit and meaning of Chinese medicine, nonetheless, at the end, the original Chinese medicine will not be maintained and it will develop in the same way as Western medicine. Isn't this kind of promotion useless? In order to investigate herbs, especially the efficacy of certain herbs combined together in a formula, we don't need to hope or urge the medical education bureau to add a new compulsory subject "Chinese herbs" to Western Medicine Schools. The more we use the herbs, the better we can discover their various efficacies.

Some say that not allowing Chinese Medicine Schools to be included in the education system is giving up Chinese medicine and destroying our own culture. But can't we see the fact that many diseases that could not be cured by Western medicine doctors can be cured by Chinese medicine? I think these kinds of reasons are self-explanatory. Not only Chinese medicine can do it, but credit also goes to Zhang 張 the Celestial Heaven priest, Wang 王[98] the Daoist recluse, Christians and Buddhist nuns that many diseases have been cured. These things always happen. The following example is interesting and worthy of research. Have a look!

> In the fall of 16th year (1927) Mr. Jiang 姜 invited me to see his son. During diagnosis, the patient is in a state of languishing. He cannot sleep well at night. His eyes are white and slightly red. His lips and tongue are dry. He is thirsty but doesn't drink much and prefers hot drinks. His abdominal region is in pain like there is something pushing out. He doesn't like palpation against his abdominal region. He has a slippery pulse. The coating of tongue is grey-black. According to the patient's family, he feels that the disease stems from his diet. He had seen two doctors, and used several doses of Xiao Dao Lou Zhi Yan Zi Bu Wan 消導蔞枳燕子補丸 but the condition has not improved. At that time, the patient's family was grinding Rhinoceros horn into small pieces to put it in water to drink. However, the patient frowned and refused to drink. …I could not see the reason so did not prescribe.

[98] These names are simply generic name like one would say Mr. Smith in English.

I have heard that the family invited a Western doctor in the afternoon, who diagnosed the patient with enteritis, enema was performed and Western drug was given to the patient. …

The symptoms were worsening and there was no improvement. There is no other way, the family could only seek help from God. …in a shamanistic way they received a prescription from someone, and the patient took it. Naturally, his heart sincerely sought it, as if guarding a baby. Two hours after he took the prescription, the abdominal pains were severe, there was great urgency and in the toilet many pieces were expelled, half an hour later everything became normal.

Later on I met again Mr. Jiang and asked him for the prescription. …The prescription included 2 Qian 錢 of Huangqi 黃芪, 3 Qian of Danggui 當歸, 2 Qian of Zaojiao 皂角, and 1 Qian of Gancao 甘草…

Normally this prescription is applied externally, rarely is it taken internally. Now this met heads on with the patient's emotions, the efficacy was miraculous, if there was help from spirits one can consider. The patient's two eyes were slightly red, at night could not sleep well. That he couldn't sleep well was caused by the stomach pains. The tongue was dry, his diaphragm and chest felt obstructed, and so fluids would not rise upward. These symptoms all belong to this syndrome, but one can mistake true causes with false ones. Because of this one would use Xi Jiao Rhinoceros horn to generate fluids and clear heat. The heart is engaged with the fake heat and therefore the doctor will not use warming and unobstructing herbs.

Aside from me disliking to drink Xi Jiao Rhinoceros horn and rather like warm unobstructing herbs, there was no other reason for me to prescribe herbs. The other doctors preferred cool purging and so used Lou Zhi etc, this hardly had an effect. Now that the shamanistic prescription used Huang Qi, this helped strengthen the Qi, Dang Gui was agitating and increasing fluids, Zao Jiao is warm and moving around, this all helped expel the

> feces. Gan Cao is sweet and mellow, it harmonized the center and generated fluids, this all conformed to the patient's disease.
>
> I am not encouraging superstition, but I am amazed by the miraculous effectiveness of this prescription, so I wrote this down.

This article, which is from first volume of *Xiandai Mingyi Yan An* 現代名醫驗案, is by Ye Jingqiu 葉勁秋. Whether it is reasonable that Mr. Ye 葉 explained it in this way, remains a question. If we are sincere about academic research, first we should deduce from the diseases, second explain the pathology and not have wild guesses, third the ingredients of each formula and the changes occurring after mixing herbs together, how does it impact body cell etc should all be thoroughly researched.

Can young or old Native medicine doctors solve these kinds of complex problems? What tools can they use to seek answers? If one can only use a vague explanation for marvelous and unpredictable phenomena then it is better to advocate theory of ghosts and Gods.

For example, the statement "lower back pain uses Eucommia ulmoides Du Zhong 杜仲 and headache uses Ligusticum Chuan Xiong 川芎 is the essence of Chinese medicine" is not correct. In conclusion, efficacy of herbs and medical science are two different things. When Chinese medicine has progressed, it will be little different from Western medicine. Chinese medicine is experience-based knowledge of herbs. Advocating Chinese medicine before understanding the relevant pros and cons will restrict the progress of Chinese medicine. Chinese Medicine Schools entering the educational system will become its early demise. This is my conclusion.

> Editor's note: The author, Jin Risheng,[99] is not a Western medical physician, rather, he is a purely Chinese medicine physician to the core. Now he is regretful about the error of going astray. So he takes the meaning of, "Things in the past have died yesterday, things in the future are like alive today Jin Ri Sheng 今日生," as his pen name for alerting and encouraging himself and redeeming his previous mistakes. In a boundless sea, he turns his head to the shore. Jin Risheng 今日生 truly has this "live today" spirit.

Article end

[99] Jin Risheng is the phonetic writing. The phrasal meaning is "live today"

The issue of establishing Chinese Medicine Schools and education

By Chen Yu 陳郁

Source: *Compilation of Discussions about Chinese Medical Education* 中醫教育討論集

Pages 478–486

Since the Education Ministry does not permit establishment of Chinese Medicine Schools at this time, people in the Chinese medical community are feeling angry and wanting to cry out against this injustice. They appeal to each other for unity. Some say that the refusal reason is that the Ministry condemns Chinese medicine, while others say that it is a tactic to eliminate Chinese medicine. They cannot stop fearing and worrying. Recently, the Central Political Committee promulgated three principles for establishing Chinese Medicine Schools:

1) Specialized schools training Chinese medicine practitioners should follow the rules for other specialized professional schools, enrolling only high school graduates.

2) Educational regulations will be articulated by the Education Department together with Chinese medicine committees from the Health Ministry, following the curriculum example of specialized medical schools.

3) Our native herbs should receive special attention and investigation by research institutions appointed by the Education Ministry.

These three points clearly demonstrate a fair chance for developing both Chinese and Western medicines, and not an unfair prospect for Chinese medicine development. The first principle is also called "following the rules of schools for professional training or above in the educational system". The second principle is also named "referring to the curriculum of medical schools to draw up an educational standard" so that Chinese Medicine Schools from now on will be regulated by the *Relations Act* 關係法規 of the Education Ministry, just like other specialized schools. Since government decree must be reported, here is the *Relations Act* extracted:

A. Constituent Act of Schools for Professional Training 專科學校[100] (announced by government July of year 18 (1929))

Article 3

Schools for professional training set up by provincial governments or city governments are called Provincial or City Schools for Professional Training. Schools for professional training set up by persons or private legal entities are called Private Schools for Professional Training. To change the organization or suspend activities of the school requires permission from the Education Ministry.

Article 6

Teachers of Schools for Professional Training are categorized into full-time and part-time staff, and are hired by school principals. The number of part-time teachers cannot exceed one third of the total number of teachers.

Article 8

The entrance requirement for Schools for Professional Training ought to be graduation from public high schools or registered private high schools, or possession of equivalent level of educational history and passing an admission exam.

B. Amended Rules for Schools for Professional Training (announced by Education Ministry in August of Year 18 (1929) and amended in March of Year 20 (1931))

Article 3

The entrance requirement for Schools for Professional Training ought to be graduation from public high schools or registered private senior high schools, or possession of equivalent level of educational history and passing an admission exam.

The number of admitted students possessing equivalent level of educational history cannot exceed one fifth of the total number.

[100] "School" in Schools for Professional Training 專科學校 is equivalent to the term "College", but since the modern Chinese term for college is Xue Yuan 學院, we keep the term "School".

Article 5

Categories of Schools for Professional Training are:

Category A *(omitted)*

Category B *(omitted)*

Category C *(omitted)*

Category D 1. Medical Specialized Schools

2. Pharmacological Specialized Schools

(The rest omitted)

Article 10

The minimum cost of setup and annual operation of all types of colleges for professional training (cost of setup includes construction and equipment) are tentatively set as follows:

Categories	Setup cost	Annual operation cost
Medical schools of category D	$150,000[101]	$100,000
Pharmacological schools of category D	$100,000	$80,000

The first year annual operation cost of all Schools for Professional Training ought to exceed two thirds of the amount stated in this table.

Article 17

Graduation examination, the examination of the final semester, should include more than five categories of questions, in which at least three of them should span the entire curriculum. The graduation examination will be supervised by teachers from within the school and committee members from outside the school, dispatched by the Education Ministry, while the principal is the examination committee chairman. Examinations of every subject should involve the participation of one committee member from outside the school if possible. The Education Ministry will send staff to monitor the examination when necessary.

[101] Denomination is Chinese Yuan not dollar; here the $ sign is simply used to demonstrate currency.

C. Implementation program for a broad setup of Agricultural, Medical and Engineering Specialized Schools in all provinces and cities (Government Ordinance of Executive Yuan[102] issued in June of year 20 (1931))

b. Setup Criteria[103]

II. Setup criteria of medical schools are as follows:

1. Medical schools should follow the constituent act of schools for professional training.
2. The duration of study in medical schools is four years of study and one final year of internship.
3. Medical schools may include only medical programs or programs related to pharmacology. The latter is called Medical and Pharmacological School.
4. Medical and Pharmacological Schools should establish an ancillary hospital having at least 200 beds.
5. The cost of setup and first year operation of medical schools should follow the following criteria:

    I. Cost of medical construction and equipment not less than \$150,000. Cost of first-year operation is \$100,000. Cost of setting up ancillary hospital is \$150,000.

    II. Cost of pharmacological construction and equipment not less than \$100,000. Cost of first-year operation is \$60,000.

[102] Xing Zheng Yuan 行政院 Government Executive branch.
[103] Chen Yu quotes excerpts throughout this article—selection of numbered section is Chen's; his article here is reproduced in full.

D. Amended Rules for Private Schools (Education Ministry announced Aug Year 18, amended Oct Year 22)[104]

Chapter 1 – General Principle

Article 3

Private schools should register with an Education Executive Department 教育行政機關 and be supervised and directed by the same department. The school's programs and all other particulars should comply with current educational rules.

Article 9

If a private school is managed poorly or disobeys regulations, the Education Executive Department will cancel its registration or direct it to shut down. If a school did not register, the Education Executive Department will command it to shut down and halt operations. If that school does not register within three years, the Education Executive Department will cancel their ability to register.

Chapter 2 – School Council

Article 11

The school management committee is the representative of the established private school. The first management committee should select proper personnel for its directorship.

Article 12

The number of school council directors cannot exceed fifteen and they should elect one chairperson from among them.

Article 13

The school council's composition and limits of authority, as well as school council directors' term of duty and re-election measures, should be stipulated in the school council's statute.

[104] 1929 and 1931 respectively

Chapter 3 – Private Schools for Professional Training or Above

Article 26

Setup of private schools for professional training or above should comply with the following procedures:

1) Report of setup should be done after registration at Education Executive Department. Schools without setup permission by Education Executive Department cannot enrol students. When reporting, they should provide the following particulars, together with school floor plan and instruction leaflet:

   I. College name and its category

   II. College location

   III. State of land and building

   IV. Source of operating funds and budget table of operating funds

   V. Organization and curriculum

   VI. Reference books' and textbooks' table of contents

   VII. Catalog of all books in library and catalog and value of all apparatus and specimens in laboratory

   VIII. Curriculum vitae of principal and teaching staff

2) Application for registration should be processed following one year of operation. For application, the following particulars are required:

   I. State of funds after operation

   II. Same as IV to VIII in (1)

   III. Every rule and statute

   IV. List of students

   V. State of training and teaching

Article 28

Application for setup of private schools for professional training or above requires the following:

1) Number and categories of schools or programs in universities or independent colleges should have setup funds and annual operation funds exceeding the amount set in Article 10 of University Statute.

2) Number of professional schools and categories of colleges for professional training should have setup funds and annual operation funds exceeding the amount set in Article 10 of the amended Schools for Professional Training Statute.

Remarks: setup funds and annual operation funds should be deposited in a bank.

Article 29

Registration of private schools for professional training or above requires:

I. Items submitted have been proven to be true.

II. Practically complying with current educational statutes as well as administering a strict school statute.

III. Number of teaching staff who are competent and specialized must exceed two thirds of all teaching staff.

IV. Students must meet entrance requirements. Current students should obtain good academic results.

V. Equipment meets demand.

VI. Assets or interest of capital with other confirmed income (income from tuition fees excluded) must be sufficient to sustain its annual operation funds.

E. Medical Professional Schools' Temporary Curriculum 醫學專科學校 (Issued June Year 24 (1935) by Education Ministry)

Description:

1) This curriculum is piloted in all Medical Professional Schools across the entire country starting from year 24 (1935).

2) The teaching material syllabus of each subject is separately distributed to every medical school for reference and analysis. Every school should submit a report to describe its opinion, within one year, for reference.

3) The allocation table of teaching hours, hours of lectures, experiments and clinical practicum should be modified according to the particular situation. But

the modification range should be restricted to within 20% of the original and be approved by our department.

4) In every elementary and clinical course, preventive medicine and public hygiene concepts should be instilled so as to equally emphasize treatment and prevention.

5) In Chinese literature, the teaching time of medical terminology is one year. If extra time is needed, it should be supplemented in tutorial format.

6) Chemistry tutorials are required when students' chemistry level of knowledge is low.

7) In mathematics, statistics should be emphasized. In psychiatry, neurology should be emphasized. Psychology should be added into the curriculum.

8) In obstetrics, twelve periods of delivery observation and four periods of midwifery should be included. Obstetric models should be used to instruct students.

9) In clinical subjects, emphasize common diseases in corresponding places.

10) Tropical disease is classified as internal medicine. Orthopedics, urology and surgery are classified as surgery.

11) Medical history, medical ethics, sociology, hospital management and so on are elective subjects to be allocated to the remaining teaching hours.

12) Remaining teaching hours, other than those allocated to elective subjects as stated above, are used for clinical practicum.

13) After finishing four years of school study, students should intern in a reputable hospital for one year.

14) Medical Professional School examination principles are as follows:

    I. Examination is compulsory for all subjects.

    II. Other than the examinations mentioned above, there are former-period and latter-period examinations as well. Former-period examination examines every elementary subject. Latter-period examination examines every clinical subject. Former-period examination is held at the end of second or third academic year. Latter-period examination is the graduation examination.

    III. Examinations are classified into written and oral.

Medical Professional Schools' teaching hour allocation table of each academic year

Academic year	Subject	Total teaching hours	Year total [105]
First academic year	Party's Duties	36	1206
	National Literature	108	
	Foreign Language	144	
	Mathematics	72	
	Biology	128	
	Analytical Chemistry and Organic Chemistry	272	
	Physics	270	
	Biochemistry and Physiology	144	
	Wartime Rescue Training and Physical Education	32	
Second academic year	Anatomy; Histology; Embryology and Neuroanatomy	424	1176
	Biochemistry and Physiology	144	
	Bacteriology and Parasitology	288	
	Pathology	288	
	Wartime Rescue Training and Physical Education	32	
Third academic year	Pharmacology	144	1124
	Physical Diagnostics; Laboratory Diagnosis and Internal Medicine	326	
	Surgery	230	
	Pediatrics	152	
	Psychiatry and Neurology	96	
	Dermatology and Venereology	112	
	Radiology	32	
	Wartime Rescue Training and Physical Education	32	

105 "Total teaching hours in the academic year"

Fourth academic year	Internal Medicine	236	1114
	Surgery	230	
	Obstetrics and Gynecology	180	
	Public Hygiene	192	
	Ophthalmology and Otolaryngology	154	
	Forensic Medicine and Physical Education	32	
Fifth academic year clinical practice	Internal Medicine (including Pediatrics, Psychiatry, Dermatology and Venereology etc.)		Four and a half months
	Surgery (Urology, Orthopaedics, Ophthalmology, Otolaryngology, etc.)		Four and a half months
	Obstetrics and Gynecology		One month
	Public Hygiene		One month
	Holiday		One month
	TOTAL		12 MONTHS

Article end

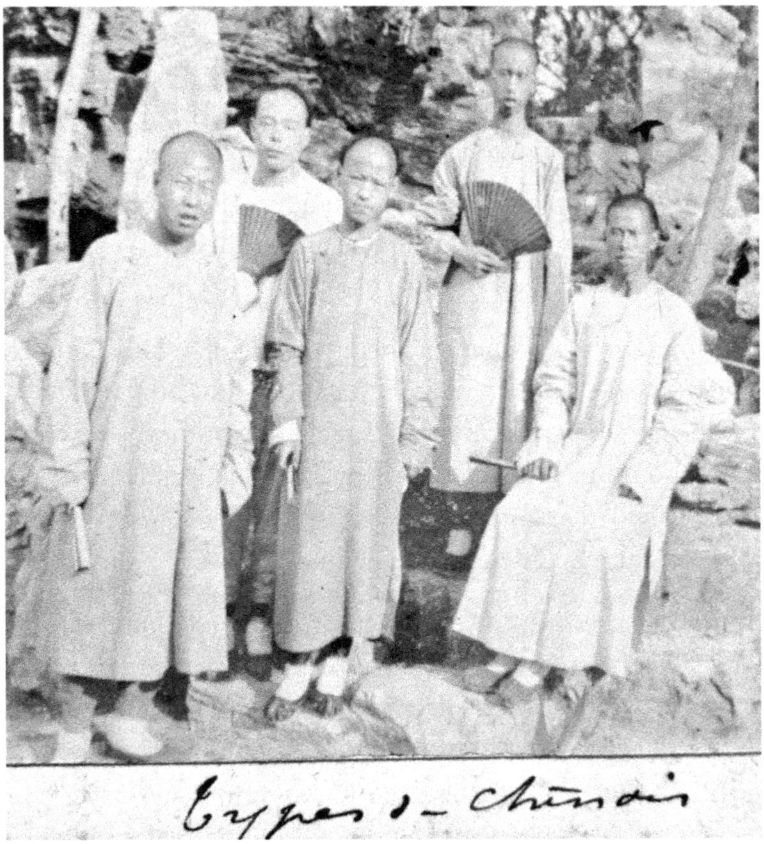

Photo by Mr P. Goux in early 1900s. "Chinese people".

Discussions comparing Western and Chinese medicines' equality

By He Xiaojun 何笑君

Source: *Compilation of Discussions about Chinese Medical Education* 中醫教育討論集

Yaron: Ouch! Here we see the reality for many Chinese medicine practitioners in the 1920s and 30s.

Pages 486–491

As scientific medicine is gradually developing, mentioning the names of Chinese medicine and Western medicine, which are opposite to each other, brings up heated debate.

The old medicine physicians call themselves "National medicine doctors Guo Yi 國醫" or "Chinese medicine doctors Zhong Yi 中醫" hoping to conserve the quintessence of Chinese culture and the knowledge passed down from their ancestors, which give them pride. They are conservative and stubborn. The new medicine doctors also include a group of little-knowing and shallow persons that call themselves Western medical doctors 西醫. In fact, both of them study but do not carefully interrogate, and they make mistakes that multiply. This greatly hinders the development of scientific medicine and the enhancement of national public health. Mr. Wang Jingwei 汪精衛 has thoroughly and clearly criticized the ridiculous name calling:

> "After a few times of being invaded, our country had adopted and emulated the tangible military weapons and other machinery of foreign enemies, rather than saying our primeval weapons had a few thousand years of history and are still usable now. We have never divided scientific weapons into Chinese and Western ones. But we largely divide medicine into Chinese and Western."

Without a doubt, the progression of science has stimulated change in every kind of human knowledge, thoughts and life. For example, the "eyes seeing thousand miles" and "ears hearing voices a long way off", depicted in our country's *Investiture of the Gods Feng Shen Chuan* 封神傳, describing enhanced sight and auditory faculties of people. Can it be compared with a telescope, telegram and wireless telephone? Wooden ox and horse carriage also aimed at increasing mobility, but can it compare to cars, planes, trains and steamship? Therefore, the evolution of things must all pass considerable phases before success. "Eyes seeing thousand miles" and "ears hearing voices a long way off" are only imagination, while wooden ox and horse carriage are musings. It is clear that they are useless. Today, the ones who call themselves National Medicine doctors are like this. Their intentions are to save people, yet they have not progressed for thousands of years, sticking to their wrong theories, simple and crude techniques, unclear observation, shallow thinking and lack of progress. This is so called "benevolence with no skills, then quack kills."

Nowadays, the names of Chinese and Western medicines not only appear in ordinary discussion, but also central government committees suggest "Equal Treatment of Chinese and Western Medicine" and "Chinese Medicine be Added into Educational System" in the Third National Congress. These people lack medical knowledge and therefore propose these kinds of valueless suggestions. But we cannot fully censure them. The most contemptible ones are the old medicine practitioners behind them who instigated them to make these proposals. They do not observe the worldwide trend of progressing toward a bright future; instead, they still work hard to set us back. In fact, there is adequate basis for scientific medicine in our country. Since the Nationalist government has set Jinling 金陵[106] as the capital, the national medicine level and health facilities have grown remarkably and are now at a considerable extent. If we are now set back, what will be the consequences?

1) Inequality of old medicine and scientific medicine in the theoretical aspect

Medicine in Greece, which has 2000 years of history, is detaching from abstract because its theory has not developed. It is the same situation with the old medicine now. What is the difference when comparing Yang excess, Yin inadequate, five elements and functional activity of Qi, with water, fire, earth and air in the Greek classical elements? What is the difference when comparing it to Pythagoras's Microcosm and Macrocosm? These kinds of abstract theories existed in every ancient society. Their names are different but their meanings are the same. Why is it the essence of only Chinese culture? Such theories have been in the history of other countries and they treat them as ragged shoes, whereas our country treats them as a golden rule and precious precept and is complacent about it. The theory of scientific

[106] Equals today's Nanjing 南京

medicine must be based on facts and experiments and not on shooting at random. For example, bacteria are the cause of many diseases. But it is found because it has passed "Koch's postulates". Koch said:

> "(1) The microorganism must be found in abundance in all organisms suffering from the disease
>
> (2) The microorganism must be isolated from a diseased organism and grown in pure culture and the cultured microorganism should cause disease when introduced into a healthy organism
>
> (3) The microorganism must be re-isolated from the inoculated, diseased experimental host and identified as being identical to the original specific causative agent."

Then, it can be known that a certain bacterium can cause a certain disease. But the old medicine is not like that. They say liver-fire, kidney-asthenia, lung vacuity, ...Yang excess and Yin inadequate. If I ask, "What is Yin? What does Yang indicate? To what extent is it excess? To what extent is it inadequate?" They are not able to answer. A simple saying, the formation of feces and urine, its pathological changes and biological components is thoroughly understood in scientific medicine. But old medicine is still guessing the good effect of using feces and urine. For instance, *Chinese Medicine Dictionary Encyclopedia* 中華醫學大辭典 says, "the character of feces is bitter, cold and non-toxic, can cure pandemic disease, severe heat, typhoid fever-heat toxins, ...can cure abscess, hemorrhoid, smallpox not grown. Fecal ash, fecal liquid, meconium and liquorice soaked with fecal liquid is specially prepared fecal medicament." And it also states, "the character of urine is salty, cold and non-toxic. Effect is promoting vision, benefit voice. Can cure cold, headache, malaria, red eyes, deaf ears, gum bleeding, consumptive lung disease, retention of placenta, detoxify and destroy intestinal worms." When reading this, I cannot help sighing. The so-called essence of Chinese culture of the old medicine is silly to the greatest degree, but they still treat it as a classic. The consequence is inconceivable. In these two years, I have seen many cases of using whitish urine to wash eyes but still without recovery. This is surely a "no skill". For this reason, all the books of old medicine should be treated as harmful and should be burnt and then thrown into the sea. In old medicine the amount of old things did not exceed that of ancient Greece. However, about their respective evolution, there is no equality to be mentioned.

2) Inequality of old medicine and scientific medicine in technical aspects

Diagnosis in old medicine only includes inspection, auscultation, inquiry and palpation. "Inspection" is only confined to color of face, "inspect forehead knows heart, inspect nose knows spleen, left cheek liver, right cheek lung, cheekbone kidney." Following this theory, how then does one inspect the remaining organs in the body? Inspection in scientific medicine is not like this; they use x-ray to inspect pathological changes and physiological phenomena of every organ. Using disparity of mirrors to gain detailed insight into ear, nose, throat and eyes. Using microscope to inspect microorganisms in feces and urine, changes in blood cells, bacteria and parasites. Inspection of things as tiny as hair down to toes of patients. The inspection of scientific medicine does not use ears to replace eyes and mouth to replace anus. In other words, inspecting ears cannot know eyes, similarly, inspecting forehead cannot know heart. The so-called "auscultation" only hears sound at one end, which is not reliable. The "auscultation" of scientific medicine, in contrast, uses the stethoscope to hear heart and lung sounds. For example, hearing the breathing sound of a drowned and dying person solely by ear, one may think he was dead. But using a stethoscope at the cardio area, the heart sound can be heard. Undergoing artificial respiration can raise the dead. The so-called "inquiry" in old medicine only asks the ten things. In contrast, scientific medicine asks everything related to the disease. For example, having liver abscess one must ask medical history of dysentery, having inflammation of both eyes one must ask medical history of gonorrhea, having lung tuberculosis one must ask family history of tuberculosis… Concerning "palpation," old medicine says pulse at different positions can diagnose diseases from different organs. All people with knowledge know that it is absurd. There are also percussion, palpation, bacterial reaction, biochemical experiment and pathological examination in scientific medicine.

The treatment of old medicine is mostly using herbs. The number of types of herbs in each prescription is at least ten, which is similar to ancient Greece. The so-called "multiple bombs prescription" includes so many herbs that its make efficacy inconspicuous. What is more, they do not know which herb treats which disease. On the contrary, scientific medicine uses drugs as minor treatment. Its main point is to assist the body's natural recovery ability. With efficient drugs, one drug is already enough. There are predicted effects and no adverse effects from multiple drugs. Herbal products in our country lack technique. For decoction, put herbs in water and boil without restriction of time and checking of temperature. If there is an element that is easier to dissolve at low temperature, then why put it in boiling water? If there is an element that is insoluble in water, it does not dissolve in water no matter how long the boiling time is. So, is there any effect of taking this herbal drug? Even if it really shows effect, it is certainly not the anticipated one.

3) Equal treatment should not exist between old medicine and scientific medicine

According to the above facts, old medicine has straggled far away. As old medicine and scientific medicine are not equal, it is clear that no equal treatment should exist. The President has divided equality into true and false; saying that within the old medicine putting sages and the foolish as equals is a false equality. Scientific medicine is crystallisation of every scientific branch today and the result of accumulation of wise and great medical scientists. In contrast, old medicine is still wandering between the *Neijing Suwen* 內經素問 of Huang Di 皇帝 and Qi Bo 岐伯 four thousand years ago. They have no contribution to make, because the ancient people had restricted observations, lack of knowledge and obstructed minds, making medicine mediocre and silly. Now, since someone wants the wise scientific medicine and silly old medicine to have equal treatment, then that must be false equality. Some of the old medicine practitioners overestimate their ability, act as great persons and beg for pity from politicians and vainly attempt to get equal treatment. This act is not worthy of a sneer from a person of good sense.

4) Old medicine cannot enter educational system

Education is a product of thousands of years of this country's history and cannot be changed rashly. The education of our country today, from kindergarten to university, is neatly arranged and strictly organized. All the subjects, grading of schools and academic theories are deduction of science. Today's secondary school's students with moderate understanding of science would not believe Yin Yang and Five Phases theory. Though they do not know about medicine, they would ask when talking about medicine "where is your evidence?" and "is it visible, touchable, able to be smelled? …"

Today, the already established so-called National Medicine Professional School 國醫傳校 only includes superficiality of physiology, pathology, biochemistry and pharmacology, and then the old medicine subjects are also added. This kind of curriculum is nondescript, neither horse nor ox. How can it be called National Medicine? In their teaching, most people just try to make a living, however, they harm other people by doing it, so they are guilty, for which they deserve to die ten thousand times. The people vocal about equal treatment say, "approve the registration of these schools". The leaders of today's Education Ministry, if they possess moderate knowledge of science and modernization plan, should shut those nonsensical schools down. Our people possess too little knowledge and too weak ability to judge. From backward places to the metropolis, there are miracle drugs in temples, holy water getting back souls of Taoist priests and Buddhist monks, a so-called hospital established incantation department Zhu You Ke 祝由科 in Hunan who is teaching also martial art. Though different in names, they are similar to the old medicine. They also have their own theory and ask the government "witchcraft and medicine come from the same origin. Old medicine can enter the official education system, why can't we? Old medicine can have equal treatment with scientific medicine. Why should we be excluded?" I am not sure how the Education Ministry will respond to them.

5) Sincere advice to the old medicine community

I am not rejecting the conservation of the essence of Chinese culture. But today's old medicine is not the essence of Chinese culture. It is the waste product of Chinese culture. It is ragged shoes for other countries. Benevolence should be possessed, together with good techniques. Today's old medicine doctors do not possess good techniques. Their benevolence is enough to destroy and kill. If they just want to make a living, then they can change their career or ask their offspring to learn scientific medicine in order to complete their own unfinished aspirations, all along not harming people with bad techniques. We cannot criticize people who have learnt old medicine in past generations. But those who learn old medicine today and set up old medicine education, they cannot shirk from responsibility. Our country's herbs should be investigated by applying financial and human resources allocated by the Central Government. We should get together scientists and medical scientists and start determining herbs' properties and pharmacological traits. This is not a job the incompetent old medicine community can do.

Conclusion

Today's medicine is the collection of wise medical scientists' achievements in each country. Japan has its contribution. Our country has its contribution. Italy and France have their contributions. Britain and America also have their contributions. It can neither be called Eastern medicine nor Western medicine. It can only be called scientific medicine. Old medicine cannot be compared and is not equal to scientific medicine in academic, technological and theoretical aspects. They are not equal; how can it have equal treatment? Old medicine's academic system totally betrays today's educational system. Today's education is all deduction of science. The theory of old medicine is false and abstract. How is it worthy of entering the educational system?

Moreover, the so-called National Medicine Professional Schools have mixed into their curriculum superficiality of scientific medicine, and yet failed to form their own subject. Why does our education system need a new subject—National Medicine? Even after this motion of hindering cultural progress has passed in the third national congress, how many people with clear minds will let their offspring learn old medicine? I know for a fact that many committees, who have supported this motion, consult scientific medical doctors when they get sick. So, did they support this motion just for the sake of conserving the essence of Chinese culture?

(*Changsha Root Out Newspaper Medical Special Edition* 長沙掃蕩報醫學特刊)

Article end

Reply to a friend's question about special training course of sanitation

By Ye Jingqiu 葉勁秋

Source: *Compilation of Discussions about Chinese Medical Education* 中醫教育討論集

Yaron: Humor was also a way to deal with the grim reality. The author makes good points on behalf of Chinese medicine, asking to maintain its uniqueness.

Pages 492–493

Concluding everything in the world with ideals, is never denied but always appreciated by scientists and philosophers. I remember a secondary school teacher saying in a meeting that, "Some people are now doing research on love education. How weird is that!" Later, this teacher recognized how wrong he was. He declared it to everyone he met and even became a propagator of love education. Chinese people do a lot of speculation about ideals, which is a clever step. What is sad is that most people stop there. Or maybe some did lots of covering up after finding that their speculation, at the end, was a mistake. They saw the covering up as a kind of amendment, which is an even bigger mistake. This is why we can't help admiring the secondary school teacher who recognized and showed his own mistake.

In these two or three years, I often hear or read about the special training course of sanitation 衛生特別訓練班 offered by Jiang Su Province Medical College 江蘇省立醫政學院. A lot of people criticized it without having knowledge of the course itself. Nevertheless, the facts are different from their imagination.

The aim of this course is to improve the knowledge level of Chinese medicine practitioners and to train them in terms of physiology, epidemiology and bacteriology so that Chinese medicine practice may become more scientific. Jiang Su Province Medical College was very clear, when advertising for general students, that students should accept the assigned service workload, except for those taking the special training course of sanitation. It was like a rat opening its eyes and eating the rat poison.[107] The people participating in this training, aside from learning some clever tricks, did not make any progress with the medical college. I, myself, ate some of this rat poison so I know its sweet and yet bitter taste; compared to ones who did not go through it, I have some personal experience to share.

There was no relationship whatever to Chinese medicine. The course was about bacteriology, physiology, anatomy, epidemiology, pathology, sanitary science (or public health), personal health, diagnostics, pharmacology and so on. As far as I remember, on the bulletin board there was once a notice, "A talk about *Cold Injury Treatise* 傷寒論 will be delivered from eleven to twelve o'clock next Monday, by Mr Du Tongjia 杜同甲, in the fourth classroom (which is the classroom for the special sanitation course)". The following Monday there was another notice, "Mr Du Tongjia does not feel well, thus the talk is postponed until next Monday". And the next Monday there was the third notice, "Mr. Du Tongjia is not yet recovered and the talk is cancelled". At the same time, there was an announcement in the advertising column of two newspapers (*Nanjing Central Daily* 南京中央日報 and *Morning Daily* 朝報) made by Mr. Du Tongjia about another talk cancellation in Zhen Jiang Medical College 鎮江醫政學院. Until today I still did not figure out the catch inside all these. There was one time that Mr. Chen Guofu 陳果夫 spoke at the Memorial Hall about the weak point of Chinese medicine, "Chinese medicine lays particular emphasis on ideals and lacks scientific experiments and research. Moreover, everyone uses

[107] Thinking it is something good, but in reality very bad.

different medicines and they believe only their own medical theories. As a result, Chinese medicine lacks uniformity, which weakens its effect."

"Making Chinese medicine more scientific" has become an increasingly popular slogan. The weird thing is that the slogan itself is expressing an idea: "Chinese medicine is not scientific". Then how do we make it on the right track of becoming scientific? First, we must give up all traditional values. Second, we have to admit the existence of bacteria and accept modern theories. Third, we must go for the knowledge attained by fundamental scientific tools. The meaning behind Mr. Chen's offering of the special course in this medical college proves that. It is essential and the only way to renovate and protect Chinese medicine. In the future, when the time comes, they will beat down those of us who tell lies and nonsense. They will not allow their lips to talk about Qi transformation. They will have to make all statements clear and well-founded so that everyone understands and believes them. Not only do they have to think and speculate, but they will have to prove their stance with evidence. Words such as "magical" and "unbelievable" should never appear in any medical dictionary. God gifted us with animals, plants and ores so of course we should treasure them and never give them up. Chinese medicine formulas with long history and proven by experience we should of course use. However, we should not be satisfied with knowing that it works but rather we should strive to know why it works. We should have new statistics to prove its efficacy and find its active ingredients. It is still a long way from maturation.

Now, as a result of this attitude, the special training course of sanitation appears to be anti-Chinese medicine in the opinion of some. They are concerned that the course will eventually replace or engulf Chinese medicine. Since they don't want Chinese medicine to change, in their opinion, Chinese medicine should never become like this. They rather see Chinese medicine go back to the time of the Han 漢 and Qin 秦 dynasties or even the three Dynasties[108] era 三代. They also think that since it is called Chinese medicine (not Western medicine), we should never admit the existence of bacteria. They think that recognizing bacteria is no different from surrendering to Western medicine. According to them, Western medicine is opposite Chinese medicine. How can a school of Chinese medicine adopt the entire course of Western medicine? Instead, it should have its own unique Chinese medicine courses and they should be different from Western medicine courses.

[108] Xia, Shang and Zhou predating the Qin and Han dynasties.

Here, I would like to state my own opinion. This sanitation special course I took was running counter to Chinese medicine, it erases Chinese medicine, because it was all about Western medicine. All the items within did not have any trace of Chinese medicine. If this special training course is assumed to be desirable, in order to improve Chinese medicine to become more scientific and, by that, be accepted into the general education system, then this is totally wrong because there was not a thing about Chinese medicine in it. The course was entirely prepared by Western medicine schools. The only difference from Western medical school is the admission age limit being discounted 20%; the cost, however, was not discounted 20%.

(As of recent times, my mother Chinese medicine school is over-poisoned and is no longer doing Chinese medicine; it should no longer recruit students.)

Article end

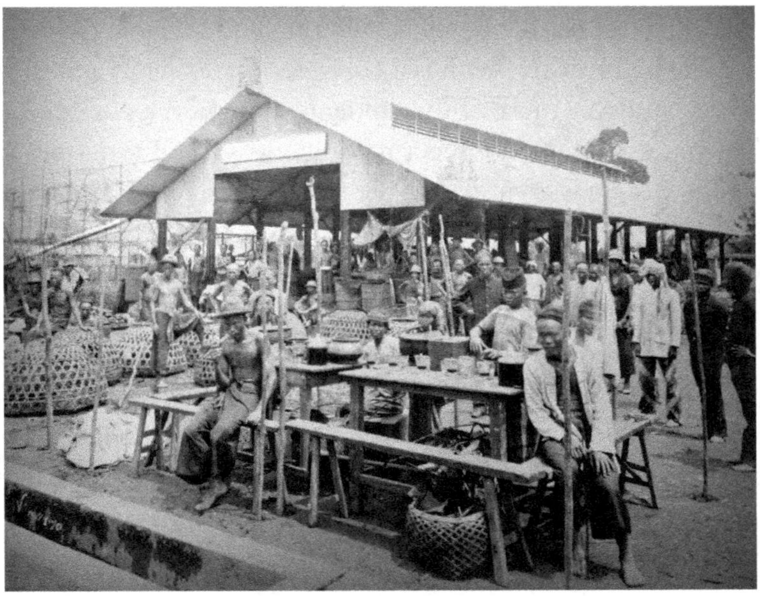

Photo by Mr P. Goux in early 1900s. "Market".

A special school and its special students

By Xu Daolai 徐道來

Source: Compilation of Discussions about Chinese Medical Education 中醫教育討論集

Yaron: Humor seemed to have been a motif in the anti-Chinese medicine group as well.

Pages 503–504

It has been several decades since the initial establishment of schools in our country. The syllabus has changed several times. But amongst the schools, the curriculum is generally the same. However, the school I want to talk about is really special, a school one of a kind. On the surface it seems to be a regular school, with ordinary weekdays and weekends, summer and winter holidays and memorial days. In addition to regular schools, it also celebrates festivals like Duan Yang 端陽 and Chong Jiu 重九. Every day at 9AM the bell rings and classes begin. After 50 minutes the bell rings again and the classes are over. Like this, classes begin and end as many as six times per day. The students seem to enjoy that a whole lot. They feel so free even during class, let alone the time after class. The professors are all so knowledgeable and experienced and talented. In happy times they have a drink and become poets. In happier times they practice inner elixir in the midst of clouds. They talk about Yin, Yang, wind, rain, night and dusk. They have thousands of books, River Picture He Tu 河圖 and Luo Chart Luo Shu 洛書, Yin Yang 陰陽 and the Eight Trigrams Ba Gua 八卦 inside their gut. Their daily task is to relieve the people's suffering and know about life and death. If one says it is not like a university, yet it is a college specializing in a profession. If one says it is a university, and yet most of the students have never attended any school, then this looks like a scam. The school recruits students several times per year and its reputation among the people is great. What the school is doing cannot be clearer than it is. However, the Government, which should be responsible for the school, turns a blind eye. The students in this school mostly come from rich families and the tuition fee seems to be no big deal for them, taking their "promising future" into account. Because the students come from the upper class, they do not have to care about their study results at all. This is why they are so relaxed during the classes and after four or five years of study they graduate. After graduating from the school, their motto is to have great benevolence, and saving the world is their banner, their ambition is to pull out the money from their patients in the name of kindness. What a special school! How special the students are!

Article end

How to learn Chinese medicine well

By Ye Jingqiu 葉勁秋[109]

Source: *Compilation of Discussions about Chinese Medical Education* 中醫教育討論集

Yaron: All through the years a struggle existed in many practitioners' minds between the useful and useless in Chinese medicine. Aside from theoretical debates about its contents, there was also the reality on the ground: the war, the money, the greed, the pride. These factors did not help one in deciding a better path.

The following article demonstrates the coercion practitioners faced regularly at that time and, to a degree, still face today. We should reflect and see if we ourselves are subjected to similar pressure from society and, indeed, the profession itself.

Pages 504–512

The income of a Chinese medicine doctor has always been impressive. The doctors in China have the same status, no matter whether they practice medicine, divination or fortune telling. That's why so many people envy doctors.

A great number of people have lost their home and place to stay since the war began on July the 7th [Marco Polo Bridge Incident]. Yet doctors can still make a living in the chaos. This profession is making more and more people jealous. Some heartless doctors have made use of the situation to illegitimately get money in the name of charitable work and saving the people. This problem can only be solved in different times, not during war. The general public find it hard even to satisfy hunger, it seems impossible to have spare money for seeing a doctor and buying medicine. The rich, however, never have to worry about their health, and of course, there will never be any problem as long as they pay. This situation during this time gets different doctors to react in opposite ways. If we care for the health of our people in this nation, then we should promote public health care. Then it is certain that diseases will not be seen so often. However, some doctors do not want this to happen. Every single person, even fools, knows that in current society this problem exists. However, this is not what I want to talk about in this article, so temporarily I will just put it aside.

[109] Ye Jingqiu 葉勁秋 1900–1955, graduated from Shanghai Chinese Medicine Specialized School 上海中醫專門學校, later served as a professor at the Shanghai China's Medicine College 上海中國醫學院教授. During the Communist era served as committee member of Shanghai Department of Health—Chinese Medicine Compilation and Editing Committee 上海市衛生局中醫編審委員.

Medicine is a good business, and being a doctor can earn a living in this chaotic day and age. This is the truth in front of us and it seems that many people are moved by this prospect and want to become a doctor. Let us have a look at where doctors really come from. In the past, Confucian sayings and the *Classic of Poetry* stated about physicians that some of them were educated since birth as Confucian scholar physicians and some used to work for the government as official medical doctors. These doctors were at the highest position, with fame and money. We cannot say anything faulty about them. However, there are those today who come from nowhere and have made a large amount of money, those who are not even doctors, and yet have a lot of patients, while doing some back-room deals, and those who are illiterate and passed the exam and became doctors. These are also facts in today's world of chaos. I think lots of people will hate me for washing the dirty linen in public. Look, it is a different world now, dear medical practitioners! We cannot think only for ourselves any more at this moment. It is not anymore the 18th century in the Qing 清 dynasty now and we must make our mind clear so that the Chinese nation can survive in this world. The national calamity did not come without a reason! We can only win the game when we know all about both our enemies and ourselves. If there is dirt at the corner, there is no way to hide it. Even if I did not talk about it, someone else will. I am very concerned about the problem that the entire field is facing now. It is like the elephant in the room. Many people wanted to turn a blind eye but one day the problem will grow so big that we cannot ignore it. There have been some articles reviewing the situation and pointing out the problem. This is a good sign.

The quality between different doctors varies too much. As long as you put in a little bit of effort you can be a famous doctor, it's so easy. It is the kind of effort you put in that matters the most. There are all different ways to get one famous.

The most common reason for people to take a job as a doctor is to make a living. Yet there are some other reasons. For example, some people are not healthy themselves so they want to become a doctor to cure themselves as well as do more good things for others (which they believe is also good for their own health). Some people just think that Chinese medicine is so mysterious that they should find out what it really is. Some become Chinese medicine doctors just to be patriotic. They (the ones who do not work as a doctor just for the money) are exactly what I want for now. The Chinese medicine teaching should be tailored for students so that each can make use of their strengths.

So, how do we study Chinese medicine? What kind of books should we read? We must have a general idea of what Chinese medicine is first. There are two goals in medicine: prevention of disease and curing of disease. The process of prevention is too broad to talk about here and a single person cannot accomplish it. So I am going to skip that part.

Lesson One

Anyone who works in this industry with a goal of curing the disease may use different kinds of tools or methods but under one condition: it must be for the patients' benefit. The tools and methods should be as affordable and effective as possible. This may not be achieved under the current situation of our society. As a result, a public health care system has been suggested for quite a long time. As a private business, if a doctor charges a very low consultation fee, there will be two problems.

Firstly, the price charged cannot represent the social status of the doctor. People will judge a doctor on how much he charges. Secondly, the price may be so low that it cannot gain the trust from patients. If the price of medicine is low, people will doubt its potency. If the procedures are not complicated enough, there is no way to make a fortune out of patients. Medical business, as a social activity, is tightly connected with other aspects of society. If a doctor follows only what he has learned and works as a scholar in front of the patients without getting to know the psychology behind what people think, it is certain that he will have only few customers. The career of a doctor depends mostly on word of mouth. A doctor is lucky (or he knows how to promote himself) if he is often talked about and appreciated. Therefore, clever doctors often get into the general public. They do not hesitate to expand their business by any means. In some cases, as long as a doctor is moderately famous, some people will have faith in him. For instance, if a patient gets worse and worse after treatment, they will not blame the doctor if they have faith in the doctor. Instead, the patient may think it is their fate, or they just deserve it.

Undoubtedly, medical science is not only complicated but also technical. Nevertheless, everyone in our Chinese society seems to know a bit about medicine. It is common for doctors to hear patients claiming that their endogenous heat is too strong and that the doctor should prescribe some antipyretics. Sometimes patients believe themselves to have Yin deficiency of the Kidney and ask for some medicine to reinforce Yin. Seldom are these patients humble and rarely do they doubt their thoughts. Whenever they have some cough or sputum, immediately they become a specialist of lung disease. Whenever they feel stiffness or soreness, immediately they know it must be rheumatic disease and ask for acupuncture. The students who study Chinese medicine must learn to cope with the situation when patients want to decide everything for themselves.

Lesson Two

"What is Chinese medicine exactly?" This is the second part of the lesson students must know. Chinese medicine is not exactly a kind of specialized knowledge. It is a combination of all kinds of common sense and general knowledge. Chinese medicine is quite apparent in terms of the way we observe a disease. Yet it is also full of crafty and even irrelevant imagination. For example, smelly nasal discharge is connected with sinusitis Nao Lou 腦漏.[110] When the anus is leaking it called crossed intestines Jiao Chang 交腸. Skin ulcer that looks like a cucumber is called cucumber carbuncle Huang Gua Yong 黃瓜癰. Disease in winter is called Winter Warmth Dong Wen 冬溫, disease in spring is called Spring Warmth Chun Wen 春溫.

The characteristics of Chinese herbs divide into only two categories: Cold and Hot. However, we cannot tell for certain if an herb itself belongs to cold or hot. Many people are certain that Chinese medicine can treat disease. It is quite true. However, we need to be clear about the concept of disease Bing 病, we need to know what does it take to understand this concept. With all that modern machinery and diagnostic equipment, some people get confused. Some people argue that Chinese medicine should not be over-criticized considering that Western medicine itself has a lot of problems. In my opinion, criticizing the flaws of Chinese medicine does not make Western medicine flawless. Being "correct" or "not correct" is the limitation of people and understanding according to what they have learned.

Many diseases need explanation yet we cannot explain it clearly. Modern knowledge cannot explain the formless origin. For example, who is there that can shorten the pathological development of a disease? Normally disease is treated only after it had occurred trying to recover the body back to its original state, after the body itself did not succeed in fighting it off. Bian Que 扁鵲 said it well, "who can revive the dead and make bare bones grow flesh, one can revive only the not-dead 誰能生死肉白，不

[110] Literal translation: discharge from the brain.

過不死者使之起耳." These are words with real principle. Disease Bing 病 has its entire story; an origination point and pathological development, and this cannot be explained by imagination alone. Diseases are difficult to understand, and therefore anyone researching medicine should treat them seriously. Those who treat disease should be humble toward everything.

Some say that Chinese medicine is a specialized and technical knowledge and not a common sense kind of knowledge. Then how can they explain the fact that there is not a single book in any library introducing and explaining diseases with specificity and detail? Chinese medicine was only common sense in ancient times and therefore, with common sense alone, one cannot be clear about the specific details of a disease. Chinese medicine can cure a disease but this does not mean that Chinese medicine has a clear concept of the disease. In the world before civilization, the only thing that cured disease was the incantation of witches. For the general public, God and bodhisattva could cure diseases. They believed that all animals have their own way to treat their own diseases and that any living body in the world has an instinct against getting hurt and falling ill. Therefore the efficacy of Chinese medicine still needs to be investigated.

Every disease entails one or more possible painful or painless symptoms which are not supposed to be. We call these symptoms Zheng 症. Having Zheng does not necessarily mean someone is sick. It may seem like a disease but it is actually physiological presentation, such as the spermatorrhea of a growing young man and sleeplessness of the elderly. Apart from these, the psychological problems that scientific machinery cannot detect or diagnose can also be treated with Chinese medicine. The trick of Chinese medicine treatment is that we can treat the "Zheng" using the experience of our predecessors and our own. Also, doctors know how to calm patients down with words of consolation. They teach their patients to be peaceful and happy. When their patients die, the doctors would say something like it is their destiny whether they live or not, just like being rich or poor is heaven destiny. All things end with just a few words. The death need not be investigated further. As the saying goes, "when someone's dead things end, why bother to look for the root of his disease then?"

A student must know about all these things before he/she learns the knowledge inside textbooks. Otherwise, no matter how hard they work, they work in vain.

Personal Education

There are countless books about Chinese medicine throughout the generations. Students who really want to learn Chinese medicine may encounter the problem of choosing which books to read. They cannot read all the books. Choosing books may be an obstacle for learning. Some say that Chinese medicine students just have to read *Tang Tou Ge Jue* 湯頭歌訣, *Mai Jue* 脈訣 and *Yi Zong Bi Du* 醫宗必讀. Some say it is just heresy to suggest that there is no need to read *Su Wen* 素問 and *Ling Shu* 靈樞. And some say that Zhang Zhong Jing 張仲景 is the most influential doctor in the history of Chinese medicine, we have to read his two greatest works, *Shang Han Lun* 傷寒論 and *Jin Gui Yao Lüe* 金匱要略 to gain the ability to cure all diseases. Others say that there is no Cold Injury Shang Han 傷寒 in the whole area in the south of Yang Zi River 長江. As a result, instead of *Shang Han*, we just need to read the work of Ye Tian Shi 葉天士, a famous doctor who lived around the area south of the Yang Zi River. A lot of people say that Chinese medicine is a mystery. It is true that some doctors are famous for using tonics, some well known for using laxatives, some become rich because of using hot herbs, while some others make a fortune using cold herbs to cure. If you don't believe my words, this is also recorded in books, see the following text as an example:

> "Mr. Jade Decoction has received the family trade of gynecological medicine. His treatment became famous for its extraordinary efficacy. One time there was another doctor thinking that Jade's treatment efficacy was too weak, so he didn't dare using lighter doses. Instead he gave large dose Da Huang 大黃 until the patient recovered. Within one year he has prescribed several hundred pounds of it. In Wu Xi 無錫 there was another teacher who liked to use Ren Shen 人參, also within one year he used several hundred pounds. The knowledgeable compares himself to others and uses it, the ignorant simply resort to arms." —From *Wu Jin Gazette* 武進縣志.

Just for the fun of it we must mention the book *Mai Jue* 脈訣. It is a must to not only read but also deeply understand. However, let me make it clear, reading this book is not for practical application. But rather, it is for dealing with patients. We have to know the jargon of a pulse like Cun, Guan and Chi 寸關尺, San Bu Jiu Hou 三部九候, names such as floating pulse, deep pulse, slow pulse, and frequent pulse so that we can talk to the patients in the language they understand.

Learning Chinese herbal medicine is the most important step for Chinese medicine practitioners in order to perform their treatment. Generally, practitioners should know a certain amount of Chinese herbs, enough for their clinical use. One way is to read through the book *Ben Cao Cong Xin* 本草從新. It is also important to study the two books *Wen Re Jing Wei* 溫熱經緯 and *Lin Zheng Zhi Nan* 臨證指南, for one's own reference on properly using formulas according to different symptoms and signs recorded in these books. If one follows the principles and use the formulas in these two books then surely there will be no big errors. If a serious medical accident has happened, and one is sued in court, it will still be possible for the practitioner to protect him or herself since they cannot be charged with using formulas in a wrong way or without a correct diagnosis of the pulse. Regarding *Tang Tou Ge Jue* 湯頭歌訣, it is a famous and well-known book nowadays, and when speaking of Chinese medicine, this book must come to mind. It seems that this book is the soul and a structural part of Chinese medicine, but why is it so? The answer for it is "believing in Jesus is a principle of its own"!

According to Chinese medicine, disease is explained the four seasons and eight solar terms,[111] disease in spring is caused by wind, disease in summer is caused by summer heat, disease in autumn is caused by dryness and disease in winter is caused by coldness. Therefore, for each of the seasons, there are one to two common formulas that could be used for any symptoms and signs in each, for instance, Huo Xiang Zheng Qi San 藿香正氣散 and Liu He Tang 六和湯 can treat the symptoms and signs caused by summer heat and dampness. Gui Zhi Tang 桂枝湯 and Ma Huang Tang 麻黃湯 treat diseases with symptoms or signs of catching cold. For supplementing Qi, the first formula you can think of is Si Jun Zi Tang 四君子湯 and for supplementing blood Si Wu Tang 四物湯 absolutely is your first choice. The abovementioned formulas are composed not only by one or two herbs, but rather more complex combinations and thus writing up different *Decoctions in Rhymes*[112] for memorization is the best way. These *Decoctions in Rhymes* are easy to read, memorizing being easier with rhymes. It is not difficult to understand why *Tang Tou Ge Jue* is such an important book in Chinese medicine after understanding the above reasons. There is always the question, what is Chinese medicine in reality? In fact, to answer this question is not difficult. When one knows the essentials of *Tang Tou Ge Jue*, and after memorizing the *Decoctions with Rhymes*, we can say that we are always more than half way getting it!

---

[111] 四時八氣 explaining the ancient calendar system, separating a year into twenty four solar terms with eight main ones.

[112] 歌訣, written up by the practitioners in poetic form with rhymes for easy memorization of Chinese medicine formulas.

The following is just the opinion of this paper. In order to improve one's business one must match his skill Gongfu 功夫. One of the first requirements to match one's skill is to know which hat a person is wearing. Disparity in the educational level of Chinese people is great as well as their knowledge. Some believe that malaria is caused by ghosts, some believe malaria must be caused by sputum and excessive eating. When they listen to words such as "bacteria," "cells," "nerves" or "pathogens" in Chinese, they even think that you are speaking Chinese in another form of Western languages.

...Some despise the jargon or few terms in Chinese medicine such as Liver fire 肝火 and damp-heat 濕熱 they see it as false. But other terms like Kidney-vacuity 腎虛 or Yin depletion 陰虧 they tend to accept and believe in their treatment. Therefore I have a reminder for you here to learn Chinese medicine and please pay attention to this: There is a difference between theory in Chinese medicine and treatment efficacy. It is, in fact, mentioned by the old practitioners in their books, as follows:

Li Xianruo 李顯若[113] said, "The thoughts of Xue 薛[114] in treating diseases is well-known and being admired by other old practitioners, but he always insists on using old formulas from the old books to treat patients. Though his knowledge in theories and philosophies is admired by others, his treatment efficacy is not that good compared to his knowledge."

Dong Ji Bei Yao Fang Si Ku Ti Yao 董級備要方四庫提要 mentions, "There are some old formulas not shared in public; they are used as secrets. These formulas provide good treatment efficacy; however, explaining the theories or concepts for forming these formulas even Bian Que 扁鵲 could not answer it."

Xu Lingtai 徐靈胎 said, "Secret formulas are always useful but it is not possible to elaborate on their meaning or on the concepts or theories used behind them."

Wu Shuqing 武叔卿 said, "To use it must be easier then to explain the concepts or meaning behind it!"

There is always someone insisting on finding out the reason behind Chinese medicine treatment and formulas, because they think that there should be reasons or theories to show how Chinese medicine is working so well. In the end, it is not likely

---

[113] A person whose writing is recorded in the book Leng Lu Yi Hua 冷廬醫話.

[114] Xue Lizhai 薛立齋 of the Ming dynasty.

that they will come up with a conclusion. Some think that just learning Chinese medicine is not enough, but it should be a higher level of studying Chinese medicine. To study it, one should start from the old books *Nei Jing* 內經 and *Shang Han Za Bing Lun* 傷寒雜病論 and then browsing through the books written later by the doctors in the Jin and Yuan dynasties they will become enlightened. If these were smart people, they would know that the theories behind the formulas would be too difficult for them to understand after reading those books. However, people who still insist on this kind of study definitely link Chinese medicine with the religions of ancient China such as Buddhism or Taoism. Before the war started, there were many organizations for Buddhist meditation and Taoist cultivation etc religious activities who still dared raise their heads. Many participants of these organizations were indeed Chinese medicine leaders.

Some learn Chinese medicine hoping to protect this essence of Chinese culture, however, in order to tell the difference between essence and trash we need a new understanding. Then we can avoid treading an erroneous path.

Some learn Chinese medicine for maintaining their own health or to accumulate good Karma for their next generations; these people should only read the following three types of books:

1) Different Materia Medica

2) Various Chinese medicinal formulae

3) Medical records written in note form

A prerequisite for anyone wishing to study the Materia Medica is to investigate whether its effects are the same as those stated in other books. And those who would like to study medicinal formulae should first explore the pathogenesis of diseases and accumulated experience. Those who study medical records should write in note form, as every medical case comprises the beginning, development and end. There are all sorts of varieties and clues in the records. You can investigate special effects of certain drugs on certain diseases, like the effect of Herba Artemisiae Scopariae Yin Chen Hao 茵陳蒿 on treating jaundice and Radix Dichroae Chang Shan 常山 on treating malaria. This is the right way forward for people to study Chinese medicine.

Article end

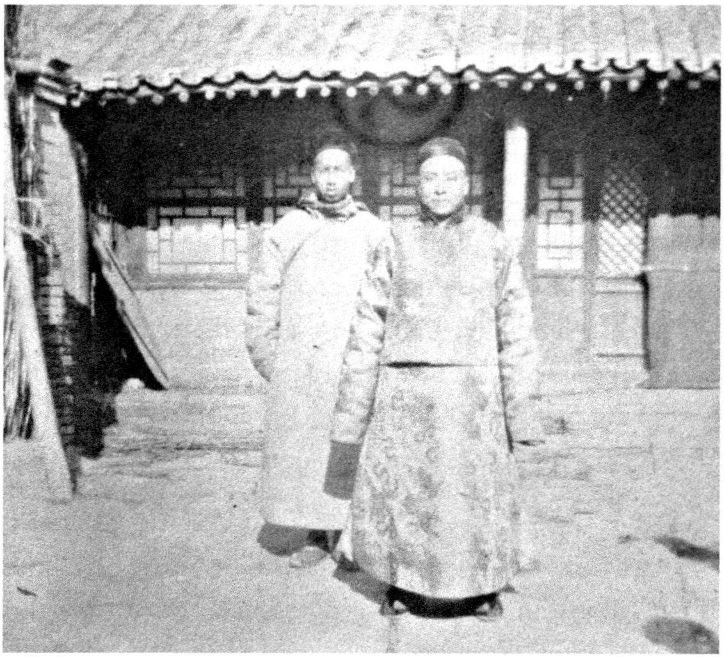

Photo by Mr P. Goux in early 1900s. "Mandarin from Tien Tsin Shien".

Chinese medicine doctors thereafter

By Ye Jingqiu 葉勁秋

Source: *Compilation of Discussions about Chinese Medical Education* 中醫教育討論集

Yaron: Sean Lei states:[115] "Although practitioners of Chinese medicine were pursuing professional interests newly created by the state, they were not simply being forced to accept policies issued by the state. On the contrary, they actively participated in initiating, negotiating, and even designing the policies, regulations and reform programs for Chinese medicine... One crucial finding of this study is that their scholarly efforts of reforming Chinese medicine were inseparable from their political objective of assimilating Chinese medicine into the state."

Lei goes on to explain that Chinese medicine practitioners at that time served, in reality, as agents of the state, helping the state to reach deeper into rural areas. This is a fine observation helping us to understand the dynamics surrounding Chinese medicine and it can be seen clearly in this article.

[115] *Neither Donkey Nor Horse,* Page 263, Sean Hsiang Lin-Lei, University of Chicago Press.

Pages 512–517

Assuming that there are enough graduated medical doctors to be assigned to every village in the country, still no immediate changes can take effect in the current condition of our healthcare system. This is related to the collective intellect and economical situation of our society. Although Chinese herbs could be expensive, they are still much cheaper than visiting a Western medicine doctor, considering the high consultation fees of Western medicine doctors and high costs for different kinds of tests: blood tests, stool tests and all sorts of scanning. What's more, you have to pay extra for an injection and for other medical equipment. It is best if you are healed from undergoing all these tests. However, in reality, they are of not much use. Nothing can be diagnosed from these test results. The situation becomes even worse if the reports from two different doctors do not match.

In contrast, Chinese medicine doctors don't need to conduct any tests whatsoever. All they do is prescribe some herbs, and the illness that has wrestled us for years will inexplicably be gone. Such cases are not rare. Considering this impact of Chinese medicine, it is impossible for Western medicine to take over Chinese medicine overnight. The common medical knowledge that the majority of people hold has passed down over the past centuries. Repulsion and resentment will arise if these concepts and ideas were to be replaced with modern context.

For instance, patients will accuse the doctor of misconduct if he tries to undress the patient for examination. Patients may also blame the doctor for any unpleasant feelings or accidents caused by minor surgeries, anesthesia or acupuncture. Some may ask, should we then allow our medical standards to continue to deteriorate this way? No! Absolutely not! The improvement of medical standards in our country relies entirely on the government power and collective intellect. So when exactly will we see the improvement? This depends on the concentration degree of political power and the extent of growth in collective intelligence. Let's say that the authorities did a great advocacy job and so the collective intellect grows exponentially, then the wait time will be shortened. Otherwise, it will be extended. No matter how long we have to wait, we will attain the goal someday. This is so called a natural selection; the better one prevails and the weaker diminishes.

Not long ago, the provincial government sent officials to advocate hygiene and sanitation in rural areas. Not only did the villagers turn them down, but they sneered at them until they all left embarrassed. "You are all so young and have no idea how things work. Why don't you just go home, have a bottle of soda water and enjoy a scoop of icecream? For us villagers, it is nothing special to have dozens of flies or other insects ingested. We befriended them. Have you ever seen any of us die from infectious disease?" This is what the villagers told the officials. Many people nowadays still share the same opinion. Even though the phenomenon can be explained by immunology, citizens of a civilized country should not adopt such a living style. The majority of sickness and deaths are due to unhygienic habits of the villagers. Thus, it is unreasonable to accuse people of poking their nose into others' business. From cases like this, we should realize that advocating hygiene and sanitation is not as easy and straightforward as it seems.

Because of living environment and habits, Chinese people can easily relate to Chinese medicine. They have a lot of opportunity to come into contact with Chinese medicine. Thus, Chinese medicine doctors play an important role in improving public health and they should act as health leaders. They have to rectify the misconceptions and fallacies held by the general public, by instilling proper knowledge into them bit by bit. As time goes by, all humiliation that Chinese medicine once suffered will be water under the bridge. This grave responsibility rests on the shoulder of all Chinese medicine doctors. Our colleagues should not belittle the importance of your role.

Some people may worry about the life span of Chinese medicine. This is because they know nothing about medical science. The effect of Chinese medicine can never be substituted. Without doubt, science will continue to make progress and scientific analysis will go more and more in depth. Nonetheless, Chinese Materia Medica has its unique characteristics and functions that synthetic drugs cannot replace. There are surely advantages in both kinds of medicine. Western medicine doctors are desperate to isolate the active ingredients in a drug, and then examine them one by one. The most prominent effect of one ingredient would then be taken as the major drug action. However, several questions will arise. What would be the drug action if the prominent effect of one ingredient is combined with a minor one? Can we predict the action of a drug from its most prominent effect when one ingredient is combined with other ingredients? And is it possible that a crude drug with multiple active ingredients can actually counteract the side effects? The answers to those questions can affirm the infinite possibilities and value of Chinese Materia Medica.

Not only leading scholars, even Chinese medicine doctors see all too clearly that Chinese medicine theories have become nothing but worthless and obsolete antiques which will only end up on the shelf. When Sun Ke 孫科, Feng Yuxiang 馮玉祥 and other scholars proposed to include Chinese medicine into the educational system, I wrote an article, published in the "Future Education" column of *Tian Jin Da Gong Bao* 天津大公報 to express my opposition. The article was quoted in several medical journals thereafter such as *Yi Yao Ping Lun* 醫藥評論, *Zhong Xi Yi Yao* 中西醫藥 and *Yi Jie Chun Qiu* 醫界春秋. Here is my conclusion: "Education and our country's constitutional development are so closely related that one wrong move will actually affect the whole game. We must review thoroughly the character of Chinese medicine. As for the education of Chinese medicine, we should first develop a comprehensive system of Chinese medicine or else it will become very difficult to recruit teachers, prepare teaching materials and examine academic theories. It will only cause distress if we merely focus on the end without considering the means."

Now let's look at the tentative curriculum of Chinese Medical School announced by the Ministry of Education (refer to the Education column on 4th and 5th of June, 1939 of *Shen Bao* 申報教育欄). Are Chinese medical subjects included? Although they are called Chinese Medicine Schools Zhong Yi Xue Xiao 中醫學校, they are actually the same when compared with Western Medical Schools. All we have to do is add a few lectures on Chinese medicine in the curriculum of Western medicine. However, to create a new branch in medical science is not a legitimate decision.

Chinese medicine doctors thereafter have no other choices but to embrace science, including subjects like physiology, anatomy, pathology, pharmacology and diagnosis. This is a must. We should include scientific examination in our diagnosis and we should adopt every possible method in treatment. Undoubtedly, Chinese medical formulae still retain a certain value. On one hand, it is wrong for Western medicine doctors to disparage the effect of Chinese herbal medicines. On the other hand, neither should Chinese medicine doctors overrate their efficacy. An average Chinese medicine doctor normally uses no more than a hundred types of herbs. They combine them into different formulas to treat diseases. This is why many people say that Chinese medicine doctors are treating diseases from the root while Western medicine doctors are merely tackling the symptoms.

I may have to elaborate a little on this. The state when there is absence of disease is considered physiologically normal, which depends on a balance between different parts of the body. From time to time, we may encounter some external stimulation (including summerheat, cold, joy or anger). We then rely on the homeostasis of our body. We have all sorts of inborn mechanisms to prevent us from falling ill. We develop diseases when we cannot adapt to external stimulation. In Chinese medicine, it is rare to have one formula devised specifically for only one disease. Common principles of treatment include "exterior-releasing", "downward-draining", "qi-supplementing" and "blood-nourishing". Chinese medicine doctors do not focus on separated parts of your body. Instead, they focus on the human body as a whole. For instance, symptoms in the ears and eyes can be caused by liver and kidney vacuity or wounds on the skin can be due to liver fire blazing. This is also why people say that Chinese medicine doctors can treat diseases from the root. In fact, Western medicine doctors are also treating the root of a disease by identifying the pathogens and pointing out the cause of the disease. No matter what, Chinese medicine doctors will have to gradually alter their way of practice both physically and psychologically in the future. They will not continue to do what they are doing today. As time elapses, the words "Chinese medicine doctors" would only be seen in history books.

What Chinese medicine doctors can and should do is build rural hospitals across the country. This is a matter of utmost importance. I have written to Mr Chen Guofu 陳果夫, the governor of Jiangsu Province, a few years ago. Here is an extract of my proposal:

> God is casting misfortune on China, causing numerous disasters here. People are suffering. They are in desperate need of subsidies, food and clothing. It becomes very difficult to provide preventive healthcare to them and the best option is to construct urgently rural hospitals all over the country. Use in them good native drugs to treat with modern methods to diagnose and deal with emergency and infectious diseases. For thousands of years, our people had strong faith in our traditional herbs, for they can be found everywhere. If we can make use of the readily available materials, not only can we provide a place for pharmacologists to do research and practice, but we can also benefit people living in rural areas. The main arguments are as follows:
>
> First, China ranks among the top in the world for supply of our native herbs. We have accumulated numerous efficacious formulas in the past thousands of years. It is such a shame if they

gradually die out or if other people take over them and introduce them to the world.

Second, we have to improve our agricultural practices before we can improve our country. It is definitely not a blessing to our country when peasants are suffering hardship. Building more hospitals is the only way out.

Third, people who are living in poverty can hardly receive any fruits of our development in public health. Our country has long been fighting for social welfare. Thus, we should build hospitals all around the country so that everyone can benefit.

Fourth, we should, without qualm, assimilate new knowledge from time to time. We should also be aware that what we have learnt in the past is not a hundred percent indisputable. The key is to maintain a balance between the two. Medical science is categorized as natural science, where experiments are carried out all the time. Therefore, we should build more hospitals so that they can be used to conduct related academic investigation. However, much equipment is required to set up a Western medicine hospital. It will be a major hurdle to build hospitals everywhere. Often, only one or two are built even after investing a lot of effort and only the affluent people living in the city can enjoy the service. People will become increasingly superstitious if rural medicine gets more and more popular. Hence, for the sake of rural patients as well as the development of preventive healthcare, we should build rural hospitals all over the country.

As for the cost, we should first discuss this matter at the National Economic Council. We can also appropriate certain amount of money from public expenditure, solicit funds from other sources, or allot the cost from public health, national security and public welfare expenses. As for the organization of the hospital, the wards should be separated into three classes. There should be 100 beds in class A ward, 50 in class B and 10 in class

C. Doctors should determine whether the patient should be admitted into the hospital according to the number of consulting patients. There has been no such practice before. We should make such decisions based on the practicality and utilization of resources. Only in this way can we meet local demand and, at the same time, be consistent with national conditions. Chinese medicine has a long history. It is a pity that it is all based on hypothetical theories. If we continue to follow the footsteps of our ancestors, we will only be walking on a path that leads us to disaster. (I have run a similar hospital 30 years ago in rural areas, and similar articles can be seen on Ru Gao Yi Bao 如皋醫報 some 10 years ago.)

The war has damaged a lot of places and injured many people. The government should start building rural hospitals without any delay. More will be needed to heal the wounded when the country returns to peace. For the good of Chinese medicine and Chinese citizens, it is absolutely essential to build rural hospitals across the country.

Article end

Review of "*How to learn Chinese Medicine Well*" and "*Chinese Medicine Doctors Thereafter*"

By Song Daren 宋大仁[116]

Source: Compilation *of Discussions about Chinese Medical Education* 中醫教育討論集

Yaron: As curriculum-style learning became the standard in Chinese medicine approved schools, the old apprentice system was shutting down. To become a licensed Chinese medicine practitioner, one needed a proper education of a standard curriculum in a registered school.

Variations of opinion and differing notions within Chinese medicine of the past were squeezed down into a unified single path, which ultimately will become the singular path of TCM during the Communist era.

In my opinion, we now have a chance to think again of the good and bad that came out of it and—exactly as they used to say at that time—we need to keep the good and get rid of the bad.

Pages 517–524

Recently, the articles *How to Learn Chinese Medicine* and *Chinese Medicine Doctors Thereafter* written by Ye Jingqiu 葉勁秋 were published in the social service column in *Da Ying Wan Bao* 大英晚報. The points raised in the article are worth debating. Mr Ye is an experienced Chinese medicine doctor who has been teaching in various Chinese medicine schools in Shanghai. A few years ago when I established the Chinese and Western Medicine and Pharmacology Research Society 中西醫藥研究社, Mr Ye was also one of the ordinary members. He then started his research in the Provincial Medical Administration College 省立醫政學院. He doesn't hesitate to point out any mischief within the Chinese medicine community in a direct way, regardless of social

[116] Song Daren 宋大仁 (1907–1985) was born in Macau and arrived in Shanghai in 1924. Studied in Shanghai Chinese Medicine Specialized School 上海中醫專門學校 with Ding Ganren 丁甘仁. He graduated from the 8th class and helped author several books, including Medical Cases of Mr. Ding 丁氏医案 and the Shanghai Chinese Medicine Specialized School Graduation Commemoration publication 上海中医专门学校毕业纪念刊. 1927–1932 part-worked part-studied Western medicine in Shanghai Dongnan Medical School 上海東南醫學院. Received Bachelor of Modern Medicine, graduating with the 6th class. Served as a doctor in the same hospital in the Gastrointestinal department and at the same time served as professor in Shanghai Chinese Medicine College 上海中醫學院 and was shouldering the clinical teaching responsibility for Western and Chinese medicines. In 1933 became a member in the Japanese Digestive Organs Disease Association 日本國消化器病學會會員. In 1935 Chinese and Western Medicine and Pharmacology Research Society 中西醫藥研究社 formed and he served as executive manager. He was the chief editor of Chinese and Western Medicine and Pharmacology Periodicals 中西医药期刊, which has become one of the 9 major medical associations of the country exercising vast influence in the entire country. In 1937 Song established Gastrointestinal hospital in Shanghai. He was a celebrated GI specialist and often advocated the use of Western drugs with Chinese herbs.

status or relationships with others. His articles are generally accurate, though some places can cause misinterpretation. I would now like to bring them up for discussion. Below are some of my opinions, to which I think Mr Ye would also agree.

As practicing Chinese medicine doctors, we should not ignore the feelings of our patients. However, we should base our diagnosis and treatment on academic research. It is unreasonable to pander to our patients and not treat them seriously. Due to differences in the traditional culture, being a Chinese medicine doctor is very different from being a Western doctor. When dealing with obstinate and stubborn patients, or patients without any professional knowledge, you have no choice but to tell them something like qi-regulating, dampness-regulating and phlegm-transforming. The actual prescription, though, is still based on science. This is not wrong, and it can also prevent people criticizing you. However, you cannot do the same if it is someone knowledgeable and with a clear mind. You have to explain to them in detail and educate them. Otherwise, you might unintentionally become a barrier to the medical revolution.

Because of political corruption, education in China cannot be made universal and the majority of people from different social class in modern China still hold incorrect concepts that have been passed down in the past thousands of years. Therefore, every patient has more or less formulated their own view: they will tell you when to calm the Liver, dispel the dampness, regulate the qi or transform the phlegm. This is quite annoying when you are practicing. If you do something that is contrary to what the patient thought, he will totally lose faith in you. How about doing what they ask you to do? You will then have to do things that are against your conscience. What can you do then? Even though this is an inevitable phenomenon during the transition period, Chinese medicine doctors should bear some responsibility. If all Chinese medicine doctors are like Mr Ye and we are committed to fight the hardship together, then patients would still consult Chinese medicine doctors when they are sick. Then, the success of Chinese medicine doctors depends entirely on the level of their own academic ability. And so, it is acceptable to please patients, as long as you prescribe according to your own diagnosis. On the other hand, practicing according to the patients' will would be against the moral code, and anyone who does this shall not deserve to be called a doctor.

It is the educational problem of the entire society that causes people, living in rural areas, to reject preventive care education. When politics and other disciplines are not on track, it is impossible for an educational campaign to be successful. People living in rural areas do not believe in bacteria—the fact is that they know nothing about it. Indeed, they may not develop diseases even after they consume a considerable amount of flies, but according to Western medicine doctors, if one has gastric juice with exceptionally low pH, the person may not develop diseases even if they are infected by the bacteria. Yet, one cannot predict the strength of one's gastric juices. We should not jump immediately to the conclusion that this is an immunology principle just because one or two cases arise occasionally. Flies are surely vectors of diseases, but the amount of bacteria they carry varies. Let's say the amount of bacteria it carries is minimal—it may cause no harm to the host even if the person consumes the fly. Even so, bacteria are undoubtedly one of the pathogens of infectious diseases. Although precipitating factors are involved sometimes, no infectious disease can be caused without the invasion of bacteria, no matter how cold it is or how weak our immune system is. Hence, we should explain to people in detail whenever they raise their doubts during our advocacy. Only if we explain the underlying principle clearly can we truly educate them. I have seen many promoting officials lecturing the public in an affirmative tone but without mentioning any evidence or whatsoever to support their arguments. Such an attitude would only induce resentment and is not at all conducive. I admire the missionaries for their preaching skills. Their effect is amazing. They can alter the deeply rooted beliefs of ordinary people and convert them into firm believers of God. We should definitely learn from them.

It is not difficult to be a Chinese medicine doctor. All you have to do is read some books, like *Tang Tou Ge Jue* 湯頭歌訣, *Ben Cao Cong Xin* 本草從新 and *Lin Zheng Zhi Nan* 臨症指南, and then you can call yourself a doctor. Others would not deny that either. Nevertheless, for Chinese medicine doctors thereafter, a minimum requirement should be established. Mr Ye mentioned that any Chinese medicine doctors thereafter have no other choice but to embrace science, including subjects like physiology, anatomy, pathology, pharmacology and diagnosis. We must include scientific evidence in diagnosis and we should use every possible way to treat. Now that the Ministry of Education has announced the curriculum of Chinese Medicine Schools, which also incorporates various disciplines of the modern medical science, advocates of medical reform like us would absolutely endorse such a change. Nonetheless, when it actually comes into effect, problems may arise. Should we re-examine those Chinese medicine doctors currently in practice? And should we provide supplementary lectures to them so that they can attain the expected standard of practice? Those are questions for health care administrators to answer. Let's put them aside for now.

Chinese medicine doctors used to treat according to the symptoms. Diseases names diagnosed using scientific methods are nowhere to be found in Chinese medical books. Despite having a definite modern diagnosis, we still have no idea which herbs to use when it comes to treating the disease. There still isn't any book that explains the treatment using Chinese herbal medicine based on scientific principle. Whether you learn your knowledge of Chinese medicine in professional schools or through mentorship, those dated manuscripts are no longer applicable. Many formulae recorded in those manuscripts are ineffective. It is difficult to set up guidelines regarding the selection and application of these formulae. Compiling a textbook of "Chinese medicine therapeutics" is part of the literature rearrangement plan; we should treat it seriously. However, it was only started recently and this job requires collective effort. Apart from knowledge of different academic subjects, they should also be taught skills of doing literature review. This way, they can help challenge the status quo of Chinese medicine by making use of their scientific knowledge. If what they have learnt cannot merge with science, though the knowledge will be useful in clinical practice, they are still prescribing according to their own instinct instead of scientific evidence. It is then only a futile attempt to include physiology, pathology and other such courses into the curriculum. Originally, Chinese medicine should have been only a department in medical schools. All they had to do is organize lectures from time to time and do research on Chinese medicine. Only because of stubborn requests from people in the Chinese medicine sector did the government decide to allow separate Chinese Medicine Schools. This is only a transitional measure and it has already caused a lot of problems.

Since the enforcement of the Chinese Medicine Ordinance, Chinese medicine doctors have enjoyed a secure profession. It is no longer a problem for them to make a living. What's more, the Ministry of Education has recently published the standard curriculum for the program in Chinese medicine. All these suggest that the government does not hold prejudice against Chinese medicine. Now that Chinese medicine doctors enjoy equal legal status with Western medicine doctors, they are certainly obliged to promote public health. Instead of obstinately placing themselves at the opposite side impeding the progress of society, they should bear our responsibilities and fight with us together. Although there is still no clear regulation as to whether the system of apprenticeship should be abolished, such a system should be repealed sooner or later as apprentices cannot gain comprehensive knowledge and it would be difficult to obtain a practicing license that way.

From now on, the only way for those who would like to learn Chinese medicine is to receive education from Chinese medicine schools that are established and approved by the government and teach according to the standard curriculum, in order to learn about Western medical knowledge as well as traditional Chinese medical skills. In the future, people will not distinguish between a Western doctor and a Chinese one. If there were any differences between the two, it will only be in the application of drugs. One uses herbs while the other uses synthetic drugs. As time goes by, Western and Chinese medicine doctors will converge and people will not be able to distinguish the two. These new Chinese medicine doctors will no longer be picked on, as what they do has become more reasonable and detached from superstitious beliefs. As for those Chinese medicine doctors who are already practicing, they should at least know the basics of the new scientific medical theories. Otherwise, they would not be able to compete against the new Chinese medicine doctors and would inevitably be eliminated.

Now, I have attached a book list at the end of this passage, containing the books that I think are useful and easy to read. After finishing those, there are still tens of thousands of great books for you to read. You can select any book of your choice, focus on topics that you find interesting and move on to more advanced-level books after you have finished those at the beginner level. Or else, you might be frustrated when you cannot understand the content of the textbook when you first enter medical school. Every Chinese medicine doctor will know which kind of Chinese medical books to read first and would not need someone like me to comment. But I still have one more piece of advice: read more books on Chinese medicinal formulas and don't make mystery out of things. This way, we won't be stuck in superstitious beliefs and share the fate of our predecessors.

I have already mentioned the track that Chinese medicine doctors thereafter should take and I can just end here. However, there are still a few comments in Mr. Ye's writings which I found questionable and worth discussing. Mr. Ye mentioned that, "it is wrong for Western medicine doctors to disparage the effect of Chinese herbal medicine." This is what happened twenty to thirty years ago, but not anymore. Aren't there a lot of locally manufactured drugs among the new drugs? Ephedrine,

Eumenol, Sinomenine, Zinomin and Ginsenin are some examples. Those that are made locally include Ephedrinae, Pacdin, Omensal, Fancnol, Polygasol, Simalin, Gimlnor and Antihustin. These are all scientifically made Chinese medicine products commonly used by modern doctors. So how can this be considered as "disparaging the effect of Chinese herbal medicine"?

The crude drugs of Chinese Materia Medica have complicated ingredients; some may overlap with others. Without scientific research on their active ingredients and refinement by sophisticated scientific methods, their content will be inconsistent. If we cannot determine how many active ingredients are present in every gram of drug, we cannot use them any way we want. One more point that Mr Ye might have missed: the majority of Chinese medicine prescriptions are in the form of decoction. Nonetheless, many active ingredients in the Materia Medica are insoluble in water. Or the ingredients are chemically altered when they are heated. As such, even though the herbs are proven effective under scientific investigation, they might not be as effective when applied clinically. It is simply impossible for Chinese herbal medicines to exert their full effect in decoction form.

Mr Ye said that it is much more expensive to consult a Western medicine doctor than a Chinese one considering the consultation, medication and laboratory testing fees. However, new Chinese medicine doctors from now on will also adopt scientific diagnosis. In such a case, all sorts of expenses will also apply. We should be aware of the importance of scientific examination in diagnosis. This is an important step that cannot be skipped. Not only bacterial and parasitic diseases require medical tests for us to understand their pathogenesis, many other diseases also require a series of blood tests and urine tests before we can come up with a conclusion. One complete examination only costs you no more than a few dollars. In contrast, if Chinese medicine doctors diagnose using outdated diagnostics and treat using miscellaneous drugs, even if it causes no great harm, the expenses resulting from prolonged treatment would have been hundred times more than the original fee for modern medical tests, to say the least of it. It is worse if the disease is still not cured after paying all these fees.

I still remember Zhang Jianhou 張劍侯, the news editor of the *Evening Voice Ye Bao Ye Sheng* 夜報夜聲, has written the following short passage named *The death of my daughter Xiangying* 翔英: "I have learnt a lesson after the death of Xiangying—do not hesitate to consult a Western medicine doctor and conduct any necessary medical tests, whether that be X-ray examinations, blood tests or stool tests, especially when you have persistent fever. You should find out the cause of the disease, and then treat it with appropriate drugs, no matter whether you are using Chinese medicine or Western medicine." After reading this, I felt sorry. There is no better way to remind people by publishing the article. If the patient cannot afford different kinds of expenses, they would not be able to afford the consultation fee or medication fee either even if it only costs one dollar or few cents. The only solution is to build more hospitals and offer free medical service. This has already become the problem of the entire society.

The most important thing that should be done right now is to construct rural hospitals all around the country. Sadly, no one has committed to do such a thing. We do have charities establishing hospitals, but those are only Chinese medicine hospitals of poor quality. They spend a substantial amount of money on providing free consultation and medication every year. (However, nearly none of them take notice of rural areas.) Many of the physicians that work in these hospitals lack experience and knowledge. Some charities even hand out leaflets printed with Chinese medicinal formulas to patients and encourage them to try! This is totally inappropriate. They themselves don't even know whether those formulas are effective or not. Even though some may work in treating diseases like stomachache, diarrhea and vomiting once in a while, the disease causes still haven't been identified. Even if these formulas cause no harm, they may have already impeded the required treatment. This is something we all try to avoid.

Mr Ye hopes that Chinese medicine doctors in the future can participate more in the work of rural hospitals, which is wonderful indeed. Nevertheless, they should be meticulous and diagnose in compliance with principles of science. As for the treatment, they should also use modern drugs and not only decoctions, pills and powder. Only then can Chinese medicine help promote healthcare development in China. As for the organization of wards, class C wards should be equipped with the most number of beds, followed by class B and A. According to living standard of rural areas, hospitals situated there should reserve more rooms for poor patients. Urban hospitals are organized this way, so should rural hospitals. Yet Mr Ye suggests that class A wards should have the most number of beds, and class C the least. I find this unreasonable, but he doesn't elaborate on the rationale behind it.

Reference book list:

Title	Author/translator	Publisher
Basic Biology *Zhong Xue Sheng Li Wei Sheng Xue* 中學生理衛生學	Shangwu 商務 Zhonghua 中華 Shijie世界	Kaiming 開明
Principles of Physiology *Sheng Wu Xue Yuan Li* 生物學原理	Translated by Yu Xiaosong 余小宋	Shangwu 商務
Physiology *Sheng Li Xue* 生理學	Xue De 薛德	Shijie 世界
General Anatomy and Physiology 普通解生理學	Li Fujing 李賦京	Zhongguo Kexue Gongsi 中國科學公司
General Embryology *Pu Tong Pi Tai Xue* 普通胚胎學	Wu Yuandi 吳元滌	Shijie 世界
Human and Organisms *Ren Yu Sheng Wu* 人與生物	Jia Zuzhang 賈祖璋 and others	Kaiming 開明
Highlights in Biology *Sheng Wu Xue Yao Lan* 生物學要覽	Wang Rulin 王儒林	Zhonghua 中華
Miracle in Life *Sheng Ming Zhi Qi Ji* 生命之奇蹟	Xu Dalian 許達年	Zhonghua 中華
Science and Life *Ke Xue Yu Ren Sheng* 科學與人生	You Jiazhang 尤佳章	Shangwu 商務
A Scientific View *Ke Xue Guan* 科學觀	Wang Guangxi 王光熙 and others	Shangwu 商務
Slosson's Science Compilation *Si Shi Ke Xue Cong Tan* 斯氏科學叢談	You Jiazhang 尤佳章	Shangwu 商務
Interesting Chemical Stories *Hua Xue Qi Tan* 化學奇談	Gu Junzheng 顧均正	Kaiming 開明
New Realm of Physics *Wu Li Xue Zhi Xin Jing Jie* 物理學之新境界	Gao Shuke 高孰可	Shangwu 商務
Introduction to Theoretical Physics *Li Lun Wu Li Xue Chu Bu* 理論物理學初步	Pan Zuwu 潘祖武	Shangwu 商務
Chemistry and Modern Life *Hua Xue Yu Jin Dai Sheng Huo* 化學與近代生活	Zhu Renhong 朱任宏	Shangwu 商務
Outline of Physical Chemistry *Wu Li Hua Xue Da Gang* 物理化學大綱	Wu Fu 伍甫	Shangwu 商務
Biology in Everyday Life *Ri Yong Sheng Wu Xue* 日用生物學	Wu Fu 伍甫	Shangwu 商務
Physics in the Modern World *Jin Dai Wu Li Xue* 近代物理學	Zheng Taipu 鄭太朴	Shangwu 商務

Principle of Science *Ke Xue Yuan Li* 科學原理	Zhou Fangong 周梵公	Shangwu 商務
Bacteria and Human *Xi Jun Yu Ren* 細菌與人	Gao Shiqi 高士其	Kaiming 開明
Supplementary Teaching Material on Natural Science *Zi Ran Bu Chong Jiao Cai* 自然補充教材	Xu Yunzhao 許允昭	Zhonghua 中華
Self-learning Package of Chemistry Laboratory *Zi Xue Fu Dao Hua XueShi Yan Fa* 自學輔導化學實驗法	Cai Song 蔡松	Zhonghua 中華

Above are some books on natural science.

Medical Series *Yi Xue Xiao Cong Shu* 醫學小叢書	Available on different subjects	Shangwu 商務
Introduction to Medical Science *Yi Xue Gai Shuo* 醫學概說	Xu Dalian 許達年	Zhonghua 中華
Basic Medical Science *Yi Xue Chang Shi* 醫學常識	Tao Chisun 陶熾孫	Beixin 北新
Medicine and Health *Yi Xue Yu Wei Sheng* 醫學與衛生	Hong Shi 洪式	Xinya 新亞
Public Health Physiology/ Symptoms/ Emergencies *Da Zhong Yi Xue Sheng Li Pian Zheng Hou Pian Jiu Ji Pian* 大眾醫學－生理篇 症候篇 救急篇	Gu Shoubai 顧壽白	Kaiming 開明
Introduction to Chinese and Western Drugs *Zhong Xi Ying Yong Yao Wu Chang Shi* 中西應用藥物常識	Gu Xueqiu 顧學裘	Kaiming 開明
Introduction to Pharmaceutical Chemistry *Yi Yao Hua Xue Gai Lun* 醫藥化學概論	Gu Xueqiu 顧學裘 and others	Kaiming 開明
Clinical Diagnosis *Zheng Hou Zhen Duan Lu* 症候診斷錄	Wang Zhihua 王秩華	Wuding Gongsi 五定公司
Nursing in Modern Life *Xian Dai Kan Hu Xue* 現代看護學	Edited by Ding Huikang 丁惠康	Shangwu 商務
Practical Nursing on Infectious Disease *Chuan Ran BingShi Yong Kan Hu Fa* 傳染病實用看護法		Xiehe Hospital of Beijing 北平協和醫院
Organic Medicinal and Pharmaceutical Chemistry *Yao Ying YouJi Hua Xue* 藥用有機化學	Gu Xueqiu 顧學裘	Shangwu 商務
Introduction to Genetics *Yi Chuan Xue Qian Shuo* 遺傳學淺說	Chen Jianshan 陳兼善	Zhonghua 中華
Medicine and Human *Ren Yu Yi Xue* 人與醫學	Gu Qianji 顧謙吉	Shangwu 商務
Physiotherapy *Wu Li Liao Fa* 物理療法		Zhonghua 中華

Above are books on new medicine.

History of Medicine *Yi Xue Shi Hua* 醫學史話	Mu Shaoliang 沐紹良	Shangwu 商務
China's Medicine and Pharmaceutical Scientific Discussion *Zhong Guo Yi Yao Ke Xue Tao Lun* 中國醫藥科學討論	Zhang Zihe 張子鶴	Zhongguo Kexue Tushu Gongsi 中國科學圖書公司
Commentary on Zhongjing's Shang Han Lun *Zhong Jing Shang Han Lun Ping Yi* 仲景傷寒論評譯	Yan Derun 閻德潤	Wuding Gongsi, Shanghai 上海五定公司
Criticism of the Feudal Medicine of the Han Dynasty *Huang Han Yi Xue Pi Ping* 皇漢醫學批評	Yu Yunxiu 余雲岫	Wuding Gongsi 五定公司
The Meaning of Febrile Disease *Wen Re Fa Hui* 溫熱發揮	Yu Yunxiu 余雲岫	Wuding Gongsi 五定公司
The Medical Revolution of Mr. Yu *Yu Shi Yu Xue Ge Ming Lun* 余氏醫學革命論	Yu Yunxiu 余雲岫	Wuding Gongsi 五定公司
Explaining Medical Terminology *Shi Ming Bing Shi* 釋名病釋	Yu Yunxiu 余雲岫	Wuding Gongsi 五定公司
Six Medical Texts of Xu and Xi *Xu Xi Yi Xue Liu Zhong* 徐溪醫學六種	Xu Lingtai 徐靈胎	Available at major bookstores
Collection of Discussions on the Scientification of Chinese Medicine *Zhong Yi Ke Xue Hua Wen Ti Tao Lun Ji* 中醫科學化問題討論集	Song Daren 宋大仁 and others	Association of Chinese and Western Medicine Investigation
Collection of China's Medical Treatises *Zhong Guo Yi Xue Yi Shu Lun Ji* 中國醫學藝術論集	Song Daren 宋大仁 and others	Association of Chinese and Western Medicine Investigation
Chinese and Western Drugs with Annotations *Zhong Xi Yi Yao He Ding Ben* 中西醫藥合訂本	Volume one, two and three	Association of Chinese and Western Medicine Investigation

Above books are for further study.

If you have skimmed through the above books and wish to investigate even further, you can continue on the *Medical Series* 醫學小叢書 published by Shangwu 商務, Zhonghua 中華 or other great books by private publishers. This way, I hope readers won't get lost in that large amount of books and the reference book list can serve as a guide when you don't know where to begin.

Article end

The Constitution of the Association of Chinese and Western Medicine Research

Source: *Compilation of Discussions about Chinese Medical Education* 中醫教育討論集

Pages 525–529

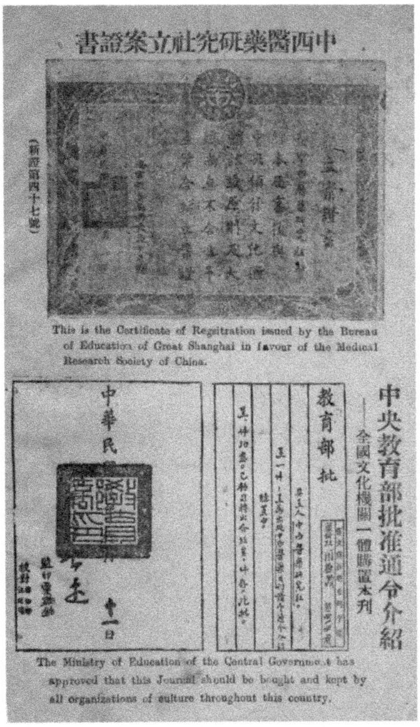

"The Medical Research Society of China Certificate of Registration". This society published the collection of articles we have translated.

(Last amended in June 1937 by 2nd Council)

ARTICLE I: GENERAL

1) The name of the Association shall be "The Association of Chinese and Western Medicine Research Zhong Xi Yi Yao Yan Jiu She 中西醫藥研究社"

2) The aims of the Association shall be:

    a. To unite talents in Chinese and Western medicine for organizing literature in Chinese medicine using scientific methods.

    b. To discuss medical-related issues based on facts and truths without bias.

c. To promote common knowledge of medicine and hygiene, promote the progress of Chinese medicine scientification, and promote healthcare and sanitation of our society.

3) The head office of the Association shall be in Shanghai.

ARTICLE II: MEMBERSHIP

1) The Association shall consist of the following four types of members:

A. Associate members 社友. Associate members shall be persons from the medical community who are interested in the purposes of the Association, and are approved by the Council.

B. Members 社員. Members shall be persons who have met the one of the requirements described below and are approved by the Council.

a. Prior status as an Associate member for at least two years, has published reports occasionally or served the Association actively.

b. Graduated from a medical school, or possesses certificate issued by the government allowing medical practice.

Those who have met the above requirements shall hand in a thesis. There is no restriction on the topic. However, the thesis shall be related to medicine or pharmacology.

C. Fellows 基本社員. Fellows shall be Members of the Association who have met one of the requirements described below.

a. Prior status as a Member for at least five years, publish thesis occasionally, and approved by the Council.

b. Distinguished scholars in either Chinese or Western medicine, published thesis that are specially recognized, recommended by two of our Executive Committees or Members and are approved by the Council.

D. Patron members 贊助社員. Patron members are persons who are experienced in medical business or skills, made extraordinary contribution to the Association, recommended by two of our Executive Committees or Members and are approved by the Council.

2)

a. In applying for membership, applicants shall submit to the Association completed application forms, resumes, and three passport photos of 2x2 inches, and shall pay entrance fees of ten dollars and annual membership fees of five dollars. Those who are applying in autumn shall only have to pay half of the annual membership fee. Incomplete application shall not proceed.

b. For Members and Associate Members who have paid fifteen dollars annually for at least four consecutive years shall be exempted from paying any membership fee thereafter.

3) All members, after the approval of the Council, shall be given a letter of accreditation and subsequently an official certificate of membership after two years, when they have paid the certificate fee of two dollars. Associate members shall be given a certificate of associate membership at no additional charge.

4) All members of the Association shall enjoy the following privileges:

a. To attend General Meetings of the Association.

b. To elect, propose and speak in General Meetings.

c. To be elected, vote and veto (Not eligible to Associate friends)

d. To enjoy all facilities provided by the Association; and to authorize the Association to assist in doing literature review.

e. To apply for the assistance of the Association in case of business dispute.

f. To enjoy free subscription of one publication and a discounted price for other publications of the Association.

5) All members of the Association shall carry the following obligations:

a. To abide by this Constitution and the resolutions of the Council; and to assist the operation of the Association.

b. To advocate the purpose of the Association and to actively recruit new members.

c. To pay the annual membership fee accordingly.

d. To assist and write articles for the publications of the Association.

e. To report academic or research findings and from time to time local medical conditions.

6) All members who satisfy one of the following conditions shall have their membership terminated, upon the approval of the Council:

a. Resign his/her membership.

b. Do not fulfill his/her obligations deliberately for at least one year.

c. Damage the integrity of the Association.

d. Acting to oppose the revolution.

e. Being deprived of civil rights.

ARTICLE III: ORGANIZATION AND FUNCTIONS

7) The General Meeting shall be the sovereign organ of the Association. Its power shall include those described below:

a. To evaluate and decide on the policy of the Association.

b. To consider and adopt the Budget and financial report of the Association.

c. To pass amendments of the Constitution and present new Executive Committee members.

d. To approve proposals from the Council or from members.

e. To approve ideas on fund raising.

f. To decide on affairs that cannot be resolved by the Council.

8) The Council shall be the executive body of the General Meeting. The council shall be formed by nine to eleven Executive Committees appointed by the Association. Three Committees selected as Standing Committees by the Council will execute resolutions of the General Meeting or Council Meetings, attend to the work of the Association and represent the Association. The term of office of Standing Committee shall be two years, which can be renewed when re-elected.

9) At least two months before the expiration of the Council's term of office, five to seven members shall be selected as Election Committee who shall draft a list with

names that is double the number of those elected and then a secret ballot shall be held. Nominees with the highest numbers of votes shall be elected. The following five nominees which receive less number of votes shall fill the vacant position in due order.

10) The Council shall include the office of General Affairs, which comprises the division of secretary, accounting, general administration and investigation. If necessary, extra standing Committees shall be selected by the Council among the Executive Committees to handle daily operation of the Association. Its organization, constitution and regulations shall be drafted by the Council.

11) The Council shall include various specialty committees. Members who have a specialty shall be selected as committee members to assist in the research, examination and publications issues of the Association.

12) The Association shall include the Board of Directors. Its constitution shall be drafted by the Board of Directors.

13) Any branches with more than fifteen members or associate members shall receive a budget equivalent to half of the total annual membership fee paid by the members or associate members at the branch. Its constitution shall be drafted by the Council.

14) A branch office shall be established at any places with members and associate members. Members or associate members may be appointed as local medical inspector. The constitution of a branch office shall be drafted by the Council.

15) The Association may take on medical professionals or professionals from other disciplines as the consultants of the Association.

16) The General Meeting shall be held annually; the date and place thereof shall be announced by the Council with advance notice.

17) The General Meeting shall be held when a quorum of at least half of the members and associate members are present. A proposal shall be passed when over half of the members present a vote for the proposal. When there is a same number voting for and against the proposal, the President shall have the right to make the final decision.

18) If members cannot attend the General Meeting due to business or other reasons, he/she may authorize other members as delegate, and shall notify the Secretariat in advance.

19) The Executive Committee shall hold meetings every three months. The meeting shall be called by Standing Executives. Chairperson of each division shall be present. If necessary, Standing Committee or one third of the Committee members may call an emergency meeting.

20) In the event of emergency, the Executive Committee may call an emergency meeting. If the meeting failed to be called or quorum cannot be formed, the voting shall proceed using letters.

ARTICLE V: FINANCE

21) The funds of the Association shall include Annual Subscription of members and income from Publications. If a large amount of money has to be drawn, the Executive Committee shall vote and decide on the method to collect funds.

ARTICLE VI: PUBLICATIONS

22) Publications of the Association shall include journals and books. Manuscripts thereof shall be approved by the Specialty Committee.

ARTICLE VII: AMENDMENTS

23) In case of any ambiguity in the Constitution, the Executive Committee shall submit an amended draft to the General Meeting. The Constitution shall be amended when the draft is passed at the General Meeting.

24) After the amendment, the Executive Committee shall submit the amended Constitution to the local government office for approval.

Article end

[Book] China's Acupuncture and Moxibustion Science 中國針灸科學

Feb 1934 by Zhou Boqin 周伯勤

Edited by Qin Bowei. Published by: Shanghai Chinese Medicine Publishing House, Published in February 1934. 校刊者秦伯未 出版者上海中醫書局

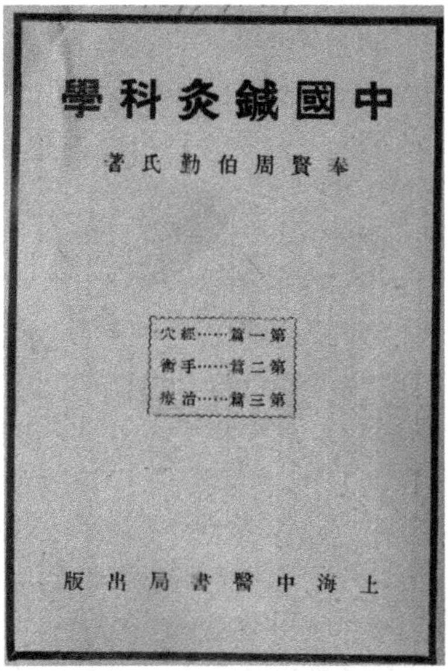

China's Acupuncture and Moxibustion Science title page

Yaron: This book had considerable influence on the practice of Chinese medicine and acupuncture during the Republic and into the Communist era.

A good number of acupuncture techniques and ideas taught in TCM schools today originate in this book or, even when mentioned in earlier books like in his teacher's Cheng Danan 承淡安, they became standard practice in China since the publication of this book. The simplification work, coming two years after Cheng's original acupuncture book, appealed to many.

The New Acupuncture and Moxibustion Study 新針灸學 by comrade Zhu Lian 朱璉, published in 1952, follows and further develops the new trend of acupuncture that sprung up during the Republic and, indeed, with this book here.

Modern scholars at times describe the new acupuncture and TCM as a Communist invention but in reality TCM, the way we know it today, started its "new" development in the Republican years, largely as an urgent response to state pressures and a survival tactic in a modern scientific environment.

This book comprises three chapters: Acupuncture Points; Hand Techniques; and Treatment.

First Preface

Our nation's medical works include an immense number of books. Yet, if you try to research the contents of any one of them, its scope is of mythology and therefore it will seem odd and strange. In order to dishonor disease, I also visited these books, and since my nation's medicine did accumulate several thousand years of experience, not necessarily does it not have any strong points. Looking at its old and decaying theory though, it is not enough to induce trust in the person. It is because, for a long time, it was lacking science. What needs to be done is to take Chinese medicine theory, rearrange and improve it. The obstacle for doing this hides within one's ability to learn. To the end of life, one should not be at leisure with this affair. In recent years, coming from the East and West, are doctors of civilized nations, who loudly sing their physiology treatment methods. They take our nation's acupuncture and moxibustion art and establish private schools, the purpose of which is entirely to research this. Their result being that this treatment method is mysteriously superior to physiology treatment methods. Now our nation has invented it first and to the contrary views it as worn out shoes. One can only sigh. The crux of the problem is with the profoundness of the acupuncture points. Most literature is not clear about this. Charts with commentaries are often confused and disorderly. In addition, treatment schemes do not differentiate clearly if one should use acupuncture or moxa. Even though there are many acupuncture books, they all follow the same pattern. Therefore, I am afraid, one cannot inquire thoroughly about it. Recently, my teacher Cheng Danan 承淡安[117] wrote a book titled *A Study of China's Acupuncture and Moxibustion Treatment* 中國針灸治療學. Within it, he considered science. The lines are organized clearly and strict order prevails. When it comes to acupuncture points being accurate and the essentials of tonifying and sedation, he might as well be the

[117] Cheng Danan 承淡安 (1899–1957) a Chinese medicine practitioner and member of China's Academy of Sciences. In 1954, he was invited by Jiangsu government to serve as the director of the Jiangsu Chinese Medicine Advanced Studies School (which later became Nanjing TCM University).

person who has rendered outstanding service to the medical profession. What a pity! The points and pathways are complex, to remember them is very difficult and it causes one to overrate their own ability. Instead, effort should be made in research and gaining experience. While considering works of other practitioners, I erased the superfluous and made the segments concise. For added benefit, I have used the most modern physiology and, altogether, pointed out 165 points. At the end there is an appendix of treatment scheme. To give it a face, I named it *China's Acupuncture and Moxibustion Science*. If, in order to discuss and deliberate on it, to save it without substitute, scholars will gather in the country and overseas and will perfect it, then this will be my good fortune, it will be our nation's acupuncture and moxibustion future path of good fortune.

September 2nd, the 22nd year[118] of the Republic of China, recorded by Zhou Boqin 周伯勤.

Second preface by Qin Bowei 秦伯未

Yue Ren 越人 punctured Wei Hui 維會[119] and the corpse of the prince of the state of Guo 虢 came to life immediately. Yuan Hua 元化[120] punctured the brain cavity and the headaches of King Wu of the state of Wei immediately stopped. This was at the spirit level. China's acupuncture and moxibustion is a medical art that truly cannot have been culminated by any other country's medical knowledge. When we consider the acupuncture principle, it does not escape the stimulation of nerves and increasing blood flow. It is a kind of simple and uncomplicated physiological therapy. It recovers the physiological systems' function and that's it. Now when China's acupuncture and moxibustion claims that there are twelve meridians and 365 points with specific locations, it seems that there is no trace of it that can be found. However, when looking at the core of these, for example Shen Ting point 神庭, one can see in front of the tendon the facial nerve and the trigeminal nerve branches as well as a branch from the anterior neck artery. The point Ting Hui 聽會[121] also has the trigeminal nerve and the facial nerve as well as the anterior artery. And so one can tell that, underneath the acupuncture points, there are nerves and blood vessels.

118 1933

119 Qin Yueren 秦越人 is said to be the real name of Bian Que 扁鵲. Wei Hui 維會 is another name for the acupuncture point 玉泉 Yu Quan.

120 Yuan Hua 元化 is another name for Hua Tuo 華佗 who has treated King Wu of Wei 魏武帝, which is the posthumous name for General Cao Cao 曹操.

121 The Character Ting in the point name Ting Hui in this text is written with an old character composed of 總 and 頁.

When nerves receive heat and physical stimulation from an object, the sensory nerves become abnormally excited. With neuralgia and nerve palsy kind of diseases, this has the ability to calm the pain and stimulate the numbness. With motor nerves the action is stronger, because the stimulation is so great, the amount of signal changes and it can adjust the disease pathology from within the central nervous system. It has a clear calming effect on the sympathetic nerves. Functions of glands and inner organs surge because there is fluctuation in the hyperfunction of nerves and locations they are distributed to. Blood vessels via neural stimulation first contract and then in further response dilate. In the blood, according to latest research in Tokyo University, Japan, white blood cell quantity increases. In rabbit experiments using moxa, within one or two hours they could more than double the white blood cell count. There is a similar result with protein injections. Since the blood white cell count has increased, the rabbit immunity increased as well, and one could see that blood vessels dilated. This may lead to an increased metabolism, which in turn may increase nourishment and growth. This is the principle of acupuncture and moxibustion. Now acupuncture and moxibustion was invented by our nation, and yet our nation's scholars only know that it works but not why it works. To the contrary, scholars of foreign countries are proving it. Today we want to guard it. My associates try to open the *Neijing* and read it. It is all about the application of acupuncture and moxibustion. When we look at later persons than Qin Yueren 秦越人 and Hua Yuanhua 華元化,[122] such as Huang Fumi 皇甫謐, Wang Weide 王維德, Dou Hanxiang 竇漢鄉 and we read their books, they are all called acupuncture and moxibustion authority, unaware that the use of herbal decoction became more involved and the study of acupuncture was neglected. When the theories of the West entered, our nation's essence perished. This, for people with feelings, is a source of sorrow and pain. Now, as for Mr. Zhou Boqin 周伯勤, in his medical work and study, he alone has the ability to reach to this dormant and perishing acupuncture and moxibustion. He uses science to explain the old theories and, with this, the old obscure meanings become clear. When compiling this book *China's Acupuncture and Moxibustion Science,* I was asked to preface it. Hence, I assembled my humble opinion and reported it here.

The year Jia Xu 甲戌[123] by Qin Bowei 秦伯未

Preface end

[122] Hua Tuo
[123] 1934

The applications and equipment of acupuncture

Pages 107–114

Section 1: The manufacturing of needles

The ancients called it "golden needle" but the material was no other than galvanized iron,[124] because iron also belongs to metal and so they wanted to beautify its name. Acupuncturists today mistake it for a golden needle and they make it out of gold. The manufacturing is not smooth and it causes the patient pains when applying it. These are nothing like the round and smooth iron needles. Therefore, in manufacturing, one should follow the ancient methods and use galvanized iron. It should be tempered twice or thrice, as well-tempered creates a very pliable quality. Firm and yielding is suitable. Hammering it makes it thin and round, like a thread and then break it, every section with a fine tip. On every section coil a copper wire, (There are people who manufacture needles for sale but they don't use medicine to boil it. One can buy these and cook himself) then boil it in medicine. Use loess and rub it on. When it is shiny then it is ready.

The method of boiling the needles: First use Wu Tou 烏頭 and Ba Dou Rou 巴豆肉 each one Liang, Ma Huang 麻黃 five Qian, Mu Bie Zi Rou 木鱉子肉 10 pieces, Wu Mei 烏梅 five pieces. Place these in the same clay pot as the needles, add water and cook it for 1 day. Remove and wash it clean. Then use Ru Xiang 乳香, Mo Yao 沒藥, Dang Gui 當歸, Hua Rui Shi 花蕊石 each half Liang, put the needles again in water and cook for one day. Remove the needles and use Zao Jiao water 皂角水 to rinse clean. Then take the needles and insert them into dog meat, insert the same as before and cook for one day. Remove it during the night and use loess or clay powder and rub it until it is shiny and the tip is pointy. At this point you can start using it.

Section 2: The shape of needles

In antiquity, they divided needles into nine types. The *Su Wen* 素問 has a treatise of the 9 needles. However, many are not used anymore. Only the fine needle type is commonly used today. But for now, we just want to explain the nine types. The first is the Chan needle 鑱針, its head is big and its tip sharp-pointed. It is used to drain heat from the head. The second is Yuan needle 圓針. Its body is round and pointy

[124] Ma Jiao Tie 馬嚼鐵.

and the tip looks like an egg, not sharp. It can prick the skin but not injure the tendon and flesh underneath. The third is Di needle 鍉針. It is sharp like lacquered grain tip, which is similar to the coarse needle used today. The fourth is Feng needle 鋒針. It is used for bleeding; it is the three-edged needle. The fifth is Pi needle 鈹針. It looks like a sword and is used to cut abscess and drain pus. It is similar to the scalpel used in surgery. The sixth is Yuan Li needle 圓利針. It looks like an ox tail. It is round and pointy. It is used to expel sudden pain. The seventh is Hao needle 毫針. It looks like fine hair. This is the kind of needle that is often used today. The eighth is Chang needle 長針. It is a little thicker than the Hao needle, and longer. The ninth is Huo needle 火針.[125] It is similar to the Chang needle, however its head is rounder. It is used for abscess in between the bones and joints where it is not appropriate to use a scalpel to cut it open. Among the nine needles, the Hao needle has the widest range of applications. Chang needle, Feng needle and Huo needle are used on occasion. The others are looked at as old worn out sandals.

Section 3: Hand techniques for acupuncture

When using acupuncture, one must determine first which points should be needled and which points use moxa. One should have the patient sit, lie down or lie on his side, or sitting and bending forward. When sitting, the back should be straight and both hands placed on one's knees, the feet should be slightly apart and one should not be slanting but, rather, upright. When lying down, the arms and legs should be stretched straight and lie horizontal. When lying on one's side, the bottom leg should be straight while the top leg should be bent. While bending forward, the hands should hug the neck and the person bend forwards horizontally. Only after the position is assumed, one then measures the points' locations, he takes the needles and wipes them clean. With the left thumbnail, he presses on the acupuncture point and uses a little force to cause the nerves underlying the skin some numbness (this can reduce pain while piercing the skin). The right hand holds the needle and pierces straight. As it is piercing, one twists it and allows it to enter. When the needle has entered few millimeters one pauses. One can tonify or sedate. One assesses the direction of the meridian and slightly twists it. Every twist can only amount to half a circle of the handle, not like a wheel turning and turning. Then, one asks the patient

[125] Huo needle 火針 or fire needle should be a typo. Other versions of the nine needles name the last one Da needle 大針 or big needle. The characters Huo and Da are very similar and often mixed in texts. However, 2 lines later the author uses again Huo needle, which makes it less likely to be a typo.

if there is a sore, heavy or scattering feeling. Ignore if the patient only feels pain, or if the patient does not feel pain or sore heaviness at all. One then inserts the needle a little more or pulls it out a little bit and then twists it again. After the patient has started feeling sore heaviness for one, two or three minutes then the needle is removed. Then one punctures the next point (if, for example, one uses even method of tonifying and sedating, then one can twist it to the left and to the right).

Section 4: Hand techniques for tonifying and sedating with acupuncture

The hand techniques of tonifying and sedating all include "if it is excessive, sedate it; if it is deficient, tonify it." Following and aiding it is called tonifying, while receiving it and capturing it is called sedating.[126] Sticking it in is tonifying, while lifting it is sedating.[127] Advancing three times and retreating one time is tonifying while retreating three times and advancing one time is sedating.[128] What does it mean, "to follow and aid it is called tonifying"? To follow means the flow of Qi in the meridian. To aid means to aid the transportation of Qi in the meridian. For example, hand Tai Yin lung, it travels from the chest to the hand. If one punctures the Jing point on the lung and follows the meridian's direction, gently twists and then gently and slowly removes the needle, he then immediately presses on the open hole, then this is called tonifying. This is the meaning of following it and aiding it. (Follow the same principle for the other meridians). What does it mean, "receiving it and capturing it is called sedating"? Receiving it means going against the direction of the meridian Qi. Capturing it means capturing its meridian Qi. For example, when sedating the lung Qi, one should go against the meridian's direction and gently twist it, then rapidly remove the needle and slowly go to press on the hole. This is called sedating. This is the meaning of receiving and capturing it (use the same method for the other meridians).

Section 5: The different types of moxibustion

Moxibustion basically uses Ai 艾[129] and burns it. Later generations invented medicinal moxibustion, which added other medicinal substances to it (Shu Huang Ru She 硫磺乳麝[130] etc) and then burned them together. They used these to help the medicinal ability. Like this, it could easily penetrate into the tendons and flesh. With more

---

126 The meridian direction.
127 The needle.
128 Inserting and pulling of the needle.
129 Chinese mugwort, a kind of plant.
130 Sulfur, Frankincense and deer musk.

potency, they could decrease the number of moxa cones needed. The method has reached a state of perfection. There is also a "thunderous fire needling 雷火針" using pungent and fragrant medicinals that move the blood and unobstruct meridians. They mix them with the Ai leaves and roll them into a bamboo tube shape. They burn it, and while separated with a cloth, they iron it against the point, or they fumigate it against the point. This allows the medicinal Qi and the heat Qi to penetrate the point and the disease can be cured. The efficacy is excellent. Compared to the Japanese moxibustion, there are some differences. There is also a Tai Yi Shen acupuncture and moxibustion method 太乙神針灸法, which is similar to the thunderous needling method. To see its preparation methods and herbs used, refer to the book *The Science of Tai Yi Shen Acupuncture* 科學太乙神針, published by the Chinese Medicine Publishing House.

Section 6: The absurdity of modern moxibustion methods

In modern times, the method of moxibustion by acupuncturists is as soon as they insert a needle into the point, they take some moxa and put it on the handle of the needle and then burn it. They have lost the true meaning of moxibustion. This method only causes the needle to become hot and that's it. It causes the local area to feel hot. It causes the blood fluid to have some change, but its efficacy is minimal.

Section 7: Three opinions on acupuncture and moxibustion treatment

The root principle of acupuncture and moxibustion is stimulating the nerves. It increases blood flow. It is a kind of simple, not complicated, physiological treatment. This method has started in the *Neijing*, was carried out by Bian Que and later by all historical records was carried on and transmitted to different persona. Its usage surged during the Yuan 元 and Ming 明 dynasties. Coming to the Qing 清 dynasty it has started declining. I, the author, have peeped through the medical works of the past and feel that the earlier virtuous acupuncturists would use acupuncture and moxibustion to treat severe diseases and cure stubborn illnesses, as easy as flipping of the palm. It was even so divine like Yue Ren puncturing Wei Hui point and bringing back to life the corpse of the prince of the Guo state, or Yuan Hua puncturing the brain cavity and immediately curing the headaches of King Wu of the state of Wei. Every single time it was a divine art, and so when I research all the acupuncture books twice and thrice, I have the following three opinions toward the current state of research and experience:

1) The person self-measuring scale for locating acupuncture points.

If one wants to quickly cure a disease using acupuncture he must first locate the points accurately. One must use the person Cun 寸 self-measuring scale. The method to do it is creating artificially an individual measuring scale. The measurement standard is the person's middle finger. The distance between the crease of the first joint closest to the fingertip and the crease of the second joint is 1 Cun. This Cun is divided into 10 Fen 分. With this in mind, one uses measurements. When measuring, one may discount the measurement if the body part is contracted or stretched out. For example, when looking for Gao Huang 膏肓 point, the location is below the fourth vertebra and above the fifth and then sideways 3 Cun. First, one establishes the measurement standard; he estimates the measurement of the patient's middle finger between the two joints. He then, let's say, estimates that the patient's length is 10% shorter of his own, and so all other measurements are discounted 10%. Therefore when the practitioner looks for Gao Huang point, when he travels sideways from the spine, he only measures 2 Cun and 7 Fen. If the original measurement showed the patient measurement to be longer 10%, then all other measurements need extra 10%, in which case, without a doubt, the location of Gao Huang point will be 3 Cun and 3 Fen away from the spine. If, for example, one looks for Jiu Wei 鳩尾 point on the Ren 任 meridian, he should use the same measurement method as mentioned above. Measuring from the naval upward it is 7 Cun or from the xyphoid process it is 1 Cun downward. One then measures the patient's middle finger distance between the two joints and he calculates and discounts the distance to Jiu Wei point accordingly. If one does not use this measurement method and only measures the distance by looking at it, then it is "veering off at the origin one millimeter, will veer of target a thousand miles". Without it, people will die left and right.

2) One must separate acupuncture from moxibustion.

The two words "acupuncture moxibustion Zhen Jiu 針灸" in a sentence cannot be separated, however, in treatment, each has its own function. When it is proper to use moxa, then use moxa and when it is proper to use acupuncture, then use acupuncture. Like this, the true meaning of acupuncture and moxibustion is not lost. Today, there are many acupuncturists who, when they treat a patient, as soon as they insert the needle they use moxa and put it on the needle handle and burn it. The acupuncturists consider this as "warm needles". Their ability is exhausted, while the patient suffers great pain without any efficacy. Because of this, both acupuncture and moxibustion have lost their ability. For example, let's take the two points Ya Men 啞門 and Shen Que 神闕. In acupuncture and moxibustion practice, it is prohibited to moxa Ya Men. If you moxa this point, the mouth becomes mute Ya 啞. Likewise, it is prohibited to pierce Shen Que; piercing it will injure the person. If one uses the needles with the burning tail and assumes them to be warm needles, then one does not know how to handle these two points. In addition, all scholars' works dealing with moxibustion explain direct moxibustion to be the norm. In general, the proper method is: use ginger and scallion juice and rub it on the point, then place on top of it a moxa ball and burn it.

3) The art of tonifying and sedating.

The earlier virtuous masters said: Follow it and aid it is called tonifying, receive it and capture it is called sedating. They also said three advances and one retreat is tonifying, while three retreats and one advance is called sedating. Advance and insertion, retreat and lifting are indeed the unchanging methods of tonifying and sedating. My sedating and tonifying methods can be summarized with the following eight words: follow, aid, receive, capture, advance, insert, retreat, lift. Each can perform its sedating or tonifying according to the meridian's path. For example, if we want to tonify He Gu 合谷 point of hand Yang Ming 陽明 meridian, on the patient's left side we will rotate the needle toward the right,[131] the thumb will go backward while the index finger will go forward. If we pierce the patient's right side then the needle will rotate toward the left,[132] the thumb will move forward while the index finger backward. As for sedation method, it is the opposite. It is only that for sedation method one removes the needle quickly but goes slowly to close the hole, while for tonification one removes the needle slowly but goes fast to cover the hole. The early virtuous ones have said: if one wants to understand the secret of tonifying and sedating, receiving and following, it is all within this principle. And so, the standard of treatment for acupuncture and moxibustion is: one tonifies for itching, numbness and deficiency and one sedates for pains, aches and excessive conditions. This, one cannot ignore.

[131] Clockwise, practitioner uses his/her left hand.
[132] Counter clockwise, practitioner uses his/her left hand.

Section 2: Wind strike 中风[133]

Yaron: In the following section we see simplification and standardization of treatment: X group of symptoms can be treated with Y acupuncture/herb protocol.

Even though there is some differentiation of causes such as heat and cold, or locations such as meridians, blood vessels and organs, emphasis is placed on treatment practicality. There is no ambiguity or mysteriousness, nor is there an attempt to explain in detail the mechanism behind the efficacy in a scientific way.

The Native medicine doctor, in the eyes of Zhou Boqin, needs to know the symptoms and then follow a protocol for these symptoms. This, too, continued as a trend in TCM formulation in the Communist era: an easy-to-learn, practical and seemingly effective treatment modality.

As we can clearly see by now, in a way several trends have continued from the Republic into Communist China in forming TCM. When I reflect back on that time I can only imagine that the TCM makers of the 1950s, by copying and continuing trends from the 1920s and '30s, may have felt themselves "traditional." Continuing the Chinese medicine scientification of the older generation but peppered with new Communist ideology and responses to political and social pressures, they may have seen themselves as developing it further. Possibly, this is why they called it Traditional Chinese Medicine.

Pages 131–134

Type 1: If it hits the meridians

Cause: Wind is Yang evil; it often enters from the outside, starting at the skin level and entering the meridians. Piercing the meridians, the *Neijing* 內經 states: if it strikes the face use the lower Yang Ming 陽明, if it strikes the neck use the lower Shao Yang 少陽, if it strikes the back then use lower Tai Yang 太楊.[134] Therefore, when wind strikes the person, then the three Yang meridians should be used.

Symptoms: The body feels cold to touch but the person feels hot, body feels heavy achy and sore, skin and muscles don't function, tendons and bones cannot be used, headaches and stiff neck, the corners of eye and mouth stretched abnormally, the disease onset is abrupt, the pulse on both sides is wiry and floating, tongue coating is thin and white.

133 Stroke, but can also mean any state of paralysis or palsy.
134 Yang Ming Stomach meridian, Shao Yang Gallbladder meridian and Tai Yang Urinary Bladder meridian.

Treatment: He Gu 合谷, Qu Chi 曲池, Yang Fu 陽輔, Yang Ling 陽陵, Feng Fu 風府, Nei Ting 內庭, Gan Shu 肝俞. Each point pierced four or five Fen deep and twisting lasts two minutes each.

Adjunct treatment: Sheng Ji Da Huo Lou Dan 聖濟大活絡丹,[135] use aged liquor to swallow one pill.

Type 2: If it hits the blood vessels

Cause: When wind evil enters the branch meridians, then the blood vessels become obstructed, heat causes tendons to lengthen, cold causes tendons to spasm, and therefore one can see a syndrome of physical crookedness.

Symptoms: Mouth and eye being crooked, or half of the body paralyzed, or arm and leg spasm, or both left and right side paralysis, wiry pulse and slippery, tongue is white or red.

Treatment: When the eye and mouth are slanting, use the point Di Cang 地倉; if the slanting is on the face left side, then pierce and moxa the face right side. For other points, follow the same principle. Use Jia Che 頰車, pierce each point five Fen deep and twist for two minutes or use moxa three or five cones. Moxa Ren Zhong 人中 three cones, pierce He Gu 合谷 four to five Fen deep, twist for three minutes, moxa Jian Shi 間使 12 cones.

If half body is paralyzed, moxa Bai Hui 百會 three cones; first pierce He Gu 合谷 on the healthy side, then moxa same point on the diseased side. Same principle applies to all other points. When piercing, enter four to five Fen, retain and then twist for two minutes, then again burn three cones moxa. Qu Chi 曲池, pierce five Fen, twist two minutes moxa three cones. Jian Yong 肩顒, Shou San Li 手三里, Kun Lun 崑崙, Jue Gu 絕骨, Yang Ling Quan 陽陵泉, Zu San Li 足三里, pierce and burn moxa. Gan Shu 肝俞 burn moxa five to seven cones.

If it is left and right side paralysis, acupuncture and moxibustion is the same as the previous.

If the arm has spasm and numbness, pierce and moxa Shou San Li 手三里, Jian Yong 肩顒, Qu Chi 曲池, Jian Shi 間使, Hou Xi 後谿, He Gu 合谷, and only pierce Qu Ze 曲澤, depth three Fen, twist for two minutes.

If the leg has spasm and numbness, pierce and moxa Xing Jian 行間, Qiu Xu 邱墟, Kun Lun 崑崙, Yang Fu 陽輔, Yang Ling Quan 陽陵泉, Zu San Li 足三里.

[135] "The sages rescue greatly invigorating the branch meridians elixir". Also called "Greatly invigorating the branch meridians pill 大活络丸" and "The great divine invigorating the branch meridians elixir 大神活络丹". A prescription from the book *Lan Tai Gui Fan* 蘭台軌范 by Xu Dachun 徐大椿, compiled 1764.

Adjunct treatment: Huang Qi 黃芪 3 qian, Gui Zhi 桂枝 one qian, Bai Zhu 白朮 three qian, Dang Gui 當歸 three qian, cook into a decoction and drink.

Type 3: If it strikes the inner organs

Cause: When there is much phlegm and damp and the body Qi is not sufficient, or from smoking, drinking alcohol and other desires, or from excessive thinking and anger, the foreign evil rides this deficiency and enters the inner organs and their meridians. It is what we call today cerebral hemorrhage.

Symptoms: The mouth closes forcefully and doesn't open, phlegm and saliva overflow, there are loud sounds from the throat, can't recognize people and situations, paralysis of four limbs, can't recognize pain, speech stuttering, bowel and urine leakage, the pulse could be felt or seem absent.

Treatment: If the mouth closes and won't open, burn moxa three or five cones on Jia Che 頰車, Bai Hui 百會 and Ren Zhong 人中.

If phlegm and saliva overflow, burn moxa dozens of cones on Guan Yuan 關元, one dozen cones on Qi Hai 氣海 and three to five cones on Bai Hui 百會.

If one cannot speak and he doesn't recognize pain, then burn moxa 100 to 200 or even 300 cones on Shen Dao 神道.

If there is stuttering, then follow the explanation for striking the meridians half body paralysis and use those points pierce and burn moxa.

Adjunct treatment: True Jilin Ren Shen 吉林人參 3 qian, cook it into decoction. Use Hei Xi Dan 黑錫丹 one qian and drink it with the Ren Shen decoction together.

Section 5: Hiccup impediment 噎隔

Pages 141–144

Type 1: Cold impediment

Disease cause: The Yang Qi in the central palace is weak, cold Qi is congealing, spleen Qi cannot ascend, stomach Qi cannot descend and then cold impediment occurs.

Symptoms: The epigastric region is bloated, vomiting of clear fluid, four extremities are cold, food does not go down, pale facial complexion, both pulses are thin and slow.

Treatment: Moxa three to five cones Shan Zhong 膻中, five to seven cones Zhong Wan 中脘, Zu San Li 足三里 pierce five to six Fen retain and twist for one minute and then burn on it moxa five cones, Gong Sun 公孫 pierce three Fen retain and twist for two minutes then burn five cones moxa, Xue Hai 血海 moxa two cones.

Adjunct treatment: Chuan Jiao 川椒, Fu Zi 附子, Chuan Lian 川連, Bai Zhu 白朮 cook into a decoction and drink.

Type 2: Hot impediment

Cause: Stomach fluid dries out, the digestive tract is dry, stomach fire surges upward and so food cannot come down.

Symptoms: Stomach and epigastric region feel very hot, bitter mouth and dry tongue, agitated, restless and thirsty, red face, pulse is fast and after eating the person vomits.

Treatment: Nei Ting 內庭, Ran Gu 然谷, Yang Xi 陽谿 and Da Ling 大陵 pierce three Fen deep retain and twist for two minutes.

Adjunct treatment: Sheng Chuan Jun 生川軍, Yuan Ming Fen 元明紛, Sheng Gan Cao 生甘草, Sheng Jiang 生薑, Da Zao 大棗, cook into decoction and drink.

Type 3: Qi impediment

Cause: Heart depression, melancholy stagnates without resolution, and so Qi becomes oppressed in the center, transportation and transformation fails, liver Qi rises adversely, the diaphragm Qi is obstructed.[136]

Treatment: Zhong Wan 中脘 pierce eight Fen up to 1.5 Cun retain and twist for one minute, Shan Zhong 膻中 moxa three cones, Qi Hai 氣海, Wei Shu 胃俞 pierce each three Fen retain and twist for two minutes, then moxa same point three to five cones, Lie Que 列缺 pierce two Fen, retain and twist for one minute, Nei Guan 內關 pierce three Fen retain and twist for two minutes.

Adjunct treatment: Ban Xia 半夏, Fu Ling 茯苓, Zi Su Geng 紫蘇梗, Chuan Pu 川朴, cook and drink decoction.

Type 4: Phlegm impediment

Cause: Stubborn phlegm retains in the midst of the digestive pipe, obstructing the pathway, whenever food and drink enter the throat they become impeded and can't fully descend.

---

[136] The character Ge 膈 repeats in this section in disease types. Like Cold Ge and Hot Ge, however it has the meaning of divide or impediment, therefore we have translated it as Cold impediment etc. In this line it states 膈氣不通 the diaphragm Qi is obstructed and Ge means diaphragm.

Symptoms: Cough and shortness of breath, phlegm sounds in the throat, chest and diaphragm feel oppression and unease, can't swallow past the throat food and drink, the two pulses are full and slippery.

Treatment: Fei Shu 肺俞, Da Du 大都, Xia Wan 下脘, pierce each five cones,[137] Tian Tu 天突 pierce three Fen deep, retain and twist two minutes then moxa five cones, Feng Long 豐隆 pierce five Fen deep, retain and twist for two minutes then moxa five cones.

Adjunct treatment: Sheng Jiang 生薑, Lai Fu Zhi 萊菔汁, Yue Shi San 月石散, blend and stew and drink warm.

Type 5: Food impediment

Cause: After hunger, suddenly eating great quantity of food, it obstructs above the stomach, it obstructs the Qi mechanism of the stomach and creates an impediment, it often happens to old people.

Symptoms: Chest pains, with pain free periods, hard to swallow food, and it is very painful, to an extreme Qi is so obstructed that it is life threatening.

Treatment: Use the same instruction as Qi impediment.

Adjunct treatment: Mu Xiang 木香, Bing Lang 檳榔, Ren Shen 人參, Dang Gui 當歸, Huo Xiang 藿香, Gan Cao 甘草, Zhi Shi 枳實, Da Huang 大黃, Hou Po 厚朴, grind to fine powder and moisten downward[138] with a little honey.

Type 6: Deficiency impediment

Cause: Because the spleen and stomach fluids parched and blood dried out, the stomach mansion is dry and cannot transform and receive.

Symptoms: dry skin, food and drink cannot descend, stools look like sheep excrement,[139] both pulses are deficient and thready, the person's body is cold and the spirit tired.

Treatment: Zhong Wan 中脘 moxa 30 cones, He Gu 合谷, Tai Chong 太沖, pierce three to four Fen, retain and twist for three minutes.

Adjunct treatment: feed often human milk, pay attention that this syndrome patient often can't eat.

Book excerpt end

---

[137] Seems to be a typo or missing characters, should be 'pierce certain depth then apply moxa 5 cones'.

[138] Swallow.

[139] Small dry pebbles.

About Chen Cunren 陳存仁 (1908–1990)[140]

Was born to a family of silk traders which then lost its fortune and at age 8 he lost his father. Chen graduated from the Shanghai Chinese Medicine Specialized School 上海中醫專門學校 and, in 1929, set up a clinic on Shan Dong Lu 山東路 in Shanghai, and reportedly was proficient in internal medicine, gynecology and acupuncture. In 1928 he established the *Health Newspaper Kang Jian Bao* 康健報. On March 17th, 1929, during the great convention of Chinese medicine doctors opposing the Chinese medicine abolition attempts, which took place at the Shanghai Chamber of Commerce main hall, Cunren was selected as one of five representatives to go to the government in Nanjing and present the petition *Opposing Chinese Medicine Abolition Attempt*. Cunren was the chief editor of *China's Medicine Great Dictionary* 中國藥學大辭典, published in 1935. In 1937, he published *A Collection of Kampo Medicine* 皇汉医学丛书, with several dozen volumes, systematically arranging Japanese Kampo (Chinese medicine transmitted in Japan). In 1947, he was elected as a member for the first national assembly of the Republic of China. In 1949, during the establishment of the People's Republic of China, Cunren left Shanghai to Hong Kong to practice medicine there. He passed away in 1990 in Los Angeles, USA.

[140] *zh.wikipedia.org*

The way to study Chinese medicine: A lecture by Mr. Chen Cunren

Cunren medical seminar, recorded by Shao Yagu 邵雅谷

1954 by Chen Cunren 陳存仁

Yaron: The following excerpts from Chen Cunren were published in February 1954 in the *Chan Yuen Medical Publication Series* volume six, printed by the Chen Chan-Yuen [141] Chinese Medicine Research Institute. Mr. Chen had a clear approach to Chinese medicine, a practical approach. In an era when modern science could prove things as fact, while Chinese medicine often relied on speculation, this was a reasonable solution.

Today, while we still may lean toward being pragmatic or theoretical or even philosophical, all positions having strong and weak aspects, I think that considering Mr. Chen's approach is worthwhile. His guiding principle, I believe, existed since the earliest times: absorb the useful and get rid of the useless. However, useful and useless was determined by the circumstances and needs of that time.

Some already-discarded Chinese medicine theories may become useful in the 21st century, especially as modern science moves beyond the "only physical reality". Other aspects—like identifying symptom-patterns and easily matching protocols to them—may not be useful anymore, since today we no longer need cheap and easy mass education of low-level medical technicians.

Chinese medicine should further develop and not only copy from the past. So adding to Mr. Chen, here I will say, in Chinese medicine not only what was useful in the past is valuable, but also what may help us develop into the future

Pages 13–26

[141] Chen Chan-Yuen is southern dialect for the same name Chen Cunren.

Recognizing clearly the correct way will prevent wasting time.

Now there are many people who feel "now that our family is wealthy we should also learn some skill" and so thinking of learning Chinese medicine there are many. Most of these people wishing to study Chinese medicine look for books they can study it from. Not only ones who didn't study Chinese medicine are like this, but also ones who have studied Chinese medicine are like this. When I traveled in many countries overseas I met many overseas Chinese and many of them have asked me what books should they read? Where should they buy these books? So in order to respond to this need I am talking today about "the way to study Chinese medicine". This will serve as a combined response.

Many people feel that studying Chinese medicine is an easy affair, however, at the beginning stages of learning, in reality when you look at Western medicine books they are much easier, because in Western medicine books they gradually progress from superficial to deep. Chinese medicine books at elementary level, however, are scarce. Books that describe Chinese medicine foundations are even harder to come by and, therefore, for the beginner student of Chinese medicine, while reading books, it is common not to understand.

From a teaching point of view, Chinese medicine is lacking systematic teaching materials. Chinese medicine schools in the entire country have teachers choose their own teaching materials and they cannot unify a standard. This, therefore, causes hardship for the readers who study Chinese medicine. In reality, people who study Chinese classical literature—history, poetry, verses—they are all lacking a progressing literature from superficial to deep. If you go look at bookstores that sell Chinese medicine literature, you get the feel that from ancient to present it is vast and voluminous. It is like buying the 24 histories, can't tell where to start. It causes people who contemplate studying Chinese medicine to feel the hardship and not know where to start.

Now, in order to point out the correct access to this medicine, we first need to resolve a problem, which is "what is the true value of Chinese medicine?" To explain this issue I divide it into three parts:

1) Chinese medicine truly has efficacy healing many diseases. With many complicated syndromes, it can show removing the root, comprehensiveness and entire body effectiveness character. With this, Chinese medicine had an era

of flourishing science. Until today, this achievement could not be eliminated through selectiveness. The key is entirely within the medical efficacy. However, the scope of medical efficacy has its limitation; being honest, one cannot claim that it can cure everything.

2) Since Chinese herbs are combined into formulas in treatment, the efficacy can reach even greater comprehensive efficacy. For example, Ren Shen 人參, Bai Zhu 白朮, Fu Ling 茯苓, Gan Cao 甘草 combined together make a formula. This formula is called the Four Noble Ingredients Decoction. Di Huang 地黃, Shan Yu Rou 山萸肉, Huai Shan Yao 淮山藥, Fu Ling 茯苓, Dan Pi 丹皮, Ze Xie 澤瀉, the six ingredients combine together to create the Six Ingredients Di Huang Pill. This is the synergy of a formula. Stemming out of the accumulated experience of medical treatment over the centuries that these formulas were developed and named, allowing practitioners to easily remember them. This was very convenient. Even more so, because the herbs are combined into a formula, the efficacy can reach to the entire body of the patient. And so the result of a Chinese medicine treatment, if one can use the efficacious formulas from the literature, accurately and flexibly target the disease, combine the herbs appropriately, then the herbs' characteristics merge together and yield an effect. This effect is severing the disease course which creates a recovery kind of effect. It is absolutely not like Western drugs that cure the east and damage the west kind of side effects. Therefore, with Chinese medicine, big disease becomes a small disease and a small disease disappears. It is unlike certain Western drugs that constantly generate side effects, the first disease is cured and then there is a second disease, the second disease is cured and then there is another disease.

3) In ancient times, Chinese medicine did not use scientific instruments for diagnosis; however, throughout the centuries in medical literature, there are many records of "subjective diagnostic methods". There were many diseases that, from a mere external inspection, were able to infer the disease origin and development. For example, one of the diagnostic methods is observing; this comes entirely out of experience. An old experienced Chinese medicine doctor, through his accumulated experience, can already forecast the development of the disease, as if he has a scientific divinity.

The above three points are the true value of Chinese medicine. Therefore, when reading Chinese medicine literature, one should select books that demonstrate the above three points. It is like panning for gold; one should hunt and collect these materials. Therefore, I hope that people who wish to study and research Chinese medicine will guard themselves from, and cast away, empty theories. There is no need to be stuck in the mud with the old five phases and six Qi theories. One should adopt a measure of reading books in order to reach an application. One must get rid of most of the empty theories. He then must recognize the true value in efficacious prescriptions and be clear about them and absorb them. This is what I point out as "the path of learning".

What, then, is an "empty theory"? China's medical "empty theories" have four characteristics:

1) The style of sticking stubbornly to reciting classics, especially the lines in the *Nei Jing* 內經, *Nan Jing* 難經, *Shang Han* 傷寒, *Jin Gui* 金匱, commentaries, explanations about them and categorizing them, all the while beating about the bush.

2) Because many Chinese herbs have real efficacy, however, there is no way to explain why, many took the task to explain them with Yin Yang and five phases. Disease etiology and pathology was also explained with Yin Yang and five phases. These have no value whatever.

3) While receiving influences from Buddhism, Daoism and Confucianism and while explaining the principle, many incorporate superstition, or they use a style of honoring the classics and venerating the Dao, they believe that the ancient records in the classics are the highest realm and that there is nothing higher than that.

4) While having some influence from natural phenomena, they differentiated Yin Yang, hot cold, deficient and excess, exterior and interior, and with this they believed that the entire medical knowledge lies with these eight words. This especially was the case during the Qing dynasty and its medical literature; everybody was arguing with each other about it, with no end.

These empty theories, after all, how did they form? In reality, it resulted from the herbs healing well the patient. The authors of medical works could not explain the disease pathology, however, they wanted to explain how the disease was cured, and so these four different characteristics of empty theories came to play. Amongst all the many books, the most popular and widely-circulated are the Yin Yang and Five Phases books. Just like charcoaling therapy—charcoaled Ce Bai Tan 側柏炭, charcoaled Di Yu Tan 地榆炭 they all have the effect of stopping bleeding. In today's perspective, it is very scientific; there is no need to make up empty theories about it. However, in those times, one could not but make those five phases theories up: "Fire restrains Water in order for the red to control the black". In reality, this is a random medical theory and there is no true value in it. Theory should only be like the *Shang Han Lun* 傷寒論 style, being blunt and straightforward, for a certain syndrome there is a certain decoction that can cure it. This is very scientific. *Shen Nong Ben Cao Jing* 神農本草經 is likewise the same. It talks about a certain herb that can remedy a certain disease. It is a work that carries a scientific spirit.

The ancient medical literature, because of era limitations promulgating theories, was just a waste of words. When we now read the ancient medical books, we should get rid of all the empty theories and maintain all the useful materials. Like this, it can become beneficial and not a waste of time.

In this discussion, when I introduce the correct path of Chinese medicine, I emphasize this style of learning and entering this school. I hope that people who study medicine will read many medical books with this style of reading books. They should absorb the useful parts and apply them in clinical setting. There is no need to talk much about theories but, rather, recognize the disease and know the method to handle it. One should remember the formulas' names, efficacy and the ingredients composing them and, if one can do it in this way then, with half the effort, the reward will be double. This is the correct access point to enter Chinese medicine, which is also the way to pre-resolve the problem.

I have also met many friends who research the Chinese medicine classics extraordinarily, or they can memorize them fluently, within Yin Yang five phases cold hot deficiency and excess they make somersaults, and yet from beginning to end they don't get at the essentials. When they see a disease, they don't know what disease it is, nor can they understand the connection between the different symptoms. When it comes to a prescription, their chests are empty; when it comes to selecting herbs, there are no herbs they can use. They have lost that part of Chinese medicine that has true value to it. To the contrary, they absorb and use the useless. This kind of learning is a grave mistake!

If one wants to learn Chinese medicine, he'd better sign up for an examination to a Chinese medicine school. According to the world medical education standard, it should be a seven-year study. In China, they have fixed the curriculum to five years. In some, even less; it takes only four years to graduate. Specialist schools also have a three-year program. At present, according to government regulations, one must have a curriculum of at least three years in order to register oneself and open a practice. However, in order to accommodate overseas students' needs, the number of years can be stretched longer or made shorter. Nonetheless, for one who is interested to learn Chinese medicine, he must first realize that to study Chinese medicine, two or three years will not suffice. One must allow at least five years of continuous study and advanced study in order to succeed. If one thinks that studying this is an easy affair, then it will surely not succeed.

Inside China, Chinese medicine schools of this scope include three in Shanghai 上海 and one in each Nan Jing 南京, Hang Zhou 杭州 and Lan Chi 蘭谿.[142] There are students who wish to do things quickly. They study half a year in school A and then switch to school B; they learn there one and a half years and then switch to school C and graduate there. In this fashion they can graduate within two or three years. However, reaching a graduation diploma does not mean one was successful with studying Chinese medicine. There are many who, after graduation, still do not know how to diagnose a patient; they cannot write a prescription. To the contrary, it shakes their own confidence. It becomes their own self-made failure. Therefore, I want to convince everyone, if you don't want to learn Chinese medicine then fine; however, if you have a desire to learn medicine, the fast way is not the correct way. We call this "study is without boundaries, and not only with one teacher". One should seek learning in many different directions, with a humble heart. For example, Ye Tianshi 葉天士 studied from 17 teachers and spent many years and then he started using herbs, also without shame he kept on inquiring, only then he started treading the path of accomplishment. No matter if it is in a distant foreign land or around the block, self-cultivation is forever the same. From antiquity what we call a Confucian scholar doctor, they all cultivated themselves and succeeded. However, self-cultivation requires much learning from many books, it requires a knowledgeable teacher to point the way; then there is a time when success arrives.

Going back to the root point: the reason Chinese medicine exists is because it can cure disease, not because it has the names Tai Yang 太陽, Yang Ming 陽明, Shao Yang 少陽 etc. In order to benefit students and prevent them from wasting their effort in vain, I would like to point out the following:

142 Also known as Lan Xi, a city in Zhejiang province.

1) One must recognize diseases and symptoms.

2) One must give a prescription for those symptoms.

3) One should analyze the prescription for the use of single herbs within it.

If the medical student can keep this objective in mind then he quickly can enter the path of medicine. There are many people who study Chinese medicine who learn thoroughly the *Nei Jing* 內經, *Nan Jing* 難經, *Shang Han* 傷寒 and *Jin Gui* 金櫃; not only do they learn them well, but even everything is clear and logical. However, as soon as they get to the clinic they feel helpless. This is the saying in the medical circles stating "even though the author has thousand words to say, but when treating a disease not one of them is effective". One need only look at people who are already practicing medicine—there are many who are very scholarly, yet they can't unravel the medicine. This is because when they study medicine, they don't use or think of practical experiments. Therefore, it is hard to blame people of the generation of Yu Yunxiu 余云岫, who considered Chinese medicine books to largely be full of empty theories and useless talk. However, at the same time, he was full of admiration toward Wang Shishan 汪石山 case studies compilation and Chen Sicheng 陳司成 records of cases. He was of the opinion that such authors had the spirit of practical experiments that medical scholars around the world have.

From ancient to the present, medical books are plenty. However, most of these books were written by people who could not treat a disease. There are books that only deal with Yin-Yang, five phases, external-internal, deficient and excess kind of talk. They are made by people who can only solve problems on paper. These books cannot be regarded as valuable and no added attention should be given to them. Because there are these books by authors who have never seen a single patient—they were a special paper warrior. For example, Ke Yunbo 柯韻伯,[143] of the Qing dynasty, a person of Ci Huo 慈豁 who never practiced medicine: He went into solitude to learn the books and so he composed *Shang Han Lai Su Ji* 傷寒來蘇集;[144] however, in reality, he never had practical experience of treating patients. Chen Xiuyuan 陳修園, of the Qing dynasty, a person of Fu Jian province Chang Le city 福建省長樂市: He compiled dozens of medical works. Jiang Qingling 蔣慶齡, who transmitted Chen's knowledge, stated that whenever Chen diagnosed a patient it would take him half a day to write a prescription. In reality, Chen is a medical author and that's it. Huang

[143] Also known as Ke Qin 柯琴 (circa 1662–1735), considered one of the three great *Shang Han Lun* commentators of the Qing dynasty.

[144] This book is a compilation of Ke's three works: *Shang Han Lun Zhu* 傷寒論註 (4 scrolls); *Shang Han Lun Yi* 傷寒論翼 (2 scrolls); and *Shang Han Fu Yi* 傷寒附翼 (2 scrolls).

Kunzai 黃坤載, of the Qing dynasty, a person of Chang Yi 昌邑: because a charlatan doctor used the wrong medicine, his eyes got hurt, and with a firm resolution he determined to cure the doctors. He composed more than 10 medical works but himself did not practice medicine. In more modern times, like Mr. Zhang Taiyan 章太炎, who composed the *New Treatise of Sudden Disease Cu Bing Xin Lun* 猝病新論 etc books, while he himself did not practice medicine. Of course he could not speak of his own experience treating diseases. Especially the absurdity of Lu Zhiyi 盧芷頤, who, being blind, composed *Finding About Shang Han Mo Suo Shang Han* 摸索傷寒 which, in its entirety, is a blind explanation. Therefore, while choosing medical books, one should first treasure applicability, and be very scarce with researching empty theories; this approach is excellent.

There are many doctors who seldom read books; some, rather, focus their effort on practical study with elder and experienced doctors; some attain prescriptions that have passed through generations and when they encounter a disease, they can immediately respond at will. They can really cure some of the diseases. People who study medicine should not err in understanding what is the task of the doctor, this somehow is in relation to one's destiny. I dare say that there are some doctors who must first truly heal a certain number of diseases and only then can they flourish.

Today, I can give an example: let's say there is a Confucian scholar doctor who has studied extensively the medical books of ancient and present, and his writings are superior. However, in a distant place there is one who's chest does not have one drop of black ink, being a kind of village doctor he can only do a kind of medicine that treats anal fistula, with a thread hanging and cutting it. After these two people have been practicing for ten years, the scholar doctor will have his clinic vacant while the village doctor will have his practice full like a market place. Between the two doctors, there is nothing related to having or not having good luck, it is rather due to who has clinical efficacy.

Therefore, when studying medicine, the task at hand should be looking for efficacious formulas and herbs and using them to treat a disease. Then one can reach the objective of serving the patient. One can be successful even by reaching one or two treatment techniques; however, if one can be versatile and knowledgeable in all books, getting to the many prescriptions and attaining the many efficacious treatment methods, he can than become a very talented Chinese medicine doctor and this is even better.

Section end

Yaron: Many Chinese medicine practitioners in the 1930s and, as we can see in the following section, even up to the 1950s, lacked basic knowledge of modern physiology and anatomy. The author points out that since some modern physiology knowledge is taught in middle schools then Chinese medicine practitioners needed at least that. Complete ignorance of basic physiology cannot exist in any medicine.

Today, of course, the situation is different; all Chinese medicine practitioners know basic anatomy and physiology. However, a push to include more and more Western medicine in Chinese medicine schools does not stop with basic anatomy, physiology and pathology but, rather, the more that TCM wishes to advance the more modern bio-medicine is incorporated. This became the established norm to advance Chinese medicine. It is a norm that started in the 1920s and is unchanged even today; advancing Chinese medicine means incorporating more Western medicine knowledge into it.

The author, in this article, has a genuine request: let's get out of ignorance. "Ignorance", for him, means not knowing modern medicine. However, if you substitute Chinese medicine knowledge with modern scientific knowledge, then does Chinese medicine still exist at all other than by name? And if it exists just by name, why do we need it? I have the opinion that Chinese medicine indeed has ignorance in certain aspects, yet nor does modern scientific medicine escape ignorance. I agree with the early TCM designers and the Communist architects, that both medicines should contribute their strong points to form a better "new" medicine which is stronger than before. However, creating this "new" medicine should not be tempered or artificially forced. It should not be influenced by political, strategic and other unrelated-to-medicine reasons.

A coerced creation of a "new" medicine and textbooks are not what we, Chinese medicine practitioners, truly want. Chinese medicine's strong points need to be developed; they need to become so compelling that modern medicine could not overlook them, and then eventually a natural merge may occur. Modern medicine is already pushing ahead with researching energy and life, why should Chinese medicine remain with the 1930s reformers' idea of "Chinese medicine is only accumulated experience of efficacious formulas"?

Study process of medicine's foundations

Now I will talk about the process of learning medical books. There are two kinds of medical books; one is foundations and the second is clinical applications. Foundation books talk about physiology, pathology, medical history, herbs etc. Clinical application books include treatment, internal medicine, external medicine, gynecology, pediatrics, case studies etc. Nowadays, a student in junior middle school reads physiology and hygiene teaching materials. They all know the common knowledge of human physiology and the proper locations of the inner organs. How is it possible that someone who studies Chinese medicine will not have this basic knowledge of junior middle school. Therefore, the first task is to learn physiology and anatomy. The level should be at least the same or better than a junior middle school student. This is the minimum foundation needed; otherwise this person does not have the most basic knowledge.

As for learning physiology, the first step might as well be buying a copy of junior middle school physiology teaching materials. This must be easy to learn. One needs to draw oneself the chart of the human organs locations three times. This is the work of self-cultivation. I especially emphasize that each person uses their own hand to do this work; the drawing must not be very detailed, it just allows this material to sink deep into the brain.

The first step

One should look at the chart in the book of the inner organs and draw accordingly his own chart. The second time one should not look in the book and draw the organs chart, and the third time one should draw freely and in a casual manner on a piece of paper the organs and write the organs names next to them, then one can use this drawing as reference in order not to forget.

The second step

Buy a more detailed and deep physiology book. One needs only to read it carefully in order to supplement the lacking of the first teaching materials. If one wants to apply external medicine or acupuncture then he needs to be better versed in anatomy knowledge.

The third step

One should understand modern physiology and anatomy and know China's ancient physiology and anatomy. He should be able to differentiate between the two and know the differences and similarities.

What is China's ancient physiology and anatomy then? In the ancient Chinese medicine books, there are many technical terms all explaining the functions of the physiology. In order to learn this aspect, one can buy a book *Essentials of Nei Jing*. In this book, there are quotes such as: "the heart is the monarch, it is where the spirit becomes clear, the lungs are the minister, it is where the rhythm is regulated, the kidneys are the official of strength, it is where agility comes about..." etc. These kinds of old theories one must know about. After one knows them he must incorporate modern physiology terminology in order to explain the old terms. This is because the old terminology appears in many medical works, and after one becomes clear about these terms, then when he reads ancient medical books he feels that they are easy to understand.

Here, I must emphasize, when researching physiology one should resolutely resort to objectivity. Using modern physiology is the main thing. The mistakes of Chinese medicine physiology one must correct and find technical terms to explain these errors. The physiology spoken of in the *Nei Jing* truly contains mistakes. In our day and age we should not be stubborn in our brains. We should not say that because we claim the classic has an error then we have departed from Dao. We should have the spirit of experiments that Wang Qingren 王清任 had—a person of the Qing dynasty who wrote *Correcting the Errors of Medicine Yi Lin Gai Cuo* 醫林改錯. In order for him to understand better the human body, he went to execution grounds to observe bodies because, at his time, other than this option, there was no way to know how things really are in the human body. However, now, this is not the case. Physiology and anatomy books are published and circulated everywhere, how can one not discuss this? One should know what the Chinese medicine person is lacking: it is physiology and anatomy. We, who research Chinese medicine, with a humble heart, should absorb the modern knowledge of physiology and anatomy. This will be then a positive phenomenon of modern times. Absorbing new knowledge is part of the principle, and Chinese medicine must embrace it and not be embarrassed by it.

Section end

Research methods of clinical medicine

Yaron: The following section has a good idea how to further develop Chinese medicine. It claims that modern medicine has a standard for names and that all diseases have been fixed and declared which is, of course, wrong. Disease names do change at times, new diseases are frequently discovered and diseases that were thought to originate from X finally are discovered to originate from Y. However, Mr. Chen explains that historical complexity often confuses practitioners more than helping them and this is a valuable assessment. Let's think together with him of how to resolve these confusing issues. We should certainly learn the need for standards from modern medicine, but I think those for Chinese medicine need not be identical.

Internal medicine is the research of diseases related to internal medicine. In the old times, doctors researching internal medicine will learn the *Shang Han*, *Jin Gui* and *Wen Bing* books. In reality, this kind of research goes into an avoidable trifling problem. It beats around the bush in a very big way. In addition, if one eats the ancient without digesting it, has the posture of believing the *Shang Han Lun* in a revering fashion, and then looks down at the Wen Bing books; believes that modern prescriptions school cannot use classical prescriptions, to an extreme only reads one family's books; some use only hot herbs while others only cold herbs or only tonifying herbs; all along himself feels like he is the best; these are all wrong. Our objective in studying medicine is to see through modern and ancient, take the middle road and not be partial, only look for efficacy in treatment, not talk about schools of thought and boast about them, all the different schools have tunnel vision looking through a peephole.

Nonetheless, when we look initially at China's numerous internal medicine books, one can feel dizzy and blurry vision; he cannot tell where to start. Here, there are two solutions which I want to explain clearly. First, is the different way that diseases and symptoms are categorized in ancient versus modern times. Second, disease names are not the same in ancient times compared to modern times. After one becomes aware of this entanglement, then learning books has a beginning point.

The first point: First, I want to talk about the different methods that modern and ancient people used for categorizing diseases. In order to explain clearly, I want to make an analogy. From earlier on, there is a joke that goes as follows: "Four blind men felt an elephant. The first blind man palpated the elephant's front two legs and so he concluded that an elephant has two legs. The second felt the elephant's trunk, he didn't know what he was feeling and he thought that he was feeling a leg. He thought that the leg is like a rod that can curl at will. The third blind person felt all four legs and the trunk, and so he claimed that an elephant has five legs. He was under the impression that the trunk was a leg as well. The fourth blind person felt the trunk and ear. He said that an elephant is like a big giant bird, it has wings that look like leaves, it is possible that it can fly."

This joke is comparable to the classical prescriptions school, the modern prescriptions school, the Shang Han school, the Wen Bing school; this likewise is a funny joke. Think about it, that the Wen Bing school claims that a true Shang Han cold injury is a disease that finds itself only in the north, and that the south has not this disease; isn't this likewise groping blindly and talking blindly?[145] Everybody in the past could not see the complete picture of internal medicine, and so Chinese medicine for 1700 years did not have one bit of advancement. Coming to medical doctors in the 300 years of the Qing dynasty, it was all "you curse me and I curse you", classical prescriptions and modern prescriptions all fighting with each other endlessly. Now, at present, we should, early on, look at the entire picture of the elephant. However, there are still people who would not open their eyes and look at the elephant's entire body. They still rely on one leg and one trunk, themselves thinking that they know with their blind talk. So, explaining fully, the Shang Han school and the Wen Bing school each follow their different methods of disease differentiation of their time; each is able to see only a part of the big picture and that's it.

Once more, giving a simple analogy between disease names and geographical names: for example, in China's geography, the earliest land unit is a Zhou 州, emperor Yu 禹 divided it into 9 Zhou 州, Shun 舜 divided the land into 12 Zhou 州, Zhou 周 divided it again into 9 Zhou 州, coming down to the first unification of Qin Shihuang 秦始皇, he divided the domain into 36 Jun 郡 and later again into 40 Jun 郡, coming down all the way to the beginning of Qing the domain was divided into 18 Sheng 省 and then later into 22 Sheng 省 and during the nationalist republic it was changed again. The categorization methods of Chinese medicine febrile diseases also changed with the dynasties; the biggest difference can be seen between Zhang Zhongjing 張仲景 representing the classical prescriptions school and Wu Youke 吳又可 representing the modern prescriptions school.

[145] This idiom means grope about in the dark and talk irresponsibly.

See the following table for further explanation:

Qin and Han	The *Nei Jing Su Wen* 內經素問 took all febrile diseases and named them "cold injuries". It states that for cold injuries there are 5 types: 1. Zhong Feng 中風 wind strike. 2. Shang Han 傷寒 cold injury. 3. Wen Bing 溫病 warmth disease. 4. Shi Wen 濕溫 damp warmth and 5. Zhong Ye 中暍 sun strike.
Han	Zhang Zhongjing 張仲景 *Shang Han Lun* 傷寒論. Zhong Jing followed the five categorization of the *Su Wen*, but separately he also added Nüe Ji 瘧疾, Huo Luan 霍亂 etc febrile diseases and recorded them in the *Jin Gui* 金匱 book.
Han until the end of Ming	Going through many dynasties who, from beginning to end, preserve "guarding the old" *Shang Han Lun* 傷寒論 realm, they could not break through this ring and were still only talking about syndromes and not talking about disease names. All febrile diseases were categorized under the 6 conformations.[146] At the same time, there were many other febrile diseases being recorded in numerous medical books. However, these were not able to overturn the six conformations categorization method.
The end of Ming till the Qing	Wu Youke 吳又可 *Treatise of Warmth Pestilence* 溫疫論.[147] Many febrile diseases point to warmth pestilence; they are categorized as initial stage treatment, external and internal transmission, evil in the chest and diaphragm etc treatment. Wu Jutong's 吳鞠通 *Wen Bing Tiao Bian* 溫病條辨[148] categorizes most febrile diseases as upper Jiao, middle Jiao and lower Jiao. It includes the following types: wind warmth, warmth heat, warmth pestilence, warmth toxin, winter warmth, summer heat warmth, concealed summer heat, damp warmth, cold damp, warmth nüe 瘧, autumn dryness etc. Lei Shaoyi's 雷少逸 *Shi Bing Lun* 時病論[149] uses the four seasons to categorize and has 24 disease names. Spring: spring warmth, wind warmth, warmth disease, warmth toxin, evening onset. Summer: cold injury, wearing on summer heat, summer heat in center, summer heat warmth, summer heat cough, summer heat Zhai 瘵 sickness, Huo Luan, heat disease. Autumn: summer heat Nüe 瘧, wind Nüe 瘧, concealed summer heat, autumn summer heat, damp injury, warmth damp, autumn dryness. Winter: cold injury, cold strike, wearing on cold, winter warmth.
Modern times and Western medicine names	Damp warmth cold injury disease (which is warmth disease), typhus (which is warmth disease with patches), cholera (which is Gua Rang 瓜瓤 warmth), bubonic plague (which is Yin Yang toxin in the *Jin Gui* 金匱), contagious cold (which is the cold injury from the *Shang Han Lun* Ma Huang 麻黃 lines), wind injury disease (which is the *Shang Han Lun* wind strike Gui Zhi Tang 桂枝湯 syndrome), scarlet fever (which is Lan Hou Dan Sha 爛喉丹痧), measles (which is Xi Zi 瘜子 and Chi Zhen 赤疹), smallpox disease (which is Dou Chuang Tian Hua 痘瘡天花), recurring fever (*Shang Han Lun* has a few lines about it), wind warmth disease (which is lung wind phlegm shortness of breath etc—pneumonia), chest pains disease (*Shang Han Lun* has lines about it—pleurisy), malaria (Jin Gui Nüe Ji 瘧疾), tetanus (which is Qi Feng 臍風), hundred days tuberculosis (which is Tao Hua Zhu Ben Ma Lao 桃花疰奔馬癆 etc), Damp Heat[150] (which is damp injury etc—gastritis), mumps (which is Yi Zhong 頤腫) , erysipelas (which is Liu Huo Chi You Dan 流火赤游丹).

[146] Tai Yang, Shao Yang, Yang Ming, Tai Yin, Shao Yin and Jue Yin.
[147] Published 1642 CE.
[148] Published 1798 CE.
[149] Published 1882 CE.
[150] Fever contracted during the humid season.

Looking at the above table, one can easily see the Chinese medicine methods for categorizing diseases. Not only the methods are not the same at each dynasty, but the disease names are also not the same. This is a fact. The first entanglement in researching Chinese medicine is the different categorization in different dynasties. Even around the same time period within the same school, like Wu Youke dividing diseases according to what transpires first and what last, where Wu Jutong uses the three Jiao to divide diseases, Lei Shaoyi uses the four seasons to divide them. This can be compared to the four blind men palpating an elephant, each person expresses the results that he has personally come by. If one did not see this table above, it is possible that he too will follow the earlier generation and will keep on palpating like a blind man for a long time.

For us now, we must go and see the entire elephant. First, find exactly how many diseases internal medicine has. In our modern age, there are Western medical books that we can refer to for corrections. As for Western medicine, not only are disease names fixed in books in our nation, but also they are publicly fixed in "the international standardized record of diseases". According to this international standard list of diseases we must find out, verify and correct our Chinese medicine diseases' names. Amongst us, there are those who perform mutual comparisons. However, no one did a thorough and clear comparison of more than a thousand years of old accounts, then create one standardized list of all disease names. For the people who study medicine, until they don't have one form like this in their hands they will never be able to be clear. Therefore, I want to make a contribution to all the students and publish such a form—a comparison chart of disease names from ancient times to present day, which will come out in Cunren medical collection the 6th volume, spread over 3 issues. After having this chart, each person will know the entire scope of internal medicine. This will make reading books much easier.

Up to here, we have explained thoroughly the issue of disease categorization from ancient times to present. In addition, we will create a standardized table comparing ancient and modern disease names. This will solve this problem.

The second point: I want to talk about the differences between the ancient disease names. This, yet again, is another huge entanglement. When we look at the above table, we can see that not only disease categorization was different throughout the ages, but also that disease names were different. For the same symptoms you could have different disease names. Let's bring an example: now, we commonly use the disease name Ban Zhen Shang Han 斑疹傷寒.[151] What does this disease call in Chinese medicine literature then? Ha! There are many, which makes it hard to find out which one is which. In the Han dynasty, Zhang Zhongjing's *Shang Han Lun* does not mention it. In the Sui 隋 dynasty, Master Chao 巢,[152] in his book *Bing Yuan* 病源,[153] called it "Wen Bing Fa Ban Hou 溫病發斑候", "Shang Han Ban Chuang Hou 傷寒斑瘡候", "Shi Qi Fa Ban Hou 時氣發斑候".[154] In the Tang 唐 dynasty, in the book *Qian Jin Fang* 千金方,[155] it is called "Shang Han Ban Chu 傷寒斑出". In the Tang 唐 dynasty *Wai Tai Mi Yao* 外台祕要,[156] it is called "Ban Lan Yin Zhen 斑爛隱疹". Coming to the Jin Yuan 金元 dynasties, Zhang Zihe 張子和 the Confucian serving the family school it was called "Ban Zhen Shang Han 斑疹傷寒". Disease names in Chinese medicine, from antiquity until today, are all like this. For the beginner student of medicine, how is it possible to become clear? Yet, Chinese medicine names, one after the other, are all like this. What a huge entanglement there is!

From a rational perspective, internal medicine should have diseases as units, not syndromes. Therefore, when researching internal medicine, one must take all the ancient disease names and find out which modern diseases do they refer to? In an early stage, these all must be spoken of, must be revealed! There is no need to take again the Tai Yang, Shao Yang, Yang Ming etc names of the *Shang Han Lun*, *Jin Gui* and *Wen Bing* and keep on using them, nor take upper Jiao, lower Jiao and try to insert them. These ones, early on, did not match with modern times.

First, we must explain why these disease names in ancient times were in such a chaotic state. In reality, Western medicine books, from ancient times to present, also use different names. It is only in recent history that they were gradually standardized and, even then, not fully standardized. Therefore, there was a need to arrange an international conference to standardize them completely. Our own Chinese history is very long, medical literature is vast and the nation has not, as yet, performed the standardization task. It is hardly untenable that, throughout history, disease names were different. For this, we can also make an analogy; for example, China's place names were

[151] Typhus.

[152] Chao Yuanfang 巢元方 (550–630 CE)

[153] 諸病源候論, also called 巢氏病源 and 巢氏诸病源候论

[154] We choose not to translate the disease names into English as the author uses the ancient and modern names similarities to draw a conclusion. Here Fa Ban 發斑 means to develop patches or macules; there is Ban "patches" in the modern name for Typhus and in ancient disease names.

[155] By Sun Simiao 孫思邈 (? –682 CE)

[156] Compiled by Wang Tao 王燾 752 CE.

also not the same from antiquity to today. For example, this place "Guang Zhou 廣州" had many different names, from ancient times to present. In the Spring and Autumn and Warring States periods it was called Bai Yue Di 百粵地. In the Qin 秦 dynasty it was called Nan Hai Jun 南海郡. In the beginning of Han 漢 it was called Nan Yue Guo 南越國. In the Three Kingdoms era, the kingdom of Wu 吳, it was called Guang Zhou 廣州. In the Jin 晉 dynasty it was called Guang Zhou Nan Hai Jun 廣州南海郡. In the Sui 隋 it was called Fan Zhou 番州. In the Tang 唐 it was called again Guang Zhou 廣州. In the Song 宋 was called again Guang Zhou Nan Hai Jun 廣州南海郡. In the Yuan 元 it was changed to Guang Zhou Lu 廣州路. In the Ming and Qing 明清 was changed to Guang Zhou Fu 廣州府. Chinese medicine disease names from ancient times to present had different names exactly like in this analogy.

What is detestable in our Chinese medicine circles is that, until today, there was no standardization of ancient and modern disease names. It only gradually became the custom with some disease names that were often used and so disease names remained the same like Nüe Ji Li Ji Ma Zhen Tian Hua 瘧疾痢疾痲疹天花 etc names. Within the formless realm, they were commonly used and so became the standard. There are a few self-proclaimed scholars of antiquity who still use, in their books, ancient names; this is laughable. It is like when someone wants to travel to Guang Zhou 廣州 and goes to buy a train ticket, but he is not willing to use the modern name Guang Zhou 廣州; instead he insists on using the ancient name Fan Zhou 番州. Isn't this the same fallacy?

Nonetheless, people who study Chinese medicine always want to read Chinese medicine books from history and so they cannot avoid meeting ancient disease names, like reading records of the three kingdoms and wanting to know the modern location names. I have already invested much effort to tackle this grand problem, however, I, as of yet, could not complete it. Look at Cunren medical collection; at each volume we publish one table, like at the back of this volume talking about Ma Zhen 痲疹 disease, summarizing clearly all different accounts throughout history and, at the end, fixing the disease name. This issue is not readily available to beginner students of medicine, however there is no need for them, either, to be completely clear about it. It suffices for them to know that disease names throughout history had this kind of evolution.

The disease, after all, is this disease; it is only that names were changed and that's it. It is like when a person becomes a Daoist and he assumes a Daoist name, let's say

Wu Dao 悟道.[157] Later on, they start believing in Buddhism and assume a different name according to Buddhism, let's say Jing Ci 淨慈.[158] The person Wu Dao and Jing Ci are, after all, the same person. So is the case with people in the classical formulas school and modern formulas school, they often make their own case and fight with each other. This kind of fighting was not a small trivial matter. When we inspect the Qing dynasty medical literature, the fight between Shang Han Lun practitioners and Wen Bing practitioners was endless. It entangled for 300 years and lasted till the last decade, where medical books still contain this fight. If we use modern diseases to categorize clearly and decide, one after the other, all the disease names, then on a fundamental level there is no reason to fight anymore. If one intentionally just wants to fight then he may lose his membership.

Excerpt end

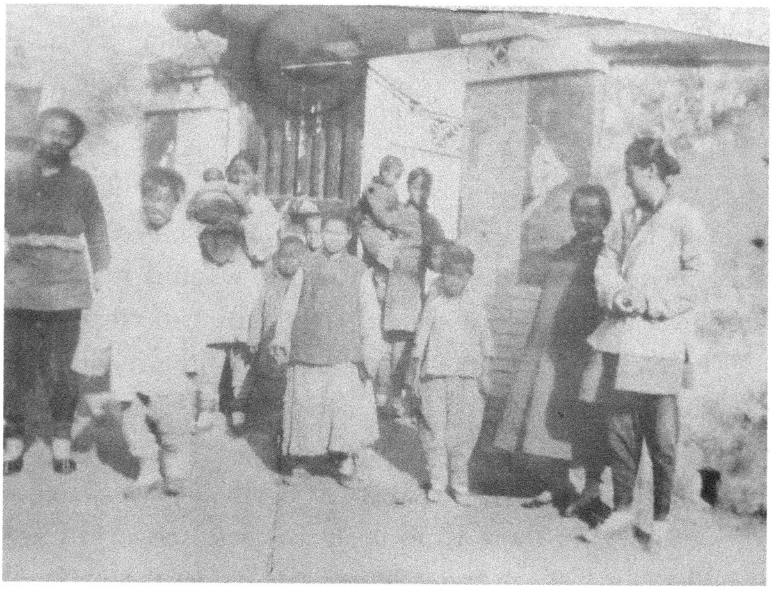

Photo by Mr P. Goux in early 1900s. "Chinese common people".

[157] Enlightened Dao
[158] Clear compassion

The spirit and methods of the apprenticeship system in the past

1956 by Qin Bowei 秦伯未

Source: *The New Chinese Medicine Magazine* 新中醫藥 第七卷第六期, June 1956

Yaron: A last faint voice before the eradication of traditional-style learning. Qin Bowei, in the 1920s, started in the Shanghai Chinese Medicine Specialized School and over the years advocated Chinese medicine modernity and standardization reform. One then wonders why, in the wake of the mightiest Chinese medicine standardization effort and the creation of government-sponsored TCM schools, education and curriculum, he would change opinion and advocate traditional-style learning? The answer, of course, I do not know. If I were to speculate I would say he feared the possible loss of traditional values—a medicine that is about to lose many of its ideals. It is also practical to think that Qin Bowei simply wanted to help the government produce many practitioners expeditiously in order to meet healthcare demands. We may never know.

Pages 242–243

Ministry of Health, Chinese medicine consultant Qin Bowei 秦伯未

The apprenticeship system is one of China's traditional education methods. In the past, the production of Chinese medicine practitioners was only partially by family inheritance; it was mainly from the inter-teaching between famous doctors. Through a relationship between teacher and apprentice, the teacher passed the knowledge and experience to the apprentice and afterwards, the apprentice passed the knowledge and experience to other people via the apprenticeship system, producing more professionals.

Everyone knows that Zhang Sangjun 張桑君 was Bianque's 扁鵲 teacher, Zhang Bozu 張伯祖 was Zhang Zhongjing's 張仲景 teacher. Later, Bianque had seven apprentices: Ziyang 子陽, Zibao 子豹, Zirong 子容, Ziming 子明, Ziyou 子游, Ziyue 子越 and Yangyi 陽儀. Zhang Zhongjing had two apprentices, Dudu 杜度 and Weifan 衛汎. Especially Bianque, following Zhang Sangjun's instruction, achieved great progress with pulse taking method. Up to Eastern Jin Dynasty, Wang Shuhe 王叔和 accomplished a book called *The Pulse Classic Mai Jing* 脉經 and it spread to Korea, Japan, Arabia and India, causing a huge impact on medicine worldwide. Zhang Zhongjing, who already knew about medicine, attained more knowledge about clinical practice through the education given by Zhang Bozu. Also, he studied a lot of case histories and prescriptions, and wrote *Treatise on Cold-Induced Disease Shang Han Lun* 傷寒論 and *Treatise on Miscellaneous Diseases Za Bing Lun* 雜病論 which was passed down to present and which became one of the medical classical books. This all suggests that the apprentice system not only passed down the professional skills and knowledge but also raised and developed Chinese medicine culture.

Family inheritance includes father and son, uncle and nephew, brothers etc. The seniors take care of the education, and this part is not much different from the apprenticeship system. Due to accumulated experience from the same lineage, the knowledge became more specific and, in this way, it has produced many outstanding people. Li Nia Ne 李念莪, the author of *The Neijing Essentials Neijing Zhi Yao* 內經知要, was learning from his uncle, and then passed the knowledge to his nephew. The He 何氏 family from Jiangsu province Qingpu county 江苏青浦县 started practicing medicine since Southern Song Dynasty, and their knowledge has passed on continuously for more than twenty generations until the present day, for example the famous doctors He Shutian 何書田 and He Hongfang 何鴻舫. Then there is the great scientist Li Shizhen 李時珍, who inherited medical knowledge from his grandfather and father and combined it with his own wisdom, studied medicinal herbs and completed the great book *Compendium of Materia Medica Ben Cao Gang Mu* 本草綱目, which scientists value all around the world. Although the scope of family inheritance is narrower, it's also an important way to produce Chinese medicine practitioners, and it should be given more attention.

Students want to have satisfying teachers, and teachers want to have proper students, so the apprenticeship system should be voluntary on both sides. Li Dongyuan 李东垣, from Jin Yuan Dynasties, admired Zhang Yuansu's 張元素 medical knowledge and offered a thousand ounces of gold for his education. Zhang Yuansu accepted this request and taught Li Dongyuan. Zhu Danxi 朱丹溪 crossed Qiantang River 錢塘江 to Suzhou 苏州, then to Zhenjiang 鎮江, then to Nanchang 南昌, and back to Hangzhou 杭州 at the end to meet Luo Zhiti 罗知悌. Luo Zhiti originally didn't accept him, but was touched by Zhu's sincerity and taught him everything. There was another story on *Records of the Grand Historian Shi Ji* 史记, Gongcheng Yangqing 公乘陽慶 had excellent medical knowledge and skills, but during that time he was seventy and had no sons to transmit his ability to. Then he met Chun Yuyi 淳于意 and passed on all his effective proven recipes. So we can see that in the apprenticeship system they respected each other. Especially Gongcheng Yangqing realized that medicine is a profession that can save many people's lives, so it should be disseminated to later generations and serve masses of people instead of being buried with the great doctors. This spirit should be followed by modern Chinese medicine practitioners.

Good apprenticeship is very important to develop Chinese medicine from the past onward into the future. The good education of the teacher and the humble attitude of the student are also necessary to learn Chinese medicine. As a teacher, Luo Zhiti used Liu Hejian 刘何間, Zhang Zihe 張子和 and Li Dongyuan's books to teach Zhu Danxi, asking Zhu to begin with studying the theory. Luo combined and extended their theories and asked Zhu to absorb the knowledge. Bianque took his apprentices to see patients together, for example, when he was treating the Prince of the state of Guo 虢太子, Bianque explained the disease condition and then asked Ziyang to do the acupuncture, Zibao to do hot medicinal compress and prescription. From these instances, we know that ancient people emphasized on the combination of theory and practice and made many efforts when teaching apprentices. As an apprentice, Hua Boren 滑伯仁 once wrote *Elaboration of the Fourteen Meridians Shi Si Jing Fa Hui* 十四經發揮 which is a famous and useful book about acupuncture. Hua Boren originally learnt internal medicine from Wang Juzhong 王居中, and then learnt acupuncture from Gao Dongyang 高洞陽 in order to enhance his skills. In Qing Dynasty, Ye Tianshi 叶天士 learnt medicine from his father Ye Yangsheng 叶陽生 when he was young. His father passed away when he was fourteen, and he felt his knowledge was not enough so he learnt from his school brother Zhu 朱. Afterwards, he went to learn from another doctor when he knew the doctor was good at treating some specific disease. In total he learnt from seventeen doctors. This demonstrates that students need to make their own efforts in addition to education from teachers.

The apprenticeship system is always carried out by questions and answers, which is now called "discussion." This kind of teaching benefits students as well as teachers. For example, in the Song Dynasty, Pang Anchang's 龐安常 father was a doctor and had taught him pulse taking but Pang Anchang thought that it was not enough, so he secretly studied Bianque's book about pulse taking. When his father examined his learning, they often had debates. There was not a specific way to do the apprenticeship, but usually it began with theoretical learning and clinical learning and carried out via discussion.

During the past twenty years, the development of medicine in our country can't be separated from the apprenticeship system of the past dynasties. Therefore, it's a correct decision of our Party and government to encourage the apprenticeship system. Some might ask, since we are going to open Chinese medical colleges and schools and also planning to organize Western medicine doctors to learn Chinese medicine, why bother to use the old way to train up Chinese medicine practitioners?

This kind of thinking is not comprehensive enough. With the development of a socialist construction, the people's demand for healthcare is increasing. The number of current medical personnel is far behind current demand. We don't have enough time and won't have enough personnel if medical staff only receive training in medical schools. Chinese medicine practitioners are, to a large degree, spread in remote farmlands and usually trusted by the farmers. So let's say there are half a million Chinese medicine practitioners—if one practitioner can take care of one apprentice, we can have another half a million practitioners in only a few years. Besides, there's no conflict between the apprenticeship system and the establishment of medical schools. Furthermore, there is abundant knowledge in the ancient medical literature; as long as we are willing to spend our time on it, we can find it out. But what was recorded in literature is just part of the ancient people's knowledge. There is a lot of clinical experience possessed by current practitioners; they can't be gathered together and then teach students, especially the old practitioners. If we don't learn from them, then the precious experience will be no longer available in the future. Therefore, the apprenticeship system was necessary not only in the past but also at present.

At present, the condition of practicing in an apprenticeship program is much easier than before. 1. The teachers regard it as an honorable job to educate the next generation. 2. Under the influence of science and the calling to develop traditional medicine, some people have made the decision to learn Chinese medicine. 3. The teaching method improved a lot compared to the past. 4. There are more teaching materials and reference books than before. 5. There is assistance from United Clinics and Chinese medicine associations. Furthermore, I especially want to point out that we can overcome any problem with the leadership of the Party and the department of health on every level. Now, Chinese medicine practitioners in Shanxi 山西 province Taigu 太谷 county have thought of many ways to train apprentices and the progress is very smooth. It's imaginable that other experienced practitioners might have been training apprentices.

The apprenticeship system is a good and quick way to train many Chinese medicine practitioners at once. Fellows should know that it's not an isolating job to lead apprentices; it's a part of the whole Chinese medicine work. I hope practitioners can be tireless in teaching and leading the new generation practitioners to surpass them and to make the biggest efforts to facilitate the development of Chinese medicine.

(Originally published in *People's Daily* 人民日報)

Article end

How To learn *The Essential of Neijing* *Neijing Zhi Yao* 內經知要

Jun 25, 1956 by Qin Bowei 秦伯未

Source: *The New Chinese Medicine Magazine* 新中醫藥 第七卷第六期, June 1956

Yaron: Chinese medicine in 1956—a time of new reality—was forming a new identity. In this article we witness an old practitioner reasoning ancient theories in a new way, adapting to a modern state and Communist ideology. Old theories might have had different meanings at their inception but here, in the new China, logic had to become materialistic and practical. This did not start in the 1950s but decisively received its final punch at this time. Here, Qin Bowei was saving tradition. In the past, as a modernizer, he believed in modernizing the medicine in the face of modern science, but now he was out to rescue its tradition. Limited by circumstances, his explanations are confined to current ideology. Overall his strategy did not change: reform Chinese medicine to a more practical art. During the Republic, however, when many practitioners wanted Chinese medicine to stay "old", he vigorously wanted reform and now, in the Communist era, as everyone was promoting radical reform (willingly or by coercion), he argued for the old—or at least for slowing down the rapid transformation. Today, times have changed and we, like Qin Bowei, must seize this opportunity and proactively move in a better direction. It is time to find what truly is best for Chinese medicine's development. The principle for Qin never changed: keep it real and do the best you can to keep it alive!

Pages 248–251

Introduction: *Neijing* 內經, *Treatise on Cold-induced Diseases Shang Han Lun* 傷寒論, *Golden Chamber Jin Kui Yao Lüe* 金匱要略 and *Herbal Materia Medica Ben Cao Jing* 本草經 are four classic books in Chinese medicine. These classic books point out the academic thought of Chinese medicine, theoretical system, treatment principle, and knowledge of formulas and herbs. This means that the four aspects of theory, methodology, formula and herbs are included in those classic books.

Chinese medicine has been working tirelessly for the laboring people in China for thousands of years. Recently in the entire country, under the correct leadership of our Party and government, Chinese medicine has been curing more and more diseases which didn't exist in the earlier medical books, such as epidemic encephalitis B, undulant fever, bacillary dysentery, hypertension, cerebral cortex fatigue, schistosomiasis etc. This achievement is no accident; there certainly exists a unique theory serving as foundation for the treatment, just as there's no way to win a battle without correct thoughts or weapons. The classic books mentioned serve as a guideline for Chinese medicine fighting disease, however using its principle for exploring the new also matters. Therefore, in order to inherit, organize and develop Chinese medicine as our country's legacy, we should continue studying these ancient texts, especially the *Neijing*. Being the core of Chinese medicine academic thought, we should learn it first.

Neijing Essentials Neijing Zhi Yao 內經知要 is the abridged edition of *Neijing*. Although it was chosen by the editor subjectively, and couldn't satisfy all people, it undeniably contains the important parts of *Neijing*, making it appropriate material for those studying the *Neijing*. Below are my reading notes from *Neijing Zhi Yao* for your reference, and any corrections are welcome.

1. The nurturing life of Dao, Dao Sheng 道生

Dao Sheng summarizes the ancient nurturing-life methods. Its central idea revolves around internal cause and external cause. The internal cause refers to strong or weak constitution, and the external cause refers to stimulation from the environment. People need to adapt to the environment, for there is no other way to live. *Neijing* emphasizes that the disease cause stems from an internal conflict within the organism. An external cause is only regarded as a condition for disease transformation but it's only due to internal cause that this transformation can take place. This is why :

> "There is a correct time to avoid the seasonal evils and thief wind, when one is calm and non-desirous; the true Qi follows naturally; if one can maintain the integrity of the mind and the control of emotions, then how can diseases arise 虛邪賊風 避之有時 恬淡虛無 真氣從之 精神內守 病安從來?"

These 24 characters are the structural frame of the entire book. They portray four levels of nurturing life accomplishment: immortals 真人, semi-immortals 至人, sages 聖人 and virtuous men 賢人. Among these, immortals and semi-immortals are imaginary, which might have been a construction of Daoists during that time. Only sages and people of virtue can be a model for people to follow. This narrative is similar to that said by people of antiquity, "learning the way from the supreme, you only get the medium; learning from the medium, you only get the inferior." If we analyze and compare these four precepts, they don't escape the two aspects internal and external, and so we know that their thoughts in reality were similar to ours.[159]

Furthermore, not only ask people to adapt to the environment, but also follow the environment to facilitate the body's constitution. This is the main idea behind *Si Qi Tiao Shen Da Lun* 四气調神大論. The main idea of this chapter is very plain and simple; it considers the natural phenomena, such as "Every natural creature is flourishing 萬物以榮", "Every natural creature is prosperous and begins to bear fruit 萬物華實" etc, [in relation] to people's life situation, and proposes precepts such as "In spring, sleep late and get up early. Stroll in large steps in the courtyard 夜卧早起 廣步于庭", "In summer, sleep late and get up early and do not get bored with longer daytime 夜臥早起無厭於日" etc. The point is to benefit the spirit and obey nature, so there are "the desire to live arises 以使志生", "never get angry 使志無怒" and other sayings. Those sayings point out that if we only take care of our physical exercise and neglect to calm the spiritual part, there will still be internal conflicts. Therefore, *Neijing* emphasized the inherent spiritual value in the natural weather phenomena. It also uses the regularity of growth and decline in human beings to explain the importance of taking care of one's physical body. These theories have the same idea as in the sentence "when essence and spirit guard inside where can disease come from?"

Ancient people called human's capability "Qi", and also called the environmental climate "Qi". There is some explanation in *Neijing* chapter *Ci Jie Zhen Xie Lun* 刺節真邪論:

> In the category of Qi there are genuine Qi, upright Qi and evil Qi. Genuine Qi is received both from the sky (referring to innate) and grain Qi (postnatal nutrition) and is replete throughout the body. Upright Qi is upright wind, which comes from one direction. It is neither excess wind nor vacuous wind. Evil Qi is vacuous wind evil and harms people. It hits so deeply that people can't extinguish it on their own.

It explains that [what refers to] the genuine Qi in ancient times is actually essential Qi and original Qi, while evil Qi is an abnormal climate. Genuine Qi and evil Qi can't exist at the same time in one person, which means if genuine Qi overcomes the evil Qi it manifests as health; the opposite manifests as disease. That is the reason the Dao Sheng article emphasizes so much supporting genuine Qi to resist evil Qi.

[159] There is no such thing as external cause of disease without pre-existing internal disharmony.

2. Yin Yang

Ancient people observed the expressions of both conflict and harmony that exist objectively in nature and produced first a body of knowledge based upon sensibility, and then developed a body of knowledge based upon rationality, and finally matured it as a unifying principle to explain all phenomena. This is the source of Yin-Yang theory. *Neijing* understood and processed all medical questions with Yin-Yang theory, mainly the aspects of inter-transformation and inter-restriction. In *Neijing*, the Yin-Yang theory presents a comparison rather than concrete notions. So in *Neijing*, many sentences such as "cultivate Yang to become heaven, and cultivate Yin to become earth," "exterior is Yang, interior is Yin," "back is Yang, abdomen is Yin," "Yin is quiet and Yang is restless"—they explain that the function and nature of Yin and Yang are different, while other lines such as, "Yang is born and Yin grows, Yang restrained and Yin concealed," "Yang transforms to Qi, Yin becomes form," "predominance of Yang generates heat, predominance of Yin generates cold," and "clear Yang emerges from upper orifices, murky Yin emerges from lower orifices," "predominance of Yin leads to disorder of Yang, predominance of Yang leads to disorder of Yin," etc. elaborate the effect of Yin and Yang. Therefore Yin-Yang is a flexible concept that can refer to many conditions and its medical usage is not simple and fixed.

Simply dividing into Yin and Yang can't solve many sophisticated and complicated problems, so Yin and Yang was further divided to make it "Yin within Yin, Yang within Yin, Yang within Yang, Yang within Yin." It should be certain, however, that no matter how Yin and Yang change, they are always relative rather than absolute, interdependent instead of separated and isolated. Specifically, there is balance between Yin and Yang. In *Neijing* it states:

> The importance of [the relation between] Yin and Yang is to have Yin securely stored so that Yang can remain soundly installed. A disharmony between Yin and Yang is like having only spring but no autumn, or only summer but no winter. Make an effort to maintain the harmony [between Yin and Yang], this is what the sages practice [as the best way to maintain good health]. If Yang is overpowering [so that] Yin cannot be secured, it will be exhausted. [The ideal situation] is that Yin remains peaceful and Yang is secured, then the mind is calm 陰陽

之要 陽密乃固 兩者不和 若春無秋 若冬無夏 因而和之 是謂聖度. 故陽強不能密 陰氣乃絕 陰平陽密 精神乃至.

This explains how the organism's internal balance can adjust to the external environment. On the contrary, the organism's internal imbalance will cause physiological disorder, which is the main reason for disease. This is the concept of integrity in Yin-Yang theory in *Neijing*. People used Yin-Yang to present the objective findings and phenomena in order to create symptom differentiation within the framework of materialism, which became the system of Chinese medicine theory.

3. Complexion diagnosis

In Chinese medicine, people usually use several diagnostic methods such as inspection, auscultation and olfaction, interrogation, pulse-taking and palpation in order to diagnose. Therefore, in *Five Organs Generation Essay Wu Zang Sheng Cheng Lun* 五臟生成論 there is "combining the complexion and pulse, then one can know everything 能合色脈 可以萬全." Complexion diagnosis is actually complexion inspection, including the reflection of internal organs on the face and eyes. For example, "blue and black is pain, yellow is heat, white is coldness," or "heavy and murky is internal, floating and glossy is external," or "regard long as short, regard white as black, then the essence is declining," these sentences are all within this scope. However the *Neijing* distribution of certain organs in certain locations of the face we cannot use it mechanically.

Except for some specific diseases that have obvious colors—for example, the main symptom of jaundice is yellow eyes and yellow skin—we don't need to regard five colors as the only principle. Mainly, we pay attention to its brightness and luster. This is why in *Neijing* it says, "inspect the luster to see if the practitioner is a good doctor", "inspect the luster to see if the patient's condition is going well." Others such as "A healthy red should be as the color of cinnabar wrapped by a white silk cloth instead of ochre. A healthy white should have the soft glow of goose feather but not the glaring white of crystalline salt. A healthy green should be as jade instead of blue hue of indigo. A healthy yellow should be as the color of realgar wrapped by silk gauze instead of yellow dirt. A healthy black should shine like multiple layers of varnish and not be matte like humus". Doctors see the extent of luster to distinguish the condition of wellness or illness. Chinese medicine cures disease in a way that regards the whole organism as a single phenomenon, meaning it combines curing disease with curing people. On one hand, it observes the symptoms of the whole body, while on the other hand, it estimates the remaining energy and strength the patient still has. We can check the patient's energy and the disease condition through complexion inspection, combined with other diagnostic methods. That's the reason complexion inspection is the first of the four diagnostic methods.

Complexion inspection isn't limited just to the face. In *Neijing*, it says, "Yellow and red is wind, green and black is pain, white is coldness, yellow and red and also greasy is pus, much red is blood, too much pain is convulsion, too much coldness is skin numbness." It obviously includes symptoms of the entire body from internal medicine and local symptoms of external medicine and traumatology. Therefore, complexion inspection includes every place that the doctor can inspect.

4. Pulse diagnosis

There are two ways to take pulse in *Neijing*; one is "nine readings on three sections." Three sections means upper, middle, and lower sections of the human body, and nine readings means three locations for each section. "One small pulse is ill, one big pulse is ill, one fast pulse is ill, one slow pulse is ill, one hot pulse is ill, one cold pulse is ill, one collapsed pulse is ill," this means that, among the nine locations, if there's one irregular pulse then this can form the basis for diagnosis. The other pulse is "wrist pulse-taking method;" it is Cun-Guan-Chi pulse-taking method used nowadays, which is the method of taking the pulse of radial artery. In later times, people mainly took the pulse from wrist radial artery and gradually gave up on "nine readings on three sections". That's what Zhang Zhongjing criticized, "take pulse on hand instead of foot".

In *Neijing*, dawn is the best time to take the pulse. It also recognizes the relationship between breath and pulse, and this knowledge accords with modern medicine. But, during that time, many of the recorded pulses only had the description of the condition without a name, so now several pulse names don't match the pulse condition. Even if some of the pulse conditions in *Neijing* are actually the same as the pulse names that we use today, we can't use the modern meanings to explain those names in *Neijing*, such as "string," "hook," "fur," "floating," "firing firewood," "spreading leaves," "occasional visitors," "mud balls," "horizontal beams," "the thread on a bow," "pouring paint" etc. There were more than thirty kinds of pulse conditions, the meaning of which was to describe how the disease progresses.

Chinese medicine always emphasizes the four diagnostic methods equally rather than solely depend on pulse. We attach importance to the combination of the symptoms and pulses, which means it requires the specific symptoms and specific pulse. For example, the pulse of fever from external contraction should be floating, tight, slippery, fast or similar kinds; the pulse for internal injury deficiency should be deep, thready, soggy, soft or similar kinds. In contrast, the pulse when external contraction meets internal injury or internal injury meets external contraction is called Yang symptoms with Yin pulse or Yin symptoms with Yang pulse, and both need attention. In *Neijing* it says, "If one's shape is big but pulse thready, one dies when lacking air to breathe. If one's shape is small but pulse is big, one dies when there's too much air in the chest."

It's best to merge the pulse, physical shape, and symptoms together, while paying attention to the disease process and the patient's lifestyle. For example, If you diagnose a disease just by taking the pulse without asking the disease progression and lifestyle situation, then it is like the saying: "If diagnosing and not asking for the origin, emotions, diet, waking and sleeping in a disorderly fashion, chance of poisoning (pointing to drug poisoning), how can one know the disease?" Therefore, Chinese medicine has been doing sophisticated clinical inspection since very early times.

5. Viscera manifestation Zang-fu 臟腑

The five Zang refers to five organs, but it includes the six Fu hollow organs. In *Neijing* it says, "five organs store up the essence and don't dispel it, while six hollow organs digest and transport the food and water without storing it," so doctors in the past emphasized the Zang organs and not the Fu hollow organs. However, in *Neijing* it also says, "a man who is eight feet tall he has skin and muscles, one can measure it from the outside by palpating along it, or after he dies one can dissect the body and see it." There are "bone measurement article," "meridians and tendons article," "pulse measurement article," "organs article," and "stomach and intestines article" etc. in *Neijing* talking about the size, length and weight of bones, tendons, artery and organs. These articles didn't omit the Fu hollow organs and they didn't regard Zang organs as a stand-alone mechanism. They had some organic connection. The *Ling Lan Mi Dian Lun* 灵蘭秘典論 compares the organs to political organization to describe the relationships between the organs. The *Liu Jie Zang Xiang Lun* 六節臟象論 divides the surface of the body to the organ's governed domains, it assumes the organs conduct the entire body. The former perspective demonstrates the internal unity of the whole body, and the latter perspective focuses on curing the disease on the surface. Chinese medicine depends on this theory to get effective results in clinical practice.

Neijing can barely explain the sophisticated physiology of the organs, so it offered a name "Spirit" Shen 神. Since this character can't represent different conditions of each organ, it got divided into "spiritual soul" Hun 魂, "corporeal soul" Po 魄 and other names, all derived from the same assumption. *Nanjing* 難經, as a supplement of *Neijing*, says, "Zang organs are where human's Shen spirit-Qi store, so liver stores Hun spiritual soul, lungs store Po corporeal soul, heart stores Shen spirit, spleen stores thoughts Yi 意 and Zhi 智, kidneys store essence Jing 精 and will Zhi 志." So we can understand that the spiritual soul and corporeal soul Hun and Po in *Neijing* are just synonyms of Shen spirit, only referring to the physiological phenomenon of one organ. Furthermore, in *Neijing* chapters *Jin Kui Zhen Yan Lun* 金匱真言論 and *Yin Yang Ying Xiang Da Lun* 陰陽应象大論 it says that the five organs correspond to four times and five directions, flavors, colors and Qi etc. The purpose of that is to sum up these unorganized things based on the logic of nature instead of physiology.

In *Wu Yun Xing Da Lun* 五运行大論 it says, "When Qi is excess, it inhibits what it can overcome and counter-restricts what it is overcome by. When Qi is deficient, then what overcomes it over-restricts it and what it can overcome counter-restricts it." It refers to Yun Qi 运气 rather than physiology. Yun means moving, Qi means the year-Qi. Ancient people observed the transformation of six Qi during the four seasons every year and regarded it as disease cause in epidemics. In this method they used water, fire, wood, metal and earth five elements as the basis. They assumed that five elements are the substance of Yin-Yang, and Yin-Yang is the Qi of five elements. The Qi can't exist without its substance and the substance can't move without its Qi. The substance resides in the earth while Qi moves in sky (as seen in *Leijing* 類經). Therefore the success and failure is derived from the strength and weakness, and the change between excess and deficiency can be observed from the restriction and generation. These changes originally were not connected to organs, but became linked to physiology and pathology later and became the five-element generation and restriction theory.

6. Meridians

The term "meridian" Jing Luo 經絡 is hard to explain in modern anatomy, but it plays an important role in Chinese clinical medicine. It mainly divides the whole body into several parts and creates the connection between exterior surface and interior organs, specifically connecting many acupuncture points to become one line. So the same line has radiation sensation when one point on it is stimulated. Undoubtedly, it is from clinical acupuncture experience accumulated since ancient times. There are regular meridians and extra meridians. Their paths have been described in detail in *Neijing*. In short, there are hand three Yin and three Yang, foot three Yin and three Yang, distributed all over the body including upper and lower, front and back, left and right, and four limbs. Hand three Yin meridians travel from organs to hands, hand three Yang meridians travel from hands to head, foot three Yang meridians travel from head to feet and foot three Yin meridians travel from feet to abdomen. In extra meridians, Dai Mai surrounds the hypochondrium like a girdle. Chong, Ren, and Du Mai start at perineum and travel on chest, back and abdomen respectively, which is called "one source, three branches". Because among the extra meridians only Ren and Du Mai have acupuncture points, these two meridians were included with the regular meridians and thus there are fourteen regular meridians.

Neijing divided common diseases according to meridians, and so we need to know the symptoms of each meridian after being familiar with the location of those meridians. Diseases recorded in *Bing Neng chapter* 病能篇 were according to the twelve meridians, identifying which symptoms belong to which meridian and to which organs. Thereupon it became much easier to treat disease.

7. Treatment principle

The symptoms' pattern differentiation in Chinese medicine is divided into four categories of Yin-Yang system: coldness, heat, deficiency and excess. We use warm nature herbs to dispel coldness, cool nature herbs to clear heat, sweet and purgative to discharge heat and nourishing herbs to supplement deficiency. These are the main methods of Chinese medicine treatment. Because the pathogenic factors are complicated, there are two kinds of treatment: routine treatment and contrary treatment. Routine treatment uses herbs whose nature is opposite to the disease progress in order to treat the disease, while contrary treatment uses herbs whose nature is similar to the disease progress. That is what we call "treat adverse symptoms with routine treatment" and "treat conforming symptoms with contrary treatment". Contrary treatments are mostly used for false symptoms, whose pathogenic factor is different from the observed symptoms, for example, dysentery with frequent bowel movements but not completed stools and tenesmus. For this situation, we can't use anti-diarrheal for frequent bowel movements. To the contrary, we should use purgation to evacuate the intestines. In *Neijing*, the clinical treatments are introduced as follows:

Routine Treatment	Contrary Treatment	Adaptive Disease
Treat cold with heat	If treat cold with heat but gets worse then should tonify yang	Cold disease
Treat heat with cold	If treat heat with cold but get worse then should nourish yin	Hot disease
Treat tiredness with warmth (warm to develop), treat dryness with moistening (nourishing), receive (astringent) the dispersing (wasting and dispersing), benefit (tonify) the damaged (loss and damaged), run (activate blood, regulate channels) the unmovable (flaccidity and impediment), calm (tranquilize) the frightened (infantile convulsion, palpitation, insomnia)	Treat stuffiness with tonic (vacuous abdomen distention belongs to slow digestion, we can tonify it.)	Vacuous disease
Cut (offensive attack) the hardness (such as lumps), remove the intruding (such as cold), disperse (eliminate and disperse) the knotted (such us goiter), attack the remaining (such as stagnated food), slow (alleviate) the urgent (such as hypersonic tendon)	Treat diarrhea with purgative (such as dysentery)	Excess disease

One of the treatment goals is to eliminate pathogenic cause of cold, heat, vacuity and excess. Also, due to the location of pathogenesis, there are divisions between superficial, deep, above and below. It is important to know how to choose the most efficient and appropriate method to deal with diseases.

Partial article end.

Chapter 3: Debating Chinese Medicine versus Western Medicine; Native versus Modern

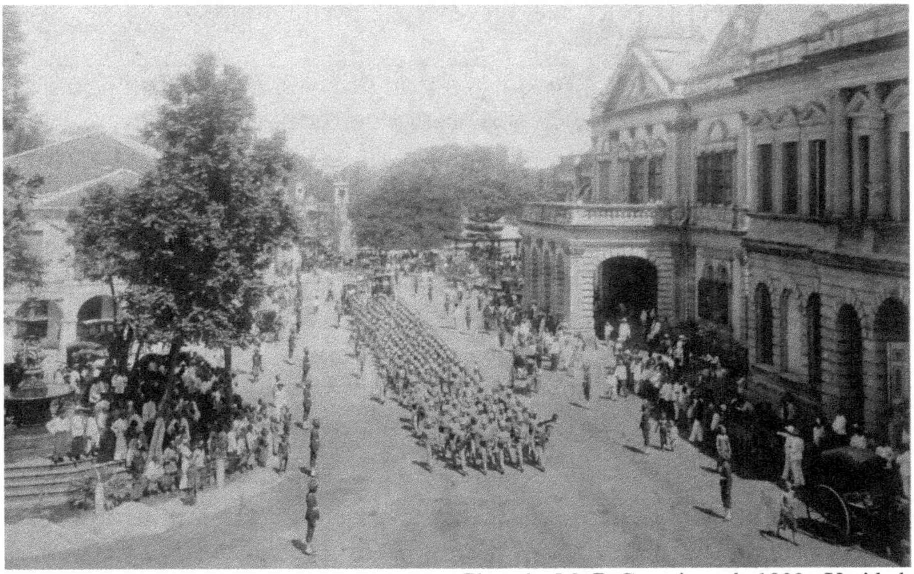

Photo by Mr P. Goux in early 1900s. Untitled.

"There was one book, *The Big Iron Spear of the World's Medicine and Pharmacology* 醫藥界的大鐵椎, which criticized the deficiencies of Western medicine and caused the skin many bruises. At the same time, there was another book published by the commercial printing house, for which a foreword was written by the famous Western medicine doctor Yu Yan 余巖 (Yunxiu 雲岫). In this book, they used Chinese medicine ancient texts to criticize Chinese medicine... In my hands I was holding these two books, reciting and reading them with speed and I was undecided... Sometime thereafter, by chance, [visiting] a Western medicine doctor that I knew well, I saw his wife taking Chinese herbs. It seemed as though I had finally struck gold. I resolutely decided to investigate Chinese medicine further."[160]

[160] *My experience with Pavlov's theories and Chinese medicine scientification.* 1954 by Jing Xiaochou

The Medical History of China 中國醫學史

By Chen Bangxian 陳邦賢

Chapter 4: Modern Medicine 現代的醫學

Subchapter 1: The Rapid Development of New Medicine 新醫學的蓬勃

> Yaron: We start first with a short historical narrative by Chen Bangxian illustrating the modernizers' view of major debates that took place at that time and we follow with the debates themselves. We must evaluate these debates for their content—and not for their socio-political narratives—as this may help our profession, even today.
>
> Pages 257–268

The medicine in China started with the Spirits and Gods era, it then developed into the Experiments era and now it is in the Scientific era. We can also say that the medicine developed from a mythical medicine, to a philosophical medicine and then into a scientific medicine. Under European cultural influence gradually coming eastward, thousands of years of Chinese philosophical medicine, with one whim, transformed into a scientific medicine. In the last thirty years, there has been a rapid development of new medicine, thousands of miles per day. This is due to the importation of Western and Japanese medicine, which transformed, with one whim, how the people in China think. The promotion of new medicine in Qing Dynasty is shown with the paragraph below.

In the preface of Ding Fubao's 丁福保 *Li Dai Yi Xue Shu Mu Xu* 歷代醫學書目序 (August 29th Guangxu Reign),[161] it says:

> Since Westerners gradually came to China and infiltrated the medical circle, their influence on medicine was so great that for four thousand years since the time of Shennong this kind of change was not seen. Our undeveloped medicine spread by simple books and songs keeping people's brains and mouths busy memorizing and reading so they didn't think about the

[161] 1904

> meanings. Gradually people were like the pigs and sheep lazily sleeping on firewood, they simply neglected others' strong sides. According to the natural law, a few decades from now, this quintessence of Chinese culture, Chinese medicine, won't be preserved anymore. Isn't it sad?

Also, in *Twentieth Century New Neijing Preface* 二十世紀新內經序 (January 34th Guangxu Reign),[162] it says:

> …in ancient theory of bones, ancient people made a connection to heaven, saying there were 365 degrees in heaven, and therefore the number of bones is also 365, reflecting heaven. Actually, there are only around two hundred bones in a human body. Even a kid would know this if he had learnt physiology. In addition, the number of bones differs between boys and girls, elders and children. As for pulse theory, since ancient time it is divided into three parts, Cun, Guan and Chi 寸關尺. Cun belongs to heart and lungs, Guan belongs to liver and gallbladder and Chi belongs to kidneys. Now, people have no idea what the pulse is for. It's permissible to examine the general body condition by taking the pulse but it is not permissible to identify a specific organ. As for digestion, people think that the movement of spleen makes the stomach grind the food inside, instead of knowing the truth—there is gastric juice and bile, and both digest food. There is no evidence to support the grinding stomach theory. As for heart, people say it has seven holes and three hairs. Wang Shuhe 王叔和 from Jin 晉 Dynasty related the seven holes to the Big Dipper with its seven stars, three hairs to San Tai (the current Ursa Major), which was totally wrong and misled later generations. Other similar mistakes he made were about the shape of the organs; for example, he claimed there were six lobes in lungs and seven in liver. As a matter of fact, there are five lobes in each of lungs and liver. About the position, he said spleen was at right and liver at left, while the truth is the opposite. He also claimed that heart transports blood to be the gov-

[162] 1909

ernor of the spirit, while kidneys govern urination and store Jing, which is totally wrong with the function of the organs. Seminal vesicles are at the back of bladder and pancreas is at the back of stomach; this kind of knowledge was not listed in books in the past. He also said some disease is related to Venus, some disease is related to Mars; or emperor fire raises up to heaven in the year of Si Hai 巳亥, Taiyin raises up to heaven in the year of Zi Wu 子午, Shaoyang raises up to heaven in the year of Chou Wei 丑未. Chen Wei 讖緯 mystical theories, which are disorganized, wrong, and cannot be explained either… in May of the year of Ren Yin 壬寅,[163] Mr. Wu Zhifu 吳摯甫, from Tongcheng 桐城 City, had told me, "The shortcoming of our native medicine is being combined with Confucianism. The classical books, such as *Neijing* and *Nanjing*, are all falsified. The positions of the five organs mentioned inside these books were totally wrong because there were new and old versions of *Book of Documents* in Han Dynasty. As for the five organs, the old version was consistent with Western medicine, while the new version claimed the liver at left and lungs at right. By the end of Han Dynasty, Zheng Kangcheng 鄭康成, who was a follower of the old version, still adopted the theory of five organs from the new version. For two thousand years since then, this mistake has been passed down and not corrected, and Zheng is liable for this." He also said, "Zhang Zhongjing 張仲景 and Sun Simiao 孫思邈 are considered the pinnacle in the ancient Chinese medicine world; however, the twelve meridians in Zhang's *Shang Han Lun* 傷寒論 were wrong upon anatomical dissection of Western medicine. The theory of five organs in Sun's *Qian Jin Fang* 千金方 was similar to the new version, which is totally wrong. That's the reason why our traditional medicine is under-developed…

Also, in *Nei Ke Xue Gang Yao Xu* 內科學剛要序 (June 34th year of Guangxu Reign):[164]

[163] 1902

[164] 1909

> Most of the old books of Chinese medicine talk about Yin-Yang Qi transformation, five elements and five flavors theory of generation and control, which are as confusing as a mirage. It's like a little mouse entering a big cow's horn: the deeper it gets, the harder it is for it to come back out.

Also, in *New Shang Han Lun Xu* 新傷寒論序 (September 34th year of Guangxu Reign):

> Alas! This precious treasure medicine from the West coming to China—we should have welcomed and learnt it. Instead, we just stuck to Confucianism and old medicine and refused to learn the new knowledge, just like a frog in a well.[165] We cannot do anything but see more and more people get ill and die. Is there anything more sad than this?

Also, in *Yi Xue Bu Xi Ke Jiang Yi Xu Yan* 醫學補習科講義緒言:

> There have been some mistakes in our nation's medicine for four thousand years, so much so that it couldn't help people's health and sometimes even might have killed them. There are five lobes of lungs but practitioners think six; same as for liver, there are five lobes but practitioners think seven. Lungs are in the center of the body but practitioners think they're at the right; liver is at the right but practitioners think it's at the left. There are four chambers in a heart but practitioners think there are seven holes. Ureters are above and connected to bladder but practitioners think bladder has no upward connection. These all are mistakes in the ancient books, there is nothing else to it. If we want to correct these mistakes, dissection anatomy should be taught. Kidneys belong to the urination mechanism while doctors think that it is storing essence Jing 精, which is, rather, the function of seminal vesicles. Heart pumps blood, yet doctors think that it is the monarch; they don't know that the clear spirit Shen Ming 神明[166] is the function of the brain. Native practitioners don't know that liver produces bile, outer kidneys (testes) produce semen, pan-

[165] That thinks that the well is the entire world.

[166] Here the author means clear mind.

creas produces pancreatic juice—because it's not mentioned in old medical books, there is no other reason for it. If we want to correct this situation, we should teach physiology. Opium is harmful to the human body but there are seven to eight out of ten native practitioners using opium; there is prevention for lung diseases but there are four to five out of ten practitioners having cold cough; it's not proper to bend the spine but there are hunchback practitioners and their chest volume becomes smaller; a house should be kept well ventilated to be healthy but some practitioners close all windows and doors and their bodies are injured by accumulated carbon. These are all habits from lower-strata of society, there is nothing else to it, and we can correct them by teaching hygiene. Gypsum Shi Gao 石膏 cannot clear heat or moisten dryness, nor is it emetic or purgative; it cannot be used as medicine. However, practitioners think it can treat stroke, cold, mania and toothache. Prepared salt Qiu Shi 秋石 has nothing but uric acid, but doctors think it can nourish kidney water, treat deficiency lethargy, dispel phlegm and clear deficient heat etc benefits. Gentiana Long Dancao 龍膽草 and Coptis Huang Lian 黃連 can tonify the body and increase appetite, so it's very suitable for deficiency conditions, yet practitioners have totally opposite opinion that they are bitter and cold and can damage the stomach. There is nothing else to it except being a mistake by Ben Cao 本草, a falsified book. If we want to correct this, we should teach pharmacology. If Salmonella typhi exists in small intestine then Typhoid fever comes up; if dysentery bacteria exists in large intestine, then dysentery happens. However, practitioners still don't know this and only follow the old sayings. Mania is brain's disease but practitioners think it's due to the blockage of phlegm. Plague and malaria are caused by microorganism but practitioners still think it's due to ghosts; Wind stroke in *Su Wen Ling Shu* 素問靈樞 and Zhang Zhongjing's books was due to the wind, however, Liu Hejian 劉河間 claimed it was due to fire, Li Dongyuan 李東垣 claimed it was due to qi deficiency with invasion of wind evil, while Zhu Danxi 朱丹溪 claimed it

> was due to phlegm and dampness. But actually, the cause of wind stroke is that blood from a ruptured blood vessel in the brain presses on the brain. This is the only cause, so the other statements, there is nothing else to them except bluffs, one after the other, from ancient people. If we want to correct this, we should teach pathology and internal medicine. Heart pertaining to fire, liver pertaining to wood, spleen pertaining to earth, lungs pertaining to metal and kidneys pertaining to water, the connection between five organs and five elements makes no sense, which is obviously clear for anyone who knows a little bit of physics. Red entering heart, green entering liver, yellow entering spleen, white entering lungs and black entering kidneys, the connection between five organs and five colors makes no sense either, which is obviously clear for anyone who knows a little bit of chemistry. The corruption of our medicine has already hit extreme."

During that time, not only medical doctors were promoting medical revolution, but also other scholars were supporting the advent of new medicine. They all said that there is no difference between Western and Chinese medicine, the only difference between the new and the old medicine is between a metaphysical medicine and a scientific medicine.

More or less, they all rejected the old medicine because of the Yin Yang and five element generation and control theories, which no one can believe in. Next, I'm listing some writings provided by common scholars[167] in late Qing Dynasty about the new medicine:

In Wang Jingyi's 王景沂 *Ke Xue Shu Mu Ti Yao Chu Bian* 科學書目提要初編—*Yi Shu Ke* 醫術科, he said:

> Westerners' knowledge is more advanced; they're good at anatomy. Since the knowledge of anatomy has been discovered, scholars can use this as a base to do deeper research. There is connection between the organs and bones, blood vessels and tendons; they are very close to each other. When a change happens, it's necessary to figure out the cause and remove it. Only

[167] Not medical doctors.

> when we understand all of this, can we confidently treat patients. Some people are not aware of this knowledge yet are still proud of their tiny skills, simply opinionated imbeciles!

In Liang Qichao's 梁啟超 *Du Xi Xue Shu Fa* 讀西學書法, he also said:

> Medicine in Western countries is set to be a special subject and only the chosen preeminent students can take the course. Medicine education in China has no system; people learn it from patchy sources including even incomplete ones in ancient books. The difference of the medical skills between these two kinds of doctors is very obvious. In *Book of Han Dynasty Han Zhi* 漢志,[168] medicine was listed as one kind of the Fangji 方伎 professions. It is a pity that we abandon it now.

In Tongcheng 桐城 City, Wu Zhifu's 吳摯甫 *A Letter Back to Xiao Jingfu Chi Du Da Xiao Jing Fu Shu* 尺牘答蕭敬甫書, he said:

> Respectful, you have been sick since last October and still not recovered in the middle of this May. You, my brother, your constitution is always strong, how come it declines so much like that? It's caused by the herbs you take. Nowadays, Western medicine is so popular, and its theory is very developed and profound while its method is very fast and simple. If one is being treated with Western medicine, as long as the treated disease is not stubborn, it won't last too long. However, most of my friends still firmly believe in the medicine of China. They follow what they are used to, can't see the damage done, peacefully err for the sake of Chinese medicine and wouldn't give Western medicine a try, while their diseases cannot recover. You have lived in Shanghai for a long time, where you can be easily well-informed. However, you rather stay with Chinese medicine and are being tortured by the disease instead of trying out Western medicine. Your valuable body is committed to a quack, isn't that improper? If you listen to me and try out Western medicine once when you're a bit ill, then you'll know that I'm right.

[168] *Han Shu Yi Wen Zhi* 漢書藝文志

Also in *A Letter to He Songpo Yu He Song Po Shu* 與何松坡書, he said:

> I heard your eye disease is getting worse and I am concerned about that so much. I also heard native practitioners say that, for those who have eye diseases, taking a hundred times Chinese herbs can bring back the original eyesight. The following lines are from Zhang Chuhang 張楚航 of a prior generation; "If it doesn't work after taking Chinese herbs a hundred times, then the person who's trying had better stop trying." That Yin-Yang and five elements theories in Chinese medicine have no connection to sick people, is a fair statement. According to Chinese medicine theory, eye disease is related to liver and kidney meridians, but the distance between liver, kidney and eyes is a thousand miles. Now, you are taking herbs to treat liver and supplement kidneys to help your eye disease, yet even if you treat the liver and kidneys it is unlikely to cure the eye disease. In addition, so called treating liver and kidneys herbs—can't they actually do damage to the real liver and kidneys organs? I'm persuading you to not take Chinese herbs for long duration. Herbs seem to be working differently for different people, some supposed to tonify but they don't tonify, some supposed to drain but they don't drain, and they can have other downsides. Followers of *Ben Cao* 本草[169] don't know about this and use those herbs. The lucky ones get the medical effect, but often people don't get rid of the original disease and instead it becomes worse. One must guard against this.

Also, in *A Letter to Lian Zhiqing Yu Lian Zhi Qing Shu* 與廉志卿書, he said:

> If your brother has pulmonary disease then he should, as soon as possible, see a Western medicine doctor and move to a place by the sea to get the iodine from the ocean wind to supplement the lungs. Although he has taken malt extract and fish oil to nourish the lungs, he still needs to be careful not to catch a cold. This is not easy to treat; Chinese medicine hasn't shown any ef-

[169] Chinese materia medica

> ficacy, not even a tiny instance. That people say Chinese medicine works on this disease is a talk lacking understanding. A Western medicine doctor uses a stethoscope to hear patient's lungs; this kind of examination is definitely more reliable.

Also, in *Correspondence Addendum to a Letter to Lian Zhi Qing Chi Du Bu Yi Yu Lian Zhi Qing Shu* 尺牘補遺與廉志卿書, he said:

> In the previous letter you said that Mr. Ke 柯 just recovered from the latest disease but still has ongoing cough. How's his condition recently? You also mentioned not applying either Chinese or Western medicine, which seems right but is actually wrong. Chinese medicine is unreliable so it's proper not to take it. But if you don't take Western medicine, then you will never know the Western medical superb skill. You still harbor Chinese medicine in your chest and can't abandon it. The wrong theory of five organs in Chinese medicine is Kang Cheng's 康成 fault. Cough is a small symptom, however, it can cause a big problem. Chinese medicine practitioners don't have herbs to cure cough, nor do they know what organs or physiological function are related to cough. These are very clear in Western medicine and if someone doesn't know about Western medicine he can't take care of himself well.

Also, in *A Letter to Ke Feng Sun Yu Ke Feng Sun Shu* 與柯鳳孫書, he said:

> Yesterday, your letter arrived from the 13th and I was very happy to hear that you had a baby boy on the afternnon of the 12th. This is big happiness and worth celebrating. For certain routines there's no need to remind you anything, but for how to take care of your baby boy, you need to confirm with a female Western medicine doctor, instead of following the old Chinese traditional ways of rearing kids. There are many unreasonable and silly routines that women follow in our country—those are really jokes, and people who follow those, although they claim they love their child, actually harm the child. So you definitely need to inquire about the Western method for taking care of

> children, this is the only secret. The general idea is outlined in the book *Fu Ying Xin Shuo* 婦嬰新說, but in this book it's too simplified.

Also, in *A Reply Letter to He Baochen Da He Bao Chen Shu* 答何豹臣書, he said:

> Medicine of Western people is very refined. I didn't know Chinese medicine is nonsense until I read Western medical books… The comparison between Western and Chinese medicine is like comparing successful warriors to little kids… So Hejian 河間, Danxi 丹溪, Dongyuan 東垣, Jingyue's 景岳[170] books can all be burnt. Yet, you still think they have unique and profound ideas, which I think is a mistake.

Also, in *A Reply Letter to Wang Hezhi Da Wang He Zhi Shu* 答王合之書, he said:

> Fu Chen's 紱臣 disastrous disease should have healed; how can one dare say it was God's workings? Based on day-to-day knowledge, we know that Chinese medicine cannot be relied upon. Since *Ling Shu* 靈樞 and *Su Wen* 素問, it was always like this. Up to the bronze man Tong Ren Tu 銅人圖,[171] it was lacking evidence. The materia medica *Ben Cao* talked strongly about herbs without knowing what they were. They are all inferior to Western medicine, which directly examines internal organs and blood vessels, with much more evidence to infer disease; there is absolutely no empty talk—the drugs are developed by chemists and work 100 percent of the time.

Also, in *A Letter to Wu Jiyue Yu Wu Ji Yue Shu* 與吳季曰書, he said:

> Your literature attainments are very high, however, your medical knowledge is just about average. You are like the person of the state of Yue 越人,[172] only guarding the way the state of Yue sees things; you don't know how the medicine in the five continents[173] has surged. Looking back at our country's old medicine

[170] Liu Hejian, Zhu Danxi, Li Dongyuan, Zhang Jingyue 劉河間朱丹溪李東垣張景岳

[171] A bronze statue showing the meridians and acupuncture points, started ca. northern Song dynasty.

[172] Also means Bian Que.

[173] Around the world.

> being full of old nonsense theories, it is not worth one coin of cash. You don't accept Western medicine, so not once have you read even one of the many Western medical books already translated. You only concentrate on *Su Wen* 素問, *Ling Shu* 靈樞, *Shang Han* 傷寒, *Jin Gui* 金匱, *Qian Jin* 千金, *Wai Tai* 外臺 and other Chinese medical books. Your belief in Chinese medicine is so firm as if concealed in your chest and cannot be removed. Why aren't you eager to seek progress? If you view Chinese medicine with no bias, are these so called Yin-Yang and five elements theories reliable? Is there no fallacy with inspecting five organs by taking the pulse? Have the herbs in *Ben Cao* already been tested and are the listed characteristics of each herb totally accurate? Is five elements pairing to five organs not a fallacy? The life or death of a human is a big thing, can we really deal with it with using some immature medical knowledge?

Also, in *A Letter to Xiao Jingfu Yu Xiao Jing Fu Shu* 與蕭敬甫書, he said:

> Xi Zhi 曦之 is able to convince Mr. Zhao 趙 to gather all chemists to examine the herbs' active chemical ingredients in *Shang Han* and *Jin Gui*, which will be a great contribution to our country. Would you please present to Mr. Xi Zhi my opinion about this?

According to the above quotes, we know that intelligentsia in late Qing endorsed the development of scientific medicine. The power of new medicine has grown bigger and more prosperous in the Republic era. In the 3rd year of the Republic,[174] Education Minister Wang Daxie 汪大燮[175] highly advocated abolishing Chinese medicine. Yu Dexun 余德壎, at that time, joined up all the Chinese medicine practitioners in the entire country, and organized a group seeking to save Chinese medicine. Their delegates delivered a petition to the State Council Guo Wu Yuan 國務院 and other Departments, applying to keep Chinese medicine and herbs. The State Council commented:

[174] 1914
[175] 1859–1929

> Chinese medicine started from ancient times and was transmitted from one to the other. This system is very clear. It became a professional subject amongst all the others and people can enjoy its benefit. The medical curriculum that the Education Ministry formulated follows the Western method. We decided that including divergences with Chinese medicine will not be beneficial, and we chose what was urgent first, therefore we didn't include Chinese medicine in the medical curriculum. Our intention was not to abandon Chinese medicine.

The following comments from the Education Ministry:

> The leader and other members of the committee organizing the group to research and preserve Chinese medicine do have very good intentions. However, the situation is such that, similar to all around the world, science has become more and more refined. The course content of any specific science should be based on its latest theory. Therefore, the curriculum of medical schools formulated by the Education Ministry includes different kinds of specialized departments such as anatomical dissection and experiments. However, without a complete scientific knowledge, there is no way to teach it. The curriculum was decided by the Temporary Education Committee, and also evaluated by the medical professionals hired by Education Ministry, before being announced. Our hope for medicine is to have a complete system of learning which follows the trend of the entire rapidly-developing world. Thereafter, we can implement the anti-epidemics sanitary policies without obstacle. All this is not due to discrimination against Chinese medicine. Also the curriculum and relevant regulations for Chinese medical schools will be announced, so there should not be more discontent.

The influence of the new medicine became even more vigorous after the change of the regime;[176] most notably was the First Central Health Committee Meeting 第一次

[176] This refers to the Wuchang uprising 武昌起義 which was part of the Xinhai revolution in 1911 that brought down the Qing government.

中央衛生委員會, where Yu Yan 余巖 proposed "*Abolition of Old Medicine to Remove Obstacles from the Development of Medicine and Public Health Fei Zhi Jiu Yi Yi Sao Chu Yi Shi Wei Sheng Zhi Zhang Ai An* 廢止舊醫以掃除醫事衛生之障礙案", his reasoning being:

> I think the object of individual medicine is the individual person and the purpose of it is to cure diseases. The prerequisite of disease treatment is illness recognition. In addition, in the modern era, therapeutic medicine has developed into preventative medicine, individual medicine has become social medicine, and the object has become the masses instead of a single individual. The health administration public health policies are now purely based on scientific new medicine plus an overlay meaning of modern politics. Those theories of old medicine now, such as Yin-Yang, five elements, six Qi, Zangfu and meridians are all falsified without truth to them, so this is the first reason that it should be abolished. Facing the patient, the pulse taken is the radial artery's pulse, which is falsely divided into three sections as Cun Guan Chi, relating to different internal organs. This is total nonsense, one cheats himself and others. The origin of it came from Wei Hou 緯候 School and astronomy, both of which are groundless. This is the second reason to abolish the old medicine. The old medicine practitioners don't know how to diagnose, they can do neither disease diagnosis, death investigation, nor plague prevention—not to mention eugenics. This can't be used for our nation's health policy and to benefit the people's livelihood. This is the third reason to abolish the old medicine. The key point in human cultural evolution is the abolition of the notion of earth and heaven being connected. This was seen again and again throughout history. What is called "abolish the notion of heaven and earth being connected" means oppose the "heaven virtue" and revere the human affairs. Get rid of mysteriousness and praise facts. The government should eradicate superstition and eliminate idolatry and, in turn, spread scientific concepts and knowledge to the masses, altering their thinking toward scientification. Now, the old medicine practitioners still follow divination and superstition to confuse people. The gov-

> ernment does disinfection and teaches the masses sanitation ideas and the knowledge about bacteria, for example, that bacteria are the source of disease. Yet, the old medicine practitioners still insist that getting a cold in winter results in the disease of warmth the next spring, getting an illness of heat in summer causes malaria in the following autumn. These theories actually block the development of science, so this is the fourth reason it should be abolished. In short, every additional day we don't get rid of the old medicine, it is another day people don't change their old thoughts, one more day the development of new medicine doesn't elevate, one more day health instructions can't be put into place. I've been researching our medical revolution for more than a decade. I know very well the old medicine and I have refuted it in detail. It is a necessary measure to take in order to improve the people's livelihood and national progress. This is the grand plan of our nation; it is not a trivial master-servant argument. Its fulcrum lies with the modern day. If we pay great attention to this, it is a good fortune.

During that time, Yu was blamed and criticized by many Chinese medicine practitioners for this statement. Among modern medical books, there are some written by people who insisted on medical revolution, such as Yu Yan's *Medical Revolution Discussion* (*Yi Xue Ge Ming Lun Ji* 醫學革命論集, the original name was *Yu Shi Yi Shu* 余氏醫述), Wang Qizhang's 汪企張 *My Humble Proposal about China Medicine for The Two Decades Er Shi Nian Lai Zhong Guo Yi Shi Chu Yi* 二十年來中國醫事芻議, and Hu Dingan's 胡定安 *Collection of Medicine Discussions Yi Shi Yan Lun Ji* 醫事言論集. Even Chinese medicine intelligentsia claims it has become a new Chinese medicine, which is extracted from ancient books but organized by scientific means. This, as well, is influenced by the trend of new medicine.

Chapter 6 : The statistics of health groups 醫藥衛生團體的統計

Pages 337–338

Subchapter 1: China Medical Association 中華醫學會

China Medical Association Zhong Hua Yi Xue Hui 中華醫學會 was established in 1915 and merged with the Medical Missionary Society of China Bo Yi Hui 博醫會 in April of 1932. Medical Missionary Society of China was established in 1886, most of the members serving in missionary medical centers. After the merge, there were more than 1700 members. The headquarters are in Shanghai, other branches are in Nanjing 南京, Shanghai 上海, Beiping 北平, Guangzhou 廣州, Hong Kong 香港, Changsha 長沙, Jinan 濟南, Suzhou 蘇州, Guling 牯嶺, Wuhu 蕪湖, Kaifeng 開封 etc. There are fourteen members in the council and one is elected to be the chairman by the others. There are all kinds of committees such as the public health committee 公共衛生委員會, the medical education committee 醫事教育委員會, the missionary medical committee 教會醫事委員會, the standard for hospitals committee 醫院標準委員會, the business guarantee committee 業務保障委員會, the publication committee 出版委員會 and the research committee 研究委員會, etc.

There are the Chinese Medical Journal 中華醫學雜誌 and Chinese Medical Guides 中國醫學指南 as publications. The range of doctors' research includes public health, tuberculosis, internal medicine, orthopedics, biochemistry and forensic medicine etc. In the library, there are about 250 journals published from China, United Kingdom, Japan, Germany, France, Italy and Russia.

Subchapter 2: Republic of China Medical Association 中華民國醫藥學會

Republic of China Medical Association Zhonghua Minguo Yiyao Xuehui 中華民國醫藥學會 was organized by people who studied medicine abroad and inside our country and are now working in the medical industry. It was established in May of 1915. The headquarters were originally in Beiping 北平 and subsequently moved to Shanghai 上海 after sixteen years and its name changed to Medicine Central Administration 總會. Originally, there were branches in Suzhou 蘇州 and Hangzhou 杭州 only; now there are branches in Beiping 北平, Nanjing 南京, Suzhou 蘇州, Nanchang 南昌, Hankou 漢口, Hangzhou 杭州, Wenzhou 溫州, Taixing 泰興, Chaozhou 潮州, Shanghai 上海 etc. There are also mail correspondence centers in other places. It has more than eight hundred members and publishes *New Medicine Monthly Journal Xin Yi Yao Yue Kan* 新醫藥月刊. Other than researching important medical and academic topics, its business also includes fixing medical terms, investigating parasitical diseases, researching our national medicine and our nation's herbs and revising medical regulations.

Subchapter 3: Other medical institutions 其他醫藥衛生學會

There are many other medical institutions, for example: National Medical Doctor Federation 全國醫師聯合會; Chinese Nursing Association 中華護士會, which has more than four thousand members; Chinese Physiological Society 中國生理學會; Chinese Microorganism Society 中國微生物學會; Chinese Pathology Society 中國病理學會; Chinese Ophthalmology Society 中國眼科學會; Chinese Antituberculosis Association 中國防痨協會; Chinese Pharmaceutical Association 中華民國藥學會; Chinese Public Health Nursing Association 中華公共衛生護士學會; Chinese Medical Improvement Society 中國醫事改進社; Shen Zhou Native Medical Association 神州國醫學會; Tropical Disease Research Center 熱帶病研究所; Chinese Health Education Society 中國衛生教育社; Mental Health Association 心理衛生學會; China Association of Native Medicine 中華國醫學會; Chinese and Western Medicine Research Society 中西醫藥研究社; and other groups.

Chapter 8 : The establishment of the Central Native Medicine Bureau 中央國醫館的設立

Pages 344–345

On March 17th, 1929, the Chinese medicine community gathered to file a petition to the government to cancel the Central Health Committee's *Extinguishing Chinese Medicine* proposal. At that time, this was a heated debate in all National Medical Associations, but then it was dismissed by the government. Until now, Chinese medicine people regard March 17th as a commemoration day. In 1930, the *Central Bureau for Native Medicine Organization Ordinances Zhong Yang Guoyi Guan Zuzhi Tiaoli* 中央國醫館組織條例 was issued. According to this document, Chinese medicine was called Native medicine Guo Yi 國醫,[177] Bureau for Native Medicine was located in the

[177] The term Guo Yi 國醫, which was already mentioned early on in the Song dynasty but widely used during the Republic, has a double meaning of "National Medicine" as well as "Native Medicine". Chinese medicine practitioners priding their culture would rather see it as the national medicine or even state-sponsored medicine, however, all who were for progress and modern medicine would rather see it as Native medicine with a derogatory connotation, meaning not modern like the rest of the world. As Western medicine gradually became dominant in China, the term "Guo Yi" was dropped and Chinese medicine

capital, Jiao Yitang 焦易堂 was elected director 館長 and Chen Lifu 陳立夫 was elected council chairman 理事長. Branches of Native Medicine Bureau were set up in all other provinces and abroad and sub-branches were set up in all counties. Also, an academic reorganizing committee 學術整理委員會 was established within the Bureau for Native Medicine. *An Outline Draft for Organizing the Native Medicine* 國醫藥學整理大綱草案 written by Lu Yuanlei, 陸淵雷 said:

> The medicine business in our nation was regarded as witchcraft since ancient times and it was given and accepted privately among common people. The government rarely managed the medical industry. Since it has been practiced for a long time, there have been more and more schools. It will be a huge task to reorganize them all, which is why the council members were so wary of starting this work. The only way is to ask advice from experienced masters from home and abroad, to draft the leading principles and then follow them. Gradually we can accomplish this task. No scholars argue about reorganizing Chinese medicine. However, there is much divergence in people's opinions. Some think we should follow the old school, some argue that we should give up old notions and follow the new things. See benevolence see knowledge,[178] each selects the essence of their choice. They treasure what they like but want to destroy what they don't like. It wouldn't be successful if we adopted everyone's opinion. So here, I draft five prerequisite questions to unify people's thoughts, four goals of reorganization to define the priority, seven provisional missions and six regular missions and set a schedule to urge and accomplish it.

Every listed rule was explained in detail and well-ordered; Yu Yan 余巖 replied in a letter: "Your thoughts surpass others' opinions in this generation, the prerequisite questions are the most important. If we follow what you say then the rubbish part of Chinese medicine will be removed and the truthful will remain, the wrong will be removed and the correct will remain, and then the scientification of Chinese medicine will have a proper path, just like the saying 'a carpenter makes his tools first and then he can build a square or round shape'."

---

was again called Zhong Yi 中醫. Throughout this book we translate "Guo Yi" as "Native Medicine" to maintain the then-prevalent distinction between old and new, native and foreign.

[178] A part of a Confucian statement; the benevolent sees benevolence in everything, the knowledgeable sees knowledge in everything.

In January 22nd, the 25th year,[179] the government promulgated *Chinese Medicine Regulations Zhongyi Tiaoli* 中醫條例. Guangdong 廣東 province, in the 24th year,[180] established the provincial Native Medicine College Guo Yi Xue Yuan 國醫學院 and its affiliated hospital. There are many private Native Medicine Colleges 國醫學院 and Native Medicine Specialty Schools 國醫專科學校 in other provinces. Jiangsu Provincial College of Health Policy and Management 江蘇省立醫政學院 organizes special health training classes and specifically recruits on-the-job Chinese medicine practitioners to train them with scientific medicine for one to two years. This is the latest situation of Chinese medicine.

Book excerpt end

The contrast between modern medicine and ancient Chinese medicine

1934 by Wu Hung Tak 胡雄德

5th Year, Medical Faculty. February 28, 1934. *The Caduceus*, Journal of the Hong Kong University Medical Society. Volume 13, Number 4. November 1934

Yaron: This article demonstrates the overall situation that Chinese medicine doctors faced, as seen with the eyes of modern educated people influenced by a Western modern world. Such a description of poor education and illiteracy among many Native medicine practitioners was also given by Chinese medicine practitioners themselves. It was a reality forcing Chinese medicine to alter its direction toward a more modern and, at that time, more respectable profession.

Pages 55–65

While modern medicine is generally accepted and practiced all over the world, ancient Chinese medicine still remains firm in the belief of most of the people in China. The very fact that this practice has existed for forty centuries and that it is so implicitly believed in by the masses is proof that there must be some good in it. Both systems have their own successes and superiority, but there are innumerable differences between them in every department. Ancient Chinese medicine started with the

[179] 1936
[180] 1935

development of the civilization of China over four thousand years ago, but owing to the conservative teaching there was practically no further progress after it had reached its so called climax, and it remained a rational, semi-scientific but dignified practice which was based upon the accumulated knowledge of centuries, and which represented the observations and experiences of many bright minds. On the other hand, though modern medicine developed only a few hundred years ago, yet owing to the rapid advances of science on which it depends, it has progressed to such a degree as to defy any other systems of medicine in the world. Thus their main difference can be summed up in two words: modern medicine is *scientific*, and ancient Chinese medicine is *empirical*.

Anatomy and Physiology

Disease is a departure from health. It is clear that it is impossible to study and know the nature of disease without a thorough knowledge of all the organs and systems in the body, and the normal physiological functions and working of them in a healthy individual. The teaching of modern medicine is based on this principle. There is a long course of anatomy and physiology for medical students before they study morbid anatomy and the abnormal functions of the body. They have to find out and learn for themselves every system, organ and structure of the whole body by spending most of their time in painstaking dissections, and aided by the microscope. The normal functions of different organs and systems are also seen, proved and studied by the students themselves in various experiments conducted by scientific methods. Having such knowledge of anatomy and physiology, they can readily detect departures from the normal.

The students of ancient Chinese medicine, however, are without any practical knowledge of these subjects. On account of the Confucian dogma which holds the body to be sacred and not to be mutilated in any way, and also because of the great reverence for the dead, it could hardly be expected that anything could be made out in anatomy and physiology, hence gross mistakes have been made and are still sometimes seen. Works on anatomy were only done a few times as recorded in old literature. The dissections were done on the bodies of robbers and criminals who had been executed. Drawings were made and descriptions of the positions and relations of different parts of the body recorded. Although some of the descriptions were accurate, they were not without mistakes and they were learned by the poor students without any chance for them to find out the errors.

As to physiology, no experiments have ever been done for the study of it. All the theories were opinions, and thoughts argued out by various writers in different periods. They never had the slightest idea of the proper functions of different organs. The brain was thought to be the abode of the spirit and energy. Thinking was supposed to be done by the heart. The blood stream was said to start from the foot and to circulate to the kidneys, the heart, the lung, the liver, the spleen, in the order mentioned, and from the spleen back again to the kidneys, thus making a complete circuit. These and many others were the absurd theories form the so-called physiology, and it is no wonder to find that pathology is so different between the two systems of medicine.

Pathology

This subject is the greatest contrast between modern medicine and ancient Chinese medicine. Whereas in other subjects we still find some similarities between them, in this subject the theories are absolutely different.

In modern medicine, pathology is regarded as the science of disease. It investigates by scientific methods the basis for disease—the changes underlying its symptoms, and its functional disturbances. It is based on anatomy and physiology. The methods of study are those of physiology, and are thus of various kinds—physical, chemical, and anatomical; and they are applied both in observation and in experiment. The etiology of disease is regarded as the abnormal state, or part of the system, of organ or structure affected by some disturbing cause from outside. These abnormal states may be (1) hereditary, depending on the abnormalities in the germ plasm, (2) congenital, presenting at the time of birth, and arising in various ways, sometimes in the same manner as in the acquired form, and (3) acquired, due to some disturbances acting after birth. The causes operating after birth are (1) improper or insufficient food and oxygen supply, (2) overwork or overstrain, (3) trauma or mechanical injury, (4) physical agencies such as heat, cold, electricity, etc., (5) invasion by microorganisms—bacteria, protozoa, and various ultramicroscopic organisms or filter-passers, (6) invasion by certain parasites, and lastly (7) chemical agents, poisons, toxins, etc. The changes in the tissue are either reactive or retrogressive as a response to these causes.

The pathology of ancient Chinese medicine is based chiefly on philosophical speculations. As has been said, the knowledge of physiology and anatomy is so poor that experimental researches on this subject are impossible to carry out, and theories of diseases have to be thought and argued out. Thus the causes of disease are attributed to supernatural agencies, atmospheric influences, and the derangement of the "two principles" and the "five elements."

The "two principles" are the "Yang" 陽 and the "Yin" 陰 which are referred to as the male and female sexes. Further they represent heaven and earth, life and death, day and night, heat and cold, positive and negative, strong and weak and, finally, acid and base.

The "five elements" are the metal, wood, water, fire, and earth. It is believed that the human body, like matter in general, is made up of harmonious mixtures of these elements. Chief representations are found in the five organs: the lungs, the liver, the kidneys, the heart, and the spleen, which are further related in a complicated manner to the five atmospheric conditions (draught, wind, cold, heat, moisture), the five planets (Venus, Jupiter, Mercury, Mars, Saturn), the five colors (white, green, black, red, yellow), the five tastes (pungent, sour, salt, bitter, sweet), the five tones, etc. Health depends upon the proper equilibrium of the male and female principles and on the right proportions of the five elements. Any derangement of the balance causes disease, which manifests itself in the pulse.

The main differences can be summed up thus. One is *experimental* and the other is purely *theoretical.*

Diagnosis

This subject is regarded by both the modern and ancient systems of medicine as the most important and difficult subject, and it requires a lot of experience and patience to make a correct one. The methods adopted by the ancient Chinese medicine are simple and limited to the so-called four methods. According to the *Nei Ching* 內經 , the medical classic, the four methods are: observation 望, auscultation 聞, interrogation 問 and palpation 切. Observation means to note the complexion and expression of the face; auscultation, to listen to the voice and sound; interrogation, to inquire into the history, symptoms, and cause of the illness, and the condition of the appetite and excretion; and palpation, to examine the pulse. In the beginning, the relative value of these four methods was in the order named, but in the course of time, the first three were gradually not so much employed, entire reliance being placed on the last. The greatest importance is attached to this doctrine of the pulse and it is universally believed by the Chinese that all internal disease can be revealed by this method alone.

The diagnostic methods of modern medicine are numerous and complicated as contrasted to the simple ones of Chinese medicine. They comprise all the four methods employed by the Chinese, and in addition, there are chemical, instrumental, microscopic, biological, bacteriological and numerous other tests. Firstly there is interrogation to inquire into the history, symptoms and cause of the disease and the condition of the appetite and excretion. Then comes next the important physical examination of every system and organs in the body to know any abnormality in position and function by the four methods of inspection, palpation, percussion, and auscultation. Special sense organs are examined with the aid of numerous instruments. Blood is examined to know the number and state of cells, to see the state of haemoglobin, and to search for parasites and bacteria. Sputum, urine, faeces, and body fluids such as cerebral spinal fluid, peritoneal fluid, etc., are examined when necessary by various chemical and bacteriological methods. Special tests such as X-rays and electro-cardiography for the heart, barium-meal and fractional-test-meal for the gastro-intestinal tract, X-ray pictures of other organs, and bacteriological tests and microscopic examinations in various disease are often necessary. All these have to be done before a modern medical man can make a correct diagnosis.

The art of pulse feeling in China is a most mysterious and misunderstood subject. Chinese physicians assert that the entire superstructure of medical practice is built upon the theory of the pulse—the nature, location, course, and treatment of every disease depends on this alone. In modern medicine, although the examination of the pulse is also of importance, yet it gives so little information as compared with that of Chinese medicine. The modern medical man only learns the rate, rhythm, force, volume, tension and the general condition of vessel wall. These only reveal part of the condition of the patient but give nothing of the nature and location of diseases other than those of the heart. As have been said, the Chinese can tell all diseases by the pulse alone, which seems absurd and illogical, but this method has been adopted and practiced for over forty centuries.

The method of taking the pulse in modern medicine is simple though certain points and rules must be observed. In all accurate records the pulse should be noted under similar conditions as regards the posture of the patient, time of day, relation to meals, etc. The radial pulse is generally taken although other superficial arteries are used equally well. Three fingers are placed along the course of the artery, the index finger closer to the heart. Rate of the pulse is counted with a watch, and the whole examination can be finished in a comparatively short time.

The Chinese pulse lore is extremely complicated and, in practice, constitutes a most detailed procedure amounting almost to a solemn rite. The examination is made upon both the right and left wrists, the physician using his right hand for the left pulse, his left hand for the right. The middle finger is first laid on the head of the radius, then adding the index and ring fingers while the thumb rests upon the dorsum of the carpus. The best time for taking the pulse is the early morning at sunrise. The physician should keep cool and collected, first noting if his own breathing is in order. One inhalation and one exhalation constitute one cycle of respiration. The normal ratio is four beats to one respiration.

According to the *Classic of Difficulties* the extent of the pulse is 1 and 9/10 of an inch, and is divided into three parts called Tsun 寸 or inch, Kuan 關 or bar, and Ch'ih 尺 or cubit, the last being nearest to the heart. Each of these divisions has two different and distinct pulses, one internal and one external, making altogether twelve pulses which correlate with twelve definite internal organs, the normal and abnormal conditions of which it portrays. Thus, according to Wang Shu-ho, the inch-pulse of the right hand reveals the conditions of the lungs and large intestine, of the left hand, the heart and small intestines. The pulse under the bar corresponds on the right to the condition of the spleen and stomach, on the left to the liver and gallbladder. The pulse felt on the right cubit shows the condition of the gate of life and San Chiao 三焦, on the left cubit it tells the state of the kidneys and bladder. Not only are the rate, character, rhythm, volume, tension, etc. minutely observed, but the age, sex temperament, constitution, weight and growth of the patient, as well as the time of day, season of the year, and influence of the constellation are also taken into consideration.

In modern medicine there are about ten types of pulse, all revealing the conditions of the cardiovascular system only. They do not as a rule interpret any abnormal conditions of other systems and organs as those in Chinese medicine. (1) Pulsus frequens: may be due to extracardiac causes such as infection besides various cardiac conditions. (2) Pulsus tarus. (3) Pulsus celer. (4) Pulsus tardus. (5) Pulsus anaeroticus. (6) Pulsus dicroticus: may also occur in high fever. (7) Pulsus paradoxus. (8) The wiry pulse. (9) Pulsus bigerminus. (10) Pulsus alterans.

In Chinese medicine there are four main principle pulses together with many minor types of less significance. (1) Fu 浮 superficial, a light flowing pulse like a piece of wood floating in water. (2) Ch'eng 沉 deep, a deeply impressed pulse like a stone thrown into water. (3) Ch'ih 遲 slow, a pulse with three beats to one cycle of respiration. (4) Shu 數 quick, a pulse with six beats to one cycle of respiration. Every variety or combination is believed to reveal a distinct disease. Thus: (1) fu, belongs to male principle, points to complaints externally connected with the six influences: wind, cold, dampness, heat, dryness, and fire. (2) Ch'eng, belongs to female principle, indicates external disease due to the seven passions: joy, anger, anxiety, worry, grief, fear, and shock. (3) Ch'ih, reveals conditions of organs. (4) Shu, reveals disease of viscera.

Chinese physicians profess to be able to predict the result of an illness by various signs of the pulse, and to tell whether or not a woman is pregnant or even to predict the sex and development of uterine foetus by these tests alone. In modern medicine the prognostic value of pulse is only limited to acute cases and it only reveals the general condition and the response of the patient, and the pulse is absolutely impossible to tell anything about pregnancy.

Materia Medica and Therapeutics

As Chinese medicine has a history of over forty centuries, it is no wonder to find that the Chinese pharmacopoeia is extremely rich in remedies. A list of 1892 different drugs are mentioned in the *Pentsao* 本草綱目, the national pharmacopoeia of China. The number of drugs employed by modern medicine is far inferior to that of the Chinese, and the list in the pharmacopoeia is only increased by synthetic compounds and various combinations and mixtures of different drugs. There is a striking contrast between the nature and source of drugs of the two systems. A greater part of the drugs in modern medicine are of mineral origin, a small portion of vegetable origin, and a still smaller portion is obtained from animals. Owing to the slow progress of chemistry, there are only a few drugs in Chinese medicine derived from the mineral kingdom. Part of the materia medica is from animals, insects, and reptiles. Practically all of the drugs are of vegetable origin. Many of these drugs are common in both the East and the West; but there are still not a few that have long been employed in China and yet which are still unknown, or have but recently been used in other countries. The Chinese claim wonder from these drugs which, owing to the crude and unscientific way of preparation, are rejected by most modern medical men. But many modern drugs, which are so effective and widely used, are really extracts from certain Chinese drugs discovered by certain research institutes. For instance, Eumenol, said to be effective in menstrual disorders, is a liquid extract from Tang Kuei 當歸, a Chinese native drug; the now famous ephedrine, which took Europe and America literally by storm, is derived from Ma Huang 麻黃, a Chinese herb that has been employed in practice for more than four thousand years.

Organotherapy, formerly much ridiculed by foreigners, but now hailed as a valuable modern discovery, has been known to every Chinese housewife. The common practice of administering kidney for backache, lungs for consumption and cough, etc., may be too far fetched but the basic idea of endocrinology exists. In recent years a great variety of glandular substance has been employed in modern medicine. Of these, the thyroid, pituitary, suprarenals, pancreas, liver, and probably the ovary, have indubitably established their therapeutic efficiency, and it is remarkable to note that many of them have been in use in China for ages past. For example, as early as the seventh century, thyroid gland was prescribed for goiter, cretinism, etc. But the way of administration is somewhat different in each system. The Chinese always take these organs wholly either as an ordinary dish, or after being treated with some vegetable drugs, whereas in modern medicine extracts or other preparations of them are usually taken while the whole crude thing is only seldom taken.

(a) *Pharmacology*: Modern medicine regards this as a science. It investigates by scientific methods the action of the drugs on the body both in health and in disease. The science of pharmacology is based upon the three sciences: physiology, chemistry, and pathology. It is impossible to decide how a drug produces an action until we are acquainted with any, or all, of the factors in these sciences which may be concerned. All the drugs are experimented chiefly on animals, and the effects are noted and studied before they are standardized and brought into use. Not only the immediate actions, local and specific, but also the remote and accumulative effects of drugs are carefully considered, so that a doctor knows how and why a disease may be benefitted by the appliance of drugs.

The Chinese pharmacology, if it exists, is simply an empirical one. It consists of the accumulated knowledge of centuries and the observations and experiences of many bright minds. No experiments have ever been done to study their action before the drugs are brought into use. Effects of the drugs are generally known after their first administration to the poor patient, and they are corrected after repeated applications.

(b) *Pharmacy*: This is another branch of science of modern medicine. It is the science and art of the preparation and combination of drugs, so as to render them fit for administration. Besides simple methods such as filtration, precipitation, etc., there are a lot of pharmaceutical processes, the more important of which are levigation, elutriation, lixiviation, aceration, percolation, repercolation, scaling, and standardizing. Drugs are prepared in various forms before administration. They are: aceta, aquae, colloidia, confectiones, decota, emplastra, extracta, glycerina, infusa, injectiones, lamellae, linimenta, liquores, lotiones, mella, misturae, mucilaguines, olea, exymella, pilulae, pulveres, spiritus, succi, suppositoria, syrupi, tabellae, tincturae, trochisci, unguenta, vina, and numerous other nonpharmacopoeial preparations such as, abstracta, emulsiones, enemata, essentiae, etc., etc.

Again the Chinese pharmacy is simple. The drugs are generally of vegetable origin: leaves, flowers, seeds, roots, barks, plus some from animals, insects and reptiles, and preparations are very crude before administration. Usually they are boiled with water for some time, and the liquid taken when hot. Essentiae and unguentum are the most important pharmacopoeial preparations. Occasionally inert media are used as the vehicles for the active principles.

(c) *Therapeutics*: In modern medicine rational therapeutics plays a much more important part than empirical therapeutics while the reverse is the case in Chinese medicine.

The prescription in modern medicine contains only a few potent drugs, and more synthetic compounds are employed. The products are elegant and refined. The dosage is small, some in drops and pills. The Chinese prescription is an exceedingly complicated one. There are one or two dozen more or less inert ingredients besides the active principle and most of them are of vegetable origin. The dosage is extremely large, usually taken warm by the bowlful.

In the olden days the Chinese had for some time some other therapeutics such as hydrotherapy, psychotherapy and vaccine therapy, but they were only employed for a short time and were gradually forgotten, entire reliance being laid on the prescription. In modern medicine there are many other methods of alleviating disease besides the ordinary prescription. General therapeutics such as diet, climate, baths, venesection, and cupping, and special therapies such as vaccine therapy, seratherapy, protein therapy, buffer therapy, X-ray therapy, radiotherapy, diathermy therapy, hydrotherapy, organotherapy, and psychotherapy are frequently employed. In fact they are regarded as more important than the taking of mixtures and pills.

Treatment

Modern Medicine: In spite of all the valuable therapeutic measures, much emphasis is being laid on prevention and public health in this subject. Indeed, preventive medicine will soon be the most important subject in the medical world. With the rapid advances of pathology and bacteriology, it is known that most of the diseases, though actual treatment is not always successful, can be prevented. The body itself may be prepared against the operation of the causes of disease, partly by judgment and matters of diet, exercise, clothing, etc., and partly by such special treatment in relation to particular diseases as is effected by vaccination and antisera inoculation. Public health involves all measures by which the community endeavours to ward off all external influences adverse to health by care of the water supply, air and ventilation, food, sewage and refuse disposal, buildings, etc.

Another important point in treatment besides the therapeutic measures is to improve the general condition of the patient so that the disease can be combated and overcome by his own vital power. This consists of rest, diet and change of environment. This measure is very useful in treatment and many cases can be cured by this method alone.

In recent years, surgery has made rapid advances, and the success may be attributed to the great help of anaesthetic and antiseptic measures. Most of the uncured cases of medicine can be mastered by this science and art. In fact, many obscure diagnoses are settled by the aid of a searching operation.

Chinese medicine: On account of the lack of anaesthetic and antiseptics, surgery in China is rarely attempted, although it was recorded in literature that wonders had been done by the renowned surgeon Hua Tuo 華陀 about two thousand years ago. Treatment is effected by the taking of medicinal decoctions and, to a less extent, pills. This is aided by the external appliances of essential oils, ointments, plasters and herbs. With only such simple therapies the Chinese claim that every disease can be cured, and this is actually the case, though it may be incredible to modern man. This may be accepted later on as more researches are being done on Chinese drugs which are so effective but unknown to the scientific world. Surgical cases such as fractures and dislocations are treated by the external appliance of herbs and other drugs after reduction and they recover in a comparatively short time.

As to prevention and public health they are not much cared. Much hygienic literature has been written in the *Chow Rituals* 周禮 and the *Analects* 論語 but they are not much believed and observed. Bad habits make the Chinese very unhygienic.

There are three accessory typical Chinese methods of treatment viz., moxa, massage, and acupuncture. Moxa is a peculiar art of the Chinese but is quite widely used by the Japanese as well. It consists of burning a tuft of soft, combustible substance upon the skin, and it cures many diseases especially those approaching death. Massage is now universally employed throughout the world and its value much appreciated. Acupuncture, which consists of puncturing certain points of the body with needles of varying size and length, is a peculiar Chinese minor operation of most ancient origin. It is considered to be a universal panacea but chiefly resorted to for rheumatism, sprains, swollen joints and deep seated pains of all kinds. 367 such points are described, each having its own name and supposed relationship with the internal organs. Owing to the ignorance of asepsis by native doctors more harm than good is done by its practice, but sometimes miraculous results are witnessed.

Training

In modern medicine, the science of medicine is regarded as one of the higher educations and is studied in college after the student has finished his middle or high school. Hence every medical man is well educated and has high moral and ethical status. They have to be carefully trained for quite a number of years in medical schools, and they not only study and attend lectures, but also do all possible practical work for themselves so as to acquire good knowledge of the normal and abnormal states of the human body before they are certified as a doctor.

The Chinese native doctors are not usually well educated. Most of them only turn to the profession of medicine when they have failed in their study of literature and classics. They take medicine as a vocation. They need not be well trained before they practice, and most of them possess only a little theoretical knowledge by reading some medical books, and no practical experience. Some of the higher grade learn more and have better experience by serving under apprenticeship. This is one great reason why Chinese medicine is not only without progress but also going backwards.

Professional Status

The modern doctorship is regarded as one of the noblest professions. A doctor is respected by the laity, his words believed, his directions carried out, and his works appreciated. On the other hand, there are strict medical ethics among the doctors themselves. A doctor is supposed to have the responsibility of saving others and work not as a vocation but for the sake of science.

In China, doctorship is classified on the same footing with fortune tellers, astrologers, and physiognomists 醫卜星相. The doctors are not much respected, and are called in or dismissed at will. Their words are not much believed, their prescriptions may be altered by patients' friends or relatives, and their works not appreciated. There are no laws or regulations governing their practice, and anybody can set himself up as a doctor. The doctors have no medical ethics among them and they work as a vocation.

Progress

There is a striking contrast in prospect between the two systems of medicine. Modern medicine is progressive and ancient Chinese medicine is retrogressive.

Even though many rapid advances have been made in modern medicine in a comparatively short time, yet researches are still carried out in every part of the world to bring this science into perfection and up to date. Within a year many alterations are made in every branch of medicine, and theories are continually accepted and rejected. The student has to get books of the latest edition if he wants to become a doctor possessing the best knowledge of the present time.

On account of the conservative teaching in China, there is great reverence for the authors of literature and classics, and none dare to question the ancient teachings. This holds well with the medical literature. Hence nobody dares to point out any mistakes and everything said by the ancients is correct. The older the book, the greater is its value. This completely bars the progress of Chinese medicine, and with lack of training of the modern medical men the science is gradually forgotten, and the art lost.

The times, however, have changed. With the introduction of modern medicine to China in 1805 a new era has been ushered in. Many medical schools have been established and every year a large number of graduates are being produced. Meantime those who are studying in Europe, America and Japan are returning in increasing numbers. Hospitals and research institutes are opening up all over the country. Works are being done to improve the ancient medical teachings by scientific methods, and we may expect a glorious future and recovery in the medical world of China.

Article end

The new medicine and its impact on old-style Chinese medical practice

1937 by Wu Lien-teh 伍連德

Source: *The Caduceus Journal*
Hong Kong Medical University Society, Volume 16 No. 1
February, 1937.

Yaron: The author of the following article is Dr. Wu, a key figure in transitioning China's medicine into modernity. He was entrusted with curbing the progression of the 1911 Manchurian plague; his success demonstrated a Western medicine superiority in treating infectious diseases. Chinese medicine practitioners were unable to cure it with Native medicine methods or even save themselves. This event—and Wu leading it, to a certain degree—paved the way for modern medicine in China. However, upon investigation one may find that modern medicine superiority actually resulted from the inferiority of the other. Modern medicine did not have a cure for the plague and mortality rate was just about 100%, yet it was able to pinpoint the transmission method; quarantine measures curbed the disease. Neither Native nor modern had a cure.

William Sommers from Yale University explained that the way Dr. Wu ordered the quarantine process was to group a certain number of people in a quarantine wagon for five days and see if any of the people developed plague symptoms, following an incubation period. If a single person displayed symptoms within 5 days, then for risk of cross infection, everyone else had to remain in the wagon for 5 more days, at the end of which everybody died. This was an extreme measure at an extreme time, and even though successful at its objective, one can only wonder at the price paid.

Chinese medicine and modern medicine both failed and, in this case, the latter failed less. For decades to come, Western medicine and Dr. Wu marched proud for their enormous success, failing to see their failure, just as Chinese medicine practitioners had marched proud into the plague, failing to see their own shortcomings. After 60,000 had perished, some even due to modern medicine measures, the lesson to be learnt is that one should look to one's own shortcomings and try to improve, not ignorantly believe one knows better or celebrate the errors of others. This, I believe, was a lesson for all.

Wu Liande and Yu Yunxiu were medical doctors who wanted prosperity for their country and were agonized by the deep ignorance prevalent among the people. In those days poverty, poor hygiene and lack of education was widespread. They wanted to change the poor conditions on the ground. Even though they are critical of Chinese medicine, we should still learn from them the spirit of change, a change toward a better and more useful direction.

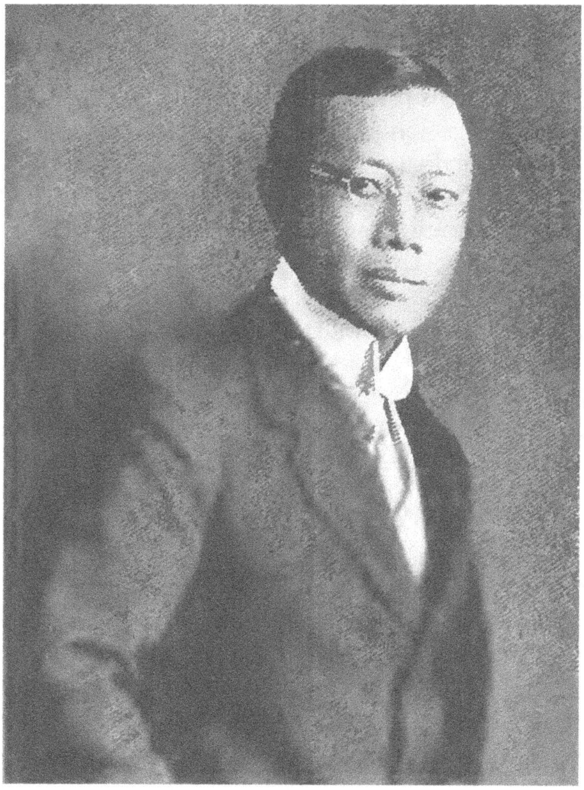

Wu Liande M.D. 伍連德 chaired the International Plague Conference in Mukden in April 1911, the first president of the China Medical Association (1916–1920) and director of the National Quarantine Service (1931–1937)

Pages 1–15

There are few places more suitable than Hong Kong to form a background for a discussion of Chinese medical history. For this was among the first cities where the early attempts to educate Chinese pupils in modern medicine were placed upon a solid foundation by the opening of a proper medical school in 1887, and it was in this colony also where the late Dr. Sun Yat-Sen, founder and First President of the

Chinese Republic, received his diploma. Not less striking is the close proximity of Hong Kong to the cradle of modern Chinese medicine in Canton and Macao. Indeed, it may be maintained that the government medical undertakings in Hong Kong form a direct continuation of the activities of the surgeons of the East India Company residing at Canton and Macao, and that the present medical stationary undertakings are a continuation of the hospital work commenced at Macao in 1838, and later transferred to Hong Kong in 1843.

The celebration of the centenary of the Canton Missionary Hospital in 1935 will have brought to your minds the fact that, before the establishment of the Macao Hospital, the new medicine had already gained a permanent foothold in South China. Earlier still, at the very beginning of the 19th century (1805), Jenner's method of smallpox vaccination had been introduced into Canton by Alexander Pearson, one of the great surgeons of the East India Company. In 1820, a dispensary for Chinese had been opened in Macao by Dr. Livingstone and the Rev. Robert Morrison, followed in 1828 by the opening of an Ophthalmic Hospital in the same city and a dispensary for the Chinese at Canton both under the guidance of Dr. Colledge who, like Livingstone, was attached to the East India Company. Though these undertakings were maintained for more or less limited periods, they benefited thousands of people and paved the way for the opening of the Canton Hospital under Dr. Peter Parker, the first medical missionary to China. It may be interesting to recall the opinions of these pioneers and their immediate followers as to the old-style practice of that time. In their view, Chinese medical art had become inadequate, being bound by the fetters of tradition. Practically no surgery was performed; indeed the knowledge possessed by the practitioners upon anatomy and physiology consisted mostly of absurd concepts, not backed by actual observation. The treatment of eye diseases was most primitive, in fact so unsuccessful that the early foreign doctors felt an urgent need to specialize in this domain. Diagnosis seemed to be based upon an examination of the pulse alone to the exclusion of other methods, a whole structure of theories being built upon this flimsy foundation. In treatment, fancies and not facts appeared to preponderate, consisting as it did partly of the indiscriminate use of acupuncture and similar manipulations, and partly of drugs which the early foreign observers believed inadequate, sometimes repulsive.

When we consider how the newcomers were hampered first by the lack of knowledge of the Chinese language and customs and then by the demands made upon their time and attention by hosts of sufferers, it is not surprising to find that those early impressions of old-style Chinese practice proved in some cases to be out of perspective, in others quite incorrect. Since that time prolonged and patient studies have been carried out, first by enlightened and erudite foreigners, later by Chinese experts, thus enabling us now to evaluate properly the strong and weak points of indigenous Chinese medicine.

Anatomy

It must be admitted that the early foreign observers erred least in their unfavourable judgment of anatomy, physiology and consequently surgery. For, although there are some early references to dissection, the traditional belief in the sacredness of the body made attempts in this direction rather sporadic. The *Filial Classic of Confucius* says, "Our body, skin and hair come from our parents; we must not mutilate them." This prohibition was lifted when the Manchus enforced the wearing of the queue with a shaved area around the head, and also since the advent of the Republic, when all men had their hair cut short. Nowadays, even women do not allow their hair to grow long but visit beauty parlours for singeing and permanent wave and sometimes indulge in the lifting of the skin to beautify the face! When needed for purposes of dissection, the corpses of bandits and criminals were secured. For these reasons, apart from some attempts to give exact measurements of the internal organs, but little useful knowledge is available in the old writings on anatomy.

A laudable attempt to replace idle speculations with careful observations was made by Wong Ching-jen who published in 1850 a booklet called *Correction of Medical Errors*. Here he describes how, during an epidemic of measles and dysentery, he had an opportunity to inspect the dead bodies of numerous children carelessly buried—thus permitting of a close examination of the internal organs. Unfortunately, he mistook the arteries for air vessels—an error he shared with the European investigators before Harvey. This is the more deplorable as there is little doubt that the ancient Chinese possessed some knowledge of blood circulation. The following significant passages can be found in the *Internal Classic (Nei-Ching)*:

> All the blood is under the control of the heart.
>
> The heart regulates all the blood of the body.
>
> The blood current flows continuously in a circle and never stops.

However, the difference between arteries and veins was not mentioned, nor were the systemic and pulmonary circulations understood—and subsequent practitioners for almost 2,000 years did not pursue the matter further.

Surgery

A similar lack of progress was present in surgery. Though we read of ancient masters, like Pien Ch'iao and Hua T'o, who knew anaesthesia and performed major operations, yet their art did not survive them. Legend has it that the manuscripts of Hua T'o were burned with the exception of a few pages dealing with castration. This is adduced as explanation why castration, performed by specialists, remained the only bold operation in old-style practice. The average surgeon was both by training and by equipment unable to carry out anything beyond the simplest interferences, like incision of abscesses and was as for a long time in Europe considered of a rather lower caste than the physician.

Eye diseases

Though writings dealing with eye diseases were abundant, practical results were not encouraging. Lee T'ao, in a recent contribution (October, 1936) summarizes that, in as much as ophthalmic diseases were considered in close relationship to the different organs, emphasis was laid upon internal medication and also on acupuncture rather than upon local treatment. However, powders, ointments and sometimes lotions were applied to a certain extent, the remedies including potent drugs like copper sulphate, borax and alum. Trachoma was recognised long ago and often successfully treated. The five kinds of operations carried out were (a) hooking or "blunt cutting method"; (b) cutting for removal of pterygium; (c) needling for removing cataracts; (d) cauterisation for ulcers and pterygia; and (e) clamping for trichiasis by shortening the lids through scar formation. This is done with a forceps made of bamboo. To judge by the Chinese proverb, "No treatment, no blindness", the faith of the Chinese in the skill of their ophthalmologists was not great. Such methods as mentioned above may still be seen in the bazaars of many crowded cities.

Pulse-lore

It would be bewildering rather than instructive, were I to give in this lecture a survey of the pulse-lore of the ancients. It was claimed that feeling of the pulse alone is sufficient for diagnosing all kinds of diseases and that it can foretell the sex of a child within a pregnant mother. More than that, by feeling of the pulse, a man may be judged noble or common, rich or poor, destined for a long life or bound to die soon!

It is clear that, just as a nostrum claiming to cure all diseases will be found useful for none, so the excessive bragging of the pulse specialists indicates the worthlessness of their method. Nevertheless, there is much truth in K. C. Wong's plea to make a distinction between the later-day absurdities of the Chinese pulse lore and the merits which this method might originally have possessed. He considers it as probable that the ancient practitioners, reduced to a few methods of physical examination, might have developed a technique in learning things from the pulse which is lost to the modern physician, who relies upon refined methods of diagnosis by X-rays, electro-cardiography and laboratory investigations.

Physical Therapy

The application of methods of physical therapy developed on lines similar to those of diagnosis. Acupuncture, practiced since the earliest times and amply discussed in the *Internal Classic*, was probably of distinct benefit so long as it was used in a judicious manner. Indeed, the late Sir James Cantlie tried to introduce it into modern practice, applying it successfully in certain cases of rheumatism. It should also be emphasised that enlightened old-style physicians, like Wang Tao in his work *The Medical Secrets of an Official*, objected to the continued use of acupuncture which, in his opinion, had become a lost art and recommended moxa in its place. However, no attention was paid to such warnings. The practice continued to be advocated and was, at the same time, debased through its indiscriminate application to all sorts of diseases and leaving it mainly in the hands of ignorant quacks or barber surgeons.

Acupuncture was only one of various methods of physical therapy in old-style Chinese practice. Besides this, ample use was made at moxa, in which cones of common mugwort (artemisia moxa) are applied to the skin at certain spots and ignited. Though this method is rather painful and the resulting wound is apt to become infected, the underlying principle of counter-irritation appears rational.

It is generally acknowledged that massage has been practised in China from time immemorial. Less known is the fact that a few of the ancients, like Hua T'o, made excellent use of hydrotherapy in the treatment of fevers. Unfortunately, this mode of treatment was not continued.

Infectious Diseases

Turning to infectious diseases, we find that in some respects the ancient ideas were quite sound. Leprosy was first mentioned in the Chou dynasty. One of Confucius' disciples, Pai Niu, was supposed to have died of it. The *Nei Ching* of Huang Ti, thus says, "Those suffering from 'ta ma feng' have stiff joints and the eyebrows as well as beard fall off; the channels being clogged, the flesh becomes nodular and ulcerates." For treatment, early prolonged medication and moderation in all things were emphasised. Chaulmoogra oil was recommended by Chu Tan-chi as early as the 14th century.

Cholera or the syndrome *huo luan*, which even in the early days was described as a sudden disturbance of the bowels and stomach, had a place in the Nei Ching, but the actual infection as we know it nowadays is believed by Yu Yun-hsiu, a living scholar, not to have been known in China until the great pandemic of 1817, since which time It has retained a more or less firm hold in this country.

Smallpox is another old disease upon which more books have been written than perhaps any other affliction. The general opinion is that it was introduced from outside, perhaps Mongolia, about 49 A.D as a result of war with the Mongols—one general, Ma Yuan, actually succumbing to the disease. An epoch-making contribution of the Sung dynasty was the discovery of inoculation against smallpox.

This happened in 998–1022A.D. when the prime minister, Wang Tan, invited a learned philosopher of Omei Mountains in Szechuan to treat his sons. It is quite possible that scientific ideas regarding inoculation were exchanged between Chinese, Arabian and Persian savants at that time resulting in its introduction into Constantinople, whence Lady Mary Wortley Montague, wife of the then British Ambassador to Turkey, introduced the method into England in 1717 by first trying it upon her own children, and then upon intimate friends of her aristocratic circle. This valuable means of prevention against a disfiguring, often-fatal disease became prevalent until superseded by the safer method of vaccination with calf-lymph, as introduced by William Jenner, in 1792. When the East India Company commenced trade with South China, its medical officer, Dr. A. Pearson, ordered the virus from India, where it had been received with favour, so that the year 1805 saw the first vaccination by cowpox vaccine of human beings in China. So rapid and universal was the success achieved, that calf-lymph vaccination became most popular, not only in Kwangtung, but as far north as Shanghai and Peking, and soon replaced the older and cruder means of inoculation with human-pox powder. This period may be termed the first stage in the introduction of scientific medicine into China. At the same time, it would be wise to withhold as far as possible the use of the word "Western medicine" when indicating modern or scientific medicine, for, as has been seen above, the first seeds were sown in the east, not in the west, and if an error was committed by early Cantonese in using the term *hsi* (western) as distinguished from *chung* or *kuo* for Chinese or national, thus bringing with it misunderstanding and prejudice, the former should be discarded, and a simpler and plainer *hsin* 新 meaning "new" or "modern" adopted. The difficulty is more evident in the Chinese rather than the English application, for true science cannot be a monopoly of the east or west, since humanity is universal and benefits all creeds and races.

Plague or *shu-yi*, as contrasted with smallpox and cholera, is not found in any ancient Chinese publication. In a book called *Ping-yuan* or *"Sources of Disease"* published in 610A.D., mention was first made of *E-he* or "malignant bubo", described as "coming on abruptly with high fever together with the appearance of a bundle of nodes beneath the tissues. The size of the nodes ranges from a bean to a plum. The skin and muscles around are dry and painful. The nodes may be felt to move from side to side under the skin. If prompt treatment is not given, the poison will enter the system, cause severe chill and end in death."

The treatise on epidemics or *Wen-yi-lun* published in 1642, introduced the word *ko-ta-wen* which has been copied into German and English books. Until the word *pesuto* (transliteration of *pest*) was introduced after Kitasaro's time, the Japanese used the character *yi* or *yeki* (meaning epidemic) for plague.

From a book of 31 pages by Hung Liang-chi (1736–1809) entitled *"Poems by Pei Chiang"* the term *Yang-tsu Ping* or glandular infection was found. Shih Tao-nan (1765–1792) a young man of extraordinary talent who died of the plague, composed a poem in which one part *"Death of Rats"* vividly described the plague epidemic occurring in a city in Yunnan in 1792. Because of Hong Kong's close connection with this disease; I beg permission to quote four of the striking verses:

Dead rats in the east,
Dead rats in the west!
As if they were tigers,
Indeed are the people scared.

Few days following the death of the rats,
Men pass away like falling walls!
Deaths in the day are numberless,
The hazy sun is covered by sombre clouds.

While three men are walking together
Two drop dead within ten steps!
People die in the night,
Nobody dares weep over the dead!

The land is filled with human bones,
There in the fields are crops,
To be reaped by none;
And the officials collect no tax!

You will notice his reference to the connection between rodents and the disease.

Syphilis is another important disease widely prevalent during the latter part of the Ming dynasty (1368–1644). No doubt, it was introduced by Portuguese sailors visiting China, who had themselves received infections from Spaniards returning with Columbus after the discovery of America. Li Shih-chen, author of the *Pen Ts'ao Kang Mu*, said that syphilis was unknown in China until 1488–1521, when patients were given pills of mercury for treatment. It started in Kwangtung, spread to the north and then other parts of the empire.

Materia Medica—The systematic use of drugs for the treatment of diseases has a history as old as that of the Chinese race. The oldest Herbal, the *Pen-T'sao Ching*, is ascribed to Emperor Shen Nung (2838–2698B.C.), though it actually appeared during the Western Han dynasty (206B.C.–25A.D.). Since that time numerous works on materia medica have been published, culminating in the Great herbal book *Pen-Ts'ao Kang-Mu* by Li Shih-chen in 1595A.D. This great classic consists of 52 volumes, the material being arranged in 62 orders under 16 classes—water, fire, earth, metals and minerals, herbs, grains, vegetables, fruits, trees, garments and utensils, insects, fishes, molluscs, birds, beasts and men. Of the 1,871 drugs enumerated, 1,074 are derived from plants, 443 from animals and 354 from minerals and other substances. Besides numerous drugs common to both Chinese and European medicine the former contained such valuable materials as kaolin, eumenol, chaulmoogra oil and ephedrine, which last is now included in most official pharmacopoeias.

In a paper read at the Congress of the Far Eastern Association of Tropical Medicine, Nanking, October 1934, *The Newer Pharmacology and its Relation to Ancient Medicine*, Prof. B. E. Read emphasised the changes that had taken place in recent years regarding the armamentarium of the modern physician, who now looks to glandular products for the treatment of deficiency diseases and to a study of the patient's diet, not so much to limit it, as to provide what is lacking in its constituents. In the place of the nine substances of animal origin appearing in the 1909 pharmacopoeia there arc now nearly one hundred, including liver extract, stomach, insulin from the pancreas, fibrinogen from the lung, vitamin A from the eye, adrenalin, thyroxin, parathormone, etc. The new conception of treatment fairly corresponds with ancient Chinese ideas, by which at least 26 parts from six different animals are used for medicine. From the pig alone, 34 parts are listed as of medicinal value. Thus pig's liver (rich in vitamins A, B, C, D and E) was recommended in the *Pentsao* for night blindness, beri-beri, scurvy, emaciation and oedema; pig's pancreas is the source of three digestive principles; sheep's eyes are used for dimness of vision and conjunctivitis; dog's brain obtained from the same animal that bites a person is applied to the wound, thus suggesting a connection with the modern Pasteur treatment of injecting an emulsion of the brain and spinal cord of rabbits infected with rabies into the victim.

With regard to deficiency diseases, it has been found that for night-blindness (due to lack of vitamin A) the addition of 5 per cent of dried yellow day lily 黃花菜 to the diet quickly cures the complaint in rats. The Chinese pharmacopoeia recommends other remedies, such as, mung beans, shepherd's purse 薺, walnut, pig's liver and others for this trouble. For beri-beri or *chiao-chi* 脚氣 89 drugs are said to be of value, and Ch'en Ts'ang-chi'i 陳藏器 as far back as the T'ang dynasty warned against the constant use of polished rice, which he said would lead to weakness of muscles, drowsiness and general lassitude. Considering that modern medicine has traced beri-beri to lack of vitamin B in polished rice, this statement by an ancient Chinese physician is almost prophetic. Vitamin E, the lack of which is supposed by modern workers to cause sterility, may, if the opinions of ancient Chinese pharmacologists do not go astray, be supplied by human placenta, rat's faeces, dog's meat, deer-horns, etc. A considerable amount of research has also been done by W. Y. Lee and R. G. Cheng in a basic analysis of common Chinese foods and drugs, varying from spinach, mustard leaves, bamboo sprout to taro, pumpkin, eggplant, cowpea, soybean and cabbage. Prof. S. Kubota of Mukden draws attention to the isolation of an active principle, called sinomenin, from the well-known Chinese drug *han-fang-chi* 漢防己 which is most useful for rheumatism; also *hai-jen-tsao* 海人草 for the treatment of round worms. From the woody part of the camphor tree two preparations, novonal and mibunol, have been extracted for the treatment of gonorrhoea. For coughs, glucosides from the root *yuan-chih* 遠志 and the seed *ch'e-ch'ien* 車前 have been obtained, while the alkaloid ephedrine derived from *ma-huang* 麻黃 is too well-known to need reiteration.

Lastly, a valuable heart tonic, *vita camphor*, has recently been recovered from the urine of dogs fed with camphor, which seems to decompose within the body of the animal and produce a strong and yet safe cardiac stimulant giving quick and accurate effects when needed.

Compare this with the isolation of *theelin* from the urine of parturient women by an American firm of biological chemists for female disorders.

Hygiene—A study of ancient Chinese medical literature also shows that the prevention of disease was placed above cure, as may be judged by the following quotations:

> The sage does not treat those who are ill but those who are well.
>
> The good doctor pays constant attention to keeping the people well so that there will be no sickness.
>
> The good physician first cures the disease of the nation, then individual ailments.

Chinese medicine attained a high degree of development during the Chou dynasty, particularly in the matter of medical organisation, hygiene and public health. *The Chou Rituals* distinguished four kinds of doctors, namely physicians, surgeons, dietitians and veterinarians. The writings of Confucius, Huai Nan-tzu, Chuang Tzu, Chou Kung and others contain numerous happy references to the performance of healthy living. Thus:

> Diseases enter by the mouth.
>
> Take deep breathing to live long.
>
> Do not fatigue your body or exhaust it and you will live long.
>
> Contentment and peace shut out all worries, giving no chance for evil to sneak into the system.
>
> Do not marry first relatives, etc.

Among other recommendations was the establishment of hospitals for the deaf, blind, dumb, lame, deformed and insane.

Ideas of a progressive nature may be detected in old Chinese medical literature, and not a few of the old-style therapeutic agents have found a permanent place in the pharmacopoeia of the modern physician. Many factors contributed, however, to reduce or even nullify the benefits of innovations, because these were often kept secret by the discoverers and their immediate pupils. On the whole, old-style Chinese medicine became more and more stagnant as time went on. In China, as in mediaeval Europe, over-reverence for ancient beliefs and traditions became a stumbling block to progress. The ingenuity of most savants was wasted in compiling subtle commentaries upon the old writings instead of being directed toward fundamental research, and the introduction of radical changes was deemed nothing short of heresy. In Europe the medical profession gradually managed to free itself from these superstitions and to give to medicine the dignity of a progressive science taught side by side with other branches of learning at the universities and practised by men of high standing. In China, on the contrary, the profession could not extricate itself from such legendary quagmire. The status of practitioners reached a deplorably low level. Though a few of the ancients were venerated as Gods the average medical man was looked upon as a kind of artisan to be called and dismissed at will. Often he could see and prescribe for a patient but once so that he had no chance to watch the evolution of diseases or obtain a thorough insight into the action of therapeutics. His prescriptions were criticised and changed at will by the family and friends of the patient, who did not hesitate to employ quacks and fortune tellers side by side with the regular practitioners. The higher the status of the patient, the greater the number of questionable advisers and therefore the fewer chances to recover.

No wonder that the medical profession ceased for centuries to attract men of good education and character. Consequently the profession was recruited from a class either unfit for manual labour, literary positions or official appointments.

Though praiseworthy attempts at proper education, holding of state examinations and registration of practitioners are on record, efforts in this direction were spasmodic in nature and ceased altogether as time went on. Would-be practitioners were obliged either to acquire elementary training in a haphazard manner or to serve an apprenticeship. It is clear that this system, even if imparting useful knowledge, was unable to provide a proper background for the pupils, who lacked adequate preparation. Apprenticeship was found to produce more promising results in cases where sons were trained by their fathers.

Proverbs like "Do not take medicine by a doctor who is not backed by the experience of three generations" explain the greater prestige of men, who besides their own skill could claim descent from noted medical families.

Beyond such family connections and the benefit to be derived from the study of a limited literature, there was little to encourage the practitioner in his professional life. Though some leaders had set high standards of conduct by their example and the laying down of ethical rules, these were never generally accepted. Medical societies, where the doctors could get guidance and where they could discuss their problems, were totally lacking. Thus each individual was largely left to his own devices.

Looking back upon this evolution we can easily understand why so many of the early foreign doctors coming to China decided that the old system of medicine was devoid of any value whatsoever. It is not surprising, therefore, that attempts by some newcomers to work hand in hand with the old-style practitioners did not lead to satisfactory results. At the Tung-Wah Hospital, Hong Kong, both systems have been maintained for scores of years; the annual medical reports of the Director of Medical and Sanitary Services provide interesting reading in this connection.

The pioneers mentioned earlier in this lecture were but the harbingers of an ever-increasing group of foreign physicians who not only continued the work in and near Canton but extended it along the coast to Swatow, Amoy, Foochow, Ningpo, Hangchow, into Shanghai, Nanking, Soochow, then Peiping, Tientsin and finally into the larger cities of Manchuria. Their work was at first largely individualistic, but gradually united efforts became possible. Some of the important milestones along this road were the establishment of a medical school in 1866 connected with the Canton Missionary Hospital under Dr. John Kerr, who published a series of textbooks in Chinese for his students, the creation of a Customs Medical Service leading to publication of a stimulating series of reports, and the foundation in 1886 of the Medical Missionary Association resulting in the issuing of a journal, invaluable equally through the articles it contained and through the opportunities afforded for the discussion of ways and means.

Whilst these labours were instrumental in bringing proper relief to thousands of sufferers, it may be stated that for a long time the new medicine developed rather side by side with the continuance old-style practice than in open competition with it.

One might almost say that their fields had become divided up. Whilst the modern medical men were usually consulted when surgical interference seemed necessary, the majority of Chinese still preferred the old-fashioned therapy for so-called internal complaints. The first serious clash of the two schools arose out of the terrible Manchurian pneumonic plague epidemic, which swept over Manchuria and North China in 1910–11, killing 60,000 persons and costing the government and people about $20,000,000. Whilst old-style medicine showed itself utterly powerless in this catastrophe, and at least 40 of its protagonists died from the infection the efficiency and heroism displayed by modern-trained Chinese physicians were instrumental in ridding the country of the plague within the short space of three months. Their work attracted universal attention and laid the foundation of systematic public health activities, thus ushering in a new (second) phase in Chinese medical history. Then followed an interval of consolidation which the Revolution and the establishment of the Republic delayed but did not stop. The inauguration of the National Government in Nanking and the establishment of the Ministry of Health in 1927 (later changed to National Health Administration) finally co-ordinated all health activities under one central organ. Under the able guidance of Dr. J. Heng Liu, a graduate of Harvard, a series of fine institutions have during the past six years been constructed and equipped in one medical centre in the capital (measuring 400 mou or 65 acres) for the treatment and nursing of patients, the investigation of disease, the analysis of drugs, and the teaching of health and auxiliary personnel. These and affiliated institutions include the Central Hospital of Nanking, the Central Field Health Station, the Nursing School, the Central Serum and Vaccine Laboratory, the Biochemical department, two midwifery schools—one in Nanking and the other in Peiping—a Child Health Station, School Health Services, Rural Health Centres, the National Quarantine Service, Central Epidemic Prevention Bureau in Nanking with a branch in Peiping and also stations in Fukien and the North-west. In order to co-ordinate activities between the Ministry of Education and the Central Health Administration, a joint Commission has been founded with a trained medical secretary in charge and having sections on medical education, midwifery and nursing.

If we contemplate the amount of work and success crowded into the comparatively short space of a century, the new medicine may indeed be proud of its record in China. But whilst these achievements encourage us to approach the work before us in a spirit of hopefulness, they should not mislead us into minimising the difficulties and rocks ahead.

In this connection let us deal first with the present status of old-style medicine. The vast numbers still practising these methods have become thoroughly alarmed through the advance of the new medicine, which now really threatens their continued existence. More than that, they have realised that their only hope of salvation lies in uniting their forces. They have been organised into a group powerful enough to secure the support of influential high officials and to prevent efforts to abolish their practice. There is no doubt that many difficulties will be met with until ways and means can be found to settle this involved problem. It is the duty of all modern practitioners to be constantly on the alert and to give their wholehearted support to their leaders and organisations. Nor should they altogether ignore the herbalists as far as their individual work is concerned. Some pertinent remarks on this point were made by Dr. Knud Faber in his 1931 Report on Medical Schools in China; he thus observed:

> When an ever increasing number of Chinese physicians is educated and graduated on modern lines, it will be more and more understood by the population that there can be different kinds of doctors but only one science and art of medicine. I have the idea that this evolution would be hastened if the students in the medical colleges and special schools had to attend a course of medical history including the history of philosophy and the content of the old Chinese medicine not for using the old methods but for better understanding what they will have to compete with in their future practice. The best manner to combat the superstitions of the old Chinese medicine is to let them come out in the daylight. The modern Chinese doctor must know them as then only will he be able to overcome them and to educate the population in this respect.

Another point I would like to mention in passing is the tendency to rely on proprietary brands of medicine rather than on Galenic prescriptions. It is true that the glaring publicity given to all sorts of patent medicine is influencing laymen in favour of the former, but it seems to me that not a few qualified practitioners also appear too willing to follow these tendencies. Rather should we insist upon the use of scientific preparations adapted to the individual needs of each patient instead of doling out ready-made stuff indiscriminately? Likewise, we should not neglect the basic methods of physical examination in spite of easy access to supplementary facilities. The danger of debasing our medical art into a craft should not be forgotten.

The vital problem facing medical administrators and educators is, however, not how to deal with individual sufferers but how to extend the influence of modern medicine in its preventive as well as curative aspects, so as to render real services to the masses. If we review this matter by comparing the number of modern-trained practitioners in China with the standards of other countries, we find the former grossly inadequate. For instance while Great Britain has one doctor for every 800 and the U.S.A. one for 1,000 inhabitants, we find in China, even admitting the maximal figure of 15,000 qualified practitioners, a proportion of 1:30,000.

This situation becomes more serious when the regional distribution of the doctor is considered. An attempt in this direction was made by Drs. Chu and Lai, who in 1935 collected data on 5,390 modern-trained physicians in China, of whom all but 13 per cent were Chinese.

It was found that these were congregated in a few large cities, 22 per cent being in Shanghai alone. Nanking and Canton are also crowded with doctors. In the former one-third of the population receives no proper attention, whilst in the latter the saturation point appears to have been reached regarding the number of physicians.

Dr. C. C. Ch'en of Tung hsien, who investigated conditions from the viewpoint of demand rather than supply, points out that China is an agricultural country, about 85 per cent of her population living in villages and small towns. On account of over-population, the average holding of a farmer's family is five *mou* (or 5/6 of an acre), producing $40 annually. It is clear that under these circumstances only a minimal sum can be spared for medical relief and indeed it has been found that the farmer spends on average thirty cents annually for this purpose.

If now $600 per annum be computed as the minimum salary for a qualified physician, 5,000 people would have to contribute 12 cents per capita to keep him alive and an addition of at least $400–500 per year would be necessary to equip him for active work. This would mean that 10,000 people are necessary to support a physician—a number which no practitioner could possibly care for.

It is obvious, therefore, that a mere increase in the output of graduates would not really remedy the present situation unless it is accompanied by measures which would direct this increased supply into the proper channels. In other words, since the vast majority of the people are unable to support an adequate number of modern trained physicians the introduction of a system of State Medicine becomes inevitable. I am glad to note that this idea is not only shared by medical educators but has been definitely adopted by the National Health Administration. Steps have already been taken to adapt the curriculum of medical schools to this new policy, and it is hoped that the teaching of State Medicine will henceforth form a prominent feature of the educational programme. The strategic position of Hong Kong University calls for urgent consideration of the establishment of a Chair of State Medicine and of post-graduate courses in Public Health.

It is quite possible that some persons may be against enlarging the powers of the state at the cost of private enterprise. They may fear that the new officials, bereft of the incentive of competition, may be tempted to do a minimum of work. It is beyond my task to deal with the general merits of this view. I feel sure, however, that it does not hold good as far as the medical profession is concerned. We medical men fortunately belong to a calling which demands the highest ethical standards and a spirit of sacrifice. We have seen that many practitioners have in times of need nobly responded to this spirit inculcated by their schools. Quite a number of promising men and women avoid private practice and prefer to receive modest salaries in working for the public weal.

The conscientious doctor in the China of the future would have to know more of preventive than of curative medicine, possessing at his finger tips accurate knowledge of the causes of such infections as smallpox, plague, cholera, diphtheria, typhoid, typhus, trachoma, tuberculosis and willing to send such patients to municipal or government hospitals for treatment rather than attempt it at his own confined or perhaps insufficiently-equipped office. He will practise partly in rural areas and probably receive an allowance from the government for keeping his district inhabitants as free from sickness as possible; in any case he will be in touch with the nearest Government health clinics where more facilities for treatment in the form of space, equipment, nurses and medicines are at hand: Through these health stations he will also take a share in advising pregnant women from the early days of conception to childbirth, which had best take place in a maternity home or the maternity department of a hospital. As the child grows up he will watch its progress step by step up to school-age, when trained school medical officers will supervise the welfare of the pupils through the toils of scarlet fever, diphtheria, measles and such like. Under constant vigilance and examination a new generation of children will develop with proper physique under a sunny clean atmosphere, immune from infectious diseases, strong against the inroads of tuberculosis, with eyes clear of trachoma and knowing simple methods of not only protecting themselves but also preventing others from being attacked. As the years go by, such a trained generation will marry healthily, possess as many or as few children as it pleases, but all being brought up with knowledge of the ordinary principles of health. From this the next step to living to a ripe old age is logical, which end can best be achieved without the purchase of old-fashioned and expensive medicaments like ginseng, deer horns, fungi, etc.

Events in other directions than medicine are shaping themselves very rapidly throughout China, and it is not too much to hope that through a proper appreciation and practice of the new medicine by both the medical and lay public a healthier and stronger generation of Chinese will blossom forth to undertake their duties for their country with greater freshness and energy, thus helping this present quarrelsome world to move along the paths of peace and happiness.

Article end

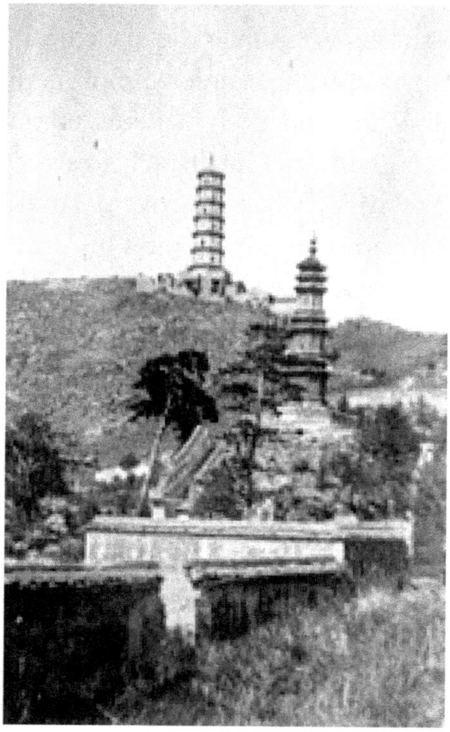

Photo by Mr P. Goux in early 1900s. "Summer Palace".

A word for Chinese medicine

1927 by Deng Xialu 燈下盧

Source: *San San Medical Publication*, 3rd Vol. 20 Issue, Published 1927 三三醫報第三卷二十期

Yaron: Beginner students too jumped into the heated public debates even before the abolishment proposal of Yu Yunxiu in 1929.

Although I'm not part of Chinese medical intelligentsia, from time to time I simply read some Chinese medical books. Recently in *Double Three Medical Newspaper* 三三醫報 there were arguments about the medical school system between Chinese and Western medical doctors. One of their debate points is Yin-Yang and five element theories. Objectively speaking, it only brushes the surface when Western medicine doctors talk about Chinese medical theories. Chinese medicine uses Yin-Yang as positive and negative points and uses five elements as pronouns. So even though these theories seem abstract and empty, they actually include a literal explanation. As for Yu Yan's 余巖 critique, it has no impact and should only be criticized. The way he ridiculed Chinese medicine as avoiding reality is like the skill of a ghost drawing another ghost.

Chinese medical theories are based on Yin-Yang and five elements theories. The fine details and comprehensiveness level is too high for Western medicine. Its strong point is way beyond a superficial level. For example, "Spleen stores nutritive Ying, while nutritive Ying houses the mind Yi 脾藏營, 營舍意" and other similar lines explain the profound mystery of physiology. Now, some Chinese medicine doctors don't care about the facts and stoutly claim that the word "spleen" in this line means a real physical spleen. Can we ask someone who has dissected the spleen already where do the nutritive Ying and mind Yi physically store?

Instead, one should start with an academic angle to promote Chinese medicine. For example, we should clarify the meaning of Yin-Yang and five elements theories to make them more reliable and based in evidence. If we can reach this level then it will cause a worldwide medical revolution. However, rejecting Chinese medicine is the worst option.

I'm new to the Chinese medicine field, and previously I was against Yin-Yang and five elements theories. But this spring I started researching Chinese medicine and since then I've learnt that it has a very profound knowledge which requires decades of learning and research. My current knowledge is just a tiny bit and originally I planned to keep learning it quietly so not to mislead anyone including myself. But now the situation made me publish this article. I'll send it to those who want this article by the end of this month. There are other articles such as *Principle of Change Yi Li* 易理, which were just finished, and I'll send them after they get published.

December 2nd 14th year of the Republic (1925)

Article end

Awakening of Chinese medicine

1927 by Sun Binggong 孫秉公

Source: *San San Medical Publication*, 3rd Vol. 20 Issue, Published 1927 三三醫報第三卷二十期

Yaron: Unifying Chinese medicine practitioners to resist government suppression, and to respond to science and modernization by standardizing Chinese medicine education, schools and textbooks, as well as by discarding old theories that cannot match the clarity of modern science.

Sun Binggong from Taicang 太倉 孫秉公

In the spring of the year Ren Xu (1922), Ministry of Internal Affairs 內務部 issued the *Managing Chinese Medicine Regulations* 管理中醫規則. Due to some objections, at the end, the proposal didn't take effect. Now there is an order for arresting fake Chinese medicine doctors; it says, "We are going to eliminate quacks in order to respect human lives." The truth is that the government prepares the ground for Western medicine to take over, and so they disrespect traditional Chinese medicine and try to destroy it. What a pity! People who have some passion for Chinese medicine should stand up and fight for it.

There are two ways to fight for it: one is internal policy and the other is external policy. Chinese medicine is being destroyed by the government and is looked down on by Western medicine doctors. All of this is caused by inferior politicians trickling in affection. However, when things rot then naturally they attract bugs. The current situation of Chinese medicine is in an extreme decline. People are stealing current prescriptions while avoiding known principles and still declare themselves doctors. They don't read the books of Qibo 岐伯 and Xuanyuan 軒轅[181] and don't consider the principles of Qi either. To an extreme, some people, who regard themselves as doctors, actually don't study any medical texts and in fact can't read, or they can just shave hair for people. Certainly the direction Chinese medicine is heading leads towards the bottom. Like this, it's hard not to have such bad reputation and contempt.

So our internal strategy should be to establish Chinese medical schools and compile uniform teaching materials, exactly the same way as other intelligentsia. This is the first priority. We should organize ourselves, Chinese medicine doctors, and implement experiments (the details of which will be published in other books). What yields good results should be kept, while what is failing should be discarded. Like this we will block the interference of the government.

As for the external strategy, we should cooperate in order to object the order from the government. However, the internal strategy should be emphasized more than the external, because the internal strategy is the solution for the root problem. Until the root is fixed the entire situation won't get better, and, in addition, this is our only way to struggle with Western medicine. The rule of natural evolution is that the good one survives while the bad one disappears. Isn't this the twentieth century, an era of scientific excellence?

As for the proposal of allowing Chinese medicine schools into the main school system, it has direct advantages for us, so we should promote that. Above is my humble opinion, if there's any mistake please correct it.

(P.S. Time is of the essence; things are pressing and urgent. I just grasped a few relevant parts to compose my article. However I still have another suggestion to Chinese medicine intelligentsia, which is to get rid of jealousy and selfish attitude. We should cooperate and help each other to develop and promote the real and profound Chinese medical theory and together prevent counter attacks by Western medicine proponents.)

Article end

[181] Yellow Emperor

"The Great Debates" between Yu Yunxiu 余雲岫, Yun Tieqiao 惲鐵樵 and Tan Cizhong 譚次仲

Includes other debates

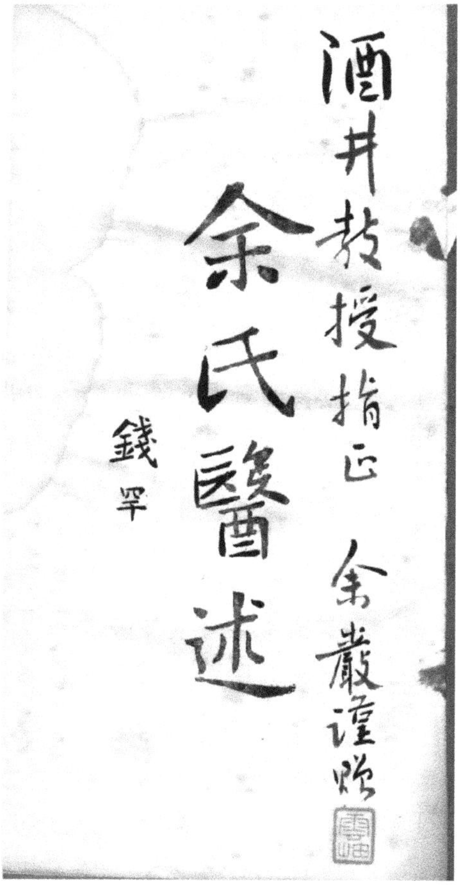

Writings from Yu Yunxiu 余云岫 (Yu Yan 余巖) 1920s—30s. Title calligraphy by Qian Han 錢罕

Our source: *Mr. Yu's Medical Narrative Yu Shi Yi Shu* 余氏醫述 is a collection of works, papers and letters by Yu Yunxiu, distributed by the Society Medical Press 社會醫報館. Publication date is not listed, however the special foreword for this compilation, written by Mr. Yu, is dated September 21st, the 17th year of the Republic (1928). Publication date is likely November 1928. This work was later renamed as *Collection of the Medical Revolution Articles Yi Xue Ge Ming Lun Ji* 醫學革命論集.

About the practitioners and a brief backdrop narrative of the time

Yu Yunxiu 余云岫 (1879–1954), style name Yan 巖, pen name Baizhi 百之, a person of Zhe Jiang 浙江 province. In 1901 attended the Xun Xi public school 潯溪公學 (founded by Pang Yuancheng 龐元澄 (1875–1945), a scholar who passed the imperial examination on the county level Xiu Cai 秀才). In 1905, at the state's expense, travelled to study in Japan. At Japan's athletic club he nearly graduated, but then transferred to Osaka medical university. Graduated in 1916 and returned to China to serve as Shanghai Hospital Medical Director. The following year he started his own medical practice in Shanghai.

In 1917, Yu published *Discussion and Deliberation on the Ling Shu and Su Wen, Ling Su Shang Dui* 靈素商兑, a book systematically refuting the ancient Chinese medical theories of the *Ling Shu* 靈書 and *Su Wen* 素問. Later on Yu (in different time periods) served as a member of the national government Ministry of Health central health committee, a member of the Ministry of the Interior special health committee, the vice chairman of Southeastern medical school board of directors, the head of China's medical research institute, an advisor to the Ministry of Education medical science state education committee, the first president of Shanghai Medical Association and the chief editor of *China's Medical Journal* 中華醫學雜誌.

Yu studied both Chinese and Western medicine and tried to find out the possibility to integrate them both. He investigated and annotated the Chinese medicine history, disease names etc; he researched and arranged Chinese medicine literature. In 1925, he traveled to Japan to attend the "Far East Tropical Medicine Conference" in which he presented his paper, *Research on China's Tuberculosis History*, pointing out that scrofula and pulmonary tuberculosis are of the same origin. He spent 15 years writing his book *The Distant Meaning of China's Ancient Disease Names* 中國古代疾病名候疏義. In his practice, Yu often used Chinese herbs as part of therapy; in his clinic he had set up a chemistry research institute and was manufacturing Chinese herbal pharmaceutical grade preparations. While arranging Chinese medicine pharmacological literature, he composed *Research of Literature about Native Herbal Production* 國產藥物的文獻研究 and *My Humble Opinion on the Production Research of Chinese Herbs* 研究國藥產物芻議.

After the communist liberation of Shanghai, Yu was already of advanced age, but he nonetheless participated in many activities. In 1950, in east China health administration conference, he proposed that medical workers should move toward collectivization. In 1953, he organized and founded Shanghai city Xin Cheng District Number 4 United Clinic 上海市新成區第四聯合診所 and served as its director. Around that time, he also served as a member of Shanghai municipal government cultural and education committee, the national health sciences research committee Chinese medicine special committee, Ministry of Health teaching materials editing and screening committee, a distinct member of China's People Republic pharmacopoeia compilation committee, and the director of China's Medical Sciences Association. Shortly after his passing, as attacks were directed at the Ministry of Health and Western medicine doctors, Yu was often portrayed as the villain—not only was he educated with the enemy in Japan, he was also a "nationalist reactionary bourgeoisie who has tried to destroy Chinese medicine of our motherland". For decades to come, fueled by Communist ideology and propaganda, Yu, who throughout his entire life tried to modernize China, became the anti-Chinese medicine iconic symbol.

Among many influential figures in the modernizing group was the physiology professor Yan Derun 嚴德潤, who invited a famous Chinese medicine acupuncturist from northeastern China to perform acupuncture on a cadaver. Thereafter, Yan dissected the cadaver and found out that some needles target nerves, while others flesh and tendons. He concluded that the practice of acupuncture makes no sense and has no real effect on the person.

At the same time, one most influential person supporting Chinese medicine was a Chinese medicine doctor Yun Tieqiao 惲鐵樵 (1878–1935). After losing his first three sons to disease, the fourth son became ill and Yun was able to cure him with a traditional Ma Huang Tang 麻黃湯 formula. He held the opinion that Western medicine should not be the only standard and that Chinese medicine should follow its own theory in order to be effective. In 1922, Yun published *Records of Widening One's Wisdom with all the Chinese Classics Qun Jing Jian Zhi Lu* 群經見智錄, a book systematically and thoroughly countering Yu Yunxiu's arguments. Yun Tieqiao and Yu Yunxiu often exchanged letters with their arguments for and against Chinese medicine. In 1925, Yun Tieqiao established the Tie Qiao Chinese Medicine Correspondence School 鐵樵中醫函授學校.

Yun Tieqiao's student Lu Yuanlei 陸淵雷 (1894–1955) served at the school as the dean of studies. Lu also studied Chinese classics and literature from Zhang Taiyan 章太炎. Lu began promoting the idea that Chinese medicine needs to be improved for the better; it needs to go through scientification. The term "Chinese medicine scientification" 中醫科學化 most likely began with Lu Yuanlei 陸淵雷. Lu Yuanlei was of the opinion that if Chinese medicine doctors believed that Chinese medicine can go through scientification, then Chinese medicine will go through scientification. Convincing Chinese medicine doctors that it is possible became the objective. In 1929 he established, with a few others, Shanghai Native Medicine College 上海國醫學院. In 1933 he served as committee member of the Central Bureau for Native Medicine Teaching Organization Committee 中央國醫館學術整理委員會委員.

In 1929, a proposal by Yu Yunxiu to effectively abolish Chinese medicine had stopped short from passing into law. Wang Jingwei 汪精衛 (1883–1944), a prominent political figure at the time, already announced that Chinese medicine is backward and needs to be changed or stopped. The measure, however, did not pass at the legislative Yuan (assembly) because of two other prominent politicians, Feng Yuxiang 馮玉祥 and Chen Lifu 陳立夫, who persuaded

Jiang Jieshi 蔣介石, the president, not to sign it into law. Even though this proposal was never implemented it was widely used by Chinese medicine practitioners as provocation in order to "rally the troops."

In 1933, Chinese medicine associations put together a draft *Chinese Medicine Regulations Zhong Yi Tiao Li* 中醫條例, hoping to push it through the legislative house Li Fa Yuan 立法院. Wang Jingwei 汪精衛, opposing Chinese medicine, became too impatient and sent a personal signed letter to the legislative house president Sun Ke 孫科 hoping to strike a backroom deal. This letter was leaked to a reporter Zhang Zanchen 張贊臣, who published it in his paper and thus made it public. This was a significant setback for the anti-Chinese medicine group as it created a public roar claiming the modernizers group to be corrupt. In 1936, Chinese medicine finally became lawful and the threat to its legal status was removed, at least temporarily.

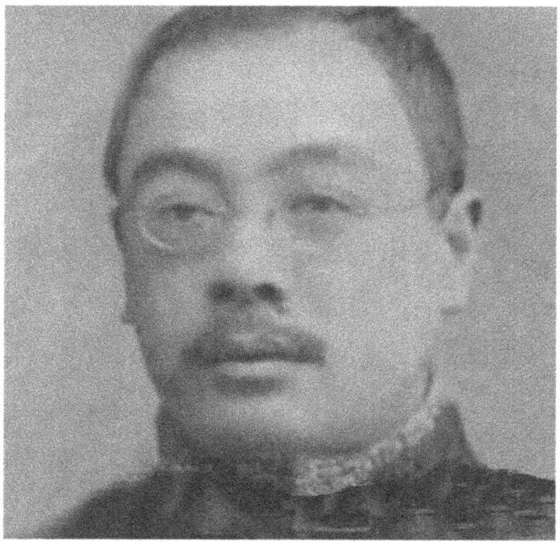

Yu Yunxiu 余云岫 circa 1917

Mr. Yu Medical Narrative: Scroll 4

A letter to the Bureau of Native Medicine about Pulse

Yaron: Points 6 and 7 are especially important for us—Chinese medicine practitioners contemplating what is proper and what may not be proper in pulse studies. One cannot ignore the fact that Chinese medicine is filled with conflicting opinions—so who is right and who is wrong? It cannot be that everybody is right in Chinese medicine if they hold opposite opinions. How can we overcome this problem?

In the 1920s–30s many Chinese medicine practitioners started a selection process of theories and ideas—what to keep and what to let go of, mostly following the principle of "only the best survives".

Mr. Yu delivers a harsh critique of Chinese medicine pulse diagnosis techniques, or at least most of its theory. During his time, Chinese medicine practitioners responded with statements such as: we have experience, we can feel what he can't, enlightened sages found these mysteries, etc—replies of inadequate scope. I think that we need to reflect on his arguments. To Yu's plea for clarity, one cannot respond with fogginess and vagueness. Let's use this opportunity to think about it again.

Chinese Medicine Association sirs, last year in an honorable letter you decided to jointly initiate a compilation of Chinese medicine teaching materials. The association, until the end of the year, had very little free time, and it only made a list of persons and a plan. It turned it over to a messenger and with the great teaching did not get involved. Until today, shamefully, I cannot forget my heart, the thoughts run for long while carrying your esteemed idea. Without appropriateness, I take an inch of spare time and briefly stretch my opinion, only you, sirs, have this to teach. I eavesdropped the affair of compiling teaching materials for Chinese medicine and that it has, aside from Yin Yang five phases and six Qi, another one big obstacle: the pulse study.

Today's doctors palpate the radial pulse, but this cannot be the topic of a class. There are 10 reasons to explain this. The artery on the Cun Kou 寸口[182] is a small

[182] Radial side of the wrist.

branch of the entire arterial system. It being fast or slow, starting or stopping, is the result of the heart movements. It has no difference then arteries in other parts of the body. Discussing its theory it is not Tai Yin lung pulse, talking about its application it is not the converging of the hundred vessels. Since the old days they have been saying it is the coming of the ancestor, it is where the 100 diseases can be known and life versus death determined. This cannot be the teaching material. This is 1.

The *Neijing* way of feeling the pulse says that there are 3 sections and 9 areas. It says that there is Ren Ying 人迎 and Qi Kou 氣口[183] and this can diagnose the entire body. There was also the saying that feeling the neck and hand is like sitting down and feeling the Cun Kou 寸口. At that time, there was already this ridiculous meaning. Towards this, Zhang Zhongjing, in the *Shang Han Lun* preface, Yang Shangshan 楊上善 in the *Tai Su* 太素 commentary had veiled criticism. But, since antiquity, unduly simple it was transmitted by only worshipping the *Classic of Difficulties Nan Jing* 難經. They didn't listen to the ridicule coming from great scholars, only transmitted diagnosis methods in medical families. This cannot be the teaching material. This is 2.

Nan Jing 難經, even though it specifically talks about palpating Cun Kou 寸口, does not contain explanatory text about sections and areas or organs there related. The 4th difficulty speaks of breathing being related to the 5 Zang 藏 organs. The 5th difficulty explains that palpating it light or heavy is related to the 5 Zang 藏. The 9th difficulty explains the pulse being slow or fast in relation to the Zang and Fu 藏府 organs. The 15th difficulty talks about the pulse being String-like, Hook-like, Feather-like and Stone-like[184] being related to Liver, Heart, Lungs and Kidneys. The 16th difficulty talks about Liver and Heart pulse. Commentators always felt that these are related to Hook-like and String-like pulses. There is no talk of left Cun 寸 or left Guan 關 positions of the pulse. Its division into Cun, Guan and Chi 寸關尺 positions were for the purpose of locating diseases in three regions, from the head down to the chest, from diaphragm down to navel, and from navel down to the feet. It doesn't have separation between left and right or one position corresponds to one organ, or statements like, "Even if the Lung's pulse is not seen, the right hand pulse should be sunken and hidden." Even though it seems that left and right are in different areas, there was never talk that the Lung pulse is at the right side, or that the Lung position should be on the right hand Cun position. However, from the olden days this was transmitted down that the left hand pulse Cun, Guan and Chi positions reflect the

[183] The pulse of the neck versus the pulse of the wrist.

[184] Xian Gou Mao Shi 弦鉤毛石.

Heart, Liver and Kidneys, while the right hand side Cun, Guan and Chi reflect the Lungs, Spleen and Ming Men 命門. Fabricated in one's head and further intensified. This cannot be the teaching material. This is 3.

The first mention of dividing left and right sides, sections and areas of the pulse as being related to Zang Fu organs is first seen in the *Mai Jing* 脈經, quoting an earlier text *Mai Fa Zan* 脈法贊. Xiao Ji 蕭吉, of the Sui 隋 dynasty, in his book *Wu Xing Da Yi* 五行大義, uses the text of the *He Tu* 河圖. It is exactly the same as in *Mai Fa Zan* 脈法贊. It comes out of the Han dynasty Wei Hou 緯候 explanations.[185] The Yin Yang and five phases theories one cannot use. The methods of dividing sections and areas to correspond to the inner organs are likewise absurd. How can one follow this? This cannot be the teaching material. This is 4.

In the *Su Wen* 素問 chapter *Mai Yao Jing Wei Lun* 脈要精微論, it states that inside the Chi 尺, there are two sides. Since the Ming 明 dynasty there are many who believe that this is related to the idea of Cun Kou 寸口 being divided into sections and areas reflecting the Zang 藏 organs. According to this, they changed the *Mai Jing* 脈經 rhymes. They started saying that inside the Chi 尺 there are two sides and that there is also inside the Chi 尺內 and outside the Chi 尺外. But the meaning cannot stick. Wang Xingu 汪心穀 challenged this. They divided Cun, Guan and Chi 寸關尺 sections, each having an upper and lower layer, which served as the inside and outside. Li Shicai 李士材 generation divided the pulse into the radial and ulnar side as inside and outside. The book *Yi Zong Jin Jian* 醫宗金鑑 stated that floating and sinking pulse should be the meaning of inside and outside. Every meaning was contradicting the previous one. "The pulse is merged as one thing, there are no two different pulses and there are no two layers." This is a statement of fact. Even furthering their discussion, how can you divide Cun Kou on its own into three sections? Where does the pulse have three layers? How can you separate it into floating and sinking? Where does the pulse have two levels where one can feel it floating or feel it sinking and with that make possible an inspection of deficiency and excess? Where from can one divide the same into areas reflecting Zang and Fu organs? This means that the pulse is actually not one unified pulse. Even their explanations are conflicting within themselves and it can't be used. Liao Ping 廖平[186] wanted to change the word Chi 尺 into Zu 足[187] and, with that, create three sections

[185] Wei Hou here means Chen Wei 讖緯, mystical Confucian prophetical works of the Eastern Han and Wei Shu 緯書 glosses of the classics that have esoteric meanings of the same time.
[186] 1852–1932.
[187] Foot. In ancient times these 2 characters could have been used interchangeably.

and nine areas that stretch all across the body. He said that the original meaning was not that Cun Kou 寸口 was divided into sections and areas to reflect the Zang organs. One can see that their theory did not resonate with him as well. Yet, from old times this has been transmitted, with no one really looking for a thorough and complete explanation. Instead, they cite and promote their favorite casually, like an amulet for self-protection saying that Cun Kou 寸口 is divided into sections. This cannot be the teaching material. This is 5.

There were two methods of dividing Cun, Guan and Chi 寸關尺 as related to inner organs. Before the Ming 明 Dynasty, most followed the *Mai Jing* 脈經. After the Ming dynasty, most people followed the *Mai Yao Jing Wei Lun* 脈要精微論 statement of "Inside Chi there are two sides". Overall, there were many separate branches. Chu Yong 儲詠, quoting the *Zun Sheng Jing* 尊生經,[188] claimed that the pulse on the right and left sides of men and women are different. Dong Yuan 東垣 claimed that the left pulse reflects external injuries while the right pulse reflects internal injuries. The book *Mai Jue* 脈訣 claimed that the right hand side Chi 尺 position reflects Ming Men 命門, while Hua Shou 滑壽 claimed that Ming Men 命門 is reflected in the Chi 尺 position of the left hand side. Li Chan 李梴 claimed that the right hand Chi 尺 position reflects the Ming Men 命門 of males, while the left hand Chi 尺 position reflects that of females. When it comes to the pulse positions of three burners, uterus, pericardium, small and large intestines they all held different views and couldn't come to an agreement. If you try to take all pulse-related books and consider them at the same time, each person's opinion is different. Chen Xiuyuan 陳修園 used *Neijing* 內經, Shu He 叔和, Bin Hu 濱湖 and Jing Yue 景岳 the four doctors[189] styles and used them together; this is already like a joke. In my opinion, there are more than 20 factions that support their own arguments as if it is logical; they explain it as if there is a principle behind it. Accepting this is following what kind of Dao 道? This cannot be the teaching material. This is 6.

Li Binhu 李濱湖[190] said, "Every time when I see doctors of my generation feeling the pulse of both hands and the six positions, they palpate it over and over again. They describe the condition of this organ being like this and that organ being like that. As if like magic, the inner organs reside in the pulse, and one can touch them and know it. There are all sorts of buffoonery. In reality, their self-deception is extreme." Xu

[188] Also known as *Mr. Shen's Venerating Life Book* 沈氏尊生書 published in 1773 CE.

[189] "Nei Jing" is not a doctor but here it means doctors who followed the Nei Jing style of *Mai Yao Jing Wei Lun* 脈要精微論. The other three are Wang Shuhe, Li Shizhen and Zhang Jingyue.

[190] Li Shizhen 李時珍 1518–1593 CE.

Lingtai 徐靈胎[191] said, "Disease names are ten thousand and pulse types are not more than several dozens. However, it is possible that one disease can appear with ten different pulse types, so how can you perform diagnosis with the pulse and know the disease? It is all guessing and chance. It is deceiving people." Chen Xiuyuan 陳修園 said, "Doctors of my generation, as soon as they open their mouth, they speak of the pulse type. One can easily know their custom of deceiving people with small tricks. The ones who study this art must be vile. Whenever medical books talk about the pulse that must be very detailed, than the readers always have great difficulty learning it. Generally speaking, it is because it does not necessarily speak the truth." These few gentlemen were all great doctors of their generation. Cun Kou 寸口 pulse diagnosis cannot be relied upon. These frank comments cannot be hidden. What is sunk deep within them, without doubt has a basis. There is nothing more than this obliterating the good heart—self-deception and deceiving others. As for the idea that one feels the two extremes[192] of the pulse, sometimes it can be relied upon and sometimes not. Upon careful inspection, there is some common ground agreed by all. For example, after blood loss, the pulse should be deep and thin; if it is floating and big, it is hard to cure. In febrile disease, the pulse should be surging and fast; if it is thin and weak, it is difficult to treat. The essence of these statements actually conforms to reality. It is extremely precious. Saying that this can reveal the difference between life and death is not an over statement. Therefore, these aspects that have experience behind them, even though they are also called pulse studies, can be relied upon nonetheless. Yet, the entirely unreliable Cun Kou pulse study being divided into sections related to the inner organs—some say that this is also reliable sometimes. This is what is called delusional thinking. This is what is called pulling a false claim, it is called "cannot tell the difference," not knowing what is right and what is wrong. This cannot be the teaching material. This is 7.

Inspecting all the literature about pulse, from ancient times to present, they all say that the pulse movement is the flow of Qi. *Su Wen Ping Ren Qi Xiang Lun* 素問平人氣象論 states, "The great collateral channel of the stomach is called Xu Li 虛里. It penetrates the diaphragm and diverges to the lung, it exits below the left nipple. Its movement can be seen at the garment, it is the origin of Qi of the pulse."[193] Here, the movement of the heart's apex cordis is mistaken for ancestral Qi 宗氣. *Ling Shu Wu Shi Ying* 靈樞五十營 states, "When the person inhales, the pulse moves twice, it progresses three Cun 寸. When exhaling, the pulse moves twice, it progresses three

[191] Xu Dachun 徐大椿 1696–1771 CE.

[192] Deficiency and excess.

[193] Here the term Zong Qi 宗氣 ancestral Qi means the origin of Qi, or the Qi originating here.

Cun 寸. Inhaling exhaling and a break in between and the pulse progress six Cun 寸. Within 270 breaths it progresses 16 Zhang 丈 and two Chi 尺. It circulates around the body when water drips two time segments. 13,500 breaths and the Qi 氣 progresses 50 Ying 營 in the body." This demonstrates the error of mistaking the pulse movement as Qi 氣 progression. And so, Li Binhu 李濱湖, even though knowing that Zang Fu 藏府 organs don't reflect themselves in the pulse, he still thought that pulse Qi is Zang Fu 藏府 organs' Qi. Regarding the pulse in Cun Kou 寸口, if it moves, it moves together and if it is still, it is all still together. Today, one uses three fingers to diagnose it. Each finger palpates the Qi of a different organ. This means that the Qi of the three different organs must arrive in succession one after the other and only then one can make this assessment. This kind of talk is implausible. The Qi of the three organs—how does it arrive in succession? The ones who try to explain this say that the left hand Chi 尺 position is the water of heaven "1". It gives birth to the Guan 關 position Liver wood. Liver wood gives birth to the Cun 寸 position Heart fire. The right hand Chi 尺 position is Ming Men 命門; it is minister fire. This gives birth to the Guan 關 position Spleen earth. Spleen earth gives birth to the Cun 寸 position Lungs metal. This kind of five phases explanation is even more so unclear and ambiguous. These people who give explanations also say that the left reflects Kidneys and the right Ming Men 命門.[194] Many ancients already refuted this notion as erroneous. Therefore, this explanation cannot withstand scrutiny. This cannot be the teaching material. This is 8.

In addition, when considering the *Nan Jing* statement, "Chi Cun 尺寸, from beginning to end, is one Cun 寸 nine Fen 分," if we average it and divide in three, then we get six Fen and a bit more. Then we get that the Qi of each organ gets six Fen and a bit more. Now the total Qi of the three organs reaching in succession must with every pulse movement[195] equal one Cun 寸 and nine Fen. Only then should the second pulse movement come into the pulse positions. Only like this can it conform to the same exact positions' locations of the first pulse movement. However, the *Ling Shu* states that every two pulse movements the Qi moves three Cun 寸; this means that within one pulse movement, the Qi only moves one Cun 寸 and five Fen. When we compare it to the one Cun nine Fen of the *Nan Jing*, it is short four Fen. In one pulse movement, it is short four Fen. In two pulse movements, it is short eight Fen. In three pulse movements, it is short 12 Fen. If the Qi of each organ is six Fen and a little bit, then after three movements of the pulse, then the amount of Qi lacking is of about two organs. So if we fix artificially, during the first movement of the pulse, that

[194] Talking about the Chi pulse position of the right and left hands.
[195] From English terminology point of view Pulse movement is the equivalent of a heart beat felt by the radial pulse.

Cun belongs to Lungs, Guan belongs to Spleen, Chi 尺 belongs to Ming Men, when we get to the second movement of the pulse then about four Fen of Cun 寸 position belong to Ming Men, two Fen belongs to Lungs, four Fen of Guan position belong to Lungs, two Fen belongs to Spleen, four Fen of the Chi 尺 position belong to Spleen, and two Fen belongs to Ming Men 命門. At the third pulse movement, the Cun 寸 position has about one Fen Spleen and five Fen Ming Men, the Guan position has one Fen Ming Men and five Fen Lungs, the Chi 尺 position has one Fen Lungs and five Fen Spleen. A disorderly chaos that cannot be managed. And, when just starting to palpate the pulse, how does one know that this is the first pulse movement, he who tries to diagnose the pulse, how can he determine that this one pulse movement he feels is the first one? This, of course, has no doable measure. In addition, with this three-finger pulse diagnosis, some people remove the third finger, saying that if the patient is short the positions get more condensed. Again, it doesn't have a proper measure. How can you then differentiate the organs' Qi? This cannot be the teaching material. This is 9.

Su Wen San Bu Jiu Hou 素問三部九候 states, "Only fast is disease, only slow is disease." Xu Xueshi 許學士, in *Shang Han An* 傷寒案, states, "The pulse is floating rapid and forceless, underneath the Chi 尺 position it is slow and weak." Lu Yuanying *Zhen Zhang En Xuan An* 呂元膺診張恩軒案[196] states, "The Guan position is slow and fast and hollow." Xue Lizhai *Zhen Gu Fei Zhai An* 薛立齋診顧斐齋案[197] states, "The Liver, Spleen and Kidneys pulse is surging, big and rapid." All these erroneous statements believe that the pulse can be partially fast partially slow. These types of medical case studies are numerous. They carry the offense of deceiving people. Coming to this point, what can benefit it solidly is the following: the reason the pulse moves or stops is rooted in a tremble of heart desire. A man has not 2 hearts, it[198] cannot move differently at the same time. Therefore the pulse of the entire body, the pulse of both hands, cannot move at different speeds simultaneously. In addition, in the same Cun Kou pulse, if there are different pulse types—floating, sinking, big and small—or that at one time there is this type and at other times another type, it is because the blood vessel itself is causing it. It is caused by a connection to skin and nerve of the same location. It is not that the organ Qi is not the same. Simultaneous fast and slow pulse movements, this logic does not exist. How come Luo Yao 羅瑤, in his *Yi Bian* 醫碥,[199] also talks about this? It was transmitted since old times and everybody sincere-

[196] Case studies of Lu Yuanying treating Zhang Enxuan.
[197] Case studies of Xue Lizhai treating Gu Feizhai.
[198] The heart.
[199] Published 1751 CE.

ly believed it without suspecting it. Also, the ones that divide the pulse into sections and areas that reflect the inner organs, they are erring as well. They say that inner organs truly have Qi and that inner organs can become diseased. This truly can cause their Qi to increase or decrease, to go faster or slower. With this, the heart recognizes the disease of the different organs and the status of their Qi. When the heart then becomes slow the pulse also becomes slow, when the heart becomes fast the slow also becomes fast. This is not the case! The beating of the pulse—1,2,3,4—is very easy to count. How can they be "so drunk during their life as if dead," transmitting this nonsense until today. This cannot be the teaching material. This is 10.

Now we have these 10 reasons why not to use this as teaching material. Dividing Cun Kou pulse into sections and areas that reflect inner organs is chaotic, absurd and reckless. It is clear to the eye. If this enters the teaching material books in order to teach with it the talented people under heaven, then this will hand down a mistake to the youngsters, which is not a small one. One cannot but think of getting rid of it. My personal view is that regardless it being Cun Kou divided into sections, Ren Ying 人迎 and Cun Kou 寸口 division method or the three sections and nine areas method, these all cannot be used. Other than that, things that are agreed by all—as mentioned earlier—these, to the contrary, have great value and should be used. Making the difference here must be weighed very carefully. One must not allow any small piece of paper or a single word which is doubtful or teaching the incorrect to enter these teaching books. If it is done like this, it will be hanging by the gateway of our national capitol, distributed to the colleges without suspicion, stored in the famous mountains; it will not harbor the swindling of self-deception, it will be transmitted to others, it will not recruit the ridicule of cheating people. After that, it will certainly be able to stand on its feet. Teaching it will be exciting.

Only raising the tip of it can't exhaust the myriads of it. Hastily set pen to paper my mistakes and deficiencies must be many, yet every compartment of my heart only wishes not to betray all the hopes of all you honorables. Sincerely contributing my hay and firewood, I do not know if it should be looked upon as wise or not. As I write this letter, I cannot help but feel alarmed. The spring's cold spell brings sluggishness.

Taking care of your health, will be fortunate indeed!

Article end

Qun Jing Jian Zhi Lu 群經見智錄

1922 by Yun Tieqiao 惲鐵樵

Published 1922 in response to the current situation of Chinese medicine and also in response to *Ling Su Shang Dui* written by Yu Yunxiu and published 1917.

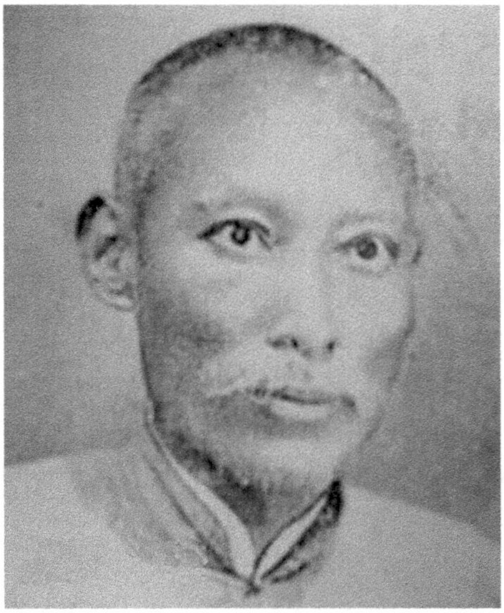

Yun Tieqiao

Yaron: Yun Tieqiao, the first to officially respond to Yu Yunxiu's arguments, demonstrates by example a humble way to study Chinese medicine. He recognizes weak aspects of Chinese medicine as well as strong points of modern science. He does not ferociously stick to his camp without logic. His willingness to learn and improve, knowing that Chinese medicine could and should further be improved, is noteworthy.

Yun, however, recognizes a distinct difference between modern science and Chinese medicine, which allows him to reconcile these medicines. Even though others, such as Tang Zonghai 唐宗海, preceded him in merging Chinese and Western medicines, Mr. Yun appears at a time when division and separation between these styles of medicine increased to an extreme and so his contribution is unique. He felt that Chinese medicine could co-exist alongside modern medicine as two separate but complementary systems, each holding its own medical principle.

Following and different from him, many new Chinese medicine schools included ever more science in their curriculum; their own medical principle being modified. For many, improving Chinese medicine meant making it more like Western science, a trend reaching epic proportions during the Communist era and, indeed, up to this day. I believe that going back to Yun's model of developing Chinese medicine is an excellent option today.

Chapter 16: *Discussion and Deliberation on the Ling Shu and Su Wen, Ling Su Shang Dui* 靈素商兌, can be discussed further

Mr. Yu Yunxiu 余云岫 used Western medicine to write the *Ling Su Shang Dui*. His knowledge of the *Nei Jing*, compared to the average Chinese medicine practitioner, is several folds. Honestly, a heroic scholar. Chinese medicine of recent years is at its bottom of all times. 99 practitioners out of 100 don't know what kind of a thing is the *Nei Jing*. In order to do scholarly research of a certain science, common knowledge of other sciences must be known first. When Westerners do scholarly research, it is like this; when Chinese people do scholarly research, it is likewise like this. Therefore, when *Qian Jin Fang* 千金方 talks about learning the grand profession of medicine, one cannot but be thoroughly clear about the principle of heaven and man; all the five classics, the ancient masters, history, heavenly bodies, the book of changes—these were all commonplace with the doctor. Here, there is not even need to mention that the doctor had to have fluency in *Ling Shu* 靈書, *Su Wen* 素問, *Jia Yi Zhen Jing* 甲乙針經, *Shang Han* 傷寒 and *Jin Gui* 金匱. Since I was born, until today, the entire nation looks at the *Ling Shu* and *Su Wen* as a lost body of knowledge. There is not one person who can explain its principle. When I was about twenty, I read the *Nei Jing* and *Nan Jing*—*Qi Xue Lun* 氣穴論, *Qi Fu Lun* 氣府論 etc chapters and I felt my head was exploding. Not only did I dread its complexity, but also I could not believe the explanations that these overall untidy meridians could be adjusted to be so uniform. When I inquired with old doctors, they would just nod their heads kindly and say they didn't know. The descendants of medical practice, like those who worship Ye Tianshi's 葉天士 case studies and *Wen Bing Tiao Bian* 溫病條辨 as if it is a concealed treasure, they force themselves to read it and what they can't understand, like the *Nei Jing*, they give up on. Since the Wuxu year,[200] all school classes and their teachers would censure five phases. From that point on, no one would open their mouth to speak for Chinese medicine and, in addition, they used shameful words to

[200] 1898

remonstrate it. I know that there are many thousands of fellow countrymen with similar experience such as mine.

After Western medicine spread out to the east, Western medicine type doctors, brave and fierce, were willing to progress, while Chinese medicine type doctors were complacent and conservative. Even good scholars wouldn't know where to start; being dispirited and disappointed they either left the profession and entered academia or talked about responding and sketched a plot to respond. Such situations, this book need not describe in detail. In summary, our nation's medicine did not see a single work that gave a complete and thorough explanation and, therefore, although many of our countrymen revere the ancient customs, only a few had the audacity to go it alone. *Ling Su Shang Dui* was written in response to the current situation. This chapter is a counter reaction to that work.

Speaking from my limited view, the *Ling Su Shang Dui* statements cannot scratch where it itches. However, its *Discussion and Deliberation Shang Dui* 商兑 can be discussed further. Now in order to evade complications and keep the plan simple, I take few lines of *Shang Dui* and extract the nucleus out. Even though I extract it, there is no dodging of problems. I would like to emphasize that the *Ling Su Shang Dui* inflicts no harm on the *Nei Jing* and here, by *Discussion and Deliberation Shang Dui*, I intend no slander upon it. As for Mr. Yu Yunxiu, my humble self worked with him together at the commercial printing house for many years. Even though we were not close friends, we never had bad feelings for each other. What is unfolding today is not personal; here I would like to emphasize it.

Ling Su Shang Dui, talking about Yin Yang and five phases, states:

> As I looked carefully from all sides at the *Ling Su* 靈素[201] book, the basis for its extrapolation is the 'assuming' guiding principle. The main thing being Yin Yang and five phases. Therefore if the Yin Yang and five phases theory is smashed, then the entire *Ling Su* standards is just like unscathed skin. Where is there then *Ling Su*? Where is there then medical science? Alas, all the sciences of our nation are poisoned blind with this Yin Yang. All who are superstitious are confined by this Yin Yang five phases malady. The appropriateness of getting rid of this fallacy is long overdue.

[201] *Ling Shu* and *Su Wen* together shortened to *Ling Su*.

As for the unraveling of this section, there is no other meaning than simply detesting Yin Yang and five phases, which includes, as well, all the people confined by superstitions. Therefore, its scope is very wide and its argument is not excessive; let's see what it says next.

It also states:

> Since the beginning of culture, in antiquity, the people revered and believed in ghosts and spirits. Therefore, in order to rule the land, people were pushed toward virtue by the threat of final retribution. Medical arts of Western Europe came from the hands of monks. Medical arts in China's Xia dynasty came out of Yin Yang practitioners. All around the globe, human evolution used this same public highway to develop the arts. Without it, this would not be possible. *Su Wen* states: "when the ancients treated disease, they could cast a spell and that's it." … The ancient Yi 醫 medicine character comes from the Wu 巫 shaman character. These are both supporting evidence that medicine of antiquity came from the Yin Yang practitioners… The origin of the *Ling Su* comes from the shamans' incantations. It was simply appropriate to observe, with great care, the Yin Yang five phases theories with any enlightenment.

This section describes Yin Yang practitioners as the shamans of antiquity. It is where *Su Wen* came out of and, therefore, *Su Wen* should not be studied. However, quoting the *Su Wen* as stating "when the ancients treated disease, they could cast a spell and that's it" means exactly the opposite.

Shang Dui also states:

> When it says Yin Yang, for an object it means exterior interior, for animals and plants it means male and female, for magnetism and electricity it means positive and negative, for chemistry it means acidic and alkaline, whatever has opposites can attain this name. Its usage, however, must stop with that; it should not have any spiritual mysterious incalculable aspects. When Yin Yang practitioners talk about it, there is a seed of something inconceivable. *Su Wen* chapter *Yin Yang Ying Xiang Da Lun* 陰陽應象大論

> states: "Yin and Yang are the Dao of heaven and earth, the principle of the myriad things, the mother and father of change and transformation, the origin of life and death, the residence of the illuminating spirit. Treating a disease must be sought after in its root." They say that Yin Yang is mystical and inconceivable; it is an obscure phenomenon that creates everything... They say that the air above the surface of the earth belongs to Yang? Or to Yin? The air, when it is close to the surface of the earth, is more condensed but when it is far from the surface of the earth, it is thinner. They say that thin is Yang and that thick is Yin, how come? This is a disorderly statement. If we look at acid granules and salt granules, do they belong to Yang or Yin? From this, one can tell that the theory of Yin Yang having the principle of encompassing the myriad things is a falsehood and an oversight. It is clear that it is insufficient to have scientific standing.

The above section describes Yin Yang as no more than external internal, male female, positive negative, acidic alkaline, or any other opposites. When Yin Yang practitioners talk about it, then it is mysterious and inconceivable, a mysterious creator of the myriad things. Also, as a principle of the myriad things it has no standard, it is a fallacy and oversight that shouldn't be taught.

Shang Dui section of five Zang and six Fu organs states:

> The *Su Wen* has a definition for the five Zang organs: "The five Zang store essence Qi and don't let it drain. Therefore, it is properly full but doesn't become excessive. The six Fu transmit and transform matter and don't store it; therefore, it can be excessive but not full." This is a fallacy. If someone knows just a little bit of physiology and dissection then they can easily know it. Let's argue with these few lines. The liver is the producer of bile, uric acid and saccharides; it also has the ability to remove toxins from the blood. If we inspect closely its anatomical structures, the bile duct begins in the liver cells and opens at the bile duct, and this is where the bile goes through to the gallbladder. Therefore, the liver assimilates materials from the intestines and creates bile, it then discharges it to the gallbladder, which then

> is being discharged to the intestines. Where is there only storage? Only drainage? They don't know the liver medical chemistry function. Instead, they try to inspect it with bare eyes; their dissection skills cannot reach to this pathway between liver and gallbladder and bile duct. Instead, they just make up that it can store but cannot drain. As for the ancient people, they were not clear about science; their instruments were crude, one cannot blame them for that. However, today, if one still silently guards the old theories, and can only say with a respectful air: "The *Ling Shu* said, the *Su Wen* said", then he did not differentiate yet the fine from the coarse, the small details; he did not differentiate right from wrong and he is only an opinionated imbecile. (The rest was omitted)

The above section uses Western countries' dissection knowledge as a proof to the wrongfulness of the *Nei Jing*. This is the backbone of *Ling Su Shang Dui* entire book. What Yu records here is even simpler then simple. This is the essence of the entire *Ling Su Shang Dui*, without leaving out anything. Therefore, it requires a statement from humble me, with my limited views and only in as much as I know to see if indeed it is so.

Recorded above are 4 sections.

The first section is anecdotal; Yin Yang five phases is a fallacy. It should have been eliminated a long time ago.

The second section states that the *Nei Jing* origin is with the shamans and incantations and, therefore, guarding Yin Yang and five phases theories is evil talk.[202] One cannot but argue with this statement. Evil is measured against uprightness. If there is no uprightness then evil cannot be seen as evil. Therefore, cheating people for their money is evil. However, if there is basis and theory behind it, there is a result to it and the intention is to benefit the economy, then it is uprightness. If we compare Chinese and Western medicines and we make Chinese medicine the evil, then uprightness means only 50 steps out of 100 steps. The following text describes it in detail.

---

[202] Evil talk means a fallacy, but here the English translation of fallacy will lose the following nuance of Evil versus uprightness.

Incantations and casting spells, the *Nei Jing* does not have it. *Nei Jing*, in chapter *Yi Jing Bian Qi Pian* 移精變氣篇, states: "The Yellow Emperor asked: in ancient times, when treating a disease, they only shifted essence and changed the Qi, they could cast a spell and that's it. Today, treating a disease, toxic herbs treat the interior, acupuncture and stones treat the exterior; some recover, some don't, how come?" It discusses here herbal treatment and acupuncture, not incantation, this is very clear. That medicine came out of shamanism, honestly speaking, does not suffice to be a disease. The *Nei Jing* originally was pure science, it did not speak of casting spells. If it did mention incantations, not likely was it evil. The ancient incantations, at the beginning, was not like modern day people who treat disease with mapping the stars and giving charms. Its true appearance was more like in the *Shang Shu* chapter *Jin Teng* 尚書金縢. In modern studies, this could be compared to parapsychology. In Liang Rengong's 梁任公[203] book, *Travel Notes in the New China*,[204] when the clergyman treated a patient one time, is also this kind of an example. Also, all the commoners who hope that some immortal prescription will have efficacy are, as well, in this category. All affairs under heaven may have a first appearance as not being a part of true principle, however, the principle's essence can be studied from it. One should not obliterate it with one stroke of a brush.

The third section states that Yin Yang are external internal, movement stillness, male female etc. It states: "When Yin Yang practitioners talk about it, there is a seed of something inconceivable. It is an obscure phenomenon that creates everything." The idea behind these statements is that Yin Yang carries along the obstruction of superstition. These words must be examined. Magical calculation and fortune telling have fault in them. Honestly, these can be called the Yin Yang that has a seed of implausible. Therefore, the *Nei Jing* is not like this.

Since antiquity, when they spoke of heaven, the first kind said that heaven has will power, heaven can see, can hear, it has authority and it can deliver punishment and reward. The Confucians had this heaven and the Daoists and Buddhists all had this heaven. This is the so-called "push people toward virtue by the threat of final retribution". We can give it a name and call it a religious heaven. The second kind was heaven without a consciousness. One that can be calculated and studied. Calamities caused by heaven's motions can be conquered by human force. Mathematicians and

[203] Another name of Liang Qichao 梁啟超 1873–1929.

[204] *Xin Da Lu You Ji* 新大陸游記 published in 1903.

astrologers, Chinese and Western both, had this kind of heaven. We can give them a name and call them scientists of heaven. When the *Nei Jing* states, "the principle of the myriad things, the father and mother of change and transformation," this belongs to the latter type. Try and see the entire book's seasonal explanations of heaven; it uses five phases, six Qi, Jia Zi 甲子 to explain heaven; it uses stars and constellations angles and degrees; it uses tones and harmonics to explain heaven, they all scheme resistance to the viciousness and cruelty of heaven motions. In the entire book, there is not one word of superstition about good fortune and bad fortune. It is clearly obvious that it is a purely scientific heaven. Whomever studies the *Nei Jing* knows that. So how come Mr. Yun alone must see it as "pushing people toward virtue by the threat of final retribution"?

When it gets to "the principle of the myriad things, the father and mother of change and transformation," it claims it as a mistake, and that it talks about the mysteriousness of life's principle. The globe has night and day, cold and heat and, thereafter, things are born and have life. If there was no night and day and no cold and heat, there would be no life. Yin Yang, honestly speaking, is day and night, hot and cold. If Yin and Yang is not the principle of the myriad things, what else can be the principle of the myriad things? If Yin and Yang is not the father and mother of change and transformation, what else can be the father and mother of change and transformation? When it comes to the principle of life, truly, there is mysteriousness to it. Today, Chinese and Western medicine both stand on the same platform, unable to penetrate this mysteriousness. An example, the *Su Wen* states: "wind gives birth to wood," *Ling Su Shang Dui* argues against it, saying: "the birth of wood comes from a seed, the birth of a seed comes from fertilization. Fertilization comes about from a stamen and pistil exchange. Stamen and pistil exchange when they are close to each other. If they are far from each other, then a bee or a bird or wind pollinates them. This wind is just one of several kinds that can do it. So how come wind is the only one that can generate wood?" The *Nei Jing* "wind gives birth to wood" does not explain it in such a way. Wind is one of the six Qi, wood is one of the five phases. They both accompany the spring in the four seasons. Therefore, it states it in such a way. Prior section has already explained this issue. Now, that the *Shang Dui* uses these words is, for us, a proof that to penetrate the mysteriousness of life, principle is indeed difficult. Now we can test it and ask: the exchange of stamen and pistil, how can it give birth to wood? The answer will have to be: it is like the animals that create an offspring; it is because they copulate, the spermatozoa and the egg merge and then it becomes a fetus. Question: what is spermatozoa made of? What is the egg made of? The two merge together and become a fetus. Is it possible to artificially create a sperm and an egg? Answer: not possible. Why not? Even though I don't understand medical chemistry, I can affirm that Western medicine, unfortunately, is not sharp enough. And so, Western medicine talks about physiology, the spermatozoa and the egg and that's it. As if I, with my Taiji 太極[205] point of view, reach to Taiji and then stop; two fives and one ten[206] allow an explanation of one step. This is also the difference of 50 steps versus 100 steps.

If we say that Western countries' medical chemistry is precise and the *Nei Jing* is unrefined, like the statements saying that Yin and Yang don't have a fixed standard and that it is a fallacy and oversight, that it is not good enough to serve as foundation for a scientific study, in reality this is not the case. The Yin Yang of *Nei Jing* expresses its cleverness in its agility. Being dead under one sentence is not the place one can find it. This is rather not easy to explain. Chinese arts all have this realm. Using an analogy in script, Western countries have grammar and stylistic, China doesn't have it. In addition, when studying Chinese script, there is no sequence it needs to be studied with, but with Western languages it progresses from superficial to deep. And so Chinese script developed on its own, as a unique writing system, and it has its own standard. If one looks at it from a superficial point of view, how is that not a fallacy and an oversight? The Yin Yang of *Nei Jing*, originally, did not take the same path as the script. However, at an initial stage, with scarce rules and regulations, it later started having its own strict standards and it has corrected itself in a similar way that the script did.

As for the five Zang organs and the Western countries using dissection to talk about it, how is this not the case? The way I see it, the *Nei Jing* arranges the rival camps as a mountain range. Because of this point, one cannot alter its foundation. The five Zang organs of the *Nei Jing* are not the dissection five Zang but, rather, Qi transformation five Zang. For example, when a patient's mouth is salty, it belongs to kidneys; when the taste is bitter, to the heart; when the taste is sweet, to the spleen etc. If the face is red, it is fire and belongs to heart; if it is black, it is water and belongs to kidney etc. When *Nei Jing* talks about a disease syndrome such as heart heat disease,

---

[205] Here, the reference is to Master Shao Yong 邵雍, of the Song dynasty, and his book *Huang Ji Jing Shi* 皇極經世 which explains a Taiji principle giving birth to heaven and earth and the myriad things.
[206] These numbers describe the center position in the He Tu river picture, where the number 10 is in the center and two 5 are above and below it.

first the person is not happy and then, after many days, there is heat, the heat then struggles and the heart feels pains, there is agitation oppression and frequent nausea, headaches, red face with no sweat. This is the disease and it is not the dissection's heart organ disease. When figuring out the disease by calculating the four seasons and five phases, then the text states the following: "When Ren Gui 壬癸 is extreme, at Bing Ding 丙丁 there is great sweat, the Qi is adverse and, therefore, at Ren Gui there is death." This is how it calculates the expiration time. This also shows that the dissection heart has nothing to do with Ren Gui and Bing Ding. Therefore, the *Nei Jing* heart disease is not Western medicine's heart disease. The good part of Western medicine is that it can treat severe diseases; when Chinese medicine uses the *Nei Jing* essence it, too, can treat severe diseases. Therefore, even with different paths, they both reach to the same place. So if one says that medical treatment without dissection is a fallacy, then I would use the same language of *Shang Dui* and say that if one does not discuss the four seasons hot and cold, the principle of Yin Yang coming and going, then this, as well, is a fallacy. I can't see that the *Shang Dui* statement is all correct and that my statement is all wrong.

The *Shang Dui* preface states:

> *Ling Su* has killed people for 4000 years... its poison was more then all robbers, wild beasts, soldiers, work accidents, disasters and wars... The Confucian callus ponders Mencius, the doctor imprisoned with Qi Bo and Huang Di, dig a hole and escape to the void, not following the evidence of facts, its poison is already of long duration. If we don't annihilate *Nei Jing* then we cannot eradicate the disaster's root... Its explanations and theories are great fallacy; there is not one section which is trustworthy... Since Qi Bo and Huang Di, there were always people explicating the *Ling Su*, Bian Que 扁鵲, Cang Gong 倉公, Zhong Jing 仲景, Hua Tuo 華佗, talking absurdities all around, they are the city wall guarding the old medicine in modern day. So how come we attack in this writing the *Ling Su* then? Answer: Bring down its capital city, block up its origin.

The above is rather vigorously exploding with anger. I would rather not answer back sarcastically. I wrote this book to have Chinese medicine practitioners reflect, first and foremost, on their own knowledge and then go and absorb other countries' new cultures. This book is not an antagonist to Western medicine and it also does not mean to say that Chinese medicine needs to be confined to the realm of *Nei Jing*. So how can I turn into the village old lady cursing at people?

Ling Su Shang Dui regards the *Nei Jing* as the enemy and so I have this one problem, I would like to discuss it with the author of *Ling Su Shang Dui*. If he does not care to give instruction, I would not dare asking. I will follow his wishes. Any logic that has one side also has the opposite side to it; it is the theory of proof. Confucius, a sage, his theories until today have room for discussion. Yang Zhu 楊朱,[207] talking about benefiting oneself, his theories in modern day, again, find research value in their midst. Therefore, the student has a common saying: "Goodness and evil are opposites, not absolutes." If one says, "there is no need to discuss Confucian theories anymore, no need to research Yang Zhu's theories," then this is an autocratic rule for a low ceiling house. The author was a foreign student in Japan; how come he is like this? How can the *Ling Su Shang Dui* only think of the not-so-good aspect of the *Ling Su*? The *Ling Su Shang Dui*, as if saying that there is no need for future generations to produce people who research the *Ling Su*. The first impression is the strongest, that he acts without much thinking and scorns it; this is not the attitude of the student. "Cang Gong 倉公 and Zhong Jing 仲景 were all shallow and unreasonable, the ancients were all impenetrably thickheaded," this kind of tone firmly announced, even without a little bit of hesitation, its excessive self-confidence cannot be matched. I say that the *Ling Su Shang Dui*, itself, can be further deliberated.

Conclusion

Nei Jing has many sections that cannot be explained; if one cannot look at those with an agile fashion, then he cannot have a satisfactory answer to them. For example, east and west have no fixed location, yet *Nei Jing* states "the east gives birth to wind"...

I say that, to become a doctor, one cannot limit himself to the *Nei Jing*. The reader may say that I am exaggerating, but in reality I am not. The physiology of Western medicine comes from dissection. The physiology of *Nei Jing* comes from Qi transformation. The analogy of it will be growing flowers and planting trees. Take the flowers' and trees' fruit, kernel, root, grass roots, bark, tree trunk, base of a fruit, calyx, ear of grain, melons and all other sections and research their compounds in order to reach at their physiology, this is the action of dissection. Learning to distin-

[207] Warring states period circa 4th century BCE.

guish the appropriate soil for flowers and trees, not offending heaven's seasonality, adjusting the surroundings' temperature, eliminating harmful pests, irrigating in a timely manner in order to follow its birth and growth, this is the actions of Qi transformation. Knowing the one, but not knowing the other, often times will yield poor results. This is the first reason why one cannot limit himself to *Nei Jing*. In addition, when speaking directly of Qi transformation, how come one may know the seasons of heaven or the appropriateness of the soil? This is because there is a study of astrology, there is a study of plants and animals, geography, soil quality, physics. This is the second reason why one cannot limit himself to *Nei Jing*. In ancient times, medicine came out of shamanism; therefore, in *Qian Jin,* it states: "in order to learn the great profession of medicine, one must be thorough with astromancy and divination 星命卜筮." Astromancy and divination are not good enough to become a science worth studying. Today there are studies like dissection, physiology, pathology, histology, embryology, psychology. The sages and superstitious people alike, even talking a million words were never able to penetrate it. If one could penetrate this fence, it would include also the sages and ancients. This is the third reason why one cannot limit himself to *Nei Jing*.

If, however, one calls himself a Chinese medicine doctor and he did not grasp the principle of the *Nei Jing*, he himself fails to clearly understand it, and instead uses one or two western drugs to show off, such as aspirin to induce sweat, Ai Mei Ding 愛梅丁 to treat diarrhea, Ka Si Ka La 卡四卡拉 to purge the bowels and the such; he himself is hungry for self-satisfaction and thinks that he can, in such a way, change Chinese medicine for the better, then he is a person that this book completely disapproves of. He is a joke for Chinese medicine. Not only that, he is a laughing stock for Western medicine. But if his entire skill is limited with that, then my Chinese medicine is not far away from being eliminated by selection.

Article end

Mr. Yu Medical Narrative: Scroll 5.

Yaron: Should one believe a theory or know it for a fact? Yu claims that if you can't prove it, don't believe it. He discounts the Chinese medicine habit of believing in the ancients—or "believing" in general. "Believing" is very much the case today as well, regardless of whether it is from the ancients or modern TCM textbooks. We should reflect on this!

Discussing the book *Records of Widening One's Wisdom with all the Chinese Classics Qun Jing Jian Zhi Lu* 群經見智錄 with Yun Tieqiao 惲鐵樵.

Subtitle: In Zhe Jiang province, Zhen Hai county 浙江鎮海,[208] by Yu Yan (Yun Xiu) 余巖雲岫

Mr. Tieqiao, about last winter I saw an advertisement for an upcoming printing of the Song version of the *Nei Jing*. I attained a copy from a friend, and in it I saw an attached advertisement for *Qun Jing Jian Zhi Lu* 群經見智錄 forthcoming circulation. In its author's[209] preface, it makes a mention of the clumsy author[210] of *Ling Su Shang Dui* 靈素商兌, as if discharging an arrow. With this, what the heart wished for was severed. The descendants, ignorant of the noblemen, the hundred small people, wish to make an appointment with victory. I accept with thanks the challenge. Like guarding a large piece of jade and, in addition, everyday gazing with hope to his reply letter to be completed. After humble me wrote the *Ling Su Shang Dui* 靈素商兌, there was not one day I didn't read our nation's medical literature. From top to bottom, from ancient to present, noteworthy discussion, I did not encounter new points of view. That one can explain the five phases and Jia Zi 甲子 theory, that there is discussion with modern scientists about the wind and rain and Ji Ming 雞鳴.[211] This is what humble me urgently desires to know more about. This is 1.

[208] In the past a county of Ning Bo 寧波, a coastal city in Zhe Jiang.

[209] The author is Yun Tieqiao, to whom this letter is addressed.

[210] The author is Yu Yunxiu, the person writing this letter.

[211] The cock crow is the second time period in the old Chinese method of recording time, the 12 Shi Chen 十二时.

Now, before *Ling Su Shang Dui* 靈素商兌 was first published, Mr. Jiang Zhuzhuang 蔣竹莊[212] spoke in a rash manner, easily scolding without consulting tactfully. I humbly said that many of today's old doctors do not necessarily read books. They don't know how to research. This is not a great cry. With pain, they administer acupuncture and absolutely there is no visible response. And so I didn't follow Mr. Jiang's words. I didn't linger in his unlucky words. The book came out 6–7 years ago and I never saw a reply from him. Your Excellency[213] has what we call "vigorous explosive anger". It is not the attitude of the scholar. And now, as if the hateful words have severed. Today, Your Excellency should rise and respond, it has been already 6–7 years. I am longing for these rare and unexpected words. I seek for it but I am afraid I will never attain it. For humble me, what he says is another thing that I urgently desire to hear and know about. This is 2.

Humble me wrote *Ling Su Shang Dui* 靈素商兌. I know very well that, for the old doctors, this is a straight-flying arrow. Now several years have passed, and even though there were one or two verbal critics, their arguments did not form any principle. There was no value for their words. Two years ago, when just beginning to write *A Study of our Native Medicinals Guo Chan Yao Wu Yan Jiu* 國產藥物研究, many science and art journals began receiving criticism from Mr. Du Yaquan 杜亞泉.[214] However, Mr. Du does not know medicine. At the same time, he was also my teacher when I was little. Even though I don't dare to obsequiously agree with what he says, I do not wish to argue as well. In today's generation, the Dao and virtue is scrapped; it is all for fame and profit. While being kindred, we take arms and separate as teacher and pupil. What the ancients supported, humble me, with sincerity, does not wish to support. This talk that does not allow benevolence is like shooting arrows at random with an expert's bow.[215] You and humble me worked together in the commercial printing house office since old times and we have the friendship of old friends. I urge you to uphold virtue of a good friendship Dao. The rocks of other mountains can be mistaken; one can have a carefree desire to talk. Zhuang Zhou 莊

[212] Jiang Zhuzhuang 蔣竹莊 (1873–1958), a famous educator, was the president of Guo Li South Eastern University 國立東南大學 from 1925 to 1927.

[213] Referring to Jiang Zhuzhuang.

[214] Du Yaquan 杜亞泉 (1873–1933) translated many Western language works about literature and science into Chinese. During the era of May 4th movement, he was an avid adversary against people who wanted to abolish or restrain the Chinese traditional culture.

[215] This line references a story from the Book of Zhuang Zi, when Zhuang Zi told his sophist friend Hui Zi 惠子, "If we don't set a target before the match, letting every player shoot at random, after the match each player will claim that he shot the target that he set himself and so he is an expert marksman. Is this the case? Shall we call him a marksman?"

周,[216] thinking of Hui Zi 惠子, said, "I no longer find an appropriate person to talk to."[217] Humble me would like to exchange with Your Excellency like the stonecutter, the uncanny feat of the stonecutter with the nose chalk. Arrange the flags and drums, be at your service and associate with all the scholars' circles. I don't kill any man nor do I hurt anyone. The happiness I attain from this is like the king facing the south. It is the refined activities of the intelligentsia. There is no injury with the Dao of friendship. If you can allow it, this is one more thing humble me would like to urgently know about. This is 3.

These days as the book[218] came out, I urgently got a copy and read it. With painstaking effort, it does have great originality. It is trust worthy, has a good study and deep thought. It is what Hui Zi 惠子 aspired for as substance. While busy with my livelihood with not much spare time, I only regret that I could not read it all immediately. However, I do have thoughts in my mind that I urgently desire to put forth, describe my humble opinion in a clear way. As soon as I saw that the great author[219] wishes to have a discussion with the author of *Ling Su Shang Dui* 靈素商兌,[220] I knew that you will not refuse me. The great author says that 360 days is one Qi Hou 氣候 [221] climatic year. This is something humble I cannot agree with. The transformation of Qi Hou 氣候 weather stems entirely from the revolution of the earth around the sun. I repeat these words. The earth revolves around the sun one cycle. Only then there is a desire to complete one year, the four seasons and the eight sections. This is proper. Therefore, when carefully instructing the farming season, one determines the day and time by the earth's orbit around the sun. This is the most important item. The calendar masters called it a Sui 歲.[222] It was the orbiting Jupiter Sui 歲. The sun traveling the sky was also said to be a Sui 歲 fullness. It was called one Sui fullness calculation. What Yao Dian 堯典[223] states 300 and six tens and six days is

[216] Another name for the philosopher Zhuang Zi 莊子, early Warring States period.

[217] This is another Zhuang Zi story about funeral ceremonies. When Hui Zi was alive he always argued with Zhuang Zi. Once, passing by his friend's Hui Zi tomb, Zhuang Zi told his students a story. In earlier times during a funeral there was a custom to draw a circle with white chalk on one's nose. At the end of the funeral, everyone would wash their nose. One person decided to ask his friend, a master stonecutter, to remove the white circle with his ax. The stonecutter, with one cry, would remove it perfectly without a trace or harm. A king heard about it and asked the stonecutter to perform the same with him, but the stonecutter replied: I can only do it with my friend. Even though I am a master stonecutter, you need the appropriate partner for this. Zhuang Zi then said, "Since my friend passed away I no longer find an appropriate partner with substance to argue with."

[218] Yun Tieqiao's book *Records of Widening One's Wisdom with all the Chinese Classics Qun Jing Jian Zhi Lu* 群經見智錄.

[219] Yun Tieqiao. Yunxiu uses "great author" talking directly (in the letter) to Yun Tieqiao.

[220] Yu Yunxiu.

[221] Qi Hou means climate/ weather, but also an ancient calculation method of the days, *Su Wen—Liu Jie Zang Xiang Lun* 六節藏象論 states: 五日謂之候，三候謂之氣 5 days = 1 Hou, 3 Hou = 1 Qi.

[222] A year, but also planet Jupiter which was used in ancient times to calculate a year according to its position in the sky.

[223] A chapter in the *Book of Historical Documents Shu Jing* 書經, an ancient Confucian classic.

exactly that. The Han dynasty Si Fen Quadrants Calendar 四分歷,[224] pointing out 365 days and one quarter, is also that. This is what I call a true year. Now your Excellency wants to calculate the weather Qi Hou and abandon this true calculation of the year, which is 365 days and one quarter. Instead, you say that 360 days is one Qi Hou 氣候 climatic year. This must be some theory that is outside of the solar and lunar orbits and the change of the four seasons. Only if there is another reason for climatic change it may be possible. Otherwise when one overly believes in the theory that five days is one Hou, three Hou is one Qi then he forgets that actually five phases and six Qi are based on the four seasons. The two conflict and therefore the theory that 360 days is one climatic year cannot stand its ground. What is called five days is one Hou 候, three Hou 候 is one Qi 氣, six Qi 氣 is one Shi 時, four Shi 時 is one Sui 歲. This as well cannot stand. What is explained as five Sui and there is an advancement to the right, six Qi goes back to the meeting point, these five and six as well have no foundation. The statement the 60 Jia Zi stems out of the two characters five and six also cannot stand ground. When You explains five Sui shift a step to the right, in the great author's addendum one cannot see anymore that he follows the short sentences of 5 characters each. Isn't it that one considers himself in the wrong already? Alas, the art of mathematics was sparse in antiquity and is abundant today. Since the San Tong 三統 and Si Fen 四分 calculations, until today, it was altered repeatedly. Since the statistics were not sufficient, only over time was the error discovered; the seasons and weather did not match and so the texts were corrected, but not according to their original principle of adjusting the calendar. They changed their calendar calculation principle not because it was good. Getting to the calendar of the Ming Dynasty it took the appearance of reform; they said it is appropriate to follow heaven in order to seek a merge, it is inappropriate in order to merge to inspect heaven. Therefore, they stated that a year should be 360 days like the truth of the *Nei Jing* in order to create one climatic year. It was a calculation scantily used in antiquity. Then they said that this was the real idea of the *Nei Jing*. You use this idea to explain this topic; claiming that, like this, you can reach the real truth of the *Nei Jing*. Maybe this is possible in reaching this kind of art. However, the calendrical history traces, their discord with heaven that was there for a long time, if one uses it to calculate the Jie Qi 節氣 segments of the year, then at the end of the year, every year one is missing five days and a bit more. If we round it up every year it misses one Hou 候. Every three years it misses one Qi, every 18 years it misses one Shi. If one continues like this, within 20 years the seasons have shifted. If you want to have

[224] Invented by Jia Kui 贾逵 85 CE.

a trustworthy explanation of the additions of the year, then you must count this into the calculation method. How can one guard the old decay, want to worship it and, with it, calculate the Qi transformation? Hold fast to a fixed method and not change with the times, this is called to merge in order to inspect heaven and one believes that he can attain truth like this—where is there such a principle? Cheng Mingdao 程明道[225] called this Qi Yun 氣運[226] theory. At the time of Yao and Shun 堯舜,[227] when they inspected the five winds and ten rains, it was still vague theory. When I saw it, I grasped this art of seeking the Qi Yun 氣運 that even at the time of Yao and Shun, even though there is talk of five winds and ten rains, resolutely there is not a sense of proper inspection. When one uses the number 360 today, we recognize it as the degrees of a complete circle. It started with the Muslims' calculations and Master Shao 邵子[228] in *Huang Ji Jing Shi* 皇极经世 also said it. However, before the Ming 明 dynasty, this was not used in China. The ancients thought that when the sun travels one day and one night this is one degree. Therefore, the sky rotation and the year rotation were not separated. In the eastern Jin dynasty 東晉, Yu Xi 虞喜[229] established the Sui year deficiency principle. After Liu Chao 劉焯,[230] the sky and the year became separated. Because of this, throughout the centuries the ancients always rounded numbers up and didn't deal with fractions. Getting to the Yuan 元 dynasty, they did not change it. Even though master Shao said it, he didn't know how to use it. That being so, the reality of the Zhou, Qin, Han and Wei 周秦漢魏 dynasties is that, with assurance, they did not have the number for the year as being 360. One can clearly consider this. When Qin Huitian 秦蕙田[231] said 360, it was the ancient method of determining the position of the sky map. He used the *Xi Ci* 繫辭傳 commentary on the book of Changes "the sun pointing to the time period 當期之日" and this is the testimony for this fact. Alas, from antiquity, when they calculated the heaven, heaven's circuit was a yearly circuit. From the time of Yao and Shun, they already knew the number to be 300 and six tens and six days. Confucius approved the book of changes, so how did he abandon the thick and follow the thin? Therefore, all commentators pointed out this deficiency. It is this point. So when he said the number 11,520 is the number of the myriad things, how could it truly be the number of the myriad things? So when we say 360, it was used to adjust the numer-

[225] 1032–1085 CE

[226] Movements of Qi or climatic changes.

[227] 2 legendary rulers 2200 BCE.

[228] Shao Yong 邵雍 (1011–1077)

[229] 281–356 CE

[230] 544–610 CE

[231] 1702–1764 CE

ous. In modern times we use it, Master Shao said it, how could it be that Confucius didn't know it? And so, when Master Shao used it, it was to mean a complete circle; when Confucius used it, it was the sun pointing to the time period. How can one attain this surplus and say it is the same? Alas, as for this generation and assessing its people, the ones who are versed with the method of reading the ancient books, whenever the ancients did not know something, it was unsuitable for one to say that he knows it. He should simply quote it. When the ancients said they knew, it was unsuitable for one to say that he did not know it. He should use it to fortify his attacks. To the contrary, with a calm heart inspect it, vastly investigate it and prove it, follow the evidence and disqualify it, this is the real attitude of the student.

The *Nei Jing* theory that five days is one Hou, three Hou is one Qi should be pointed out as lacking. That his Excellence uses the numbers five and six and explains Jia Zi 甲子 as having accurate calculation, these are deficient words. It becomes the fact of the careless and ignorant. Here, in order to teach, one criticizes a person; it is only that he loves him and therefore hurts him. The great author here also states that the *Nei Jing* 內經 discussion of the five Zang 藏 organs is the same as the five Cang 藏 storages of the four seasons. They should be five storages of Qi transformation and not five organs made of flesh and blood. This is, as well, another example that your Excellency is set out to support the words of the *Nei Jing*. How come you didn't say that man is the creation of the four seasons? If so, how come the five organs made of flesh and blood are not the creation of the four seasons? How come they don't change in accordance with the four seasons? Now, when we talk about the five Cang 藏 storages of the *Nei Jing* and we compare them to the anatomical five organs, the falsehood is evident. One cannot make it mysterious. One cannot simply make up a theory about five Cang 藏 storage organs related to the four seasons and try to demonstrate what they are not. Now, the people who discuss the *Nei Jing* talk about people who are not flesh and blood and they make them into immaterial people corresponding to the Qi transformation of the four seasons. When they talk about disease, they make disease to be not flesh and blood and they make them, instead, four seasons Qi transformation diseases. A human out of flesh and blood, five organs made of flesh and blood, disease of flesh and blood, the *Nei Jing* does not know. If it knows, it does not talk about it.

These three above are entirely not a matter belonging to the four seasons. A doctor, every day, meets with people of flesh and blood. The diseases that he treats are mostly with flesh and blood pathology. If it is not lodged in the flesh and blood, even though with hard toil, he groundlessly files a report. Basing himself on the five phases and Jia Zi calculations, he fabricates five Cang 藏 organs being related to the four seasons Qi transformation, and he can only assume the issues at hand. He combines different schools of thought, tossing about, while seeking the pathology of a flesh and blood disease. This is what his art is about. With his words, he says that disasters result from different phenomena. What kind of different phenomena? Today, when people conduct astrology and divination arts, the five phases that they use are the same five phases of the *Nei Jing* 內經. The Jia Zi 甲子 that they use is the Jia Zi 甲子 from *Nei Jing* 內經. Yin Yang 陰陽 is the Yin Yang from *Nei Jing*. The musical temperament is the musical temperament of the *Nei Jing*. What your Excellency claims to explain and use, how is this different from the five phases and Jia Zi 甲子 of that gang, discarding it,[232] as if it is not coming from the *Nei Jing*, and stating that these arts absolutely do not come from the transformation of the four seasons? Their fabrication of conforming to the generation is flying concealed; six positions, ten Jia 甲, five stars, four Qi, six kinships, nine races, fortune and virtue, punishment and killing and all these items, they merge together all kinds of schools of thought in order to seek out and forecast the good and bad fortunes of human affairs. Where is there a difference between these and the *Nei Jing* 內經 fabrication of five Zang 藏 organs, six Fu 府 organs and twelve meridians in order to seek disease pathology? In today's scholarship, if one avoids facts and material experimentation in order to get at it, and instead he relies on Jia Zi 甲子 and five phases theories, then he calculates and propagates astrology, divination, geomancy and *Nei Jing* Qi transformation theory. Your Excellence tries hard to extricate yourself from all those, claiming that your five phases and Jia Zi theory has true purpose. More so, in any kind of medical modality, if one wants to expand its foundation, how can one claim to independently elevate the *Nei Jing* and, at the same time, escape the realm of the fortune tellers and superstitious practitioners?

The two-word phrase "anatomical dissection" comes from the *Ling Shu* 靈樞; the measurement of the bones and vessels cannot be invented out of imagination. That the liver and lungs are green and white, without seeing with one's eyes, one cannot point this out. How come one thinks that the ancients only relied on five phases and Jia Zi in order to fabricate five Zang organs stemming out of four seasons' Qi transformation, and that they didn't carry out any flesh and blood investigation? When they talked about disease, oftentimes dissection was the main investigation. Therefore, in *Re Lun* 熱論 chapter, it states that the grand Yang 巨陽 vessel connects to Feng Fu 風府 point in order to explain head and neck pain, back and spine stiffness; Yang

[232] The fortune tellers' art and, in Yunxiu's mind, all the charlatans.

Ming 陽明 vessel circles the nose and branches to the eye in order to explain eye pain and dry nose; and such as these, the examples are plenty. Even in Wang Bing 王冰 commentary, whenever there was a dissection possibility to explain a disease, he used dissection to do it. For example: in chapter *Shang Gu Tian Zhen Lun* 上古天真論, explaining the face burnt and hair falling; in chapter *Yin Yang Bie Lun* 陰陽別論, explaining carbuncles, swelling, atrophy etc; these all are such explanations. These kinds of methods are truly the proper methods of medicine. It should not be discarded because their dissection methods were unrefined. It should allow following generations to follow closely behind in this realm and become honest and enlightened. And so, today's old medicine doctors, how come with the new medicine, they turn their back on it and gallop in the other direction? Like the melon farmland and the taro field, they separate it as if it cannot be merged. Today, you wish to avoid this *Nei Jing* dissection loss, and instead try to get rid of it as if not part of the Dao 道. In addition, this proper method that, for thousand generations was not pondered, he[233] finds as uncomfortable to propagate. He specifically uncovers the five phases, Jia Zi and Qi transformation theories, specifically bringing forth Wang Bing's 王冰 *Tian Yuan Ji Da Lun* 天元紀大論 and the other supplementary chapters, which are obviously not equal to the rest of the book. He believes those chapters are precious and he cannot suspect their fault. This is all "being swayed by one's emotions". One cannot, with a peaceful heart, discuss it over. Your servant here is not sharp, and has the style of retreating; when I study, I cannot get to the essence. The Qi transformation theory, until the end, I cannot believe that it is fact-based. In my humble writing of *Ling Su Shang Dui* 靈素商兌, until the end, I was not willing to accept that which I didn't know, without adding deep contemplation, scorning it like a slave. Therefore, towards your great book that contains many doubts, I know that medical matters do not come in a rush. I don't dare show disrespect. First, about the climatic Qi Hou 氣候 year and the four seasons five Zang organs theories, that their substance is so brilliant, with good fortune and calm Qi I inspected it. In case it is possible to receive your good news explaining its obscurity, I dare not honor the gift of your precious words. Overlooking the letter, I allow my thoughts to fly to an adored person; I cannot help but look forward to your reply. At the very beginning of summer, at the fourth lunar month, the good luck is only if you help yourself for more.[234]

Yu Yan 余巖 Kowtow.

[233] He means "you", a polite way to address someone directly in the third person.

[234] Said to a guest in a banquet.

A reply letter from Mr. Yun Tieqiao 惲鐵樵

Mr. Yunxiu, with a seat at the right side,[235] your honored letter of diligent worry and honest correspondence, how it helped and encouraged with goodness and richness I memorized it twice and thrice. My admiration feeling is indescribable, revering the classics and step-by-step advancing it, kind of study. How profound and vast, makes your younger brother look shallow and ignorant, insufficient to arrange the drums and bells for a debate. Only that the meaning of my humble work *Records of Widening One's Wisdom Jian Zhi Lu* 見智錄 is not the same as what is being described in your respectful letter. Your younger brother decisively and clearly knows about this historical study of earlier China, that it already has become a relic of the past. If one wishes to seek the real truth about Qi transformation, if he does not specialize in more recent astronomy, then it is not possible. Therefore, as for all the historical astrological records of the Han and Jin dynasties, when people try to reach to it with random and reckless study, not being very careful about it, these [kinds of errors] are all mentioned in *Jian Zhi Lu* 見智錄. Because the modern man denounces five phases and Jia Zi 甲子, saying that the *Nei Jing* 內經 is absurd, and directly because of that it has no bit of value, this is something that your younger brother can't do with. Because of that, I delve into this topic in the hope of explaining it and setting the records straight. The *Nei Jing* is China's ancient medical system; it is not China's modern day Chinese medicine. China's modern day Chinese medicine is preposterous. Your younger brother absolutely does not recognize it as a medical art. The recent Chinese medicine, when it states that it comes out of the *Nei Jing*, your younger brother also absolutely does not agree with that. Alas, the recent Chinese medicine absurd medical art comes from the confused *Nei Jing* commentators of the different schools. Therefore, in my humble work, I don't make even a little bit of use from those commentators' explanations. If the *Nei Jing* is used as the foundations, than this gets even closer to modern scientific view of things. If it is neatly arranged and well balanced, then it surely will create a sensible and clear medical system. It will establish a separate banner and occupy a different place from modern Western medicine. This opinion is announced clearly, time and time again, in *Jian Zhi Lu* 見智錄. In addition, your younger brother has already caught a glimpse of the deeper sense; slightly holding the handle tip of it and going forward, with hard work, will make himself advance more. With time, he will have an accomplishment, even if at present there is none; this is what led me to jeer with your *Ling Su Shang Dui* 靈素商兌.

---

[235] In ancient time the way to show appreciation and value for literature and art.

The *Nei Jing*, as a source of study, vanished into rarity. Its book is a text of stray fragments. Its principle, at the least, has no step-by-step system and so people look for its meanings by single characters. This is where its essential ideas vanish. And so, when one concentrates his mind to explore it, he often also brings back blurriness, becomes disheartened and can't grasp it.[236] When it states that being able to forecast life and death is evident in the pulse there is, nonetheless, accuracy of an iota. Every affair has its principle, and when it says "looking at complexion and inspecting the pulse, one may know life from death", it is stated not without a reason. Therefore, four years ago, your younger brother memorized that book, with much determination, and subsequently started to feel its essence. Even though he still could not penetrate the whole thing, he still carves it out without letting go. If one graduates from this book, he should go ahead and explore other kinds of sciences. And so, when your younger brother came to learn Chinese cultural studies, he saw that there are all kinds of melted keys and often brilliant people. Often, even without becoming their disciple, one could enter their school. What you mention as "jeering with *Ling Su Shang Dui* 靈素商兌" is really not such. The book name *Discussion and Deliberation Shang Dui* 商兌 is where it's at, however, its content is jeering. It is just as its name implies. It is a fair and proper sound of laughter. When it comes to the four seasons and the Zang Fu 藏府 organs, truly there is this principle. The entire *Nei Jing* book is all about this; I feel sorry that, without understanding the art, one cannot prove my words. This year, around May–June, I drafted a self-criticism of the Ming dynasty block print version of the *Shang Han Lun* 傷寒論.

This time, I announce it in this letter. I wish to prevent charlatan Chinese medicine doctors from using the *Jian Zhi Lu* 見智錄 as their excuse, hoping to avoid keeping the research of cultural studies. Whatever your younger brother was able to attain, some doubt it, while others are looking to come and learn it; it resembles the five Buddhist impurities of the world. We, the both of us, have a pure and unadulterated discussion about this art, however, your younger brother does not qualify to become Hui Zi 惠子. In addition, your kind teaching words, in regards to your thoughts not being able to stand Ji Ming 雞鳴 wind and rain, all the various safeguards of the treasure have been guarded, I very much would like to talk about it.
Your younger brother, Yun Shujue 惲樹玨, Kowtow.

Article end

[236] This is a third person statement, meaning that Yu Yunxiu could not get the essence of the *Nei Jing*.

Research on *Shang Han Lun* 傷寒論研究

by Yun Tieqiao 惲鐵樵

The preface of Zhang Zhongjing

Yaron: Mr. Yun gives valuable advice: "Only if one is dissatisfied with the current state of affairs in medicine may he worry about the disease cause, the fever of the sick, and from this angle he will begin his research. Only like this can one create 'New'."

Pages 10–11

When I read the preface of *Shang Han Lun*, I get a very special feeling. If one wishes to reach to the *Shang Han* true principle, he cannot slavishly imitate it. Getting rid of all commentaries, and plainly reading the text, is impossible. However, I am thinking, if one is tied up by the commentaries then he cannot reach his own attainment. Just as Zhongjing's medical art—if it were tied up by his generation's physicians, he would not have been able to break through the current stream, reaching to the profundities of the Yellow Emperor and Qibo. The preface states: "In ancient antiquity, there were Shen Nong, Qi Bo, Bo Gao, Lei Gong, Shao Shi, Shao Yu, Zhong Wen, in recent antiquity there were Zhang Sang, Bian Que, Gong Cheng Yang Qing and Cang Gong. From that time on, I didn't hear of anyone else worthy." It also states: "Looking at today's doctors, they don't think, ponder and seek the essence of the classics. Each follows his family's art, from beginning to end following the old." It also states: "When I reflect back on the sufferings of the past, all the people who perished with no rescue, I then sought the teachings of the ancients, extensively learned all prescriptions." From these different statements, one can know how he was different. The generations claim that Zhongjing studied medicine with his prefecture fellow Zhang Bozu 同郡張伯祖 and completely mastered his art, and so we can see that Zhongjing had a teacher. When he composed the *Shang Han Lun*, this was after he had completed his study and more or less was well familiar with his teacher's ideas. Yet this text, while narrating all kinds of life saving methods, shouts directly at his contemporary doctors for using medicine erroneously. There is not one word of transmission from his teacher. In addition, following what he unravels in the preface text, he didn't leave even a little room for his teacher there. One knows then that Zhang Bozu was no different from the rest of the doctors of the time.

He was another one of the "not thinking, pondering and seeking the essence of the classics, each following his family's art, from beginning to end follows the old." And so the medicine of Zhongjing comes without copying bare-handed. It is like a mountain on a flat ground. It is because he experienced the untimely death of the young that he sought the ancient teachings and, from there, his ability comes. It was only like this. Therefore, the very beginning stage of his thought was that people die because they get sick. When they start getting sick, they have fever. When humans become sick, how come they experience fever first? At the time, when medical doctors treated cold injuries, they must have had a set of herbs or formulas to treat this. When they used their set of herbs for this purpose, the affair was finished—they didn't labor their hearts further, this is what is called each transmits his family's art and follows the old. If one would ask "how come there is fever", the asked would be dumbstruck without an answer. 2000 years ago, the question of why there is fever could not be confronted. Therefore, one could have not but painstakingly sought the teachings of the ancients. *Nei Jing* states: "when Yang surges, there is fever/heat; when Yin surges, there is cold." It also states: "when Yang is deficient, there is cold and when Yin is deficient, there is heat". It is the key to understanding why there is fever. The *Su Wen* is the *Shang Han Lun* springing board. I feel that this statement of mine has great relevance. One must know that, in medicine and treating disease, if one is doing "copying" he absolutely cannot excel outside the present scope. Only if one is dissatisfied with the current state of affairs in medicine then he may worry about the disease cause, the fever of the sick, and from this angle he will begin his research. Only like this can one create 'New'.

Let's take today for example, my fellows. Regardless if one follows *Ye Tianshi Case Studies* 葉天士醫案言 or *Wen Bing Tiao Bian* 瘟病條辨 or *Wen Re Jing Wei* 溫熱經緯, if not this then follows the four masters of Jin Yuan, otherwise follows Zhang Jingyue 張景岳 or Zhang Shiwan 張石頑, or otherwise follows Chen Xiuyuan 陳修園 or Yu Jiayan 喻嘉言, it doesn't matter what path they follow, when they enter deep it is like a donkey rotating the millstone or a frozen fly entering the paper.[237] With utmost effort, they are energized to the end of their lives; they exhaust their years, with their head already of white hair and until the end they can't escape this scope. If one gives all this up and directly learns *Su Wen*, then if he can't get it, then so be it, but if he can get it, then there is an overwhelming clarity, as if one has climbed mount Taishan

[237] Forever they can't get it.

and now can see clearly all the mountain tops. All the scholars since the Jin Yuan are like the lower mountains. They know that there is the medicine of Zhongjing but they don't know that the underground water is dry, that the seaport is without a river link to the interior. This is why one needs the spirit of new creation. That I talk like this, people today look at me as if I am crazy, but really my words are only to seek goodness. At present times, one cannot attain an intimate friend; in the past there were Yu's words of approval. Now, in modern times, if one wishes to merge Chinese and Western medicines, absorb the essence of them both, but does not meticulously investigate the essence of *Su Wen* and *Shang Han* then their Dao is meaningless.

The six conformations of *Shang Han Lun*

Pages 12–17

The most important thing from the *Shang Han Lun* is the six conformations; the most difficult part of it is also the six conformations. Everyone reading the *Shang Han Lun* struggles with this. Anyone making commentary on it, as well, struggles with this. However, able to reach at the true essence of this, there is almost not a single person. If one cannot resolve this issue, then the entire book is unclear; where can one talk of medicine then? I remember once a famous person saying: "In China there are some excellent physicians, but they are unable and unwilling to transmit their art to others". These two lines together are extremely unintelligible and yet it is the reality. Alas, when medicine becomes good the principle is to transmit it. However, the heart must be able to understand it. If it cannot be understood then this is when it cannot be transmitted. When this happens, it is not because the fine subtleties cannot be explained but rather it is because the knowledge is not thoroughly understood. If the knowledge is not thoroughly understood, even if he (the doctor) can heal the sick flesh and bones, this still can be defined as not very good. That my humble self is able to explain this to myself and then explain to others without the smallest ambiguity in its midst, this I am short of self-confidence. Following step by step, I will develop this discussion.

All commentators say: "Tai Yang rules the body's exterior", "Yang Ming rules the interior" while "Shao Yang rules the half exterior half interior". I would like to grasp the meaning of this claim.

When Tai Yang is diseased, often there is aversion to cold. Aversion to cold is something one feels at the skin and skin is the most exterior layer of the body. Therefore, "Tai Yang rules the body's exterior" can be explained like this.

When Yang Ming is diseased then the stomach family is full, in Yang Ming organ syndrome there is heat, unconsciousness and delirious speech, one uses Cheng Qi Tang to purge it, when the dry feces come out then the heat resolves and delirious speech also stops. The cause for heat and delirious speech is the dry feces in stomach and intestines. The stomach and large intestines are inside the body and therefore "Yang Ming rules the interior" can also be explained with that.

"Shao Yang rules the half exterior half interior": when Shao Yang is diseased there is cold and heat, first cold and then heat. Explaining this, one says: "When evil disease exits from the interior outside, it reaches to Tai Yang then there is aversion to cold. When evil disease sinks from the exterior inwards it reaches Yang Ming and then there is aversion to heat." Shao Yang's exterior layer is Tai Yang while the interior layer is Yang Ming, there it is said that Shao Yang is half at the exterior and half at the interior, this possibly also can explain it.

However, even though it can explain it, it has already a part that is unexplainable. Tai Yang has a disease with aversion to cold and there is disease that has fever, so how come, when Shao Yang exits to the exterior, there is only aversion to cold? In addition, if the exterior is skin and body hair and the intestine and stomach are interior, is this half interior half exterior Shao Yang in between the skin and stomach and intestines?

When it comes to the three Yin, their explanations cannot be fathomed. Tai Yin is ultimate Yin and so it cannot have fever, Jue Yin is where the two Yin come into extinction, Shao Yin is the bottom of Tai Yang, therefore Tai Yang disease can transmit directly to Shao Yin.

When one looks over all the commentators' explanations they are more or less uniform. They all talk the same talk. If the three Yang have exterior, interior and half exterior half interior, then the three Yin should also have a physical place to be described. Tai Yin is ultimate Yin and if we follow the idea that Yang is outside while Yin is inside, then it means that Tai Yin is in the most interior position. Jue Yin is the place where the two Yin come into extinction, it is the finishing place of Yin, when compared to Tai Yin position this should be even deeper. Shao Yin is the place where one Yin[238] is born, its position closer to Tai Yang. It seems that Shao Yin should be the exterior of three Yin.

If Shao Yin is exterior, Jue Yin is interior, how is then Tai Yin half interior half exterior? Looking at all scholars, none has talked about it. Some quote the *Nei Jing* "Tai Yang is opening, Yang Ming is closing, Shao Yang is pivot. Tai Yin is opening, Jue Yin is closing, while Shao Yin is pivot." Following this discussion, if Tai Yang is opening and is exterior, Tai Yin opening should also be exterior. If Yang Ming closing is interior, then Jue Yin closing should also be interior. Shao Yang being half interior half exterior is pivot, then Shao Yin pivot should also be half interior half exterior. However, all scholars don't mention that as well. How is that possible?

Kidneys and urinary bladder are interior exterior related, liver and gall bladder are interior exterior, spleen and stomach are interior exterior. And so urinary bladder foot Tai Yang is exterior, kidney foot Shao Yin should also be exterior. Gallbladder foot Shao Yang is half-interior half-exterior, liver foot Jue Yin should also be half interior half exterior. Stomach is foot Yang Ming interior, spleen foot Tai Yin should also be interior. While appraising circumstances, this explanation seems feasible; however, all scholars did not say this.

How come they all talk about the three Yang with certainty while not voicing a word about the three Yin? Uncovering the false mask of it, all scholars, even though they labored greatly at the six conformations, they all could not come clear about the six conformations' three Yin. Master Zhu Zi 朱子 has a saying: "When I read a book, if I didn't finish the page, I do not dare go to the next page. If I didn't finish a scroll, I do not dare go to the next scroll." What we call 'exhausting it' means exhausting and understanding the meaning of it. Up till now, all the scholars could not exhaust the meaning of three Yin, and yet how come they have all sorts of developments. For example, Yu Jiayan 喻嘉言 followers, not only do they boast about it, at great length they keep on pricking at it without an end, and still can't come to terms with it!

Recently, from the eastern land[239] I came across *Shang Han Explained Meanings* 傷寒疏義 by Kitamura 喜多村.[240] In its preface, there is one section that explains the six

[238] This should be a typo; Shao Yin is where one Yang is born.
[239] Japan
[240] Kōsō Kitamura 喜多村 1804–1876.

conformations quite clearly, something that our own nation's commentators were not able to do. Following, I record his words to be a helping mountain here.

> Kitamura says: "This classic doesn't have the words 'six conformations' in it. What is called three Yin and three Yang express artificially the idea of external and internal, cold and heat, deficient and excessive. It is not the pairing of meridians and organs. Upon investigation of this treatise, this meaning becomes evident. Earlier commentators entangled the one with the other, greatly turning their back on the essence of the classic. This discussion[241] talks about the different discussions on the six diseases. It does not dare attack the earlier people. This discussion, talking about three Yin and three Yang, talks about disease positions. Yang is hard, Yin is soft; Yang is hot, Yin cold; Yang excessive, Yin deficient; this is the normal principle. When disease belongs to Yang to heat to excess, it is called three Yang. When it belongs to Yin to cold to deficiency then it is called three Yin. If we investigate it more carefully, then when evil is in the exterior and heat is excessive, then it is Tai Yang. When evil is half exterior half interior and heat excessive, then it is Shao Yang. When evil enters the stomach and heat is in excess then it is Yang Ming. And again, when evil is at the exterior and it is cold and deficient it is Shao Yin. When evil is half exterior half interior and it is cold and deficient then it is Jue Yin. When evil enters the stomach and it is deficient and cold then it is Tai Yin. Only when the exterior heat is extreme and the interior therefore is also hot, even if the interior has started heat but disease did not enter the stomach, this also belongs to Tai Yang. When the exterior is extremely cold and, therefore, the interior also started to be cold, if the disease did not enter the stomach this is still Shao Yin. Shao Yang and Jue Yin as one entity [is the situation of] the disease remaining at half exterior half interior. Yang Ming and Tai Yin as one entity describes [the situation of] evil attacking the stomach. Therefore, not talking about external or internal hot and cold, whenever disease enters the stomach it is called Yang Ming

[241] Pointing to *Shang Han Explained Meanings*

and Tai Yin. The sequence of the six diseases: when at Yang it is Tai Yang, Shao Yang, Yang Ming; when at Yin [it is] Shao Yin, Jue Yin, Tai Yin. However, at Yang, it can move and transmit; at Yin, it is still and does not transmit. Now, about its transmission and changes, Tai Yang and Shao Yin are externally-internally related, Shao Yang and Jue Yin are externally-internally related, Yang Ming and Tai Yin are externally-internally related. When Tai Yang is deficient, it is Shao Yin. When Shao Yin is excessive, it is Tai Yang. When Shao Yang is deficient, it is Jue Yin. When Jue Yin is excessive, it is Shao Yang. When Yang Ming is deficient, it is Tai Yin and when Tai Yin is excessive, it is Yang Ming. This is the fixed principle of disease transmission and transformation. It is the general outline of three Yin and three Yang.

The classic[242] three Yin three Yang sequence comes from the *Nei Jing Re Lun* chapter. I don't dare say there is a mistake, the meaning of it must be this. Only when it comes to disease transformation and transmission, one cannot restrict the transmission to this sequence. Earlier generations were not clear of this meaning. It caused people to try and feel the shadow in the dark. They did not explain it like this.

Mr. Zhang Taiyan 章太炎[243] comments: "The great work of Kitamura states 'When Tai Yang is deficient, it is Shao Yin. When Shao Yin is excessive, it is Tai Yang. When Shao Yang is deficient, it is Jue Yin. When Jue Yin is excessive, it is Shao Yang. When Yang Ming is deficient, it is Tai Yin and when Tai Yin is excessive, it is Yang Ming.' This meaning comes already from Mr. Ke 柯.[244] Ke said that Tai Yang is heart and now we can examine this. Tai Yang disease is at Ying and Wei, Ying is blood vessels and belong to heart, internally it belongs to heart and it is the exterior of the heart. Shao Yin is properly the heart organ; when Tai Yang is deficient, when blood vessels are defi-

[242] Points to *Shang Han Lun*
[243] Zhang Taiyan 章太炎 1869–1936
[244] Ke Qin 柯琴 1662–1735

> cient, they cannot resist guest evil, and so it forces itself directly upon the heart. When disease is seen at arm and leg it means that arm and leg go through atrophy. If the heart is full, then evil can only reach to the periphery blood vessels and cannot reach to the heart organ; this is when one sees heat only at the exterior of Tai Yang. Ke also said that when the stomach family is not full, it is a Tai Yin disease; it is also a similar idea to Kitamura. Only Shao Yang and Jue Yin, Ke did not discuss. Shao Yang disease often points to San Jiao and just a little to gallbladder organ. Jue Yin often points to the liver organ and little to pericardium. The principle being that you cannot mix them both together. Now when Jue Yin disease has the symptom 'heart center has pains and heat' it means the disease is in the diaphragm area, it is Shan Zhong 膻中 Jue Yin area, it also matches the San Jiao. Only when San Jiao is deficient, the fluids are not distributed, and so Jue Yin disease must have Xiao Ke 消渴 unquenchable thirst. It fits exactly what is called 'when Shao Yang is deficient it is Jue Yin'.

According to Kitamura, indeed there is this principle. My generation doesn't understand the six conformations. At a very beginning stage, one feels a little ashamed, but after some time this fades from memory. After one treats patients for a while, he doesn't pay attention to it anymore. Not only does he not pay attention to it but, finally, he also forgets that he did not understand it. Himself, he thinks that he understands it. This leaves great difficulty for future generations. Many quibble biased statements, allowing themselves to sink into the thick fog of the forgone virtuous people. This is what is called "the excellent doctor cannot transmit his art to others". This situation can only be described as "deceiving oneself as well as others". The brain is muddleheaded and careless as if inconceivable. May we ask, since Cheng Wuji 成無己,[245] Pang Anchang 龐安常, all the way through scholars of Yong and Qian,[246] who could escape the blame of feeling the shadow in the dark?

Article end

[245] 1063–1156

[246] Yong (Zheng 雍正 1723–1735) and Qian (Long 乾隆 1735–1796)

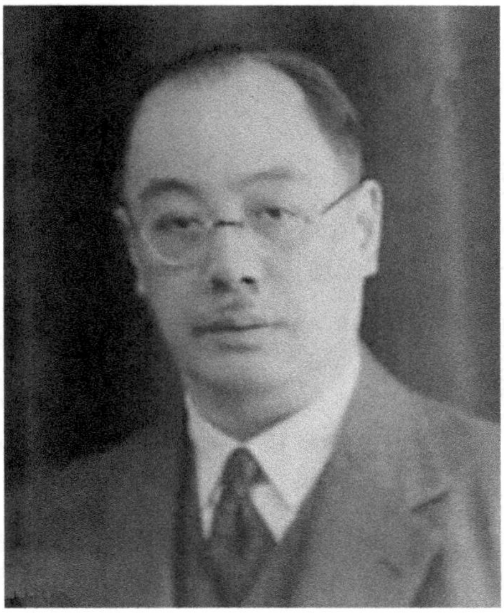

Yu Yunxiu 1930s

Arguing the *Shang Han Lun Yan Jiu* 傷寒論研究辨惑

by Yu Yunxiu 余雲岫

Yaron: By the following article, one notes the emotional escalation as time goes by. Just as debates between Yu and Yun escalate, so are the emotions throughout the country. From a courteous debate it becomes a fight.

The arguments in general have scholarly value, but in the following article Yu points out very well that Chinese medicine opinions throughout history were often conflicting and if one uses ancient quotes to justify one's own theory then there will be many other ancient quotes refuting this same theory. Thus quoting ancient classics as a testimony for accuracy is a flawed methodology.

In modern TCM, one often uses modern science to clarify and verify a Chinese medicine principle or substitute it.

I, much like Yun Tieqiao, believe that Chinese medicine can have its own methodology developing further its own principle. The debate is about modern scientific principles and methods versus Chinese medicine principles and methods. Here, in the following article, Yu points out well a few Chinese medicine shortcomings. It seems that Yu is specifically and personally attacking Yun yet, in reality, he is attacking the traditional Chinese methodology. Today, we should distance ourselves from emotions and reflect on the problem.

I have written two books to critique *Qun Jing Jian Zhi Lu* 群經見智錄 written by Yun Tieqiao 惲鐵樵. Recently, he published *Shang Han Lun Yan Jiu* 傷寒論研究. I read it when I had free time this summer. Yun Tieqiao 惲鐵樵 mentions me several times in it, so I have to express my opinions about this book.

Compared to *Qun Jing Jian Zhi Lu* 群經見智錄, *Shang Han Lun Yan Jiu* 傷寒論研究 seems to have made some progress. Firstly, it doesn't discuss five phases and Qi movement. Secondly, it doesn't talk about theories of *Yi Jing* 易經. Thirdly, it knows that the theories, far from universal, are not acceptable and tries to remove ambiguities out of the book. However, this book still keeps the theories of Four Seasons and Five Organs, which cannot possibly be proven by science. But Yun Tieqiao 惲鐵樵 hasn't given clear and detailed explanations on these theories. It is acceptable if it's only the author who is not clear about them. What I am really worried about is if other ancient medicine doctors might follow the author's way without thinking. It is really a big problem for the future of medicine. So I am going to discuss these theories, in order to reveal the truth to the people.

Shang Han Lun Yan Jiu (SHLYJ): What I want to say are the things that never have been discussed by the ancients, and there is no book to prove such things.

Yu Yunxiu (YYX): It is better to consider the historical background when reading ancient books. Confucianism in the Song dynasty was good, but it was inferior to Confucianism in the Han dynasty because Song Confucianism didn't respect the old traditions, and it explained the ancient books using Song language and individual thoughts. I don't dare to readily believe these plausible explanations, in order to avoid the misunderstanding of the ancients' original meanings. Yun Tieqiao 惲鐵樵 says he wants to say things that have never been discussed by the ancients, which means he reads the ancient medical books with modern thoughts and personal opinions. It is really not the right way to research the ancient books because it will cause misunderstanding of the ancients' original meanings.

SHLYJ: The Five Phases and Six Qi originated from the Four Seasons theory, which has a close relationship with living things.

YYX: It is acceptable to set Four Seasons for temperate countries. But the theories of Five Phases and Six Qi are unreliable. All the studies and theories related to natural disasters and immortals must rely on natural phenomena to gain universal trust. In the book *Zhou Yi Can Tong Qi* 周易參同契, Wei Boyang 魏伯陽 used the method of Ba Gua Na Jia 八卦納甲 to polish the alchemy as means of indefinitely prolonging life and said, "The words are based on facts, and the statements are presented with evidence." Yun Tieqiao 惲鐵樵 is doing exactly the same as Wei Boyang 魏伯陽. The scientific method should be serious, without being careless and sluggish. Otherwise, the hypothesis cannot be proven as true.

SHLYJ: Nowadays, the Chinese youth wear Japanese hats, Western leather shoes, and traditional Chinese long gowns. How can we call them Chinese style clothing? The Chinese style clothing must have a coherent system and independent organization. Buddhism was gradually imported to China during Wei, Jin, Qi, and Liang dynasties 魏晉齊梁. It was combined with Chinese inherent philosophy and formed Lixue 理學 in the Song dynasty. This is a good example of such fusion. In my opinion, this is not necessary for the evolution of the Chinese medicine. Otherwise, it could absorb the advantages of Western medicine and form a new Chinese medicine.

YYX: This opinion is quite specious and confused. Assimilation, fusion and evolution are inevitable phenomena in nature. Japanese hats, Western leather shoes and long gowns are the results of assimilation, fusion and evolution. What is the meaning of Chinese-style clothing? Does it refer to skullcap and mandarin jacket? They were imported from the regions outside of Shanhaiguan Pass 山海關 three hundred years ago but now they are quite common in the whole country. So Japanese hats, Western leather shoes and long gowns will also be popular and become Chinese style-clothing after a long time. If someone thinks imported clothing cannot be called Chinese-style clothing, then the clothing style created by Huangdi 黃帝 in ancient times was the only pure Chinese style of clothing. Unlike the opinion of Yun Tieqiao 惲鐵樵, I think Lixue 理學 in the Song dynasty cannot be called Chinese studies, because it was combined with Buddhism, which was imported from foreign countries. The books of Yun Tieqiao 惲鐵樵 cannot be classified as Chinese books, because there are some Western things in them.

Any person with knowledge can be our teacher. Regardless of where the knowledge came from, it can be our own knowledge if acquired by us. Chen Liang 陳良, who was from a southern province called Hubei, studied in the north of China. Afterwards, he became the most famous of all scholars in the north of China. Mengzi 孟子[247] had never sneered at Chen Liang 陳良, who had turned from the southern school of thought to the northern one. But Mengzi 孟子 derided Chen Xiang 陳相, who turned from the northern school of thought to the southern. Why? The criterion for the road to learning is based on the road itself, without regional prejudice. China is a republic now, which is different from ancient government forms, but we are still the descendants of the Yan and Huang emperors. The politics, religions and social customs are completely different from the past, but we are still the descendants of the Yan and Huang emperors. Japanese medicine, which originated from Chinese medicine, followed Western medicine in recent years and now became an independent medicine. It is possible to compete against Western medicine. So it depends on our own attitudes. Yun Tieqiao 惲鐵樵 pays more attention to the appearance of things than to their inner meaning. In a sense, he must be an old adherent of the Qing dynasty.[248] Otherwise, he should have emigrated to France or America.

SHLYJ: Two thousand years ago, if asking why heat was unavoidable in diseases, most doctors couldn't answer, so it was quite necessary for these doctors to study hard the medical theories.

YYX: Yun Tieqiao 惲鐵樵 knows that Zhang Zhongjing 張仲景 was forced to study hard the medical theories. Up until today, his theory holds the finest of the ancient teachings, naturally one need not seek diligently the ancient teachings anymore.

SHLYJ: Regardless if one follows *Ye Tianshi Case Studies* 葉天士醫案言 or *Wen Bing Tiao Bian* 瘟病條辨 or *Wen Re Jing Wei* 溫熱經緯, if not this then follows the four masters of Jin Yuan, otherwise follows Zhang Jingyue 張景岳 or Zhang Shiwan 張石頑, or otherwise follows Chen Xiuyuan 陳修園 or Yu Jiayan 喻嘉言, it doesn't matter what path they follow, when they enter deep it is like a donkey rotating the millstone or a frozen fly entering the paper. With utmost effort, they are energized to the end of their lives; they exhaust their years, with their head already of white hair and until the end they can't escape this scope. If one gives all this up and directly learns *Su Wen*, then if he can't get it, then so be it, but if he can get it, then there is an overwhelming clarity, as if one has climbed mount Taishan and now can see clearly all the mountain tops.

---

[247] Mencius

[248] At that time anti-Qing sentiment was rather common.

YYX: I would like to say that if one starts with *Su Wen* 素問 and becomes enchanted by it, then he will never achieve great success in Chinese medicine. Yun Tieqiao 惲鐵樵 only considers 360 days in a year, fabricates theories of Zangfu organs with four seasons, makes improper comments on Yi Li 易理,[249] makes up diagrams of Taijitu 太極圖.[250] All these show that he is not proficient in *Nei Jing* 內經. Yun Tieqiao 惲鐵樵 thinks that mastering *Su Wen* 素問 is essential for learning Chinese medicine. But, in my opinion, the one who masters *Su Wen* 素問 becomes more bewitched by it. Yun Tieqiao 惲鐵樵 exaggerates the importance of *Nei Jing* 內經. He regards himself as a great master of Chinese medicine. Judging by the books written by him, he is not worthy of this title because there are many misconceptions.

SHLYJ: Six Conformations is not only the most important, but also the most indigestible theory of *Shang Han Lun* 傷寒論. All readers or annotators of *Shang Han Lun* 傷寒論 make great efforts to research the theory of Six Conformations. However, throughout history, none of them could get its real meaning. Without completely understanding this theory, we are not able to completely understand *Shang Han Lun* 傷寒論 and achieve great success in Chinese medicine.

YYX: I think Six Conformations is not only the most unreliable, but also the most meaningless theory in *Shang Han Lun* 傷寒論. Actually, there is no Six Conformations in the field of Shang Han 傷寒; it is Zhang Zhongjing 張仲景 who forces this theory on it. Probably Zhang Zhongjing 張仲景 only aims to preserve the old theory, without other further purposes. But the theory of Six Conformations is highly esteemed by the later scholars, who make many unreliable explanations. Yun Tieqiao 惲鐵樵 greatly admires the views of Kitamura 喜多村, a Japanese scholar. In my opinion, his views are no better than those given by other scholars.

SHLYJ: My theoretical books are not only accessible to myself, but also to other researchers. I don't keep any confusing things in my book.

YYX: Compared to the *Qun Jing Jian Zhi Lu* 群經見智錄, I feel Yun Tieqiao 惲鐵樵 has made some progress in his new book. However, there are still some influences of *Qun Jing Jian Zhi Lu* 群經見智錄 on *Shang Han Lun Yan Jiu* 傷寒論研究. It is not difficult to know the problems, but quite difficult to act on solving them.

[249] Principle of the *Yi Jing Book of Changes*.
[250] Yin Yang Taiji symbol.

SHLYJ: Zhu Zi 朱子 said, "I do not dare to read the second page or scroll if I haven't completely understood the meaning of the first one."

YYX: It is really unnecessary to quote Zhu Zi 朱子. As for what Zhu Zi 朱子 said, it is not possible to completely understand the truth of a book only by using this method. The books written by Zhu Zi 朱子, such as *Zhou Yi Ben Yi* 周易本義, *Shi Ji Zhuan* 詩集傳 and *Si Shu Ji Zhu* 四書集註, etc., have lots of mistakes and unclear things. How can Yun Tieqiao 惲鐵樵 be better than Zhu Zi 朱子?

SHLYJ: Kitamura 喜多村 said, "It is a Taiyang 太陽 disease if the pathogenic factor is in the exterior with excessive heat, Shaoyang 少陽 disease if in the half exterior and half interior with excessive heat, Yangming 陽明 disease if in the Stomach with excessive heat. It is a Shaoyin 少陰 disease if the pathogenic factor is in the exterior with deficient cold, Jueyin 厥陰 disease if in the half exterior and half interior with deficient cold, Taiyin 太陰 disease if in the Stomach with deficient cold."

YYX: It is completely wrong to divide the body as three levels, i.e. exterior, half exterior and half interior, and interior. It shows Kitamura 喜多村 is ignorant of anatomy, physiology and pathology. Yun Tieqiao 惲鐵樵 thinks it is not proper to point out where is Taiyang 太陽 or Yangming 陽明 in a healthy body. But in his book, he says, "Taiyang 太陽 disease refers to the disease in the superficial part of the body… Cold damage passes from the exterior to the interior. The exterior means the beginning of the disease… Six Conformations are about the location of the disease, while transmission refers to the pathogenic flow from one Conformation to another. It begins in Taiyang 太陽, ends in Yangming 陽明. Taiyang 太陽 is in the exterior, while Yangming 陽明 is in the interior. The transmission direction is always from exterior to interior… According to *Neijing* 內經, the top doctors are the ones who can treat superficial diseases, the following ranks are the ones who can treat subcutaneous diseases, muscle and bone diseases, internal organs' diseases, which occurs from exterior to interior. It is the rule for all heat diseases… The transmission direction of the disease is from exterior to interior. There are specific methods for the disease in the exterior. If these methods are effective, the disease can be cured before the transmission to the interior… If the pathogenic factors gather in Taiyang 太陽, releasing the exterior is the essential method for treatment, which can dispel the pathogenic factors outward." So, according to what Yun Tieqiao 惲鐵樵 said, we know he divides the body in three levels. This is why he believes the external part communicates with the large intestine. Taking typhoid fever as an example, I can prove it is really a false theory. The bacteria are in the blood at the beginning of typhoid fever, but most of them move to small intestine after the first week. So, at the beginning, i.e. in the Taiyang 太陽 level, the bacteria are in the blood. The blood circles everywhere in the body and, therefore, bacteria can be seen everywhere. In that case, how can we divide the body into exterior and interior? Mr Zhang 章先生[251] followed the theories of Mr. Ke 柯氏,[252] thinking Taiyang disease is in the nutrient and defensive aspects. The nutrient refers to the blood vessels, which interact with the Heart and act as the manifestation of the Heart. In my opinion, Mr. Zhang's 章 theories are much better than Yun Tieqiao's 惲鐵樵. After all, realistic words are quite different from the empty and crafty.

Mr Zhang 章 said to Yan 岩,[253] "It is reasonable to say Bladder is the Taiyang 太陽, because all heat patients have dark urine and bladder is where the urine is stored. So the ancients believed bladder was the first affected organ." Yan 岩 argued that, "Most of the ancients believed the urine was produced by Small Intestine, so the Small Intestine can also be called Taiyang 太陽. The ancients attributed the dark urine to the Bladder and Small Intestine, this is why they are called them both Taiyang 太陽." Mr Zhang 章 finally agreed.

SHLYJ: Where exactly are the Six Conformations in the body? Doctors have to research deeply and try to solve all unclear things. In the book *Yi Xue Qun Jing Jian Zhi Lu* 醫學群經見智錄, I have simply explained the Five Phases theory of *Nei Jing* 內經. I will repeat it in this book, in order to explain the Six Conformations theory of Shang Han 傷寒. If doctors can totally understand the contents of *Shang Han Lun Yan Jiu* 傷寒論研究 and of *Jian Zhi Lu* 見智錄, and are able to combine them with the theories of Kitamura 喜多村, they can perform well and become more confident in taking the pulse in clinical practice.

YYX: I have written two books to query Mr. Yun's 惲 *Qun Jing Jian Zhi Lu* 群經見智錄 but he has never answered a word. I suspect his theories are not tenable. I don't think that what he says has any relationship with the Five Phases theory. The Six Conformations theory is not related with taking the pulse; how can he say doctors will become more confident with taking the pulse after mastering the theory? Yun Tieqiao 惲鐵樵 exaggerates the importance of the Six Conformations theory in order

251 Zhang Taiyan 章太炎
252 Ke Qin 柯琴
253 Yu referring to himself.

to mislead the common people. People who are interested can have a look how he makes research for this theory.

SHLYJ: Where is the Six Conformations theory from? It is from Six Qi. Where is the Six Qi from? It is from the Four Seasons.

YYX: Yun Tieqiao 惲鐵樵 regards the Four Seasons as the origin of the Six Conformations theory. Why does he insist on that? In my opinion, he is conscious of how absurd and unreliable his theory is; in order to convince people, he has to explain his theory under the guise of the Four Seasons. This trick has no real difference with the Najia 納甲[254] of *Zhou Yi Can Tong Qi* 周易參同契. I have argued that before, so I don't want to repeat it here.

SHLYJ: People are influenced by the Four Seasons. Each season has different characters, for example, the spring and summer are warm, while the autumn and winter are cold. If the seasons are abnormal, people will suffer from illness.

YYX: There are two meanings. Firstly, it talks about the weather, the spring and summer should be warm, while the autumn and winter should be cold. The unusual situations, as the *Yin Yang Da Lun* 陰陽大論 says, spring is not warm but cold, summer is not hot but cool, autumn is not cool but hot, winter is not cold but warm. All of these may lead to illness. Secondly, it is related to the body's feeling. Usually, people feel warm in spring and summer, and feel cold in autumn and winter. It is abnormal if people feel cold in spring and summer and feel warm in autumn and winter; these people are suffering from illness. In my opinion, the second meaning is the symptom of the illness. Only when people are ill can we see these situations. About the first meaning, Wu Youke 吳又可 has argued, in his book *Wen Yi Lun* 瘟疫論, the following, "Normally, spring is warm, summer is hot, autumn is cool and winter is cold. They are slightly influenced by the windy, rainy, cloudy or sunny day. If the spring is not warm but cold, there must have been many rainy days. If the autumn is not cool but hot, there must have been many sunny days. These phenomena, which are quite normal in the four seasons, don't necessarily lead to epidemic diseases. The epidemic pathogenic factors are particular substances, which are different from cold, hot, warm, and cool temperature." Wu Youke 吳又可 offered a great argument; he found out that the diseases are caused by particular substances, which are different from

[254] A method of divination

cold, hot, warm, and cool temperature. At the time he lived there was no concept of bacteria, so he had to call them as epidemic pathogenic factors.

SHLYJ: The six Qi refers to wind, cold, summer-heat, dampness, dryness and fire. These concepts are not common, for example, 'wind' is not the natural movement of air, 'cold' is not the feeling of low temperature by the human body, and 'fire' is not the flames, light and heat produced by burning things.

YYX: Yun Tieqiao 惲鐵樵 is in a confused state of mind. He has said that six Qi are caused by the changes of the four seasons, i.e. the changes of natural phenomena. But, according to what he says here, the wind, cold and fire of six Qi are not the natural phenomena. And he hasn't pointed out what exactly they are. These behaviors are really ridiculous; he just does whatever he wants to do. He hides the things that cannot be proven. If there is something that can be proven, he will boast a lot about it. In my opinion, Yun Tieqiao 惲鐵樵 is really not qualified to write books.

SHLYJ: *Nei Jing* 內經 says, "Predominance of wind causes tremor, predominance of cold results in pain, predominance of summer-heat produces swelling, predominance of dryness leads to dehydration and predominance of dampness brings about watery diarrhea." Wind, cold, dryness and dampness are weather conditions, while tremor, pain and watery diarrhea are the body conditions. So the body conditions are greatly related to the natural phenomena.

YYX: The words from *Nei Jing* 內經 are completely wrong and easily disprovable. Tremor is a slight tremble. People will tremble if they wear thin clothes in the cold winter; can we call it predominance of wind? People will tremble if they are extremely frightened; can we call it predominance of wind? People will feel pain if they are burned by fire; can we call it predominance of cold? Sores, which are associated with fire and heat according to *Nei Jing* 內經, usually cause pain; can we call it predominance of cold? People who suffer from chilblain must have swelling of the hands or feet; can we call it predominance of summer-heat? People whose main food is white rice easily suffer from beriberi with swelling, which can be cured by taking bran; can we call it predominance of summer-heat? People who suffer from heart valve disease and nephritis are usually accompanied with swelling. According to the old theory, Heart is associated with fire, while Kidney is associated with water; they are completely different in nature but present the same symptoms; can we call it predominance of summer-heat? Mild dryness Cao 燥 leads to severe dryness Gan 乾; when mild dryness is dominant then there is severe dryness Gan 乾, only saying that "when Cao 燥 mild dryness dominates, it will create Cao 燥 mild dryness" is a wrong way of saying it. People who suffer from cholera have many symptoms related with loss of water, such as emaciation, ocular emargination, dry mouth and viscous blood. They are related to the condition of dryness. Are vomiting and diarrhea caused by predominance of dampness? No, there are three pathological conditions for watery diarrhea; I have discussed that in my book *Ling Su Shang Dui* 靈素商兌. Yun Tieqiao 惲鐵樵 says wind, cold, dryness and dampness are weather conditions, which are caused by changes of the four seasons. Wind is the natural movement of air, cold is the feeling of the low temperature by the human body. Yun Tieqiao 惲鐵樵 says tremor, pain, watery diarrhea are body conditions, which are human body phenomena caused by changes of the four seasons. They are the body's response to the four seasons' changes, i.e., the symptoms of diseases. Wind, cold, dryness and dampness are the causes of tremor, pain and watery diarrhea. Tremor, pain and watery diarrhoea are the body responses to wind, cold, dryness and dampness, which are Yun's 惲 definition of Six Qi. Yet he changes the definition of Six Qi in the following lines, why?

SHLYJ: Six Qi are symptoms of the human body caused by climate changes.

YYX: We can understand Yun Tieqiao's 惲鐵樵 words like, "climate changes may cause illness for people, and the illness manifestations are called Six Qi." Is this statement reasonable? Diseases are caused by changes of climate, so we can understand this as, "Six Qi are the symptoms of diseases." Is this statement reasonable? I think readers already know the answer. Besides that, a conclusion is made according to the foregoing paragraphs. The contents of the foregoing paragraphs are completely wrong; could the conclusion be right? It is really not difficult to answer this question. Could climate conditions be symptoms of diseases? That is of course not reasonable. Furthermore, it is obviously different from the Six Qi of *Nei Jing* 內經.

SHLYJ: Someone asks what exactly are the Six Conformations? I always directly answer, "Six Conformations are the categories of disease symptoms."

YYX: This statement is quite strange, because Yun Tieqiao 惲鐵樵 provides nothing to assist or prove it. According to what he said, the Six Conformations theory is associated with Six Qi. If Six Conformations are the categories of symptoms, I am not able to find out any relationship between Six Qi and Six Conformations. Yun Tieqiao 惲鐵樵 hasn't provided detailed explanation. It is really a big puzzle. He should explain more in order to prove his statement. According to what he wrote here, I think he is falling into a hopelessly confused state.

SHLYJ: The channels and collaterals are products of the disease. *Nei Jing* 內經 thought that channels and collaterals were related with Yin-Yang. Qi Bo 岐伯 said, "Yin and Yang can be extended from a thousand to ten thousand. They continually circulate, but have one principle in common." Spiritual stability is the primary principle of health preserving. There is no obvious evidence for the existence of Yin and Yang before the onset of a disease. In that case, do the channels and collaterals exist?

YYX: This statement is quite strange, Yun Tieqiao 惲鐵樵 must haven't read *Nei Jing* 內經. *Yin Yang Ying Xiang Da Lun* 陰陽應象大論 said, "Yin and Yang is the beginning of birth and death. Yang ensures growth while Yin promotes development. Yang is responsible for killing and Yin for storage." Aren't they the same with the growth, development and storage of all things on Earth presented by Yun Tieqiao 惲鐵樵? Humans are living beings on Earth. If there is no Yin and Yang before the onset of the disease then people will have no birth, old age, illness and death. *Nei Jing* 內經 says, "The Clear-Yang moves upward into the body's upper orifices while the Turbid-Yin moves downward into the body's lower orifices. The Clear-Yang permeates through muscular interstices Cou Li 腠理 while the Turbid-Yin enters the Five Zang-Organs. The Clear-Yang fortifies the four limbs while the Turbid-Yin enters the Six Fu-Organs." Do Yin and Yang exist after or before the onset of a disease? If it is as Yun Tieqiao 惲鐵樵 says, then there are no upper orifices, lower orifices, Cou Li, four limbs, Five Zang-Organs and Six Fu-Organs before the onset of the disease. *Jin Kui Zhen Yan Pian* 金匱真言篇 says, "In terms of Yin and Yang in the human body, the external is Yang and the internal is Yin. In terms of Yin and Yang concerning the human body parts, the back is Yang and the abdomen is Yin. In terms of Yin and Yang concerning the Zangfu-Organs, the Zang-Organs pertain to Yin and the Fu-Organs to Yang." If it is as Yun Tieqiao 惲鐵樵 says, there are no external and internal, back and abdomen, Zangfu-Organs in the human body. *Bao Ming Quan Xing Lun* 寶命全形論 says, "Humans are born with a physical body and cannot exist without Yin and Yang." If it is as Yun Tieqiao 惲鐵樵 says, then the human has no physical body before the onset of the disease. *Tiao Jing Lun* 調經論 says, "Yang gets Qi from Shangjiao 上焦 Upper Jiao to warm the skin and muscles." If it is as Yun Tieqiao 惲鐵樵 says, then there are no Yang, Qi or temperature in the human body; the body surface is as cold as ice and snow. *Tian Yuan Ji Da Lun* 天元紀

大論 says, "In nature there exists the Wuxing 五行 Five Phases that govern the five directions to produce Cold, Summer-Heat, Dryness, Dampness and Wind." Can we call Cold, Summer-Heat, Dryness, Dampness and Wind the symptoms of human disease? *Tian Yuan Ji Da Lun* 天元紀大論 says, "Shen 神 manifests as wind in the heavens and as wood on earth, as heat in the heavens and as fire on earth, as dampness in the heavens and as soil on earth, as dryness in the heavens and as metal on earth, as cold in the heavens and as water on earth." Can we call Wind, Cold, Summer-Heat, Dryness and Dampness the symptoms of human disease? *Tian Yuan Ji Da Lun* 天元紀大論 also says, "Cold, Summer-Heat, Dryness, Dampness, Wind and Fire represent Yin and Yang of the heavens." Can we call them the symptoms of human disease? *Ling Shu Sui Lou Lun* 靈樞歲露論 says, "All kinds of wind can bring down houses, break trees, lift up sand and stones, cause the body hair to stand up and open up the Cou Li (muscular interstice)." Can we say that they are not caused by the air movement? So what Yun Tieqiao 惲鐵樵 says is completely wrong if compared with the *Nei Jing* 內經. He doesn't respect the original meaning of *Nei Jing* 內經, but freely understands in his own way. Respecting the original meaning of ancient medical classics, though the theories may not be applicable for present, then we are able to avoid the loss of their true meaning and see the thoughts of that time. Freely understanding in one's own way means that there must have been cases of falsifying the original meaning of the ancient books to support his own statements. Although some of those modified theories may be correct today, in fact they are far from the ancient original meaning. Actually, Yun Tieqiao 惲鐵樵 gives his own academic opinions under the guise of ancient people. Is there any respect from him to the ancient doctors? He is totally depraved. I am really worried about the fickleness of the world.

SHLYJ: *Ling Shu Jing Mai* 靈樞經脈 can be proven by symptoms. But it is incompatible with contemporary knowledge of anatomy. For example, Yangming disease manifests as dry nostril, soreness of eye sockets, headache, swelling and aching of gingiva, suppurative infectious cheek, pain around umbilicus. *Ling Shu Jing Mai* 靈樞經脈 says, "Yangming starts from the lateral side of the ala nasi. It ascends to the bridge of the nose (the reason behind nostril dryness), where it meets the Bladder Channel of Foot-Taiyang. (Foot-Taiyang starts from the inner canthus, that's why eye sockets are sore.) Turning downward along the lateral side of the nose, it enters the upper gum. Winding around Jiache (ST 6) (that's why there are swelling and aching of gingiva, and suppurative infectious cheek), it ascends in front of the ear and traverses Kezhuren (GB 3). Then it follows the anterior hairline and reaches the forehead. (That's why there is headache.) The straight part of the channel arising from the supraclavicular fossa runs downward, passing through the nipple. It descends by the umbilicus. (That's why there is pain around the umbilicus.)" Other channels are similar to Yangming, but the channels are quite different from the arteries in anatomy. So channels and collaterals, like the Six Conformations of cold damage, are seen after the onset of the disease.

YYX: According to what Yun Tieqiao 惲鐵樵 says, *Jing Mai* 經脈 and other chapters in *Ling Shu* 靈樞 are all organized subjectively by the symptoms, such as nasal cavity dryness, soreness of eye sockets. I don't believe the ancient doctors would have organized knowledge like that. I will debate what Yun Tieqiao 惲鐵樵 says. Why doesn't he say the nasal bridge is dry? Why isn't the nostril sore or painful? Why not say the inner canthus is sore? He says there are swelling and aching of gingiva, and suppurative infectious cheek—why doesn't he say pain of the lateral side of the nose, or dryness of the gingiva? Why doesn't he say the headache is limited in the anterior and posterior hairline and the forehead? Why doesn't he say soreness of the head? He says the pain around umbilicus, why doesn't he say the pain of the supraclavicular fossa and the nipple? And why he doesn't say the soreness around the umbilicus? Yun Tieqiao 惲鐵樵 has to research these questions seriously and answer them without vagueness. If he omits to do this, I will suspect that he is not able to answer them. In my opinion, there were four probable sources for the contents of the *Jing Mai* 經脈 and other chapters in *Ling Shu* 靈樞, the anatomical findings, physiological normality, symptoms and contemporary thoughts. The obvious physiological normality and symptoms were possible to be understood by the ancients. However, the anatomical findings in that time were not accurate enough, which originated differences with nowadays findings. The principle is very clear, how can one not ponder the meaning within? Natural science is based on findings of natural phenomena, which help people understand the laws of nature. Therefrom people have experience with changes of natural phenomena and they understand why change occurs. People, who have thoughts and wisdom, are not satisfied with what they find, and so they will imagine based on their findings, in order to explain the natural phenomena. This is the general rule for academic progression. Take astronomy as an example; the moving of sun and moon and the alternation of winter and summer are phenomena of nature. Sun going and moon coming, moon going and sun coming, winter going and summer coming, and summer going and winter coming, these are observations of natural phenomena. A year (365.25 days) is the orbital period of the Earth moving in its orbit around the sun, a month (around 29 days) is based on the moon's orbital period; these are the experiences gained by observations. The 28 constellations and fixed stars move to the left direction; sun, moon, and five planets move to the right direction. And the universal theories, such as Gai Tian 蓋天, Hun Tian 渾天, Xuan Ye 宣夜, Xin Tian 昕天, Qiong Tian 穹天, and An Tian 安天, etc., were the explanations made by the ancient people. Nowadays they are called the eight planets that orbit the sun. The theories of astronomy have changed a lot since the ancient times. The ancient people rely on experience, whereas modern people rely on experiments. Instruments enable people to detect things that cannot be seen or heard, providing objective evidence. So advanced astronomy is based on scientific methods and precise instruments. The natural phenomena of sun and moon, winter and summer have never changed since the ancient times. The situation of diseases is just like with the natural phenomena; the nature of diseases has never changed until now. The difference between theories is caused by different methods of experiments and precision of instruments. The theories from the *Jing Mai* 經脈 and other chapters in *Ling Shu* 靈樞 were not able to be perfected, because there were no precise instruments and scientific experiments in that time. So the error of these theories is permissible. It is really not necessary to misrepresent the ancient theories to support one's own theory. I don't want to criticize the mistakes of ancient theories, but want to criticize the present people who don't change with the times. Yun Tieqiao 惲鐵樵 is just a person of that kind, with babyish thoughts.

SHLYJ: The waste materials of blood are collected in the Lungs, transported to Small Intestines through specific passages, and excreted from the body.

YYX: These words are completely ridiculous and extremely imprudent. The nutrients absorbed by the small intestines are transported to the blood. Actually, the waste materials of blood become air if secreted by the Lungs, become sweat if secreted by the sweat gland, and become urine if secreted by the kidney. But Yun Tieqiao 惲鐵樵 uses the concepts of new medicine to explain the theories of the ancient medicine, which is more ridiculous than the Japanese hat, Western leather shoes, and Chinese long gown.

SHLYJ: It seems there is no exterior-interior relationship between the Large Intestine and Lung. However, Ge Gen Tang 葛根汤 in *Shang Han Lun* 傷寒論 provides a different opinion. Headache, neck stiffness, aversion to wind are symptoms of

Taiyang disease, which has a relationship to the skin and body hair. Combination of syndromes of Taiyang 太陽 and Yangming 陽明 will surely bring diarrhea, which is related to Large Intestine disease. Taiyang 太陽 governs skin and body hair, in other words, the Lung governs skin and body hair. The *Jing Bie* 經別 chapter in *Ling Shu* 靈樞 says, "The separate branch of Yangming 陽明 channel descends to the Large Intestine and enters the Lung. The separate branch of Taiyin 太陰 channel enters the Lung, spreads in the Large Intestine."

YYX: There are at least three mistakes in this short paragraph. Actually, Yun Tieqiao 惲鐵樵 aims to prove the interior-exterior relationship between the Lung and Large Intestine, which is not acknowledged by the new medicine doctors. Yun Tieqiao 惲鐵樵 is motivated by a need to achieve fame and fortune, that's why he distorts the truth. According to what he says, headache, neck stiffness, aversion to wind are the symptoms of Taiyang 太陽 disease. Zhang Zhongjing 張仲景 had the same statement about that, but he never said they were related to the skin and body hair. It is reasonable to say aversion to wind is related to the skin and body hair. Neck stiffness is related to muscles and bones, not to skin and body hair. Headache, which is caused by a viral invasion of cerebral vessels, has no relationship to skin and body hair at all. Therefore, we know that ancient Chinese medicine is quite different from modern science. The inferences of ancient Chinese medicine are usually far-fetched; for example, Ge Gen Tang 葛根湯 syndrome belongs to Taiyang 太陽 disease; if Taiyang 太陽 disease is related to skin and body hair, then all symptoms of Ge Gen Tang 葛根湯 are related to skin and body hair, i.e. headache, stiffness are considered to have relationship with skin and body hair, though actually they have no relationship with the skin and body hair. Scientific approach is entirely different, being more exact and reliable; that's why many ancient theories are easily proven wrong by science.

Yun Tieqiao 惲鐵樵 says Taiyang 太陽 governs the skin and body hair. This is not only unreliable, but also ridiculous. He also says that Lung governs the skin and body hair, but doesn't provide any evidence. What Yun Tieqiao 惲鐵樵 says is not clear enough for people to understand, and I suspect he is also confused about these theories himself. Yun Tieqiao 惲鐵樵 is not able to find textual evidence to prove the exterior-interior relationship between Lung and Large Intestine. He has to select Ge Gen Tang 葛根湯 syndrome to prove that. However, Ge Gen Tang 葛根湯 is specialized for treating Taiyang 太陽 disease, so he has to say the Lung governs the skin and body hair, in order to get a relationship with the Large Intestine through diarrhea. He uses deceitful methods to get what he wants. According to what Yun Tieqiao 惲鐵樵 says, we can deduce that Taiyang 太陽 disease is equal to Lung disease, that the combined disease of Taiyang 太陽 and Yangming 陽明 is equal to the combined disease of Lung and Large Intestine and that Ge Gen Tang 葛根湯 is not only for treating Taiyang 太陽 disease but is also for Lung disease. But these conclusions are completely wrong. Yun Tieqiao 惲鐵樵 works hard to conceal the truth, but his efforts prove unavailing. Is his behavior beneficial to spreading *Ling Shu* 靈樞 and *Su Wen* 素問?

SHLYJ: Aversion to cold and diarrhea are completely different symptoms. However, Zhang Zhongjing 張仲景 succeeded in treating both with the same prescription Ge Gen Tang 葛根湯. For that matter, there is an obvious evidence for the exterior-interior relationship between the Lungs and Large Intestine.

YYX: How absurd this view is. There are many other examples that one herb or one prescription can treat several different kinds of diseases. Do all the affected organs have the exterior-interior relationship? Wu Mei Wan 烏梅丸 can treat both ascariasis and lingering dysentery, is it suitable to say ascariasis and dysentery have exterior-interior relationship? Di Dang Tang 抵當湯 is used to treat both women's menstrual disorders and men's blood stasis of bladder, can we say women and men have exterior-interior relationship? Or bladder and uterus have exterior-interior relationship? In *Shen Nong Ben Cao Jing* 神農本草經, some herbs can treat more than ten diseases. I really want Yun Tieqiao 惲鐵樵 to explain to me their exterior-interior relationships.

SHLYJ: It is quite effective to needle Hu Kou 虎口 for the treatment of toothache. Hu Kou 虎口 is called He Gu 合谷 in *Ling Shu* 靈樞. The *Jing Mai* 經脈 chapter recorded, "Hand-Yang Ming starts from the tip of the index finger. Running upward along the radial side of the index finger and passing through the interspace of the first and second metacarpal bones known as He Gu 合谷 (LI 4). The branch from the supraclavicular fossa runs upward to the neck, passes through the cheek and enters the gums of the lower teeth." What *Ling Shu* 靈樞 said is completely right. According to the physiology, both arteries and veins are connected to the heart, and nerve fibers are connected to the spinal cord. Capillaries distribute blood to the whole body. According to the findings, we know that Hu Kou 虎口 has special relationship with the gums; besides that, skin and hair are connected with the Large Intestine. Although *Ling Shu* 靈樞 failed to clearly explain the location of the Zang and Fu organs, it often achieved miraculous clinical effects, which remains an unsolved mystery. The excellent theories of *Su Wen* 素問 and *Shang Han Lun* 傷寒論 can find problems that are beyond the ability of today's Western medicine view of anatomy and microscope. It is not possible to know the functions only by knowing the location of the Zang and Fu organs, that's the main defect of Western medicine anatomy. How illogical and absurd this is!

YYX: There are many phenomena of human life and syndromes that cannot be explained by today's anatomy, physiology and pathology. Such as, when edema of nephritis occurs, it first appear as puffiness of the lower eyelids, and the nail clubbing usually seen in chronic lung diseases, and so on. Besides the relationship between gums and Hu Kou 虎口, there are far more examples. The ancients had handed down some written materials about these things, which can be used as the examples of Yun Tieqiao 惲鐵樵. It's a pity that he is not able to provide more such examples. The relationship between gums and Hu Kou 虎口 is a fact that was discovered by humans and *Ling Shu* 靈樞 recorded it; actually it is not a mystery. There are many facts or knowledge obtained from observing natural phenomena by human beings that cannot be proven by today's science. Such a situation exists not only in medicine. In my opinion, if there are some phenomena that haven't been properly explained by the ancients or proven by today's science, we can wait for the following researches to prove them later. It is not proper to choose far-fetched explanations from ancient books, and exaggerate the wisdom of the ancients.

SHLYJ: *Ling Shu* 靈樞 was written after *Su Wen* 素問. Some scholars thought it was quite different from *Su Wen* 素問 in literary style, and considered Wang Bing 王冰 as the compiler of it.

YYX: There were many scholars who thought *Ling Shu* 靈樞 was written after *Su Wen* 素問. However, according to the preface of *Huang Di Nei Jing Jiu Juan Ji Zhu* 黃帝內經九卷集註 by Huang Yuantong 黃元同, it was not a correct conclusion. The following are excerpts from this book:

"*Han Shu Yi Wen Zhi* 漢書藝文志 included 18 volumes of *Huang Di Nei Jing* 黃帝內經. Nine volumes were selected and entitled *Su Wen* 素問 by doctors, while the other nine volumes were not given a specific name. In the preface of *Shang Han Lun* 傷寒論, Zhang Zhongjing 張仲景 named the other nine volumes *Jiu Juan* 九卷. *Mai Jing* 脈經, which was written by Wang Shuhe 王叔和 in the Jin Dynasty 晉, also called the other nine volumes *Jiu Juan* 九卷. In the preface of *Jia Yi Jing* 甲乙經, Huang Fumi 皇甫謐 followed the view of Zhang Zhongjing 張仲景, i.e., *Huang Di Nei Jing* 黃帝內經 consisted of two parts; namely, *Jiu Juan* 九卷 and *Su Wen* 素問. Because *Su Wen* 素問 also had nine volumes, in order to avoid confusion, Huang Fumi 皇甫謐 suggested to call the other nine volumes *Zhen Jing Jiu Juan* 針經九卷, because *Zhen Jing* 針經 was the first chapter of the other nine volumes. However, *Zhen Jing* 針經 was not the real name, so Jia Yi Jing 甲乙經 still called those other nine volumes *Jiu Juan* 九卷. *Tai Su* 太素, which was compiled by Yang Shangshan 楊上善, also named the other nine volumes *Jiu Juan* 九卷. Wang Bing 王冰, who revised *Su Wen* 素問, called the other nine volumes *Ling Shu* 靈樞, based on the name of *Jiu Ling* 九靈. And he also used the name of *Zhen Jing* 針經 according to the preface of *Jia Yi Jing* 甲乙經. Lin Yi 林億 revised *Su Wen* 素問 in the Song Dynasty 宋, and said that, "according to Wang Bing 王冰, *Ling Shu* 靈樞 was the other name of *Zhen Jing* 針經, but the book's contents were not complete. He rearranged both *Su Wen* 素問 and *Ling Shu* 靈樞. So his *Ling Shu* 靈樞 was not the original one." Shi Song 史崧, a doctor of the Southern Song Dynasty 南宋, divided *Huang Di Nei Jing* 黃帝內經 into 24 volumes and 81 chapters. During the Yuan Dynasty 元, *Su Wen* 素問 was rearranged to 12 volumes, which had combined the volumes of *Ling Shu* 靈樞, hence the name of *Jiu Juan* 九卷 disappeared, and some scholars thought *Ling Shu* 靈樞 was written after *Su Wen* 素問. According to my research based on *Jia Yi* 甲乙 and *Tai Su* 太素, *Ling Shu* 靈樞 and *Su Wen* 素問 were written in the same period. And some scholars thought *Su Wen* 素問 was more difficult to understand than *Jiu Juan* 九卷. In my opinion, that's because *Nei Jing* 內經 was written by many different doctors. It is possible that some contents from *Su Wen* 素問 are more difficult to understand than *Jiu Juan* 九卷; however, some contents from *Jiu Juan* 九卷 can also be more difficult to understand than *Su Wen* 素問. After all, *Jiu Juan* 九卷 and *Su Wen* 素問 belong to *Nei Jing* 內經. In *Su Wen Tong Ping Xu Shi Lun* 素問通評虛實論, Huang Di 黃帝 had queried about bone measurement, pulse taking, and tendon lengths, but there was no answer. Wang Bing 王冰 thought the answer should be within the contents of *Ling Shu* 靈樞. Huang Fumi 皇甫謐 said *Nei Jing* 內經 had 18 volumes, and it was composed of *Jiu Juan* 九卷 and *Su Wen* 素問. His claims are credible and provable. Actually, the contents of *Zhen Jie Pian* 針解篇 in *Su Wen* 素問 originated from *Jiu Juan* 九卷; Lin Yi 林億 also said the same in his revision. In *Fang Sheng Shuai Lun* 方盛衰論[255] he states that the contents of combining five diagnostic methods and regulating Yin and Yang were in *Jing Mai* 經脈, which actually was a chapter of *Jiu Juan* 九卷. Wang Bing 王冰 also said this in his revision. In that case, it is even possible that *Su Wen* 素問 was written after *Jiu Juan* 九卷. Since *Su Wen* 素問 followed *Jiu Juan* 九卷, how can we say that *Jiu Juan* 九卷 is inferior to *Su*

[255] One chapter of *Su Wen* 素問

Wen 素問? In the preface of *Jia Yi Jing* 甲乙經, Huang Fumi 皇甫謐 said *Su Wen* 素問 and *Jiu Juan* 九卷 were subtle and should have equal status. In his book, he quoted more from *Jiu Juan* 九卷 than from *Su Wen* 素問. Yang Shangshan 楊上善 wrote a book called *Tai Su* 太素, which combined *Jiu Juan* 九卷 with *Su Wen* 素問.

SHLYJ: There was no discussion of anatomy in *Su Wen* 素問, but *Ling Shu* 靈樞 mentioned some things related to anatomy. Even if the ancient knowledge did not transmit down completely, there must be some indications in the ancient books. The literary style of books written by scholars in the Zhou-Qin Dynasties 周秦 is quite similar to *Su Wen* 素問. However, we are not able to find anatomy contents in these books. Therefore, we can conclude that some parts of *Su Wen* 素問 were written by scholars in the Zhou-Qin dynasties 周秦, and consequently there was no study of anatomy in that period.

YYX: Si Maqian 司馬遷 said, "Many scholars think the words of Huang Di 黃帝 are not refined and elegant, and the officials are ashamed to talk about Huang Di 黃帝." Medicine, which is a specialized subject, has no relationship to the studies of scholars in the Zhou-Qin dynasties 周秦. So the similarity between the texts of *Su Wen* 素問 and the books written by scholars in the Zhou-Qin dynasties 周秦 is not related to medicine. It is reasonable that there is no discussion of anatomy in these books. Human beings have an insatiable desire for knowledge. I don't believe that ancients in that time were completely indifferent to the research of internal organs. Bian Que 扁鵲 was able to see the internal organs after taking some medicine with dew. And there were some texts related to bone measurement, pulse taking and channels in *Ling Shu* 靈樞. So actually, the ancients were quite interested in anatomy, and they had made great efforts to research it. Due to the limited conditions in that period, the ancients were not able to develop the anatomy in a deep way. They obtained anatomical knowledge mainly based on experience. Though there were many mistakes, they deserve our respect. How can Yun Tieqiao 惲鐵樵 say that there was no study of anatomy in that period? How can he argue with the chapters of bone measurement, pulse taking, and small intestine and stomach in *Ling Shu* 靈樞? There were many anatomical descriptions of the internal organs in the ancient medical books; can we say they are just the imaginations of the ancients? Moreover, in addition to anatomy, *Ling Shu* 靈樞 and *Su Wen* 素問 have many other things that scholars of the Zhou-Qin dynasties 周秦 didn't discuss in their books. Actually, *Ling Shu* 靈樞 and *Su Wen* 素問 have very few texts similar to these books. According to Yun Tieqiao's 惲鐵樵 view, except for these similar texts, all the others are not reliable. And we can also say they didn't exist in that period. I don't know whether Yun Tieqiao 惲鐵樵 will admit his mistakes or not. There was no biography for Zhang Zhongjing 張仲景 in history and the name of *Shang Han Lun* 傷寒論 was not seen before Liang Dynasty 梁. Sun Simiao 孫思邈 was not able to get the full version of *Shang Han Lun* 傷寒論 while writing *Qian Jin Fang* 千金方. He only got it when he wrote *Qian Jin Yi* 千金翼. Zhang Shoujie 張守杰 quoted *Mai Jing* 脈經 in his *Shi Ji Zheng Yi* 史記正義, but he never mentioned *Shang Han Lun* 傷寒論. Judging from this, *Shang Han Lun* 傷寒論 appeared quite late, and its contents were not reliable. Can Yun Tieqiao 惲鐵樵 admit that? He made an excuse saying that the difficulty understanding *Shang Han Lun* 傷寒論 was caused by the doctors' concealment of it. In *Qun Jing Jian Zhi Lu* 群經見智錄, Yun Tieqiao 惲鐵樵 also said *Nei Jing* 內經 was hidden by doctors during the Spring and Autumn Period, thus it was not quoted by other medical books. Dismemberment was a form of punishment in ancient China. It was recorded in many ancient books, such as *Zhou Li* 周禮, *Zheng Yi* 正義, *Lü Shi Chun Qiu* 呂氏春秋, *Han Fei Zi Shuo Nan Pian* 韓非子說難篇, *Han Shu Jing Ji* 漢書景紀, *Gong Yang Xi San Shi Yi Nian* 公羊僖三十一年, *Shuo Yuan* 說苑 etc. Therefore, it is really reasonable for *Ling Shu* 靈樞 to have anatomical contents. *Yue Ling* 月令 discussed the sacrifice of the internal organs in chronological order, i.e. Spring–Spleen, Summer–Lung, Late Summer–Heart, Autumn–Liver, and Winter–Kidney, which were quite similar to the Lung–Wood, Lung–Fire, Heart–Earth, Liver–Metal and Kidney–Water in *Gu Shang Shu* 古尚書. Zheng Xuan 鄭玄 said, "It is ordered by the sequence of the four seasons and the location of the five internal organs." In order to know the location of the five internal organs, the ancients had to dissect the body. So it is certain that anatomy existed in ancient times. In my opinion, there were two ancient ways to define the relationship between the five Zang organs and five phases. One was based on the location; *Gu Shang Shu* 古尚書 and *Yue Ling* 月令 followed this way. Another one was based on color; *Shang Shu* 尚書 and *Nei Jing* 內經 followed this way. These two ways were used by doctors and were suitable for both livestock and human beings. Actually, the ancients not only knew the location of the five internal organs of the human being, but also knew that there was no difference in the location of the five internal organs between human beings and livestock. Besides human anatomy, the ancients began to develop the comparative anatomy in that period.

SHLYJ: *Su Wen* 素問 is a mysterious book. But the pathological contents in *Su Wen* 素問 and the channels, points, and bones chapters in *Ling Shu* 靈樞 are quite similar to psychology of Western medicine. However, psychology is the study of the mind, whereas the pathology of Chinese medicine is the study of the body's natural response to illness. *Ling Shu* 靈樞 is the research result of the human body by the psychological methods. The psychology of Western medicine researches the substance to figure out the capacity Shi Li 勢力. *Ling Shu* 靈樞 and *Su Wen* 素問 research the capacity Shi Li 勢力 to deduce the substance.

YYX: The symptoms—such as cold, heat, pain and itching—are the starting points for medical research. The symptomatology, as a part of medicine, researches the diseases by observing the symptoms. With knowledge unavailable yet and poor research methods, the ancients had to research illness based on visible symptoms. Therefore, research was quite superficial and non-specific. Mistakes are inevitable if we research diseases and channels based on them. The ancients should not be blamed. But the doctors of today should be blamed if they still follow these research methods, because material conditions and research methods have been greatly improved.

People who have a rudimentary knowledge of psychology are able to know whether *Ling Su* 靈素 are quite similar to psychology or not. Actually, Yun Tieqiao 惲鐵樵 knows little about psychology, but he tries to deceive people with specious words. We will know the truth if we compare his theories with psychology.

SHLYJ: *Ling Shu* 靈樞 was written after *Su Wen* 素問. Its truth remains unknown. If it is a real classic that is similar to *Su Wen* 素問, then its contents should have been proven for thousands of years, and the channels and points should be the research results of the pathology.

YYX: Yun Tieqiao 惲鐵樵 only knows the importance of experience. He ignores research methods, which are more important. How immature his methodology is! Experience is subjective and usually not reliable. A phenomenon is usually influenced by many factors. Something that is subjective is based on personal opinions and feelings rather than on facts. For example, Yun Tieqiao 惲鐵樵 credits the efficiency of Ma Xing Shi Gan Tang 麻杏石甘湯 to Ma Huang 麻黃. Such fallacies are based on personal opinions rather than facts. They are just his personal experience and haven't been proven by experiments. Science thinks highly of experiments, which is able to find out the truth from a variety of factors. However, a few mistakes are still inevitable because the experimental methods are not perfect. People will improve the experimental methods to make progress in medicine. In my opinion, the acquired experience which is provable by experiments should not be widely advocated. We have to find experimental methods to explain and prove it first. Psychology is also based on facts, and thinks highly of experiments, so it has made great progress. It is not possible to achieve progress by relying only on personal experience.

SHLYJ: There was a patient called Zou Yuwen 鄒聿文 who suffered from throat syndrome, which manifested as strong fever, foul breath and an adherent membrane on the throat. After taking pulse, I had abnormal sensation and aversion to cold in my whole body, so I knew he was developing an infectious disease.

YYX: What Yun Tieqiao 惲鐵樵 says is rubbish. Infection begins when pathogenic bacteria enter the body. The symptoms are not possible to appear at once. Only after several days' growth and reproduction of pathogenic bacteria, the symptoms—such as chills, fever, etc—will appear. So the infectious diseases have their specific latency period—the time between exposure to a pathogen and when symptoms first become apparent. Diphtheria usually begins to exhibit symptoms from two to eight days after exposure. It is absolutely ridiculous that Yun Tieqiao 惲鐵樵 thought himself to be infected during clinical duty according to the symptoms.

SHLYJ: The premonitory symptoms of all acute infectious diseases, such as chills and fever, can be considered and treated as a Taiyang syndrome 太陽證. If the Taiyang 太陽 disease has been cured, the bacteria are no longer able to harm the body. That's why Ma Huang 麻黃 can cure both throat syndrome and cold damage. So we know all bacteria will die if the Taiyang disease 太陽病 is cured.

YYX: According to Yun Tieqiao's 惲鐵樵 opinion, Ma Huang 麻黃 is omnipotent, sweating is omnipotent, and treating Taiyang 太陽 is omnipotent. We know he is completely wrong, based on the contents of *Shang Han Lun Tai Yang Pian* 傷寒論太陽篇, which said, "Taiyang disease 太陽病 with fever and thirst but without chill, is termed Wenbing 溫病. After adoption of sweating, if the patient feels a scorching heat in the body, it is termed Fengwen 風溫." So Fengwen 風溫 is a Taiyang disease 太陽病 that cannot be cured by sweating. It also said, "Taiyang disease 太陽病, which has been treated by sweating for three days, if the syndrome is still not gone after treating by emetic, purgative, or moxibustion with a warm needle, then it turns to be a worsened disease." "After the promotion of sweating, the body has pain and the pulse is deep and slow." "After the promotion of sweating, a jumping sensation below the umbilicus like running piglets starting to move, this is called Bentun 奔豚." "After the promotion of sweating, the patient feels abdominal distension." "After the promotion of sweating, the syndrome is not gone and the patient is restless." "After the promotion of sweating, the pulse is floating and rapid." Based on above examples, we know that the promotion of sweating is not able to cure all Taiyang 太陽 diseases. *Shang Han Lun* 傷寒論 discussed clearly the situations of improper sweating, incomplete sweating, excessive sweating. But the above quoted statements were not included in these situations. So treatment failure was caused by the progression of the disease, not the improper use of sweating. The chapter of Taiyang 太陽篇 said, "After using the promotion of sweating in a Taiyang disease 太陽病, profuse perspiration will exhaust the Stomach fluid. Consequently, the patient feels restless, unable to fall asleep, and thirsty." What can we get from this sentence? "After using the promotion of sweating in a Taiyang disease 太陽病, the patient has perspiration, but the syndrome is not gone. He still suffers from fever, palpitation, vertigo, muscle spasms, trembling and shivering which are likely to cause him to fall down." What can we get from this sentence? "After using the promotion of sweating in a Taiyang disease 太陽病, the patient has fever and chills." Fever and chills are not the original symptoms of Taiyang disease 太陽病, they are the symptoms caused by the promotion of sweating. "After cold damage is cured by the promotion of sweating, the patient may still suffer from Stomach disharmony, epigastric fullness and rigidity, belching, fetid breath, water stagnancy below the costal region, gurgling sound in the abdomen and diarrhea." The symptoms of Taiyang 太陽 have been relieved, but the disease hasn't been cured. In a word, there are many different varieties of Taiyang syndromes 太陽證候, some may be cured by the promotion of sweating while some may not. They are different in characteristic and pathology, so we should treat them in different ways. We cannot use the promotion of sweating in all Taiyang syndromes 太陽證. Yun Tieqiao 惲鐵樵 thinks Ma Huang 麻黃 is the only effective herb in the Ma Xing Shi Gan Tang 麻杏石甘湯. It is totally unfounded. He also has some fallacies in regards to the treatment of Taiyang disease 太陽. He neglects the true meaning of *Shang Han Lun* 傷寒論, and overstates the importance of relieving the Taiyang syndrome 太陽證. So Yun Tieqiao's 惲鐵樵 views are completely wrong, totally unreliable and deliberately misleading.

SHLYJ: There will be no survivors if an earthquake happens. Likewise, all bacteria will be killed if the exterior syndrome has been relieved and the sweat has been excreted.

YYX: The earthquake itself cannot kill living beings. It will cause the break of electric wires and gas pipes, house's collapse, tsunami and landslide, that's why living beings die. It is quite different to the situation of killing bacteria by sweating. He always mistakenly thinks that the bacteria are in the body surface, in order to make the relationship fit with Taiyang syndrome 太陽. If what he said is true, why cannot we use the method of killing bacteria to treat chills and shivering?

SHLYJ: I dare to doubt the things that were proven by theories of Western medicine. Do the bacteria cause the Taiyang diseases 太陽病? Or the Taiyang diseases 太陽病 produce bacteria? Are the bacteria the real cause of the diseases? If we plant bacteria in a patient, and that patient suffers the same disease, we can say that the bacteria are the cause of the diseases. But it is artificial rather than natural. For example, a throat syndrome that was caused by planted bacteria is artificial, whereas being caused by severe climate change is natural. The natural throat syndrome can be treated by relieving Taiyang 太陽, because the bacteria are the product of Taiyang 太陽, the bacteria will be killed if Taiyang 太陽 syndrome is cured.

YYX: It is completely wrong to say the bacteria will be killed if Taiyang 太陽 syndrome is cured. If a person doesn't have Taiyang 太陽 syndrome, according to Yun Tieqiao's 惲鐵樵 opinion, even if we plant bacteria in his body, he will not suffer from this disease. Yun Tieqiao 惲鐵樵 thinks the bacteria are not able to survive without Taiyang 太陽. But actually, this person will suffer from disease based on the planted bacteria, regardless of having Taiyang disease 太陽病 or not. Are there any differences between artificial and natural infection of bacteria? The bacteria used in the experiments are from patients with natural throat syndrome. The nature of bacteria will not change in the process of planting the bacteria in another body. It is quite similar to spreading of a disease by airborne droplets and oral contact. Yun Tieqiao 惲鐵樵 certainly will deny the existence of infection. The infectivity is caused by a particular substance, and it has no relationship with climate change. Wu Youke 吳又可 named this particular substance Li Qi 戾氣, which is called bacteria in Western medicine. Yun Tieqiao 惲鐵樵 accepts the existence of infection, but he denies the existence of bacteria, and insists that the climate change is the cause of the disease. Mr. Yun 惲 has never made bacteriological examination before and after the onset of a Taiyang syndrome 太陽证, so his views are not trustworthy. It also shows his disrespect to the rules of creating new theories. It is impossible to make so many mistakes without his deliberate intentions. These mistakes can be easily found out if paying enough attention.

SHLYJ: In my opinion, it is not reliable to treat disease only based on its type. The types of typhoid in Western medicine are classified by its treatment.

YYX: Yun Tieqiao's 惲鐵樵 views are internally inconsistent. He thinks all doctors of Western countries use the same method to treat typhoid, while the ancient Chinese medicine doctors use different methods. If that were the case, I would agree that it is not reliable to treat disease only based on its type. Unfortunately, there is no specific treatment for typhoid until now. Different doctors may use quite different methods for the treatment of typhoid. However, the fever types of typhoid are exactly the same in different countries. So it is wrong to say that the types of typhoid in Western medicine are classified by its treatment. Somebody told Yun Tieqiao 惲鐵樵 Western medicine doctors use calomel to treat typhoid; he then supposes that all Western medicine doctors use calomel to treat typhoid. Moreover, he criticizes Western medicine doctors based on that. How insane he is! Meng Zi 孟子 said "we have to know well the person who we are going to criticize." Is it suitable to publicly criticize persons or things that we only know little or based on hearsay? All these indicate that Yun Tieqiao 惲鐵樵 has a superficial mind.

Book chapter end

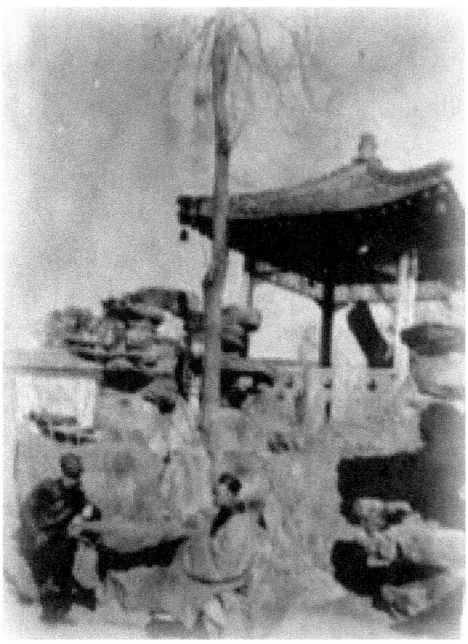

Photo by Mr P. Goux in early 1900s. "At the Ladies' Palace".

Yu Jianquan's "Meridians and blood vessels are not the same" theory 俞鉴泉经脉血管不同说

Note: Mr. Yu Jianquan's article was published in Hang Zhou's *Double Three Medical Report*, Series 1 issue 12, November 23rd year of Gui Hai (1923).
杭州三三醫報第一卷第十二期癸亥十一月二十三日出版.

Yaron: Yu Jianquan and Yun Tieqiao both responded to Yu Yunxiu on similar footings; they argued that Chinese medicine theories, such as meridians, are beyond the scope of Western medicine and therefore should maintain their unique system and not merge but, rather, co-exist with Western medicine.

The principle is: if you look for silk, one must seek it in the fine threads, if one wants to raise a net, he must lift it from the guiding rope. Therefore, any affair and its theory must attain its truthful and proper ropes and threads. The affair then can start having a principle, the theory can start being examined. If one would ask where are the threads and ropes of my medicine's theory? There is the distribution of the meridians and vessels, the temperament of the Zang Fu organs. In the realm of the new medicine there is this book *Ling Su Shang Dui*. Its words toward the *Ling Su* are of such an attack, wishing to leave for it no ground to stand on. The intention of the author is harsh. I would not describe it here in detail. Generally speaking, it claims that there is not one useful word in the *Nei Jing*, that it is a book that killed people for thousands of years. There are many colleagues of my medicine who have read it.

I also know that thousands-years-old medicine cannot be slammed to the ground. Why to embrace making people worried, argue and contend on every little matter? More so, with this I have experience of more than a year. I will make his main points and compare them here. I will clarify a little the true value of my medicine, this is my bound duty.

What the new medicine community is most unhappy about, when it comes to our medicine, is the entering and exiting beginning and end of the meridians. One should also know that when we say Jing 經, in Jing Mai 經脈, it is the Qi going in the 12 meridians. Mai 脈 of Jing Mai 經脈 is also not tubes. We can see that the *Shuo Wen* 說文 explains the character Mai as blood circulation spreading in the entire body. *Yu Pian* 玉篇 also explains as blood circulation. *Zheng Zi Tong* 正字通 says Mai is the Qi of five Zang and 6 Fu organs that flows to the four extremities. What is called "blood circulation" means the Qi of the Zang Fu. Clearly it is the Qi of the meridians. It is not blood tubes (vessels). Blood vessels are like the frontiers of the tree branches, if one merges it as one with Jing Mai then it is like "a southward bound cart travelling north". It is like horses and oxen that can't mix together. So how can one blame his attacks?

When Western medicine treats a disease, the blood vessels are the main key (fishing rope). They have capillaries, returning blood vessels, fixed vessels, veins, arteries, big arteries, big veins. They are all tubes. Therefore, Western medicine gives great importance to blood vessels. They give importance to the physical form. What I call "Jing Mai" is the Jing 經 of Qi. It is not a tube. There might be some places where blood vessels merge together with it, however, the blood vessel is still a blood vessel, the meridian is still a meridian. Therefore it is not called Mai, nor is it called a tube, nor a blood vessel, it is called a Jing Mai 經脈.

Jing Mai is where the Qi of the five Zang and six Fu travels. It is the outer boundary of the Zang Fu organs. I will use a "residence" as an analogy. The residence of a person always has an entry and exit path. For example, the inner residence of the kidneys is like the place where one keeps his treasure, the secret room. The urinary bladder is like the outer hall where one meets other people for a chat. The Tai Yang meridian has the outer path of the residence, therefore it is called Jing Mai. It is where the Qi of the Zang Fu go and spread to the four extremities.

Therefore, Qi and blood adjunct to the Tai Yang meridian belong to Tai Yang. Qi and blood adjunct to Shao Yang meridian belong to Shao Yang, the other meridians likewise. Whenever there are blood vessels in proximity of a certain meridian then they belong to that meridian. The 12 meridians distribute all over the body like heaven's garment without a seam. If you look at it you can't see it. The ones who knew it are the saints and sages of antiquity. And so, one can rely on meridians and use it for treatment. This explanation, I know that one may not necessarily believe it right away, or think that the curved is perfectly rounded.

As for blood, it does not only flow inside the tubes without coming out, it circulates between the skin and muscles, and permeates as well outside the tubes, and so it can reach to muscles and flesh. One can try to test it: when needles and blades pierce the skin a little bit, blood immediately permeates out. One clearly can ask: from which blood tube branch is this blood coming out? Jing Mai meridians, however, circulate all over between skin and muscles, partially revolves with the muscle cracks, some deep some superficial, therefore there are differences between Jing Shu 井俞 points and Ying and Wei 營衛 Qi. And so when blood surges, Jing Mai also surges; when blood declines, Jing Mai also declines, one can palpate the Jing Mai and estimate the surge and decline of blood, in addition he may know the surge and decline of Zang Fu.

The human body left and right, arms and legs, above and below, front and rear are all different. It is like borders of different countries. Weather has different Qi of hot, cold, cool and warm. Residing inside are the Zang Fu, distributed outwards are the meridians. When Jing Mai meridians are diseased, it prevents it from entering into the Zang Fu. If Zang Fu have disease, it also impacts the meridians. The one who wants to treat it needs to differentiate between Jing Mai and Zang Fu, hot cold warm or cool. One may use the Zang Fu to treat the meridians or use the meridians to treat the Zang Fu. These meridians follow the principle that one can use them to inspect outside and know the inside, or inspect the inside and know the outside. The ancient sages tested it already for a long time. Be it an internal syndrome or external inflicted injury, it all follows this ancestral principle.

The importance of Jing Mai is exactly this. What we call blood and blood tubes, do we have to ask about it? No. Blood is still water principle. Substance and quality of water is everywhere. Jing Mai connects to the Qi of Zang Fu, it distributes to the flesh and muscles. It enters and exits with Qi and blood, majestic just like the different frontier borders. And blood is like the substance of water. It spreads everywhere. Now Jing Mai is Qi. Qi can transform into blood, while blood in each body section follows each meridian's Qi transformation. The meridian of foot Tai Yin begins in the foot and goes straight upward, circulates on the back and head, it is most notably departing on a path far from blood vessels. This meridian being separated from blood vessels is one testimony. Tai Yang is the meridian of cold water. When one uses herbs (for it), it is proper to use warm herbs, while cool herbs are prohibited. This is another testimony how blood follows the meridian's Qi and transform. Foot Shao Yang meridian has a lot of Qi and little blood, when using herbs it is appropriate to use clearing heat herbs while hot herbs are prohibited, the blood is also following the meridian's Qi and transform, this is another evidence. Shao Yang meridian circles the ear and reaches to the hairline corner. When the human hair becomes white, most often it starts from the two hairline corners, it is one evidence for the "lots of Qi and little blood". If one merges the knowledge of the meridian with the correct knowledge of herb application then it is like a raft and drum acting in response (work in perfect coordination).

Western medicine is good with instruments, with the dissection method, with using microscope to narrowly see the little blood vessels progression. Therefore, when they treat a disease, using the blood vessels is their principle. This principle, as well, contains the possibility of reaching a disease cure. Now meridians, which are invisible to the eye, and on the grounds of dissection are being contested, not one of them is suitable. What we call five Zang temperament like joy, anger, sadness and fear, even more so belong to the absent minded. They are all artificial fallacies not worthy to be based on. It seems that, with all this, *Ling Su* has no value whatever.

I came across *Ling Su Shang Dui* unexpectedly. It is scornful to antiquity just like this. Furthermore, and unexpectedly, it came out of the offspring of the same parents. And so, Mr. Yu Yunxiu wantonly used his sharpened pen, saying that he himself in the past likewise participated in the killing of people (patients). People, to the end, cannot believe this. Why must I talk on and on about it and try to make sense of it? One item after the other battle it? It is because I am worried that future students will read his book and become perplexed. Therefore, I lightly explain here what is similar and what is different between Jing Mai meridians and blood vessels. I only hope that profound scholars will further this discussion.

Article end

Refuting Yu Jianquan's "*Meridians and Blood Vessels are not the Same" Theory* 驳俞鉴泉经脉血管不同说

Yaron: Yu Yunxiu crushes Yu Jianquan in this argument because Jianquan cannot substantiate his claims, at least not in a physical manner. Yu's critique, as before, simply points out that substantiating one's theory cannot simply rely on previous claims—claims which, themselves, do not have adequate proof.

This critique points to Chinese medicine's vulnerability: how to build a theoretical building with a solid foundation. The modernizers of Chinese medicine during the Republic and Communist eras used modern science as a foundation. This may have been the only way, if one chose to follow noted Republican era reformers such as vice president of the Bureau for Native Medicine Shi Jinmo 施今墨.[256] He believed that modern science is the only possible truth and there could be no two truths for one single item. Despite Yu Yunxiu exercising a harsh criticism against Chinese medicine building blocks such as meridians using a physical fact-based scientific model, we should still use it to reflect and build a stronger house.

During a long Chinese medicine history, at least so I believe, some people found amazing things, while others had an exaggerated and vivid imagination. To discover a true thing is rather difficult, while to imagine things is easy. There are those who say that first you need to imagine something then you can discover it; one may ponder this principle as well.

Scroll 3 pages 19–22

I have written the *Ling Su Shang Dui* in the 6th year of the republic (1917) in order to expose the falsehood of the *Nei Jing*. In the past 6 or 7 years, more and more people have read it. Each one felt deep heartache about my book; they all thought to attack it very happily, and for a period of time I thought that one should not do it like this. However, laying out the truth, there is no alternative but doing it. And so, some smart people have thought to alter the old sayings in order to dodge quickly the sharp blade of my knife. Last year, Mr. Yun Tieqiao wrote his *Qun Jing Jian Zhi Lu*. He adopted an idea that, in the *Nei Jing*, when it speaks of the 5 Zang organs it speaks of 5 Zang of seasonal Qi transformation, that these are not flesh and blood organs; it was a move of trying to dodge. Today, Mr. Yu Jianquan's treatise is still an attempt to dodge. However, what they know and their theories flee not into a safe haven. Why must I pursue endlessly and demand explanations from them? In addition, the *Ling Su Shang Dui* that I wrote does not have great enmity with the *Nei Jing*. It does, however, make a clear distinction between this and the truth. It does not obsequiously agree with the ancients. It does not have blind faith in the ancients and that's it, it cries out with loud voice: wake up from superstition and idiotic dreams. It is like lifting the child's ear up to teach him a lesson. It teaches them straight on a lesson to not advocate mysterious talk, embrace and rely on fantasy. One must seek the truth from facts, thoroughly explore things in order to understand the art's truth. I just hoped that they could become enlightened and that's it.

[256] 1881–1969

As for the saying that the meaning of my words are too harsh, I fear that Yu Jiayan 喻嘉言, Cheng Jiaoqian 程郊倩 scolding Wang Shuhe 王叔和, Ye Xiangyan 葉香嚴 scolding Zhang Jingyue 張景岳, Xu Lingtai 徐靈胎 scolding Zhao Yangkui 趙養葵, Lu Jiuzhi 陸九芝 scolding Yu 喻 and Cheng 程, compared to myself, are much more excessive. Recorded in the classics of the old medicine, these kinds of "scolding" are too numerous to count, and yet only the meaning of my *Ling Su Shang Dui* is too harsh. My guess is that, when they think of Yu and Cheng scolding, it is like between brothers and that this does not have any impact on the future of the old medicine; however, the critics of *Ling Su Shang Dui* compare it to foreign aggression. They feel that the foothold of the old medicine may completely collapse. This is the reason for the deep-rooted hatred against me. In reality, this is all sectarian bias; it is not arguing about the science itself.

In all earnest, I want to tell Mr. Yu, it is not that I can't hang out my shingle and become a doctor. If I would choose to be a Chinese medicine doctor, quoting authoritative works, not necessarily will I not match you, grasping in my palm high talk, not necessarily will I lag far behind you. If I chose to be a Chinese medicine doctor and would contend with you an argument, likely I would be able to keep pace with you all, certainly not gap far behind you. Therefore, in my position today, if I wanted to be an old medicine doctor then I could; if I want to be new medicine doctor then I can. Going in and out, I settle in a place where I feel my freedom. There is no high enough pile of rocks or deep enough gully that can stop me. If I would do things only for the sake of my livelihood, then I will hold in my hand ambiguous, difficult-to-understand rationality, I will speak in a shilly-shally attitude and I will now-sink, now-emerge, with the customs of the world. How is that not a better strategy? Even so, knowing it and yet not doing it like this, being able to do it and yet deciding not to do it like this, it is because Yin Yang five phases explanations, Zang Fu and meridians theories are absurd and strange. One cannot believe and comply with them. It is because I got the guidance of true principle, my conscience would not let me let go of it. Therefore, I wrote the *Ling Su Shang Dui.* It was in order to clarify true principle and that's it! There is no sectarian bias there. How can the sect of the old medicine limit itself to (targeting) myself? Me, myself, I want to understand the truth and yet the old doctors start sectarian controversies. Judging the difference between people here is just too big.

Mr. Yu's "*Meridians and Blood Vessels Are Not the Same*" *Theory*, on its own, is not worthy of repudiation. Pitifully, he is very confused, and if there are still people in the world that may believe in such things, momentarily I will leave it for everyone else to decide. Today's old medicine doctors ask patients to stretch forward their arms; with three fingers they feel their pulse, what they feel at the tip of their finger is the blood vessel. Isn't this a blood vessel? Obviously it is the up and down movement of the blood vessel. I know that he cannot but force himself to answer it is a Jing Mai 經脈 meridian. The ancients, in *San Bu Jiu Hou* 三部九候, explained that the artery in front of the ear and on both sides of the forehead are Jing Mai 經脈, but isn't it a blood vessel? Clearly, it is the up-and-down movement of the blood vessel. I know that he cannot but force himself to answer it is a Jing Mai 經脈 meridian. Also, when the old medicine doctors diagnose the pulse being floating, sunken, slow, fast, surging, wiry, stopping and knotty, is this a meridian or a blood vessel? Obviously it is the up and down movement of the blood vessel. I know that he cannot but force himself to answer it is a Jing Mai 經脈 meridian. From this, one can see that when the old medicine doctors diagnose a disease, this thing they say is Qi transformation of the 5 Zang and 6 Fu organs, it is all coming from the blood vessel, and yet they have the air on them to tell people that meridians are meridians and blood vessels are blood vessels. They believe that what *Ling Su Shang Dui* strikes is irrelevant to the old medicine theory of meridians. Alas, who can they swindle?

Let's use the *Nei Jing* again as a proof:

Su Wen Mai Yao Jing Wei Lun 素問脈要精微論 states: "Mai 脈 is the residence of blood." How does Yu explain this? *Ling Shu Ying Wei Sheng Hui* 靈樞營衛生會 states: "Middle Jiao merge at the stomach, after exiting from upper Jiao, this is where Qi is received, it secretes the waste matter, steams the fluids, it transforms its essence and moistens the Mai of the lungs. Then it transforms into blood in order to serve the entire body, there is nothing more precious than this, there it alone gets to circulate in the midst of the Jing Sui 經隧, it is called Ying Qi 營氣." Look here, Jing Sui 經隧, not only is it Jing (like in meridians) it also has Sui 隧 tunnel. If it is not a blood vessel what else can it be? There is only blood flowing in its midst, if not blood vessel what else is it?

Su Wen Ping Ren Qi Xiang Lun 素問平人气象論 states: "under the nipple, the movement reaches the clothes then ancestral Qi leaks." Here, the *Nei Jing* clearly describes the heart movement and yet the *Nei Jing* says it is Qi.

Ling Shu Wu Shi Ying 灵枢五十营 states: "The Human Jing Mai meridians above below left and right front and rear are 28 Mai, in the entire body their length are 16 Zhang two Chi 十六丈二尺, which corresponds to the 28 lunar mansions. The water leaks 100 Ke 刻 and it separates day from night. Therefore, when a person inhales, the Mai moves twice, the Qi advances three Cun. One exhale and the Mai moves again twice, the Qi advances three Cun." Here there is a clear description of the artery beating and the blood wave movement. The *Nei Jing* thinks that the movement inside Jing Mai is Qi moving. Can Mr. Yu still argue that movement of Qi in Jing Mai is entirely unrelated to blood flow in blood vessels like Horses and Oxen that cannot mix?

Ling Shu Jiu Zhen Shi Er Yuan 灵枢九针十二原 states: "Jing Mai 12, Luo Mai 15, together 27 Qi go up and down. Where it comes out is Jing 井, where it retains is Ying 滎, where it irrigates is Shu 俞, where it progresses is Jing 經, the 27 Qi advances are all in the Shu 俞 points. Where the knots Jie 節 cross, these are the 365 meetings. Knowing its essence can be summarized with one sentence; not knowing its essence will cause one to scatter endlessly. What is called Jie 節, it is where the spirit Qi travels in and out—not skin, muscles, tendons and bones."

Here, the assumption is that not only Qi travels in Jing Mai but Qi also travels in Luo Mai 絡脈. When you look at the human body and you see these greenish lines like a net under the skin like tree branches, does Mr. Yu think that these are blood vessels or Luo Mai? I know that he will have to dodge it and say "well, these are blood vessels!" So may I ask, when the ancients spoke of Luo Mai being smaller and superficial and closer to the surface and are often seen, other than these veins blood vessels, what else can one see? How come Mr. Yu doesn't think this carefully? In addition, this thing they call Spirit Qi, *Ling Shu Ying Wei Sheng Hui* 灵枢营卫生会 explains as follows: "Blood is spirit Qi." From this, one can see that when *Jiu Zhen Shi Er Yuan* 九针十二原 states "Jing Mai 12, Luo Mai 15, it is where spirit Qi travels in and out" it is nothing other than blood flowing in and out. How does Mr. Yu explain this?

Mr. Yu says: "the 12 Jing Mai distribute to the entire body, like seamless heaven clothing, if you look at it you can't see it." This statement is false. *Ling Shu Jing Mai* 灵枢经脉 states: "Jing Mai are 12; hidden, they travel between the cracks of the muscles." It means that Jing Mai are submerged deep inside the muscles, they hide from view so one can't see them. They are not like Luo Mai which are superficial, at the surface and can be seen. If one uses dissection then he can see it, it is not hidden anymore. Even without dissection, when it gets close enough to the surface one can see it. Therefore, *Jing Mai* 经脉篇 chapter states: "What commonly can be seen is foot Tai Yin going by the medial part of the ankle. It is not hidden there, and then one can see it." Mr. Yu thinks that it is like heaven clothing without a seam, you look at it and you can't see it. The only ones who could see it were the ancient sages. It is a clear-cut attempt to make Jing Mai a vague concept. He turned his back on the classics and ignored the ancients. His great slander of the *Nei Jing* goes too far.

In my words, what I use as evidence is not my own fabrication; it is reproduced from the *Nei Jing* one line after the other and one can compare. Mr. Yu invents all kinds of absurd statements, he even didn't penetrate deeply the *Nei Jing*. I don't know how he nominated himself to be "a person who has studied and read the classics intensively for many years", where did everything he read disappear to?

In general, Mr. Yu's sectarian bias is very deep; he hates my *Ling Su Shang Dui* to the utmost degree. He wants to attack it but has no way of doing it; in a flurry he flees, hurriedly he wants to find a place to place his foot, but he lingers there on a steadily worsening condition, with this he is too late to plan having the whole situation in mind. Carefully pondering the *Nei Jing*, he has no choice but to deliver theories of half explanation, list one and omit thousands. Enthusiastically talking rubbish, he is ignorant of the fact that he cannot fool singlehandedly the eyes of everyone under heaven. His other odd statements such as "When Western medicine treats disease it uses blood vessels as guiding principle", or "blood does not travel in the blood vessels, it also permeates outside the vessels"—these are all idiotic nonsense not worth one laugh. More so, one can say that these are the layman words of the ignoramus, one should not be too critical of these. It is only that he calls himself "a person who has studied and read intensively the old classics for many years." He is still rusty and superficial, his mistakes absurd and reckless make this kind of shape, really one can say that he is such a dude that boasts shamelessly!

Article end

The new book of protecting newborn babies 保赤新書

Original title: Pediatrics Teaching Materials 原名幼科講義

1928 by Yun Tieqiao 惲鐵樵

Published April 1928, Printed by Huafeng Printing and Cast Type Shop

Available in the Clinic of Yun Tieqiao at the following address: Shanghai San Ma Lu Yunnan Lu Zengleli Sannong Erjia

中華民國十七年四月出版 華豐印刷鑄字所 發行處上海三馬路雲南路曾樂里三弄二家惲鐵樵醫寓

Yaron: Yun Tieqiao confronted the anatomy debate: is modern dissection and anatomy the only true way to look at one's body? He argued that Qi transformation is different from the physical body and believed that a living human being has more than just a physical body.

Another difficult issue facing him was the introduction, by modern medicine, of germs and bacteria as disease agents. It contrasted the old medicine notion of heaven Qi transformation being the disease cause. Before the advent of antibiotics, Western medicine had little success with treating bacteria—as Tieqiao correctly points out—however, they used this knowledge with great success during the Manchurian plague and with hygiene, sterilization techniques etc. Yun Tieqiao became well aware of the situation and oftentimes, as is the case here, was learning modern medical knowledge.

The traditionalists, Tieqiao being one of their figures, learned some modern medicine in order to define better their own medicine, i.e. they wanted to set the difference clear. Their aspiration was to integrate the two medical models into the society by separating them—a state of coexistence, where one can supplement the other's shortcomings. As modern medicine progresses, so can Chinese medicine; they can be separated and complementary. Yun Tieqiao explains his view in the following book excerpt. Within his arguments, some are outdated while others are still valid a century later. Tieqiao uses modern medical knowledge to advance his own, all along maintaining a distinct principle: separating the two so they can coexist.

Chapter: Smallpox vaccination

Pages 8–10

In all kinds of pediatric diseases one must have a proper nursing method. When a doctor uses herbs well there is never a problem, only with smallpox it is hard to tell. Where do small kids get smallpox from? According to ancient Chinese medical texts, the burning desire of father and mother in the pre-heaven state, the father's essence and the mother's blood smelt together Yin Yang and create a fetus. As this fetus is being created there is a smallpox seed imbued within. In foreign countries' medical literature measles, smallpox, chicken pox, scarlet fever, typhoid fever etc diseases are all considered acute infectious diseases. In all of them one can see red spots on the patient's skin. However the disease etiology is not well understood. More or less the claim is that they are all caused by microbes, however is it a bacteria or a protozoan? Nobody really knows for certain. When a virus enters the body mostly it enters via the respiratory system.

One sees here that Eastern and Western medicines are completely different, such as the two very different explanations of burning desire versus microbes. Each has their opinion and that is how they carry it out. According to the burning desire theory it is an internal cause. It is something which is naturally concealed within one's body. It begins inside one's body and it comes out to the exterior. According to the microbes' theory it is an external cause. It is a virus coming from the external world and invades inward. What Chinese theory says is the cause Western theory contradicts, and what Western theory says is the cause Chinese theory contradicts.

My humble opinion in this matter is as follows: if we say that this is an entirely internal cause, so how come there is a smallpox virus epidemic and one sees that there are many cases happening exactly at that time? So looking just at this one fact, even if we say that this is an internal cause, there must be an external factor instigating it and only then the disease acts up. If one claims that it is entirely an external factor, this assertion is also wrong. How come a person will contract only one time smallpox in their lifetime? In addition, most people who receive the cow pox vaccine will not get infected, how come? Isn't it the case that the person himself has this disease within, and after the disease expressed itself one time, the seed within was used up completely? Therefore it cannot express itself again. Western medical books say that after the disease is contracted one time, the person has immunity for the rest of their lives. They also say that people who did not receive the cowpox vaccine are prone to contract the infection.

So this is it! One uses pox from the outside and instigates the seed from the inside to come out. Through the cowpox, one's own toxin is being expressed outward and there is nothing left within. Even though there are still viruses outside in the world, when they enter the body the inner cause is already absent and disease cannot come about. This is a much better and complete theory. Even though all you gentlemen may laugh at me, mocking me for merging Chinese and Western, thinking that I am an opportunist, the butterfly party. Humble me would rather have an affable discussion towards both Chinese and Western medicines. What I will say, everyone will appreciate.

The medicine of China, judging by the *Neijing*, is a kind of doctrine describing heaven and man join their virtue. Even though it talks about night and day, birth, growth, decline and storage, things based on evidence, yet it also contains other things characterized as mystery. Flatly not like the accuracy of science. In addition, Western countries' medical science has researched things already in very fine details, really paying attention. It reaches to the smallest of things like red blood cells, white blood cells, tiny nerves, cell nuclei as well as bacteriology. These certainly cannot be ascribed to the two words dissection and anatomy. It is also something that could not have been found with a mere imaginative thinking of heaven and man join their virtue.

Now, when we speak about the Western medicine principle of pathology, certainly it is with profound ability, yet treatment methods, aside from blood serum, sterilization and special effect drugs, there is nothing other than treating symptoms or prevention. Often they have an attitude of looking onward unconcerned. They hear that the virus has invaded and their efficacy is the same as if the patient takes no drugs at all. Only when the disease has entered deep then they adopt methods such as strengthening heart, guarding lungs, protecting the brain, which are methods slightly short of "fighting fire after setting the field ablaze". Unavoidably, the patient is in a terrible mess. Special effect drugs, even though invented daily, they treat a disease and most often can't clear the toxin completely. It stays inside and on another occasion it surfaces again as an internal root of yet another disease. This, one cannot claim to be a perfect treatment modality.

Truly, China's Ma Huang 麻黃,[257] Gui Zhi 桂枝, Ge Gen 葛根, Chai Hu 柴胡, Bai Hu 白虎, Cheng Qi 承氣, Tong Mai Si Ni 通脈四逆, when a disease is superficial they can eliminate it quickly and when the disease is severe they can raise patients from their death bed. Today, people who know both Chinese and Western medicine surely understand what I mean. It is not my hobby to be partial. Nonetheless, Chinese medicine time and time again displays this special aptitude. With this point one can certainly be self-satisfied. However, these days, Chinese medicine doctors able to deliver this kind of effect are still only one out of a hundred.[258] Therefore increasingly by comparison it looks insufficient. My humble opinion is that Chinese medicine should always be a simultaneous treatment together with Western medicine. It can supplement the deficient parts in an indirect way. Therefore with great enthusiasm I compile this book. Readers and Gentlemen, I will receive gratefully any criticism you may have toward my discussion here. When I print this book again I will include it as a pool of wisdom. I will conclude the small gossip here and return to the main theme.

Chapter: Herbs that can't be used during measles and the reason why

Yaron: Tieqiao does not shy away from modern medical knowledge but he constantly strives to develop the new in his own medicine. Developing the new in Chinese medicine while maintaining a distinct medical logic is a perfect model for the 21st century. In my opinion, if we blend Chinese medicine into modern medicine, like the Communists envisioned, it will simply disappear—becoming a chapter in the history of medicine.

Pages 23–25

There are a few herbs that should not be used during measles. The first is Shi Hu 石斛, the second Yuan Zhi 遠志, third Yu Shu Dan 玉樞丹, Bao Chi San 保赤散, Hui Chun Dan 回春丹, Zhi Bao Dan 至寶丹, Niu Huang Wan 牛黃丸, Mr Wan's Niu Huang Wan 萬氏牛黃丸, Jin Shu Shi 金鼠矢. Aside from a few other herbs allowed according to *Ben Cao Gang Mu* all the others as well should not be used. If one asks what is the reason for this prohibition? It is because I have often seen kids that have

[257] These are shortened names of herbal formulas; Ma Huang Tang, Gui Zhi Tang, Ge Gen Tang, Chai Hu Tang, Bai Hu Tang, Cheng Qi Tang, Tong Mai Si Ni Tang.

[258] This can mean both one doctor out of 100 doctors or treating 100 diseases and succeeding with only one disease.

used these and the harm done to them was great. So I bring this discussion here on purpose to allow doctors who have humble hearts to take note how to take care of little kids.

Why do they want to use Shi Hu 石斛 then? People who use this herb of course have their own reason to do so. They say that since the child fever is high, they are most worried that the kid's Yin fluid will be burned dry by the strong heat. When Yin fluid is dry then the disease cannot be saved. If the patient's tongue is very dry and Shi Hu is used then the tongue immediately turns moist. If the tongue is moist then the Yin fluid is not dry, even if there is strong fever there is no real reason to worry. This is the argument for using Shi Hu. Also among all the Yin-nurturing herbs only Shi Hu is not sticky, therefore one feels at ease in using it. There is nothing else to worry about.

Humble me wants to bring this statement into discussion. One needs to realize that when fever is high and Yin dries out this is an affair of Shao Yin meridian. In other words, when there is high fever that still did not transmit inward, more or less the ancients would use herbs like Tian Dong 天冬, Yu Zhu 玉竹, E Jiao Ji Zi Huang 阿膠雞子黃 etc, during this time using Shi Hu is also possible. This is, so they say, when the disease is still in three Yang one can use Shi Hu. This shows that the understanding of Zhang Zhongjing theory is entirely wrong, the *Neijing* understanding is entirely wrong.

When *Neijing* states "when disease is warm, deficiency extreme, then there is death." The word "deficiency" here means Yin deficiency. It shows that when the disease is at three Yang there is never the principle there of Yin deficiency. I have explained this in great detail in my *Neijing Jiang Yi* 內經講義. At this time hastily nurturing Yin, one only knows that if the tongue is moist then Yin is not dry, how come one does not know that when you nurture Yin than the pathogens cannot come to the surface. When the toxin is obstructed by the sweet cool herb and then the chest feels as if there is a lump in it and fullness, the throat becomes inflamed, thrush in the oral cavity and all sorts of other problems that are hard to get rid of.

The modern doctor, who has a bit more experience, on the one hand uses Shi Hu and on the other hand tells the family about the patient "I am afraid that this kind of disease will result in oral thrush." When time comes and this thrush comes about the patient's family is impressed and falsely believes that the doctor can forecast the future, his skill must be not bad. The doctor himself being able to predict thrush feels proud of himself as if he has reached heaven and Godly level. When it comes to the patient finally dying it is as if they are too busy to ask about it. The patient has died and people still don't understand what has transpired. When other members of the family become sick they still bring them to the same doctor. The doctor himself till his last day cannot understand what has happened. When he diagnoses and treats other patients he still uses his Shi Hu. For this kind of fellow it is best to not give a name, one should only say "one who severs destiny". One cannot use Shi Hu when cold injury ties warm disease 傷寒系溫病. One cannot use it with measles as well.

These five words "cold injury ties warm disease" 傷寒系溫病 is a concept that I invented. One can read my book *Wen Bing Jiang Yi* 溫病講義 scroll 4 and get to the meaning of it; there is no need to further explain it here. Most importantly is that if one doesn't understand the pathology behind measles then his herbs' lack of efficacy demonstrates just that. If the patient has no sweat then one uses Ma Huang 麻黃 to resolve the exterior, if there is sweat one uses Ge Gen 葛根[259] to push and resolve the exterior, which conforms to cold injury *Shang Han* 傷寒 formulas.[260] Via a shortcut this disease is also a cold injury tied to warm disease with no doubt.

So when it comes to measles, why is it a must to push it out via the exterior? With this I have a new discovery. After carefully investigating specialized articles, in regards to why not use Shi Hu, I found out that this herb helps stimulate gland secretion. On a secondary examination one can see that when the stomach has dryness the mouth has no fluids. Saliva comes from the salivary glands. The salivary gland and the stomach gland must have a very close connection. Therefore when the stomach receives water this can stop thirst of the mouth.

Fresh Sheng Di 鮮生地 even though has some similar action to Shi Hu, yet its ability to clear heat from the blood and increase fluid in the blood is very different. Therefore when measles has turned into dryness, but it did not come out yet, then it is proper to use Sheng Di and not Shi Hu. If one uses Shi Hu then the measles that did not break out is obstructed from breaking out, the hot disease has no escape route. The Yin becomes exhausted and the fluids dry out. This is what I described in my book *Mai Xue Jiang Yi* 脈學講義 as "Yin deficiency and heating it disease" 陰虛而熱之症. The saliva dries out, the tongue is dry without fluid, the blood dries extremely, heat blazes and the nerves are deprived of nourishment. Even though one uses a method trying to treat it, the Yin deficiency is too extreme and no herbs can be used

---

[259] Ma Huang Tang and Ge Gen Tang, respectively.

[260] Formulas that treat cold injury, but this also means formulas that come from the *Shang Han Lun* treatise of cold injury.

for it. Even if one uses both fresh Sheng Di and Shi Hu together there is not the slimmest chance of saving this. (Few words to supplement here, one cannot overlook the disease dynamics. When there is external evil and one uses resolving heat, there could be only the faintest of clue showing if there is Yin deficiency that one may think can warrant the use of Shi Hu).[261]

Today's doctors, as soon as they see a dry tongue, immediately use Shi Hu. To an extreme, sometimes even if there is no dry tongue they still use Shi Hu. Their malady is not knowing the meaning of deficiency and excess of Yin and Yang. This causes me to deeply dislike and feel painful about it. The two books *Tiao Bian* 條辨 and *Jing Wei* 經緯 have many false points. But the most false among these texts is the treatise *Wen Re Lun* 溫熱論 and *Case Studies of Mr. Ye* 葉案. Using Shi Hu for hot diseases indeed started from Mr. Ye 葉.[262] Seeing oral thrush in ancient books also started from Mr. Ye. As a persistent person looking for the correct herb, after encountering this book, my humble self has suffered a few skin shallow defeats[263] and therefrom my experience stems. Western people now call this disease acute Suli tuberculosis 急性粟粒結核 (for more details read my book *Shang Han Ji Yi An* 傷寒輯義按).

Chapter: Infantile Convulsion Formulas

Pages 62–63

Having fever is something that can't be prevented with children. The ancients called it "become steaming Bian Zheng 變蒸". Measles can also not be prevented. Smallpox has "planting seed Zhong Dou 種痘" vaccine, but measles cannot be prevented. Cold injury is also something that can't be avoided. Also, as for diseases being easily transmitted, not easily transmitted or completely not communicable, each has the appropriate age. Little kids suffer many communicable infectious diseases, old people however completely don't transmit.[264] Therefore seldom are there old people who contract cold injury, completely not like kids who do contract cold injury, which then changes to steaming and easily recovers.

[261] This comment is in the text in small fonts.

[262] Ye Tianshi 葉天士.

[263] The book has misled me several times.

[264] It seems that the author's meaning of transmit a disease means both transmitted from one person to the other, but possibly also has the meaning of being transmitted inside the body as in the *Shang Han Lun* from the interior to the exterior and vice versa.

In our world, one needs to supplement the medical books with these unnoted formulas. This will be helpful. Measles is also easy to cure. If the student trusts what I have written in *Bao Chi Xin Shu* 保赤新書 first and second scrolls, then he will be more than equal to the task. Treating cold injury is also easy. If the student only sinks his heart and researches what I wrote in the books *Shang Han and Wen Bing Jiang Yi* 傷寒溫病講義 as well as the cold injury case studies within the book *Yao He Yi An* 藥盒醫案, there is no need to look anywhere else.

Then the curative success rate is no more like what the Jin Gui describes as "the excellent practitioner cures six or seven out of ten". This is not me wanting to be arrogant, but rather this is the reality. It is unlike the contemporary doctors' curative success. Patients seeking cure from Western doctors increase daily. It is so impossible that the entire world is catching up to this. In their clinic, as soon as they meet upon cold injury disease, they don't hesitate a bit, immediately they open their mouth to say "one must allow this disease 21 days." They claim that this disease does not have a specialized drug. One can only listen to their explanation that this will resolve on its own. (What Western medicine calls target the symptom therapy here means just listen to an explanation that it will resolve on its own).

Alas, waiting for it to resolve on its own for 21 days, such a lengthy time period, this is an affair involving danger. One cannot bear digging with a finger.[265] If heat is fierce the stomach becomes constipated and it can always impact the brain. When these happen they use ice pillow and enemas as a treatment method. This is for them the unbreakable "only course of action"[266] one can take. This "only course of action", not only can it not cure the disease, but when you compare it to Zhongjing method of treating the same, the difference is incalculable beyond imagination. When it comes to using this "only course of action" with little kids then the danger[267] is higher than 90%. If at this time one uses Chinese medicine then the outcomes are not the same.

There is however, a perverse outline, among mediocre Chinese medicine practitioners, about the Shang Han 傷寒 cold injury concept. They think that all kinds of cold injury are all warm diseases 凡傷寒皆溫病.[268] And so to treat warm diseases they also

---

[265] One cannot bear such a slow recovery process like trying to dig a hole with a finger.

[266] The "only course of action" means you let a cold injury resolve on its own; if it didn't resolve and instead there are complications, then you treat the complications, such as constipation, brain damage etc.

[267] The danger of complications.

[268] They misunderstand the *Neijing* line that states: All cold injuries are febrile diseases.

have one "only course of action". They say that in warm disease "resolving the exterior" is prohibited, and so when the disease is at Tai Yang they don't use Ma Huang 麻黃, Gui Zhi 桂枝 and Qing Long 青龍.[269] Instead they only use Qing Shui Dou Juan 清水豆卷, Dan Dou Chi 淡豆豉 and expound on those for many days. They cannot make the difference between what is warm disease Wen Bing 溫病 and what is cold injury Shang Han 傷寒. Even more so they can't tell what is measles. In addition to Dou Juan 豆卷 and Dou Chi 豆豉, other demonic herbs like Zi Bei Chi 紫貝齒, Lu Lu Tong 路路通, Tian Jiang Ke 天將殼 etc with a whim of the pen come flowing down. They write beautifully and neat nine herbs in a prescription, each herb name has three characters, this makes it a famous doctor's prescription. They use this prescription with measles, they use it with warm disease, and they use it with cold injury as well. After many days the disease transforms into dryness, the lips are dry and the tongue is purple. They don't waste any time thinking further, again they wave their pens and bring on Xian Shi Hu 鮮石斛, Chai Shi Hu 釵石斛, Huo Shan Shi Hu 霍山石斛, Tie Pi Shi Hu 鐵皮石斛, Er Huan Shi Hu 耳環石斛[270] etc famous brands. With this the disease toxin is obstructed by the sweet cool herbs and cannot exit to the surface. The internal heat blazes more, the nerves are being roasted. An adult will fall unconscious with delirious speech while a little kid will wail without tears, his fingers tremble, there will be a sound of phlegm in his throat, breathing will be hurried and his nostrils flutter. Those doctors at this time, will not think twice, again with a stroke of a pen will bring upon Ling Yang Jiao 羚羊角, Bao Chi San 保赤散, Bao Long Wan 抱龍丸, Tai Yi Dan 太乙丹, Niu Huang Wan 牛黃丸, Ting Li 葶藶, Hou Zao 猴棗 etc medicines. These kinds of doctors like torrents are all like this. They only embrace this kind of trick and they gather substantial profit. They entirely rely on crafting this kind of art.

What do I mean with "this kind of art"? Being a quack and that's it. In my opinion, these kinds of people, what in the past they thought was their fortune on a future day will be the outlined plan for them entering hell. There is nothing to admire there, there is no accountability. What a pity it is that China's medicine was ruined to such an extreme because of this generation. So how come these herbs Shi Hu, Ling Yang, Bao Long Wan, Bao Chi San can cure a disease? What I dislike about these herbs is that people misuse them. Cold injury and measles at the initial stage are a Tai Yang

[269] Ma Huang Tang, Gui Zhi Tang and Qing Long Tang.
[270] The herb Shi Hu was so popular that seemingly different types were harvested or prepared differently or harvested in a specific location. The following are in this quote: Fresh Shi Hu, Hairpin Shi Hu, Huo Shan Mountain Shi Hu, Iron Skin Shi Hu, Earing Shi Hu.

disease. They should use a method of resolving the exterior. Not daring to resolve the exterior and yet for many days use elaborately cool sweet herbs, thereafter use purging, it means that from beginning to end Tai Yang did not resolve. If Tai Yang did not resolve and one purges than the heat sinks in and the disease aggravates. How can it be that the nerves will not be destroyed? Because of using these wrong herbs that it creates infantile convulsions Jing Feng 驚風.

Final page announcement

Yaron: Many Western medicine advocates accused native practitioners of being swindlers. The following is an announcement at the book's end, showing the fee schedule and office hours for Yun Tieqiao, a rather successful Chinese medicine practitioner in Shanghai 1928. Just for comparison purpose in 1928 One Chinese silver dollar = US$0.50. In the USA in 1928 a trolley fare would be $0.05 and lunch would cost $0.10. Compared to today it should be a factor of x 35.

Yun Tieqiao clinical cases

Mainly treating: cold injuries, warm disease, throat, measles, malaria, dysentery, epidemics, cholera, cough, exhaustion, stroke, vomiting blood, female menses, leucorrhea, pregnancy and labor, pediatric measles, pox and convulsions.

Hours: In clinic from 9:00am to 2:00pm.
Home visits in the afternoon from 3:00pm to 7:00pm.

Clinic address: Shanghai, San Malu, Yunnan Lu, Hui Leli, San Nong Er Jia
上海三馬路雲南路會樂里三弄二家

Tel: Central 5932

Costs:

In clinic: 1 Yuan 2 Jiao, with a number double this.
Home visit: 5 Yuan. If the road is far then need to consider separately.
Second opinion: 1 Yuan.
Altering the prescription: 1 Yuan.
Creams: 2 Yuan 2 Jiao.
Diagnosis via correspondence: 4 Yuan.
Visit outside of the regular times of clinic and home visits the fee is double.

Book excerpt end

Discussion with Zhou Yuxi 周禹錫 about his *Arguing with Yu Yunxiu's* 余雲岫 *Argument*

1927 by Zou Zhihen 鄒趾痕

Source: *San San Medical Publication*, 3rd Vol. 22 Issue, Published 1927, 三三醫報第三卷二十二期

Yaron: There were native practitioners who believed that fighting against modern science advancement with paper tiger articles may fix the problem. These articles Yu Yunxiu claimed as not worthy of repudiation. Indeed, self-exaggerating is not a good idea and certainly does not help in developing the new.

Dear Mr. Yuxi 禹錫, I just got your letter. I read it many times and was inspired. I memorized it over and over and got the conclusion that your knowledge and wisdom is great. Your aspiration is so high and broad seemingly with no end. If you can keep doing this diligently, one day when you have reached a great academic achievement and became a medical sage, then your talent and ability will shine in the medical field, and help people get rid of diseases and extend their lifespan. This will force other quacks to give up quackery and start learning Chinese medicine. This great mission can only be done by you.

Every character in Mr. Shoufu's 壽甫[271] great book is from experiments and experience, so how can I look lightly at it? Nonetheless, I can't be satisfied with medical books post- Tang and Song dynasties with their modern contemporary prescriptions Shi Fang 時方, because the good ones intermingle with bad ones indistinctly. Although the good prescriptions don't have true Dao (knowledge) of a medical sage, they still have a proven recipe and words of experience to support them, which I respect. These strong points can't be overshadowed by their shortcomings. However, bad prescriptions don't have any experiments to support them; people simply made them up, such as Shu Tai Yin 束胎飲, Shou Tai Wan 瘦胎丸, Hei Xi Dan 黑錫丹, Gun Tan Wan 滾痰丸 and others. Some formulas were developed for greed, such as Yang Ba Wei 陽八味, Shen Rong Wan 參茸丸, Gui Lu Wan 龜鹿丸, San Bian Wan 三鞭丸, Wu Bian Wan 五鞭丸, Zhong Zi Wan 種子丸 etc. Some did not have a logic, such as hot herbs reinforce Yang, cool herbs reinforce Yin, before birth one should keep cool, while after birth one should keep warm, use hot herbs to regulate men-

[271] Zhang Shoufu 張壽甫 also known as Zhang Xichun 张锡纯 1860–1933.

struation in order to be ready for the fetus, use Yang Ba Wei 陽八味 to treat all kinds of diseases. Others false theories include ones like Wang Haizang's 王海藏 theory about pregnant ladies have cold damage disorders, Xue's 薛氏 Qian method for cold damage disorders 傷寒鈐法, Shu Chiyuan's 舒馳遠 six meridians definition and methods, Li Shizhen's 李時珍 mutual restraint, mutual assistant and antagonism. Books that have these fake theories yield more and more fake doctors who don't have real knowledge. Ones who can only try out formulas on a patient, to see which one works and then guess which disease it is. These kinds of fake doctors are abundant all over the country, and people who believe in those fake doctors are also abundant all over the country, so the fake doctors can make good money and enjoy a good reputation yet the real medical principle is not known. The origin of this problem lies with those fake medical books. This is why I'm unhappy with those bad medical books of contemporary prescriptions.

Mr. Zhang Shoufu's 張壽甫 contemporary formulas book is amongst the finest books of contemporary formulas and it can save people's lives. This can win a good reputation and add value to Chinese medicine and I am, therefore, very happy about it. Knowledge is boundless, and although you are doing fabulously in medical field, there is another level of "cured" beyond Mr. Shoufu's current level of "effectiveness". What is the difference between "effective" and "cured"? "Effective" means the condition is currently safe while "cured" means the body is totally recovered from a disease. None of the books about contemporary prescriptions reaches the level of "cured"; only the books of medical sages are at this level. If you ask me did I reach this level yet? I would say no for my current situation, but maybe in thirty years. Today since I have not reached it yet, I don't have the posture to criticize Mr. Shoufu 壽甫. However, the Dao of medical sages is way beyond his level. It can make old people still appear young or a 100-year-old person still able to give birth. This is why in the medical classics it says, "People who know their end can keep their body and spirit merged, they exhaust their heavenly years until they are 100 years old and then they depart." The "depart" in the sentence actually means "die". The reason this text doesn't talk about dying is that people who know Dao cultivate a skill keeping them alive in this world. If they cultivate it well they can become immortals. "Depart" is due to the lack of life maintaining skills, so that people may live long without being healthy, they dispose of their physical body and then they depart. Now, grasping the principle of nature and Yin-Yang is in order to live as long as nature without an end. But compared to the vast Dao of medical sages, our knowledge is limited, just like a mouse drinking water from a river—it can't drink it up, it stops when it's full. So how dare I ask to know about the superior level? Should we even mention those arrogant people who act like in their chests there is a different heaven and earth from the Dao of medical sages.

I got the news that Jiangsu Province Chinese Medicine Federation 江蘇全省中醫聯合會 suggested to establish Chinese medical schools and that this suggestion was objected to by Yu Yunxiu 余雲岫. In his objection, he criticizes *Inner Canon of Huangdi* 黃帝內經 to be vulgar and mediocre and Zhongjing's 仲景 book to be a reckless division of six meridians and in messy disorder. I carefully contemplated his words just in case he is beyond the level of a medical sage. Then I realized that Yu Yunxiu 余雲岫 has only learnt Western medicine and anatomy and he is only able to treat parenchymal diseases. He doesn't know that Chinese medicine treats diseases following the principle of nature, dividing four seasons and categorizing diseases by Yin-Yang. Although these rules look the same, yet they can treat all different kinds of diseases and make life last for a hundred years. With his little skill Yu Yunxiu 余雲岫 dares to criticize Chinese medicine, and therefore I know he is just a ludicrous man. This arrogant man only admires Western medicine. He is like a frog at the bottom of a well seeing partial sky and thinking that it's the real size of the sky. The way he undervalues the books of medical sages is exactly like the frog's vision of the limited sky, and so he dares to say those arrogant words. I feel sorry for him! With his intelligence, if he had seriously learnt the knowledge of medical sages and had a good instructor to teach him, then he would have reached the Dao of medical sages and he would certainly regret his words. Since he refuses to learn Chinese medicine, it's like he is just standing outside of the palace looking at it from the outside. Even being told that things happen inside the palace he still doesn't believe it. If people try to tell him that Western medicine has more downsides than advantages, he will argue with it madly.

Trivially he keeps on claiming that anesthesia is the true nature of Western medicine, going around it by mouth and tongue and not letting go. Today I only hope that he can change his disrespect for Chinese medicine back into harmonious peace. The only way to accomplish this is with experiments. Diseases such as stroke, multiple arthralgia, hemiplegia, convulsion, atrophy flaccidity, impediment, bone steaming fever, tuberculosis, phlegm with blood and dyspnea, numbness, fearful heart palpitations, amnesia, tinnitus, hemorrhoids, sclerosis keratitis, suppurative lymphadenitis of neck, axillary abscess, anal fistula, abdominal mass, metrorrhagia, metrostaxis, lung abscess, intestine abscess etc. we should skip the incurable ones and talk about the ones that can be cured. Regardless if we treat them with Chinese or Western medicine, we should not regard it as successful if there is only a temporary effect but rather, wait until the entire disease disappears and the body recovers to its original state. This is the final goal. Our Dao of Chinese medicine sages can reach to this goal, but I don't know if Western medicine can reach it too. These diseases all start with accumulations in the five organs, and we can tell which organ has the accumulation by observing which symptoms are more obvious.

Nowadays electronic tomography is available to see the image of five organs inside the body and surgical skill is advanced so either dissection of the body or cutting off an injured foot or replacing with a new organ is reachable by Western medicine. This is why he is so proud of Western medicine and disrespects Chinese medicine. He thinks that it's much easier to cure a disease with those magical skills and techniques, so why bother keeping Chinese medicine to maintain longer life with an ill body? However, I'm afraid those skills and techniques are actually not beneficial to diseases. I have yet to see any of them cure abdominal mass. I don't think that they know the etiology of abdominal mass. Since it was treated with Chinese medicine, our medical sages already told us the origin of abdominal mass and passed us the knowledge of how to dispel a mass and return to a healthy condition. There is no need for any other techniques. Whichever one works I'll call it magic. If those fancy light and electronic techniques can't actually get rid of a disease and get the condition back to normal, how are they helpful? There's no need to argue, we can directly experiment with it. If Yu Yunxiu 余雲岫 can cure the disease and make the condition back to normal with Western medicine, then I'll agree with him. Chinese medicine's position will be taken by the ones who are experts at the Dao of medical sages, and I can help them. As for Western medicine, Yu and those Western medical experts at anesthesia, who often look down at Chinese medicine, they will be in charge of their side assisted by the best Western medicine doctors. Then we choose a couple of serious diseases such as tuberculosis, arm atrophy flaccidity and leg paralysis, and use both Chinese and Western medicine to treat them and see which one can cure them fully. The one who can cure most fully will be chosen as the most valuable and the other one will be ranked below. We should also record the patients' information including name, age, condition and recovery in detail and then make it public to let people judge which treatment is better. This is my opinion of Yu.

I want to discuss this with Chinese medical experts and if you guys agree with me then I would like you and Mr. Zhang Shoufu 張壽甫, as the representatives of Chinese medical group, to publish it. When publishing this, we need to add some comments next to the original text[272] to make Mr. Yu understand. I know that the content itself is very easy to understand, so I'm wondering why Yu can't get it. In addition, I found out that in his objection there are some ignorant parts, for example, he cited Yu Quyuan's 俞曲園 *Abolishment of Chinese Medicine Discussion* 廢醫論 as a support for his argument. However, Yu Quyuan 俞曲園 is an expert of Chinese literary classics but he doesn't know much about Chinese medicine. His opinion to abolish Chinese medicine is completely wrong due to his lack of Chinese medical knowledge. I can tell this from his article where he claims, "Those who healed after taking herbs would heal anyhow without herbs, while those who take no herbs and do not recover wouldn't recover even after taking herbs", which exactly shows that he knows nothing about Chinese medicine. People who know Chinese medicine know that there are two different levels describing patients' treatment and recovery, one is effective Xiao 效 and the other is cured Yu 愈. Being effective means that the medicine is working temporarily, which might be for months or years but then the disease still comes back. Being cured means that the disease is totally removed and the condition is completely healthy, this is called complete cure Quan Yu 全愈. So for patients who don't have serious illnesses, both mediocre doctors' and true doctors' herbs show efficacy. True doctors' medicine makes the evil removed entirely so it shows efficacy. When efficacy is present then cure is present. Mediocre doctors' medicine pushes the evil deep inside the body and locks it in so it doesn't come out and so it seems effective. It's a temporary effect and the evil will definitely come out in the future, and if it is treated with mediocre doctors medicine again then the evil will accumulate into a bigger disease deep inside the body.

When a disease is deep inside the body, applying medicine from a true doctor could show either efficacy or no efficacy. If the medicine dispels evil which lingers close to the surface but doesn't shake the deep lying evil then it seems effective. When the medicine is fighting the deep lying evil, it seems as if ineffective. When a disease is deep inside the body, applying medicine from a mediocre doctor may as well seem effective or ineffective. The medicine pushes the evil inside so it seems effective, however, the evil can't be eradicated by the medicine so it will be ineffective eventu-

[272] The text Yu was objecting to, Jiangsu Province Chinese Medicine Federation's suggestion to include Chinese medicine schools in the main school system.

ally. Therefore, what Yu Quyuan 俞曲園 calls "cured" really just mean "effective" and not "cured". He doesn't have a medical background so it's reasonable that he mistook one for the other. However, Yu Yunxiu 余雲岫 considers himself knowledgeable in medicine, yet he regards a wrong theory as if it were correct, which shows how little his knowledge is. Since he's so ignorant, why does he have the posture to criticize Chinese medical classics?

In addition, Jiangsu Federation's proposal to add Chinese medicine schools to the Department of Education school system is very reasonable. Furthermore, not only Chinese medicine intelligentsia should learn the Dao of our Chinese medical sages, but all medical intelligentsia from other countries should do so as well. Chinese medicine is the most important school within the Department of Education school system. Chinese medicine theory is as profound as Confucianism and the knowledge of natural law. Confucianism and the knowledge of natural law aren't easy to comprehend, not because the sages are hiding them but rather current scholars did not reach the appropriate level; although they have learnt it yet it seems like they have not. The knowledge of Chinese medical sages is in *Plain Questions Suwen* 素問, *Divine Pivot Lingshu* 靈樞, *Cold Injury Treatise Shang Han Lun* 傷寒論 and *Synopsis of Golden Chamber Jin Gui Yao Lüe* 金匱要略. There are many talented people who have studied those books and yet they can't attain this knowledge.

Yu Yunxiu 余雲岫 doesn't realize that his understanding is too minute to attain the knowledge of the medical sages and so he dares to criticize Chinese medical classics and object to the proposal of instituting Chinese medical schools. It's just like an ant trying to topple a giant tree, he's overestimating himself. Today, if we don't let him grasp the difference between "effective" and "cured", Mr. Yu certainly will mistake the "cured" in *Abolishment of Chinese Medicine Discussion* 廢醫論 with the real "cured", which means getting rid of the disease entirely and going back to a healthy state. We should explain it clearly to him.

In his objection text, Mr. Yu doesn't assess whether the treatment is good or bad in regards to the disease being cured or not, but rather he directly assaults Chinese medicine describing it as an unintelligent doctor's opinion. I think it should be assessed first if the disease was cured or not and then judge the treatment for being proper or not. This is the kind heart of the good doctor. As long as it can cure the disease, no matter if it is Chinese or Western, it is the right medical treatment. If it doesn't cure it then it's not. Why did Mr. Yu only use "unintelligent doctor's opinion" to describe Chinese medicine? In my humble opinion, I think Mr. Yu regards Western medical treatment as the only correct treatment, other kinds of treatment being by default wrong. That is why he agrees with the treatment of dissection using electronic or light or sound techniques, which is actually just killing people while using a better knife. I therefore called it an absurd thought.

Also in his objection text, Mr. Yu claims that the *Yellow Emperor Inner Canon* was not written by the Yellow Emperor and claims that nor is the content of this book the Dao of the Yellow Emperor and Qibo. The first claim is reasonable, however, I don't get the second claim. He explains that the phrasing and formatting of the *Inner Canon* is similar to articles written by Qin 秦 natives during the Zhou 周 Dynasty and not during the time Yellow Emperor was around, which is debatable. The Dao in this book describes the principle for every thing in the universe. People who get this Dao can govern properly and discipline themselves, and they also can pass down their virtue to their descendants. People who don't get this Dao have nothing to follow in their lives. Basically Mr. Yu suspects that the content of the book is forged just because the article style doesn't fit the time attributed to its composition, which means that he doesn't understand the true meaning of the book. The Dao of medical sages is like a palace, if one is merely looking at it from outside without entering it, then he has no posture to criticize. Only those who have entered the palace of medical sages' Dao know how valuable and profound this Dao is and so they don't dare comment on it audaciously.

I am not knowledgeable enough to offer important words, but I hope that modern day leading medical experts can prove Mr. Zhang Shoufu's 張壽甫 words. Mr. Zhang Shoufu 張壽甫 is the chief of Cang Zhou Lida Hospital 滄州立達醫院 and has published *In Medicine Treasuring Chinese while Consulting Western Yi Xue Zhong Zhong Can Xi Lu* 醫學衷中參西錄 and *Commentary on Medicinals Yao Wu Jiang Yi* 藥物講義. Zhang expounded on many things that were never explored before and in our medical circles he is a famous doctor. I admire him very much. Zhang explained that *Suwen* 素問 talks about treating disease with herbs while *Lingshu* 靈樞 talks about treating disease with acupuncture and moxibustion. But because it has been a long period of time since their composition, the books are not complete. In the old days, people often instructed or taught students orally, which easily led to loss of knowledge, and that is why Huang Fumi 皇甫謐 from Jin 晉 Dynasty and Lin Yi 林億 from Song 宋 Dynasty suspected that some parts of these books were forged. However the essence of these books was surely from the sages themselves and not from others. For example, it says that acupuncture can cure disease, which is acknowledged today by both Chinese and Western medicine. If this idea of acupuncture had not started by an ancient sage, then would later generations be able to make it up? Would Westerners, who deal with anatomy, be able to make it up? The valuable part of *Neijing* is attained by careful investigation. The false parts might have been added by others and can be ignored; this is exactly what Mencius meant by saying, "One cannot believe the book in its entirety".[273] Today, people emphasize Western medicine more and refuse to research the valuable parts in *Neijing*; instead, they criticize the false parts until seemingly the entire work is composed of false parts. As Huangdi's 400 million descendants, we Chinese people don't cherish—and even abandon—the old classic, it's a real pity. So Yu Yunxiu's 余雲岫 opinions that *Neijing* was not Huangdi's works should stop. Above is my humble opinion of Yu Yunxiu's 余雲岫 objection.

The experiments I suggested he do and the examples I gave of diseases before cannot be cured with sonic or light or electric techniques or cutting limbs or dissecting the abdomen. The sonic, light and electric techniques of surgery can only cure pure physical diseases. If the disease is caused by Qi transformation that results in physical problems, then surgery alone can't fix it, nor can simple Western medicine drugs. Only treating it with the theory of our medical sages, such as Yin-Yang theory, can we get rid of the disease and cure the condition back to a healthy state. Although I'm not smart and don't have much medical attainment, I can try my best to make it happen. I here hope that you, talented fellows, can do this job and I'll follow you. So far the best Chinese medicine doctors who also have the best reputation are you and Mr. Shoufu 壽甫. I sincerely hope that you can help me convince Mr. Shoufu 壽甫 to do this. If he consents to do these experiments then we, in Chinese medicine, can win. If other Chinese medicine experts would like to devote their time and do similar experiments on our behalf in other parts of the country, they are welcome.

As for Yu Yunxiu's 余雲岫 objection, the reason I brought it up is because his words systematically use Western medicine in a way to put our Chinese medicine in danger of extinction. One has no choice but to rise against this. It is a day that we must come out and shoulder the legacy of our sages. Since Western medicine has advanced eastward, physical diseases of the body have been addressed with surgery. There was no consideration of Qi transformation and, like this, there was an effect.

[273] The Book in Mencius quote refers to the *Book of Historical Records Shang Shu* 尚書.

However, those who had Qi-transformation type diseases which resulted in physical diseases, I do not know how many of them have died after those surgeries? Now, since Yu makes the mistake of knowing the physical body but not Qi, our Chinese medicine has the courtesy of "being stern with oneself but forgiving to others". How come he is not modest, and comes upon us with vigor?

Not long ago there was a Chinese fellow who had graduated in Japan and wanted to initiate a domestic management regulation for medical affairs, similar to the Japanese wanting to destroy Chinese medicine. Even though people wanted to extinguish Chinese medicine, we still survive today. Now, Yu Yunxiu 余雲岫 directly rejects Chinese medicine classics and wants to break our system, just like a foreigner coming into my house, accusing me for being guilty and wishing to expel me out of my own house. This is why I suggest doing experiments. I say that not because I know nothing about the results, I already know what will happen. Those fancy sonic or light or electrical surgical techniques cannot cure the serious problems such as paralysis, convulsion, or mass in the inner organs, because those kinds of disease are due to blockage of Qi which, only therefrom, results in physical diseases.

People who know Chinese medicine know things like the Six Qi Decoction 六氣湯方 that can really make Qi spin and transform. Ma Gui Qing Long 麻桂青龍, those kinds of formulas, disperse spring Yang, just like a dragon flying in the sky. Zhu Ling Bai Hu 豬苓白虎, those kinds of formulas, purify and descend the atmosphere, just like a tiger's excitement. Xie Xin Zhi Chi 瀉心梔豉, those kinds of formulas, have characteristics of flaming upwards, just like a red bird flying. Long Mu 龍牡, those kinds of formulas, have diving and descending characteristics, just like the guardian spirit of the north concealing in winter. After understanding the main principle behind the knowledge of our medical sages, we know how to correctly use these formulas in order to treat diseases such as paralysis, convulsion and tuberculosis. Chinese medicine can ascend the descending Qi, contract the dispersing Qi, unblock the blocking Qi and clear the stagnating Qi. When Qi moves then blood moves, and then water distributes everywhere in the body, the five fluids nourish the body and so masses in the five organs can vanish on their own without cutting it out, limbs atrophy can recover back to normal on their own without being replaced. These are examples I've seen with my own eyes. We, in Chinese medicine, have this tremendous power to cure diseases, how come we are scared instead of proving it with experiments? This is my suggestion and I don't know if you Sir agree with me. If you do, I hope you can add this into your own article and delete inappropriate parts if there are any, or add some other needed lines. I hope that after you correct the article, it can be agreed by Mr. Shoufu 壽甫 as well, and then you publish it in the newspaper and share with everyone. On the one hand we can directly, officially and academically fight with Yu Yunxiu 余雲岫. If he realizes that he is clueless then he will be silent, and this will attack the pride of Western medicine. On the other hand, if he doesn't realize that he is clueless and he dares to keep on arguing with us, then this battle between Western and Chinese medicine will be a good chance for us to reveal to the world that Western medicine has no clue on how to treat internal organs' diseases. It will be a good time for Chinese medicine to cheer up after it has been treated unfairly for so long. The unified fellows of the Chinese medical intelligentsia are the ones undertaking the great enterprise under heaven of the Dao of medical sages.

I'll be waiting for your reply; please let me know your opinion about it. In my diary there is also a reply from Mr. Hao Zixin 郝子信 from Henan, and our Society's reply to him, but it wasn't published yet. I cannot use it as I am obstructed by the Society's agenda. The idea conforms to mine so later I will use it, here I simply hand copy it in its entirety. Please review. Here I give praises for a happy new year.

Tiannian Medical Society office, Sichuan, Chongqing, no.22 Peide Tang Alley 天年醫社處四川重慶培德堂巷二十二號

Article end

About Tan Cizhong 譚次仲

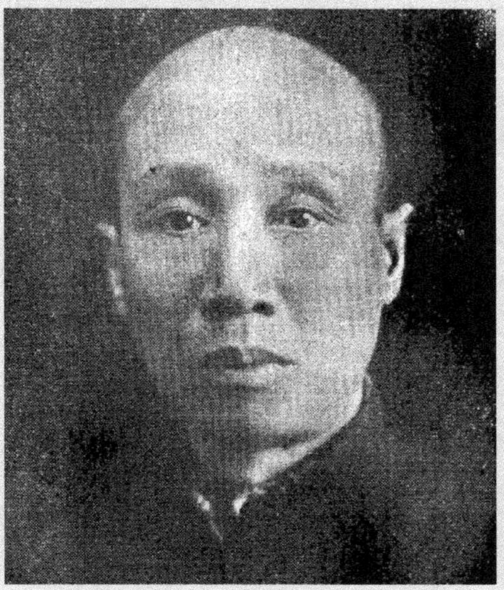

Tan Cizhong 譚次仲 was born in Zhang Cha town Foshan city 佛山市張槎鎮 [southwest of Canton] in Guangdong province in 1887. He was a celebrity Chinese medicine physician in Foshan and well known all around China. Tan graduated in his early days from Liang Guang Xue Tang 兩廣學堂 majoring in English and then became an English teacher. He then immersed in self-study of Chinese medicine theory and history. In 1933 he passed the required examination of the time for Chinese medicine licensure and started his career as a practitioner of Chinese medicine. On the eve of the war against Japan, he moved to Guangxi province and practiced Chinese medicine there.

In 1933, Tan compiled a book titled *The Medicine's Revolution Debate* 醫學革命論戰 in which he argued that no matter if it is Chinese or Western, they are both crystallization of wisdom. Chinese medicine is thousands of years old and provided, over the centuries, great benefit for the Chinese people. But he also acknowledged that Chinese medicine had its deficiencies. He promoted a notion that old Chinese medicine needed advancement through the use of science, its essence extracted and the superfluous eradicated. He advocated that scientification of Chinese medicine is the only true path of development. He pointed out that Western medicine is likewise a medicine derived from experience with its own unique principle and it is well worth studying. He opposed the notion of "keeping Chinese medicine pure" and instead advanced the idea that Chinese and Western medicine need to learn from each other in order to advance, creating a new Chinese and Western medicine merged together kind of medicine 中西醫結合, a notion well adopted in later years during the Communist era. Consequently, after becoming proficient with Chinese medicine he started learning from his Western medicine colleagues. In 1951, during the early years of communist China, he passed the official examination of Western medicine licensure. In 1952, he was invited by the National Health Scientific Research Committee 全國衛生科學研究委員會 to become a committee member. In 1953, he was elected by the Nan Hai county People's Congress as their representative. Tan passed away in 1955 at the age of 68.

Tan compiled nine works during his lifetime and wrote many articles. His first book, *The Medicine's Revolution Debate* 醫學革命論戰, which was published in Wuzhou, Guangxi and was widely read among medical circles, soon sold out. It was printed again in Guangzhou province and was sold out again. The third time printed in Chongqing, Sichuan and it became the best seller of the time.

During the time that Chen Jitang 陳濟棠 (1890–1954) headed the government of Guangdong from 1929 to 1936, he returned to Guangzhou and advocated teaching Chinese medicine. He started to offer teaching by correspondence and face-to-face. Within five years he had around 200 students, some of whom later became famous physicians.

The Medicine's Revolution Debate 醫學革命論戰

1931 by Tan Cizhong 譚次仲

Source: 4th edition of *The Medicine's Revolution Debate*.[274] The original working title of this book was *An Initial Collection of Writings about Chinese Medicine and Science* 中醫與科學首集. First publication 1931.[275] Fourth edition printed 1952 in Hong Kong by Qiu Shi Chu Ban She 求實出版社.

Tan's preface to the first collection

Humans are all alike. There are no two principles. Medical science is not separated by mountain peaks of Chinese and Western, being correct or incorrect like water and fire that clearly can't mingle together. Today's vast gulley establishes two rival camps, one defends to death the misleading notion of "Yin Yang Pillars", doesn't hesitate to exaggerate its self-standing and confer its ancient manners to be today as it has always been before. The other, their way of doing things is to falsely believe and use a scientific prejudicial inclination as an excuse, like the common speech of an old scholar dancing around empty words and forgetting the true reality, as it has always been before.

Now when you look at the Central Bureau for Native Medicine 中央國醫館 introduction, they often announce the objective of arranging the medicine according to science. Or often seeing the Central Bureau of Science's 研究院[276] blazing articles, the arrangement of Materia Medica and their appeal to a scope that cannot be supported in modern day. And so one country has two kinds of medicine—who wins and who loses? Who to follow and who not? How does that conform to the people's sufferings? Unifying what these medicines can't tolerate in each other becomes ever clearer. How shall we unify them? By using science. In other words, advancing Chinese medicine scientification and that's it! However, scientification of Chinese medicine is the responsibility of both East and West and not only of one side.

The way I see it, Chinese pharmacology and science are not two different branches. It is experience accumulated over thousands of years; history tested it with accuracy,

[274] Tan Cizhong wrote this preface to his original collection of papers that later on was divided into two separate books; *The Medicine's Revolution Debate* 醫學革命論戰 and *A Summary of the Nature and Types of Chinese Pharmaceuticals* 中藥性類概說.
[275] Tan's official biography states that he has authored this book in 1933, yet the 4th edition copy that we used as source states first publication in 1931; we have kept the discrepancy.
[276] Established in 1928 in the capital Nanjing.

much like modern experiments, and then arranged it perfectly. Only the absurd mysterious theories need to be eradicated, which then allows medicine and science to match together and be masterfully studied. This is really the only problem Chinese medicine has. Western medicine's only problem is trying to ignore the accumulated experience highlighting the pharmacological qualities of herbs, and instead only relying on chemistry, natural sciences, bacteriology and animal testing to discover it. What should be paving the way to unify the medicines into one is all within this discussion. Cizhong is not so sharp, with the aforementioned my entire ignorance is demonstrated. I drafted a manuscript about Chinese medicine and modern science containing roughly one million words. This book fully describes the task of making Chinese medicine scientific. However, under current circumstances, publishing this book is greatly needed. I therefore lovingly sought out the most essential and created two books: *My Opinion for the Scientification of Chinese Medicine* 中醫科學化之我見 and the other *The Preliminary Scientific Reform of Chinese Pharmacology* 中藥科學改造之初步. With about twenty thousand words, we neatly organized and made it ready for publishing. Even though it just begins to spin the wheel and it cannot encompass everything, those to whom it aims are the prominent persons on both sides who will enter this arena and teach it [Western and Chinese medicine]. Then, how could it remain only the trivial good fortune of a single person?

On the first month of the twentieth year of the Republic 民國二十年 (1931)

Foreword to The Medicine's Revolution Debate 醫學革命論戰 4th edition

By Tan's disciple Liu Dechen 劉德臣

My teacher Tan Cizhong 譚次仲 has advocated for the scientification of Chinese medicine for over twenty years. The one conservative Chinese medicine group promoted the idea that Chinese medicine needs to be kept pure while adhering to the old ways. The other Western medicine group advocated to completely discard the old medicine. For a long time these two groups were in a state of warfare. Fierce and extraordinarily difficult debates were unfolding. From beginning to end the science orthodoxy was erroneously considered to be the archery target, as the anti-science group carried their last-ditch life-or-death battle. Going through these twenty years of struggle, today, both sides gained complete victory. The so-called True

Principle cannot be extinguished. Public debates being free and unrestrained in one's heart, this is not the case! My teacher used great toil and wise judgment; the reader can see his great summary.

This book's original title was *My Opinion for the Scientification of Chinese Medicine* 中醫科學化之我見, which is the first half of the book *An Initial Collection of Writings about Chinese Medicine and Science* 中醫與科學首集. At present, we have changed the title to the current one. The complete *Initial Collection* was first printed in Wuzhou, second print in Guangzhou, the third print in Chongqing, and all were sold out. At present, by Qiu Shi publishing house in Hong Kong, the 4th edition is published.

Guide to using the book

1) The meanings behind the name of the book are three:
   a) Chinese medicine must become scientific.
   b) The substance of Chinese medicine must have the possibility to assimilate with science.
   c) With a wish to have Chinese medicine reach to science there must be a proper path to follow. It is like creating a vessel. First there needs to be the objective, second there needs to be the material, third there is a need for the procedures, methods and techniques to craft this material to reach this objective and become the vessel.
2) All medicines of the world have these three historical developmental steps. First they come out of religion and then from philosophy and after philosophy they become scientific. Therefore Chinese medicine must catch up to science.
3) Chinese medicine, even though very complex, can be categorized into three main aspects: abstruse theory; accumulated experience; and medicinals. Abstruse theory is the obscure philosophy, which naturally does not mingle with the scientific thought. Only medicinals have material object and accumulated experience has its real appearance. The two have been carried onward since antiquity with treating disease and have experience; these must have scientific principle contained within.
4) Considering that the importation of scientific thought has a history of one hundred years and more, and the two nations China and Japan still seem to not be able to merge and assimilate it, how is this so? This is because the path se-

lected is mistaken. In this book we use the three aspects as our starting point, yet the first section centers around the discussion and research of the path needed.

5) Around ninety percent of this book discusses and references publications by the *Shanghai Society Medical Gazette* 上海社會醫報 first, and later on by other provinces' medical gazettes and daily newspapers. It includes praise words and constructive critiques by famous persons in the fields of Chinese and Western medicine. Will this suffice to dismantle the obstructions Chinese and Western medicines were facing thus far?

6) Today the masses all hope that Chinese and Western medicine will merge into a common path, discovering cures for our sufferings and preserving our longevity. Some say master them thoroughly, some say integrate them, the bottom line is that this can take place after Chinese medicine becomes scientific.

7) This book is divided into two main sections; the first is the theoretical aspect and the second is the methodology. However, overall, it advocates for scientification, persistently using the scientific principle as the archery target. As for the antagonists of the scientific view who wish to fight it to death, who absolutely can't tolerate the boundary between Chinese and Western merging, there is very little of that in this book.

8) The Bureau for Native Medicine 國醫館 also advocated scientification of Chinese medicine. At its founding, Cizhong repeatedly had contributed suggestions, which ignorantly were not accepted. I was never, despite slight discouragement, disloyal to the heart of our nation's medicine, but rather I cared for it till my last day. My accomplishment today is inferior and not sufficient to serve as the Dao, and because of this lacking probably is not able to complete the task at hand; it is then all my own fault!

The Medicine's Revolution Debate Table of Contents

1) A Proposal to the Bureau for Native Medicine Guo Yi Guan 國醫館: How to arrange the nation's medicine by first establishing a standard.

2) Present the Academy of Sciences a discussion on how to resolve the key disputes of medical science.

3) Present again the Bureau for Native Medicine explanation: *The medicine's guiding principles are the ten principles.*

4) A Proposal to the Academy: Discussion on the importance of experience in herb research.

5) Responding to *Shanghai Society Medical Gazette* 上海社會醫報 director Yu Yunxiu 余云岫. Attached his reply.

6) A response to Hong Kong Native Medicine Magazine editor He Peiyu 何佩瑜.

7) Another reply to Mr. Yu Yunxiu's 余云岫 discussion of ancient prescriptions. Attached his reply to my response.

8) A letter from the medicine organization committee of the Bureau for Native Medicine, Mr. Lu Yuanlei 陸淵雷. Attached, a revision of the initial plan summary for the organization of the medicine.

9) A response to Zhejiang's Mr. Guo Ruoding 郭若定 questioning of the article *A New Chinese Medicine Perception* 新漢藥覺.

10) A Sincere Advice for Scientification and uniting the entire Chinese medicine community. Attached, a warning to Western medicine.

11) The must-have discussion with the entire population about the scientification of Chinese medicine.

A proposal to the Bureau for Native Medicine Guo Yi Guan 國醫館: How to arrange the nation's medicine by first establishing a standard

By Tan Cizhong

Yaron: Yu Yunxiu and Yun Tieqiao were not alone. Adding Tan Cizhong to our documents reveals three main trends in Chinese medicine during the Republic:

1. Tieqiao: a total separation of the two medicines so they can co-exist and contribute to society.

2. Cizhong: merging the two medicines and taking the strong points of each to make one strong scientific medicine.

3. Yunxiu: assimilating some aspects of Chinese medicine into modern medicine in order for it eventually to perish.

Tan Cizhong follows Yu Yunxiu in a modified manner. Yu wants to modernize China and discard of the old medicine while Tan believes that keeping them both is better.

Tan, like Yu, separates theory from practice claiming that native theory is primitive and absurd whereas accumulated experience and herbs have experimental value.

Both Tan and Yu emphasize the value of herbs but it appears that Yu is simply using "herbs" for gaining political points and possibly calming the opposition. Tan and Yu have different opinions reaching to a similar conclusion.

Their conclusion, using treatment efficacy as a standard, became the gold standard for developing TCM in the 20th century. In the Republic, Chinese medicine scientification leaned toward Yu, while during the Communist era it shifted toward Tan's model. It is not until the 1980s and '90s that a trend resembling Yun Tieqiao and other old practitioners, such as He Peiyu 何佩瑜, emerged: developing and re-discovering a unique style of Chinese medicine to exist separately alongside modern medicine.

In this document, Tan incorporates *Shang Han Lun* theory into a modern practical efficacy model. This is where Tan is different from Yu Yunxiu, who could have not considered this as valid scientific evidence. Yun Tieqiao, like Tan, also merged some modern medicine ideas but, at the end, used science to justify his own theory. Tan uses *Shang Han Lun* lines to demonstrate the old medicine's scientific nature with an objective being to bring it closer to science. It is another subtle difference between Yun and Tan, both using similar methods with different objectives.

Pages 2–12

What is the meaning of "True Principle"? Today, the world's medicine pathology and pharmacology building blocks are derived from modern scientific anatomy, physiology, bacteriology, physics and chemistry kind of experiments. Therefore every department of modern medicine, anatomy, physiology, bacteriology, physics and chemistry are getting extremely close to the Truth. Now the theories of Yin Yang, Five phases, root and manifestation Qi transformation, open closing and pivot of six conformations, their advance [from one conformation to the other], heavenly trunks and earthly branches, eight trigrams, Leading Heaven and In Spring theory, these are purely philosophical remnants coming from ancient times. They stand in sharp contrast to science's natural principle of experiments. The principles coming out of science are recognized unanimously by the entire world, it is hard to refute the scientific truth. Establishing a separate medical principle in China is a big problem. It must mean that the organs and bodily systems of people in China are different from those of people in other countries. Like earth worms that carry both sexes and can reproduce, or a lizard that hibernates for many months and doesn't eat, like a frog that covers its skin with mud and immediately dies, like a snake that can be strangled without breath and still not die, like tetanus that does not transmit to chickens, or Tuo Pi fungus 脫脾菌 that does not become parasitic on birds, or horses nasal ulcer that can't be contracted from white mice, like Ox that is not effected by Qian Luo toxin 謙洛毒, or horse that cannot be effected by arsenic toxin, and rabbit not effected by opium, hedgehog not effected by snake venom, worms living on tobacco leaves not affected by nicotine. The reason that the pathology and physiology of the above animals is different from humans is that their organs and bodily systems are entirely different from humans. Then how can they behave exactly the same. Humans do not have these differences amongst themselves and so how can medicine be different across different borders. [The scientific] medicine of the world is a crystallization of the Truth. And so whatever it finds to be true, is not even the slightest not [true], whatever it finds to be not true, is not even the slightest true. Erring from being true, or not true, is not tolerated even a hair width.

In countless generations [in history] there were many outstanding brilliant scholars. With gray hair they researched thoroughly and chiseled these foundations, yet their accumulated experience was inaccurate scientific principle. All in all, they believed that it needs to be preserved without being doubted. Today, they wish to collect the ancients' assumptions, build their walls on stilts and, with that, protest ahead. How do they try to differentiate mole crickets and ants, which follow heaven, versus mayflies and earthworms, which follow earth? Even if presenting this to a fool, he knows that this is not possible. Therefore there is a need to follow medical sciences common path in order to attain the native medicine advancement. In this fashion, one may look forward to its development. Keeping the obstacle of "departing from science and carrying our native medicine independent banner", will surely lead to a fast demise. Being sincere and yet using empty words cannot be victorious over experiments. The general rule of evolution determines it. It is the explanation of true principle; a point that must be considered.

So what is efficacy then? When there is a treatment method, only when there is efficacy it conforms to true principle. It is like nutrients relation to life, these both have the same idea. When one eats he cannot be limited only to potatoes and wheat. The native medicine treatment method had its own discoveries, which comes from natural ability of humans. As testimony, one can see that, as of today, most of the native population still believes in it. Today, in all countries, other than seeking to develop modern equipment, all look for medicinals. Native medicine medicinals' efficacy is clear, even though they have been neither arranged nor statistically studied. Amongst them there are medicinals able to supplement lacking of the international pharmacopeia. This may establish a unique banner for our native medicine, similar to special effects drugs 特效劑 such as ones for broken bones and severed tendons, bubonic plague, etc drugs that are well known in the medical community. Even if the effect can't be exactly calculated for those special effect drugs, the prize will be sought after by using it and seeing its efficacy. It is like, for example, formulas that have efficacy towards certain diseases of like the eyes, wherein after taking them inflammation reduces. Herbs taken internally that help the eyes include Qing Xiang Zi 青相子, Shi Jue Ming 石決明, Bai Ji Li 白蒺藜, Guan Sha Wan 關沙宛 etc. Herbs that can help the blood, blood vessels and circulation and that can be taken internally or applied externally for external injuries, regulating menses, calming fetus, reduce inflammation and stop pains are Dang Gui 當歸, Di Huang 地黃, Dan Pi 丹皮, Chi Shao 赤芍, Xiang Fu 香附, San Qi 三七, Hong Hua 紅花, Tao Ren 桃仁, Ling Zhi 靈脂, Pu Huang 蒲黃 etc. Or like warm herbs that have exciting effect or cool herbs that, even though they can't reach anesthesia, still have sedative effect, where these can treat many different diseases or they can be used in formulas that treat various diseases and increase the curative efficacy of those formulas, such as Huang Qin 黃芩, Shi Gao 石膏, Gan Jiang 干姜, Fu Zi 附子 etc. The above mentioned herbs not only are not used by modern medicine, but either modern drugs are not as effective as those herbs, or they even don't have any drug that has a similar effect. Even if modern medicine has a similar drug its efficacy if often not as good, for example, drugs used for nerves and blood like Strychnine, Liao Si De 了斯的[277] and iron, can't match the effect of the native herb Huang Qi 黃耆. Or drugs used to ease and calm pulmonary diseases like Yi Bu Ge 衣不格, Xin Yi Jia 辛衣加 and Ya Lu Jian 亞綠監 are not necessarily as good as the native herb Ma Huang 麻黃. Or like drugs that impact different people differently at different times, for example, reducing fever drugs, so even if the world's medicine has Aspirin, An Zhi Bi Lian 安

[277] Names of Western drugs from the 1920s we were not able to locate a translation for we have left untranslated.

知必連, Cinchona, this does not mean that the native medicine's herbs Chai Hu 柴胡, Shi Gao 石膏, Gui Zhi 桂枝, Zhi Zi 梔子, Yin Hua 銀花, Lian Qiao 連翹, Jiang Huo 姜活, Fang Feng 防風, Di Gu 地骨, Yin Hu 銀胡, Shi Hu 石斛 can be discarded of. Or if modern medicine has tonics like Strychnine, Liao Si De 了斯的, iron, iodine and phosphorus this does not mean that native medicine tonics need to be discarded of like the herbs Huang Qi 黃耆, Ren Shen 人參, Fu Zi 附子, Yu Gui 玉桂, Dang Gui 當歸, Bai Zhu 白術, Gu Zhi 固紙, Lu Rong 鹿茸 etc. Even more so there are herbs used in both world medicine as well as native medicine, yet each medicine does not know of the other's claimed effects. For example, the world's medicine does not know that Dan Cao 膽草 can cure eye disease, that Da Huang 大黃 has effect on the blood, and native medicine does not know that She Xiang 麝香 can recover the pulse, Lu Hui 蘆薈 can help the menses, likewise all of them have research value. These sort of examples are simply too many to count. Even though native medicine curative method is not limited to herbs this is its one most significant aspect. If one were to take this herbs' efficacy and make it publicly available around the world, then after people of the world suffer a broken bone, for example a broken arm, and they will try this medicinal and it works, than this kind of talk about eliminating our native medicine will significantly subside. And so when the sand bag will be used with hands and feet in order to set the broken bone and stretch the muscles, and the pain associated with this therapy will be completely alleviated with herbs, then they even more so will have nothing to argue against. In such a manner, wouldn't native medicine herbs reach all the nations of the world? Loving life and wanting to get rid of disease is something shared in common by all humans. One cannot ignore this.

There are many diseases that can be diagnosed, or that the principle is clear but they have no remedy, for example adults with malaria, when you treat it how come people develop black canker only around the equator? With blood serum being used for immunity, why is it only called a special effect drug for tetanus and diphtheria? Or scoliosis of little kids, acid reflux and stomach atrophy of the aged, how come there are no special effect drugs for those to fix the physical body and get rid of the acidity? Similarly, there are many diseases where the principle theory is clear but there is no cure. This kind of lacking in world medicine is plenty. If we speak of remedies that have efficacy but the principle is not clear, then all of Chinese medicine belongs to this category. It is not that they entirely can't be explained, it is just that the vague explanation of Qi transformation must be discarded of. One must not be infatuated with seeking "deep" and, with that, ignore the truth while seeking the distant.

This is exactly the scope of our native medicine winning or losing. Let's use an example that will firmly clarify my words, encompass and explain the topic. Today diseases of heart, lungs and brain are considered the three most deadly diseases. Symptoms of pathological changes with breathing, pulse, body temperature and brain activity, are the biggest precepts which world medicine considers for its experiments, diagnosis and treatment. And for the one whom no-one surpasses, we look back to our nation's medicine sage Zhang Zhongjing 張仲景. When contemplating what he stood by, how is this not the case that he sought after the same things? First let's discuss the outline.

Within the three Yang, Yang Ming 陽明 has death syndrome while Shao Yang 少陽 and Tai Yang 太陽 don't. Yang Ming has delirious speech, and its fever is steaming. Within the three Yin, Shao Yin 少陰 has many death syndromes, Tai Yin 太陰 doesn't, while Jue Yin 厥陰 has few. In Shao Yin the pulse is thin and small and there is desire to sleep etc heart and brain symptoms. Also when speaking of sweat, Yang syndromes should have sweat, as Yang syndrome must have fever. This is the result of the body's own temperature scattering and so it is appropriate. For Yin syndromes it is adverse, as many Yin syndromes don't have fever, this "having sweat" may be the predicting sign of collapse and therefore it is adverse. In Shao Yin section it states: "The patient's pulse both Yin and Yang are tight, if to the contrary sweat comes out it means the Yang perishes. This belongs to Shao Yin." Or it states: "Shao Yin disease the pulse is small, one cannot sweat it, as the Yang will perish." Jue Yin section states: "with great sweat if one greatly purges it and there is adverse cold, then Si Ni Tang 四逆湯 dominates it." These quotes all explain this same point.

Or gasping for air, for example—cough with gasping for air is a physiological reaction. Even though Zhongjing attaches importance to it he is not careful enough. When there is gasping with no cough one suspects a connection to the heart organ. It can be caused by a feeble heart as one of the associated symptoms. The following should be considered, things Zhongjing did attach importance to. For example, "Yang Ming [disease] gazing straight forward, delirious speech, gasping for air and fullness there is death, if there is diarrhea also death." And, "Shao Yin disease six, seven days, breathing is high then death." And, "diarrhea and adverse cold of hands and feet, no [palpable] pulse, [patient] doesn't warm up with moxa, if the pulse does not return, to the contrary there is slight gasping, then there is death," etc sections they all explain a certain point. Also when Zhongjing prohibits purging, sweating and vomiting, as these three easily descend into the feeble heart, we can see he pays attention to certain things.

If we further analyze this, then we find many more examples describing this pattern. Like: "Shao Yin disease, diarrhea stopped, the head is dizzy and at times in vertigo, then there is death." This is because body fluids are lost and it creates brain hemorrhage. Or: "Shao Yin disease, vomiting diarrhea and agitation, the four adverse [cold hands and feet], then there is death", "Shao Yin disease, four adverse, aversion to cold, and body curled, pulse does not arrive, no agitation but there is anxiety, then there is death" and: "diarrhea and pulse is minute, use Bai Tong Tang 白通湯 for it. If diarrhea doesn't stop, adverse with no pulse, dry belching and anxiety, then Bai Tong Tang jia Zhu Dan Zhi 白通湯加豬膽汁 treats it. After drinking the decoction, if the pulse is minute and continuous then there is life, if the pulse comes out explosive then death." And: "after diarrhea the pulse is vanishing, hands and feet cold, at night the pulse returns and the hands and feet warm then there is life, the pulse does not return then death." These quotes explain that when diarrhea is excessive blood pressure decreases and body temperature naturally drops. Also: "Cold injury, diarrhea lasting more than ten days, if the pulse to the contrary is full then there is death." This happens when the heart is overly stressed and so it lands in paralysis (I suspect that this presentation is caused by arteriosclerosis). Also: "Shao Yin disease, diarrhea, if diarrhea stops on its own, there is aversion to cold, and the person lies curled, the hands and feet are warm, then this can be cured." And: "Shao Yin disease, aversion to cold and [the person is] curled, sometimes agitated, the person wants to remove the clothes and blanket, this can be cured." This reflects that the body temperature can preserve its normal state. Also: "Shao Yin disease, vomiting and diarrhea, hands and feet not adverse cold, to the contrary there is fever, there is no death." This shows that body temperature increases, and the blood pressure does not decrease…

If we get rid of the distant and take on what is close then the standard for arranging the medicine is close at hand. To advance this, consider the following: experiments are the scientific principle, statistics are the fact. If one uses both of these then he can get to a complete picture. Medicine all over the world has attained this. Today, our native medicine is at the preliminary stages of being put in order and so the scientific principle and the facts are both important. Now, if native medicine accumulated experience is proper and correct, even though some of it does not conform to science, but most of it can demonstrate applicability and usage, then it contains this valuable point and will not be easily discarded for not conforming to science. Therefore, native medicine should not claim its core to be absurd and nonsensical beautiful sounding statements. The fate of this medicine's reform cannot be accomplished by one person within a brief moment. Only by following a developmental curve with science may it have discovery and advancement one day in the future.

In the past, "life" was inconceivable and placed in the spiritual realm; today we know that it exists within the medulla oblongata or enzymes or "life" glands.[278] The fetus was considered to have endless transformation that cannot be investigated, but today we know that the embryo goes through the tube and after it straps tightly it grows on its own into male or female, and its gender is not determined by the hormones secreted by the ovaries. Scurvy and beriberi cause was not known, but now it was discovered that nutrients and vitamins deficiency cause these.

In the past, one thought that it was formless cause, but now we know that the cause does have a physical form. Science of materialism and its associated powerful influence are tightly connected. Being in the physical realm is definitely the Truth. Only in such a way can medicine progress day after day and become promising. This point cannot be summed up with one or two examples.

Now, in many instances, what native medicine calls Qi transformation can be converted in reality to physical terms such as: Blood means the blood fluid, Qi equals the nerves, Yin Yang is heart, Wind is brain, Damp is stomach and intestines, Water is body fluids, Fire means excitation of the body, deficiency and excess are treatment standards, external and internal mean the depth of the disease symptoms—these all can be attained by the four diagnostic methods.[279] Where is there formless? Where is there Qi transformation? If one continues in this physical fashion then the principle naturally becomes clear, there is no need to wait one more day. In addition, when looking at disease like this there is no difference between Chinese and Western—one may advance until things become so clear like the sun and moon illuminating the clear sky. Everything will come out into the open!

To sum up all what I said, these points demand scientification of native medicine, which is its only available path. If one wishes to arrange native medicine properly he cannot avoid this. If one follows this Dao then immediately effect will come about and the principle of both medicines will become the same, Chinese and Western can collaborate and divide tasks. The disorder will be put in order and, in the future, experiments and statistics will be shared and benefited by both. Then the arrangement that we do today will not be crooked.

---

[278] Endocrine glands.
[279] Hearing and smelling, seeing, palpating, asking.

Quietly, I am looking at your esteemed Bureau[280] establishing the standard for this art that will advance our medicine. With this standard, attaining or losing something will not be fake—not even by an iota. In addition, the ones who are knowledgeable will know it, while the ignorants will not know it without a way to pretend. This will open a future path for scientification of native medicine. It will sever the thus-far superstition and guessing of illusions. This will be the great fortune of our people; its benefit will be immeasurable.

Restraining myself from saying many words I would like to share with the esteemed Bureau the following: Medical science in modern times relies heavily on specialists. You have been faithful with this endeavor for a year, with numerous plans hoping to create a complete strategy. When the cave is illuminated by the essential then every word is right on target and every action reaches an accomplishment. Moreover, medicine is profound and complicated. The new and old need be concise and comprehensive. How can one reach this objective without specialization? Therefore the reorganization plan of the old medicine requires assistance by capable specialists. I wish that the esteemed Bureau will gather talented people who have mastered both Chinese and Western medicines. These specialists should pursue the suggested path and arrange and progress the art to walk a similar path to Western medicine. This art should seek the new and not bring back the old, such as when one doesn't obsequiously agree with the ancients then he is immediately being looked at as against the classics and the sages. Like this, it is no different from following and abiding by the old ways—where can there be progress? I wish for the esteemed Bureau to embody the spirit of progress and have, as a principle, "correcting the errors of prior generations". Native medicine literature is like a jade coin and precious gem that needs to be explored and collected. There is nothing to wait, at present, everything is fragmented and conflicted. Where should one follow? I wish that that the esteemed Bureau will establish a long-term vision, bring in literature and systemize a consistent standard.

Man treasures and feels deeply convinced about Dao and Virtue. Medicine is like this too. The essence of medicine's virtue is the serving of others. To advance goodness, one must be courageous. If one wishes to serve, then he must first eradicate the self-exaggerating empty talk. If one desires to advance goodness then it is proper to remove the terrible feeling of personal prejudice. What I said above are common sayings of science. If one talks about progress by scientific methods then his understanding is already halfway there. However those who still shout and argue and

[280] The Bureau for Native Medicine.

make a speech, aloof talk about present day native medicine opposite scientification, all their words are adverse to the essence of science. They don't understand the true meaning of science. These people act like a curtain preventing the light and sound from entering the eyes and ears of the esteemed Bureau. I am afraid that they don't stop, like a sensualist after precious jade, their voices chaotic like geese and ducks. Aren't they nothing but extreme obstruction to the progress of native medicine? Using these words looks shabby, it will be my luck if you pardon my presumptuous manner. If your system appraises and accepts my words then truly it will be the benefit of the public.

Attached: Critique from Chinese and Western medicine publications toward Tan's proposal

Pages 12–20

1. Critique by the director of the *Shanghai Society Medical Gazette* 上海社會醫報, in the 143rd issue, Mr. Yu Yunxiu 余雲岫 said: Mr. Tan 譚 is clever and upright. In this text the idea is very proper. It allows the Bureau for Native Medicine to pick up on a few things how to reach to X, Y and Z academic circles. The speaker is devoted, while the listener is contemptuous. Truly there is a sense that the yellow bell is ruined and abandoned.[281] It is just that in the discussion about herbs and diseases there are places requiring more cautiousness, yet its main points are outstanding. The reader may as well ignore these minute flaws. (The above text, following the suggestions by the director of *Shanghai Society Medical Gazette* 上海社會醫報 Mr. Yu Yan [Yunxiu], was corrected.)

2. From Guangzhou *Yue Hua daily newspaper* 廣州越華日報 medical matters column director Mr. Xu Xiuwu 許修五: Mr. Tan Cizhong 譚次仲 of Wu Zhou 梧州 and Mr. Yu Yunxiu 余雲岫, of Hu Bin 滬濱,[282] both proposed this year a medical revolution. The writings by these two gentlemen, to a large degree, were recorded by this column. Through this I got to learn that these two gentlemen are thoroughly proficient with Chinese traditional studies as well as properly versed with modern studies.

[281] This is a part of an idiom 黄钟毁弃，瓦釜雷鸣 *"The yellow bell is ruined and abandoned, while the earthenware and cauldron make a big noise"*. It means: Capable and talented people are ignored while mediocre people are held high.
[282] Shanghai

In China today they are a couple of the very few highly talented people. Because they know the truth and their insight is profound, these two gentlemen can reach the same goal by different routes. (This comment can be found in the medical affairs and public health column of Mr. Xu in the above mentioned newspaper printed on November 4th of the 21st year [1932].)

3. From the head of Chinese medicine section of the *Bei Ping Arts and Literature Weekly* 北平藝文週報, Mr. Hao Yuyun 郝裔雲: The four words: "principle; truthful; efficacy; reliable"[283] are the backbone of this text. Being or not truthful and reliable, relies upon the two methods: experiments and statistics. Solid reliability of a theory comes from this. Even if someone can talk like Su and Zhang,[284] it can't be broken. In this text the style of writing is powerful and unrestrained, the versification is elegant and simple. The finale especially is with much tonal patterns and rhyme schemes, with a clever modulation in tone. It seems if one is not versed with the Qin 秦 and Han 漢 dynasties and is not a talented person then he could not easily have attained such an accomplishment, such an excellent text. Being on target with the new and the old medicines is a rarely-found accomplishment.

4. A comment by the medical affairs columnist of the *Yue Hua Bao* 越華報 newspaper, Mr. Huang Zhipeng 黃志鵬: I, amongst my peers, occupy an unimportant place from the standpoint of science. I maintain an objective and strict attitude about it. If one has a method conforming to science, which he adheres to and doesn't let go, then how can he tolerate the destruction of its true principle? Like Mr. Tan Cizhong 譚次仲 of Wu Zhou 梧州, truly an outstanding Chinese medicine practitioner. My colleagues in this column all admire his personality. Therefore all his writings we have published. This serves to show that with my different colleagues there was no scope distinction. It was all about the struggle differentiating scientific and not scientific. (This comment can be seen in the issue printed on September 24th of the 21st year [1932] of said newspaper, in an article by Mr. Huang titled *Arguing Colliding Red with Yu Youwen* 與余友文論撞紅.)

5. In a personal letter from Bureau of Native Medicine, member of the Arranging of the Medicine Committee Mr. Lu Yuanlei 陸淵雷 wrote (Mr. Lu also published his

[283] Li Zhen Xiao Que 理真效確.

[284] The tongue of Su and Zhang 蘇張之舌, refers to Su Qin 蘇秦 and Zhang Yi 張儀, two political strategists during the warring states period 475–221 BCE, who became famous for their ability to achieve their goals only by using words. The idiom talks about a person who is very skillful with words.

opinion about this text in the *Shanghai Society Medical Gazette*, in its 157th issue in the news report column as follows): Mr. Yunxiu 雲岫 kindly read the following: Recently I have read your letter *Give to Director Wu*[285] and Mr. Tan Cizhong's 譚次仲 *Explain to the Bureau of Native Medicine Item by Item*, of which all points I gladly accept. It is as good as if out of my own mouth. Mr. XX[286] of the Bureau of Native Medicine contacted certain venerable sirs to elect XXX to make the draft. At that time we did not yet look at it carefully and hastily sent it to press. When I looked at it I proposed to correct it, but Mr. X was not happy about it. Finally, I came across Mr. Tan's calling people to account, which is widely heard by everybody in the Chinese medicine community. This had me even further away from Mr. X and at this point there is not much I could do. I have been practicing Chinese medicine for a long time and truly believe that this method is able to cure diseases. In addition, there are many Western methods that we haven't acquired as of yet, and if we arrange them this will allow going on the scientific tract. If we accomplish this it will allow great progress to world medicine. But to start with, one should not be stained by the notion that the ancient sages' accomplishment is synonymous with preserving the nation's treasure. That people today have little skill and ability, and not much to show for, is not the sages' offense along the banks of the river—it has, rather extensively, become a contemporary dishonor. At this moment, the Arranging of the Medicine Committee of the Bureau of Native Medicine is urged to look over the synopsis of my draft; attached is a copy I sent to the secretary. Listening to your kind instruction, the first five items, to a large degree, confront contemporary problems; these can only be reformed by the entire assembly. I am not sure to what degree these can be adopted. Like the ignorant admonitions that, at times, are published as criticism, this text should also be published. But please note clearly that this is a suggested draft and not the official Bureau for Native Medicine definitive edition. With special respect and a praise praying for your literary health! Lu Yuanlei touch the head to the ground.

6. From the assistant director of registration of the Hong Kong Native Medicine Association Xiang Gang Guo Yi Xue Hui 香港國醫學會 and the editor of the *Native Medicine Magazine Guo Yi Za Zhi* 國醫雜誌, Mr. He Peiyu 何佩瑜: This work by Mr. Tan 譚 shows that his study is profound, while his explanations are liberally given. It is a shame though that he doesn't understand the meaning of Chinese medicine.

[285] The letter full title is 上五院長論國醫館書 A Letter to Director Wu discussing the Bureau for Native Medicine.

[286] The text mentions several people anonymously, each distinguished as Mr. X, Mr. XX and Mr. XXX; we have kept the Xs as in the original.

While he reveres the materialism of Western medicine he should know that Chinese and foreign medicines are not the same. Their difference lies between physical form and ability. Foreign medicine talks about the material of the organs. The material is a fixed entity, each person has it and so they call it a scientific method. Chinese medicine speaks of the ability of the organ's Qi. The ability changes according to different factors. This is a fluid state but it has its principle and the invisible too can be assessed. This seems as if it is not conforming to the scientific method. It is this point of difference that creates the fighting between the new and old medicines.

Leading directly to this century where modern science is surging ahead, whenever there is a scientific discovery it is often looked at as an inconceivable miracle. It is therefore named the all-powerful science. Normally, people follow it blindly and when it comes to the medicine's principle, physiology and pathology they are all convinced about the organs' physical anatomy because you can see it. However, when it comes down to seeking it via the organs' Qi, which cannot be seen by the eye, then even though there are a hundred benefits they all propose together that Chinese medicine is not conforming to science and that its theories of organ Qi ability, Yin Yang and Qi transformation should all be abolished. They think that the scientific method of dissection anatomy is all that is required, which is a huge mistake.

A human being is different from a dead object. No matter what objects we look at, they all can be dissected into parts by a scientific method. Human consciousness, however, and one's life and death, even though can be connected to different physical systems of the body, still rely on a certain kind of life Qi for their existence. This kind of life Qi, because the human himself comes in contact with heaven's Qi and earth's Qi and there are all kinds of connections and influences, where time and location is different, how can one solely rely on the scientific method of dissection to get the entire picture? If this could have been solved in its entirety, look at foreign countries these days inventing a robot, it can walk and do actions just like a person, however why doesn't it have feelings, why can't it talk? Machine can mimic the four limbs and hundred bones, and yet the nervous system cannot be man-made. This is a point to think about.

In reality, Qi transformation is part of science. The meaning of the word "science" is "a certain understanding that leads to a certain theory". If it is interlinked logically without changing then this is a kind of science. For example explaining the principle of sound is called acoustics or sound science, explaining the light principle is called optics or light science, explaining material interactions and transformation is called chemistry transformation science and electric science, explaining the physical systems inside the human body is called dissection anatomy science, explaining the actions of the different systems is called physiology. Everybody knows this, so how come Chinese medicine Qi transformation is the only one unlike the others. It explains the organs' Qi and its relation to heaven and earth and the four seasons' Qi and they create Qi transformation. No matter what transformations there may be, they all have the change between hard and soft. For example, if the sun is fierce during daytime or the night is pitch dark during nighttime, since the phenomena are not the same then the reaction created has either hard or soft expression. One simply uses the two words Yin Yang to summarize it. Categorically they are all the same, but each one of these roots can divide into endless manifestation and at the end these endless manifestations go back to this one root. How is this not an everlasting and unchanging interlinked logic? This is why it can become a Qi transformation science. This is why a theory can form and not because people decide what science is.

However, Chinese medicine explanation of physiology and anatomy is closely connected to the understanding of Qi transformation but is lacking in regards to physical anatomy. Therefore, forever it was leaning to one side and incomplete. In addition, in the past when the ancients wrote books, they often mingled the flawed with the precious. For example, in the *Neijing* 內經 they talked with great fine detail about heaven and man connection, but mixed within were five elements control and generating, heaven Qi transportation, additions of the year and all kinds of absurd talk. Thus they did something very clever and then turned around and did something clumsy. They taught people these loopholes. When Zhongjing 仲景 composed *Shang Han* 傷寒 and *Jin Gui* 金匱 the understanding was entirely of Qi transformation. There is no talk of heaven Qi transformation and five phases anymore. One should understand deeply why this is so.

One must understand that Chinese medicine needs arrangement. It cannot escape taking the strong points and supplementing the weak points, discarding the stray and preserving the truth. However, one should not ask to discard its essence, which is Qi transformation, and instead stubbornly linger on the materialistic aspect, which then will cause the entire Chinese medicine to become Western medicine. One should not claim this to be "an arrangement". In addition, not only Chinese medicine needs arrangement, but Western medicine also must go through arrangement. That Western medicine doesn't understand Qi transformation also makes it incomplete. Therefore, it is often inadequate in treating diseases resulting from interaction between heaven and man [weather related], seven emotions and six desires. If they can help each other's arrangement, each contributing its strong points and melting in one furnace, then it can be called a complete medicine.

Mr. Tan esteems Western medicine materialistic view but when it comes to Yin Yang Qi transformation, which is the key element of Chinese medicine, he merges it erroneously with five phases, heavenly stems and earthly branches, leading the year and in spring etc false theories all in one pot, claiming all of them to be an empty talk from remote antiquity. Now, he does not carefully investigate the topic and yet painfully he adds destruction. Alas! Himself considered not a stray dog, so how come he barks and bites. If this is the arrangement of Chinese medicine, how is it different from beating down Chinese medicine? His kind of discussion is exactly the same as Wang (Qizhang 汪企張) and Yu (Yunxiu 余雲岫) etc group of people. Therefore we especially published in this magazine this article, to take his errors and refute them one by one. This will allow the readers of Tan's extensive work to know its errors and not be led astray by them. With the brilliance of Mr. Tan, why didn't he research further *Shang Han* 傷寒 *Jin Gui* 金匱, as well as the *Neijing* 內經 and *Lingshu's* 靈樞 essence, and carefully come to a clear understanding—and only then voice a discussion about the ancients, so he doesn't laugh at the medical community and bring error to future generations. How can Mr. Tan call himself an admonitory friend of ours?

Tan's text claims that the world's modern science is the crystallization of truth. Thousands of years of outstanding scholars investigated thoroughly till they reach old age, and only then they could get at the scientific truth. He doesn't know that today, doctors in all countries around the world rely solely on science to explain the many problems in medicine and medicinal substances, which is insufficient. In addition, in the long history we had, with many outstanding and talented people researching all their lives and accumulating this experience, we too got to our standard of Truth. Chinese medicine has already 4,000 years since the Yellow emperor till today; the number of outstanding scholars over this history is many more than tenfold all the modern outstanding scholars of the other countries. The science of world medicine, however, was discovered over the past several hundred years, so how come one scorns only the one and not the other?

In addition, world medicine expounds on disease but it keeps on changing. For example, regarding malaria, the English Mr. Benjamin Hobson[287] thought that it started from the poisonous gas emitted by rotten grass and grains and that wind blew away the gas, infecting people. In the second half of the 19th century, Western medicine

[287] 1816–1873 CE

thought it was caused by miasma and it forms miasma. In recent days it is said to be caused by a tiny parasite living in the body of a mosquito, and when the mosquito stings the person the parasite is transmitted into the human body. Within one hundred and some years the principle has changed over and over. What they call Truth crystallization was first this truth and then the other truth. Other examples such as this one are abundant. Mr. Tan seems not to have been exploring those.

Tan's text also states that, in addition to all sciences being unanimously acknowledged by everyone around the world, if one establishes a separate medical principle coming out of China then this means that Chinese people will have to have different organs and systems from people from the rest of the world, and only then would it be possible. This section points out that Chinese medicine is the only one that has the concept of Qi transformation and that, since the organs and bodily systems of a Chinese person are no different from other people around the world, one should not use a separate Qi transformation principle in order to treat the same organs and systems. The same organs need the same treatment principle and methods. However, one here should ask if these methods have efficacy or not, not if they are of the same kind or not. Chinese medicine utilizes Qi transformation to evaluate and treat. For 4,000 years, if a method was ineffective then the people of China would have extinguished it already a long time ago. How is it that today, when looking at populations all over the world, amongst people who reach old age the majority of them are in China?

In addition, regarding the difference between Chinese and Western medicines, it is not an overstatement to say that it lies within a physical theory versus a functional one. Western medicine emphasizes dissection anatomy and it explains the physical form. Chinese medicine emphasizes Qi transformation and so it explains the functions. The first one explains the form but not necessarily can explain the ability; therefore, when they create a puppet in a human image, how could it live? Qi transformation and physical form, if we only utilize one of them, how is this not perverse? These two cannot be separated. However, Western medicine in its research has attainments, but these attainments when used to treat human diseases all around the world often have poor effect. How is it so that Japanese doctors research Chinese medicine like this in a hurry? The way Mr. Tan talks about this topic cannot stand.

In Tan's text when we get to the large section talking about native medicine and its sage Zhongjing 仲景 and his treatment of disease, it seems that Mr. Tan also knows the *Shang Han Lun* 傷寒論. The pathology he mentions is described properly and persistently. He recklessly claims that, while the efficacy gets close to truth, the principle does not make sense and that the entire native medicine is like this. If saying that Zhang Zhongjing in Chinese medicine is one person unparalleled, and yet his principle doesn't make sense, then how does the *Shang Han Lun* principle fill Mr. Tan with admiration? Mr. Tan's heart-filled admiration for Zhongjing comes from the common understanding of world medicine that heart, lungs and brain diseases are deadly. Change in breathing, pulse, body temperature and brain activity, these 4 things are the great tenets for modern experiments, diagnosis and treatment. Zhongjing's explanations happen to coincide with these and so here it is called proper experience. But sadly, how come Mr. Tan's knowledge ends here? Why doesn't he know that Zhongjing's proper experience comes from understanding Qi transformation?

Just to give one or two examples to demonstrate what I mean: How come Yang Ming 陽明 has delirious speech? In addition, when there is fever why is there steaming? It is because evil enters the stomach and intestines, stagnates and transforms into heat. Western medicine calls this "typhoid fever". Typhoid fever is a cold injury that enters into one part of Yang Ming. If one claims that cold injury is typhoid fever then this is untrue. If it is in Yang Ming then it transforms into heat but if it is in Tai Yang 太陽 then it does not transform into heat. May we ask: between the two situations, isn't this Qi transformation? In Shao Yin 少陰 there are many deadly diseases; when they enter Shao Yin it goes deep. The changes in Shao Yin are severe. When it transforms into heat, it becomes a severe "set on fire syndrome" requiring Huang Lian E Jiao Tang 黃連阿膠湯. When it transforms into cold then it becomes a dangerous syndrome of extinguishing requiring Si Ni Tang 四逆湯 and Bai Tong Tang 白通湯. How can one state that these diseases are simply brain and heart diseases? May we ask, isn't this because of Qi transformation?

When it says that Yang syndromes have sweat, this means that evil is in the exterior skin and flesh. This stirs up the sweat glands. And so when sweat comes out it is the way it should be. It means that there is evil Qi and it is not related to body temperature scattering.[288] When Yin syndrome has sweat then it is adverse. This happens when evil is in the interior Yin, it cannot steam and excite the sweat glands at the exterior flesh. Therefore there is not this principle of sweat. If one does see sweat [at this level] then he must guard from collapse. Explaining a syndrome that belongs to Yin or to Yang immediately allows one to know if evil is at the exterior or in the interior. If this is not about Qi transformation what else is it about?

[288] As Tan claimed.

Cough that has gasping associated with it, means that there is evil there. When evil is expelled the gasping naturally stops. Therefore he[289] didn't attach much importance to it. If there is no cough but there is gasping, then it means that there is no exterior evil [attack]. This means the person's own upright energy is deficient. If this energy is extremely deficient then a collapse follows. How can this merely be about the heart being feeble? Therefore he attaches great importance to it. Having cough or not having cough, while gasping, determines if there is evil or not, which can tell the difference between life and death. Again, if this is not about Qi transformation, what else is it talking about?

Tan's text states that China's medicine is not correct; he points out that concretion Zheng Jia 癥瘕 means a tumor inside the abdominal cavity. This is one mistake. He says that Nüe Mu 瘧母[290] misleads people to believe that the spleen is swollen, a second mistake. Zheng Jia 癥瘕 is caused entirely by blood solidifying and Qi condensing. Its origin cause is often the seven emotions being entangled and thus the organs' Qi can't flow smoothly. How is that related to tumors? Nüe Mu 瘧母 is caused by malaria that lingers for a long time and then the evil congeals within the blood. How is that involving swollen spleen?

Mr. Tan only knows that there are physical organs but he doesn't know about organs' Qi.[291] It follows then that he thinks Qi transformation diseases are physical diseases, resulting in one pointing to a donkey and saying that it is a horse. He says that there are many organs within the abdominal cavity and that there are different types of tumors, therefore reaching the root cause of a tumor is very complicated. He puts forth the example of females that may have different tumors in the ovaries, fallopian tubes and uterus, each carrying different symptoms. So how does one undergo preventative treatment?

There are even finer more precise modern diagnostic and treatment methods, which are evenly considered without distinguishing if they are harmful or not. Only in a sweeping rash he recklessly attacks Tao Ren 桃仁 Hong Hua 紅花 etc. Claiming that out of 100 treatments 100 patients will die. With these kinds of statements one needs only one glance to know that Mr. Tan has read very few Chinese medicine books. In the *Ling Shu* chapter *Yong Ju Lun* 靈樞癰疽論 and in *Jin Gui* chapter *Fei Wei Fei Yong*

[289] Zhang Zhongjing

[290] 瘧母蒙混脾肿 Nüe Mu, literally "mother of malaria", means that after one has malaria for a long time he may experience a lump in the abdomen that feels as if the spleen is swollen.

[291] In Chinese there is a play on words, he only knows Zang Qi 臟器 but he doesn't know Zang Qi 臟氣, where physical body and Qi are phonetically the same.

Pian 金匱肺萎肺癰篇 the meaning is profound and the principle deep, yet Mr. Tan is unable to understand these. Books such as *Wai Ke Zheng Zhi Quan Sheng Ji* 外科證治全生集[292] and *Wai Ke Jin Jian* 外科金鑒[293] distinguish Yin Yang deficiency and excess. Indeed they point to the physical organs and different types of tumors and disease etiology. The description is detailed, while the diagnostics are excellent and treatment is full of goodness. In a bright way it is well prepared. How can it be compared to his medicine where they see chest pains and they diagnose it as emphysema, if they happen to see rib pains then it points to a liver abscess and other such general assumptions? Mr. Tan has likely never set eyes on such specialized books, yet still in a rash he recklessly makes jeering comments. How is he different from one having tunnel vision? When it comes to the treatment of tumors, his medicine can only use surgery to excise it while Chinese medicine uses herbs and it is always effective. Everybody can see that. Which method is good and which is bad? If one follows it, he will know.

Tan's text berates the *Shang Han Lun* "six urgent purging" section 傷寒論六急下節 as blurred and wandering back and forth aimlessly, superficial with strained interpretations. The meaning of the words is stiff, he quotes: "if one doesn't apply these [purging methods] there is no life principle remaining and there is no proper treatment." Tan says, "if one erroneously gives one large dose of purgative formula following a suspicious diagnosis, assuming the patient has a strong healthy heart and rising fever while at the same time food remains in the intestines as constipation, then out of ten patients, quickly two or three will die. For example, when there is a similar presentation of symptoms with appendicitis, peritonitis etc. conditions that are severe and purging is prohibited. With other patients who have heart conditions one dose of purging immediately will make them sink into a dangerous situation that can't be saved, probably more than five or six will die."

Now, when I look at Mr. Tan's praise of Zhongjing's *Shang Han Lun*, saying that the accumulated experience is accurate, I thought that he too could read the *Shang Han Lun*. But when I got to this section and his scorn of the "six urgent purging", I realized that he can't really understand the *Shang Han Lun*. Alas, the knowledgeable with a thousand good thoughts may have one error. Therefore, in the book of poetry and in the six classics there are mistakes. Myself, I don't think that Zhongjing is error free. If it was not for Mr. Tan's one-sided blind trust to his medicine, then he would not have

292 Published 1740 CE.
293 Published 1742 CE.

scorned what he thinks is correct. During the discovery process of science this is something, which was not done, yet Mr. Tan's words and intention are doing it.[294]

When I read Zhongjing's lines I do not read it like Tan. In the *Shang Han Lun* six urgent purging section 傷寒論六急下節, it only describes excessive conditions with heat blazing inside and, if the sincere doctor does not purge urgently, than the patient cannot be saved. Only when one purges urgently can one save the body fluids. Truly, "without this there is no life principle left and, even more so, there is no other treatment possible." This is Zhongjing's true meaning. The meaning of the words is firm. Mr. Tan points to "blurred and wandering back and forth aimlessly, superficial with strained interpretations" and "if one erroneously gives one large dose of purgative formula following a suspicious diagnosis" then it is like Shu Sun Wu Shu 叔孫武叔[295] destroying Zhong Ni 仲尼.[296] Like it was in ancient times, this is still the case today. In addition, the *Shang Han Lun* distinguishes clearly between cases where it is allowed to purge and other cases where it is prohibited. It warns about it with great detail. Where is there this logic that one can purge even in severe cases where purging is prohibited?

Tan's text talks about Cun, Guan and Chi 寸關尺 pulses as divided into six pulses[297] being negligible and absurd. He also claims to have a thorough understanding of the native medicine and that he does not oppose it. If one is not clear about the pulse principle then sincerely he may find it odd. He does not know that the pulse method is truly one of Chinese medicine's marvelous methods. The pragmatic side of it is that when one feels the Cun, Guan and Chi positions of the pulse, one can diagnose the disease. If one's experience is insufficient please read the article we have published in the *Native Medicine Magazine* 2nd issue.

If one divides the Cun, Guan and Chi into three sections of the pulse then one can readily understand it. In addition, *Shang Han Lun* talks about the three positions Cun, Guan and Chi often. For example, In *Tai Yang Pian* 太陽篇 it states: "When Cun pulse floats and Guan pulse sinks then this is called knotted chest." Or, "If the Chi pulse is slow, one cannot induce sweat." Mr. Tan self-proclaims to thoroughly know

---

294 He scorns without checking the facts.

295 Shu Sun Wu Shu 叔孫武叔 is Minister of War of the state of Lu 魯 during the eastern Zhou dynasty.

296 Zhong Ni is Confucius. The following quote is from the Analects 19:23 "Shusun Wushu decried Zhong Ni.
Zi Gong said: "It is labor lost. Zhong Ni cannot be cried down. The greatness of other men is a mound that can be overleaped but Zhong Ni is like the sun or moon that no man can overleap. To run into death a man may be ready, but how could he hurt the sun or moon? His want of sense would show the better!"

297 Three pulse positions on each of the hands.

Zhongjing's native medicine and that he does not oppose it—I don't know where this opinion is coming from and why he says it.

In Tan's article there is praise for Chinese medicine's herbs. But it seems he knows that they work, but not know why they work. For example, he praises Chinese herbs that can heal bone fractures and severed tendons, but he only knows that these formulas have a special effect. He doesn't know that the miraculous effects of herbs for bone fractures and severed tendons find their root in the mysteriousness of Qi transformation. Their effect of healing bones and tendons no-one in the entire world of medicine can explain [with modern science]. They only know to cut and remove it so they can replace it with something else. It creates [an impression] as if China's [medicine] doesn't have the ability to address broken bones and severed tendons. I am afraid it makes the cheap straw sandals rise in value. Even more so, it brings the realm of the duke Jing of the state of Qi.[298] Chinese medicine treating broken bones and severed tendons has, with hundred trials, hundred cures. It never cut away in any one single person, how come?

It is because his medicine sees the person like a dead body. When they encounter a broken bone they view it like a rotten leg of a table, if you don't cut it right away and instead consider long about healing the rotten, then it must all decay. This is a kind of materialistic explanation. Chinese medicine knows that humans are living beings. Even though one part may sustain an injury, yet its life mechanism didn't decease. Therefore, one determines that it can be irrigated and may recover its original form. If the bone broke but bone tissues are not severed, tendons may sever but the tendon ending are still attached, therefore Qi and blood can circulate there and cause it to reunite. To help it, one uses herbs and so the broken becomes connected again and decayed is not decayed any more. When tree branches break, yet their skin is still attached to the trunk, they can recover. It is because it has life Qi and water can irrigate there. A plant has life mechanism still attached and man does not? This principle is all about Qi transformation. This is our Chinese medicine's strong point. Nonetheless, medicine was designed to save the people. Therefore, it does not hesitate to make a contribution to the world. Even if there is smallpox and bubonic plague, they are all strong points of Chinese medicine which, as well, comes from the clever understanding of Qi transformation. Mr. Tan painfully severed the science of Qi transformation. He should examine carefully its many aspects and consider it diligently.

[298] Duke Jing was installed to power by Cui Zhu 崔杼 who, in turn, was sharing the power with him. In this paragraph it means that Tan uses Western science to validate Chinese medicine and in turn Chinese medicine becomes powerless.

A second letter to the Bureau for Native Medicine explaining ten points of having no difference between Chinese and Western medicine

By Tan Cizhong

Yaron: Tan Cizhong and Yu Yunxiu both believe that Chinese medicine has to become scientific and that this can only happen by discarding its old theory. Both gentlemen, as we saw in Yu's *Ling Su Shang Dui*, and can see in the following letter, have gone to great lengths to research classical literature. Yu refutes every single Chinese medicine theory, while Tan claims these theories to be scientific—just not scientific enough. More specifically, Tan explains that *Neijing* and *Shang Han Lun* treatment related theories were always experiment-based but simply lacked modern scientific knowledge. He asserts that, by using modern science, Chinese medicine treatment will maintain its original experience-based character and will become more efficacious.

The difference between Yun Tieqiao, who wanted a unique Chinese medical principle, and Tan Cizhong's use of modern medical knowledge can be evaluated in the following article. Tan's model was favored later on during the Communist era and formation of modern TCM schools. It was due to the Communist Party's exaggerated need to drum up national and cultural identity while rejecting both old feudal values and foreign bourgeois influences. Chinese medicine had a unique native science not imported from the West and it served the purpose well.

The three trends represented by Yunxiu, Cizhong and Tieqiao influenced and created modern Chinese medicine. Today, the situation is not much different. Some Chinese medicine practitioners believe that ancient theories are nonsense, others think that old theories were a kind of science, an accumulated treatment experience that needs to become improved by modern science, and others still borrow modern scientific knowledge and develop their own unique medical principle.

During the Republic years, modern science was used by the state to gain power and establish authority; there was very little space for antiquated theories. During Communist China, there was a great need for manpower in socialized healthcare and Western medicine could not handle the job.

Today, Western medicine is in control and is handling comprehensively the healthcare system. There is no shortage of doctors, at least not in developed countries, nor is there an urgent need for governments to use science for power, at least not as drastically as during the Republic years in China. Nowadays, Chinese medicine is seen as a popular alternative to modern medicine. Now is a time where becoming "like" modern medicine is already outdated. Creating a unique alternative to modern medicine is what our patients want.

Pages 27–46

I present this letter to explain that there are no obvious differences, in principle, between Chinese and Western medicine. I have presented a letter before with a conclusion that Native medicine cannot develop independently, because all people in the world are the same in anatomy, physiology and pathology. But there are still many complicated issues that I haven't mentioned in that previous letter, which may cause many doubts. So I am going to give ten examples to prove that there are no differences in principle between Chinese and Western medicine.

Firstly, I am going to discuss blood and Qi Xue Qi 血氣. In my previous letter, I said "Xue 血 refers to blood, Qi 氣 refers to nerves". How can we know that? People lose blood from their body as a result of injury or illness. It is a fact that even ancient people knew. So there is no doubt about the statement of "Xue 血 refers to blood". About "Qi 氣 refers to nerves" I have to discuss more. In Native medicine, the concepts of Yuan Qi 元氣, Da Qi 大氣, Qi Hua 氣化, etc., all reveal that Qi 氣 is the main thing dominating internal body activities. So the function of Qi 氣 is the same as that of the autonomic nerves. The concepts of Qi Li 氣力, Qi Po 氣魄, Shen Qi 神氣, etc., all reveal that Qi 氣 is the main thing dominating external body activities. So the function of Qi 氣 is the same as the nervous system in animals. Qi 氣 refers to the nervous system. In Native medicine, Qi 氣 is always discussed together with blood.

For example, the *Ben Zang* chapter 本臟篇 of *Ling Shu* 靈樞 says:

> Channels and collaterals can move Qi and blood, nourish Yin and Yang, moisten tendons and bones and smooth joints.

The chapter of *Wei Qi Shi Chang* 衛氣失常篇 of *Ling Shu* 靈樞 says:

> Blood and Qi flow in channels and collaterals. If they stagnate, then excess 盛 will appear.

Channels and collaterals are blood vessels in Western medicine. *Jing Mai chapter* 經脈篇 of *Ling Shu* 靈樞 says:

> The twelve channels are distributed along the crevices between muscles, which are in deep locations and invisible. The superficial and visible ones are called collaterals.

The *Jing Shui chapter* 經水篇 of *Ling Shu* 靈樞 says:

> Channels carry blood and provide nutrients to the body.

Ying 營 is related to blood, and Wei 衛 is related to Qi. The chapter of *Ying Wei Sheng Hui* 營衛生會篇 of *Ling Shu* 靈樞 recorded:

> Huang Di 黃帝 asked, "Where do the Ying 營 and Wei 衛 come from?" Qi Bo 岐伯 answered, "Ying 營 comes from Zhong Jiao 中焦". Huang Di 黃帝 said, "I would like to know the details." Qi Bo 岐伯 explained, "The Stomach in Zhong Jiao 中焦 excretes the waste material, produces body fluids, transforms the essence, and finally produces blood."

Ke Xie chapter 客邪篇 of *Ling Shu* 靈樞 says:

> Ying 營 secretes body fluids, which turns to blood if transferred into channels.

There are also many discussions about Wei 衛. *Wei Qi chapter* 衛氣篇 of *Ling Shu* 靈樞 says:

> Qi 氣 comes from five internal Zang organs, and links the external limbs. Superficial Qi that doesn't move along the channel is called Wei 衛. Essence that flows inside the channels is called Ying 營.

In a word, Wei 衛 floats outside the channels and greatly relates to Qi. Ying 營 flows inside the channels and greatly relates to blood. *Tiao Jing Lun* 調經論 of *Su Wen* 素問 says:

> Acupuncture is taken along the channels, which obtains blood from Ying 營, and Qi from Wei 衛.

It also says:

> Regulate the Wei 衛 if the disease is related to Qi disorders.

So it is quite clear that Ying 營 refers to blood, and Wei 衛 refers to Qi 氣. *Nei Jing* 內經, *Nan Jing* 難經 and *Shang Han* 傷寒 all mentioned that Ying 營 flows inside the channels, and Wei 衛 flows outside the channels. In my opinion, Ying 營 (Xue 血) and Wei 衛 (Qi 氣) in Native medicine are quite similar to the blood and nerves of Western medicine, because they all circulate inside or outside the channels and connect the entire body. They stay where they should stay and they are all responsible for nourishing, moistening and smoothing.

Jing Mai chapter of *Ling Shu* 靈樞 says:

> Xue 血 and Qi 氣 circulate well only when channels are unobstructed.

In anatomy, if vessels are blocked then blood and nerves in this body area cannot function properly. Besides, the book written by Chu 褚 recorded:

> Though Xue 血 belongs to Yin 陰, it is only able to circulate normally when Yang 陽 is in harmony.

Yin Yang Ying Xiang Da Lun 陰陽陰陽應象大論 of *Su Wen* 素問 says:

> Yin 陰 and Yang 陽 are just like the male and female of Xue 血 and Qi 氣.

From this statement, it is clear that Yang harmony is related to Qi. It also says:

> Xue 血 is responsible for transporting, and Qi is responsible for governing.

So it is quite clear that blood and nerves work in coordination with each other and that blood vessels are pillars for the central nervous system. In pathology, loss of appetite is caused by deficiency of Stomach Qi, and it also can be ascribed to paralysis of nerves responsible for hunger. Breathlessness is related to deficiency of Lung Qi, and it is also considered a symptom caused by paralysis of nerves that are near the bronchi. Palpitation is caused by deficiency of Heart Qi, and it also can be considered excitement caused by neurasthenia. Beriberi is an inflammation of related nerves. There are many other examples, such as hypochondriac Qi pain is the same as intercostal neuralgia, Stomach Qi pain is the same as pain of gastric nerves, and Heart Qi pain is the same as angina pectoris. In a word, it is beyond a shadow of a doubt that Qi 氣 in Native medicine equals nerves in Western medicine.

What's more, in treatment, most herbs for treating Xue 血 in Native medicine act on blood, while most herbs for regulating Qi 氣 are just stomachics with fragrant aroma or pungent taste. Some herbs, such as Sha Ren 砂仁, Mu Xiang 木香, Bo Kou 波寇, Ding Xiang 丁香, etc., are able to stimulate the gastrointestinal nerves and other nerves, however, they cannot be called "special herbs for treating nerves". In Native medicine, there is a treatment method called "strengthening Qi in order to regulate blood circulation 固氣統血" which uses Ren Shen 人參, Huang Qi 黃芪, Gan Jiang 乾薑 and Fu Zi 附子 together with some regulating-blood herbs treating vertigo or collapse due to loss of blood. We should, however, pay full attention to the following. The Qi 氣 in Qi Wei 氣味 [property and taste] of herbs and the Qi 氣 in Qi Hou 氣候 [climate] are quite different from Qi 氣 I discussed above. I really don't know what is the exact meaning of Qi 氣 in the terms "Qi transportation in Leading Heaven and In Spring 司在之氣運" and "position of Qi in root and manifestation 標本之氣位".

Secondly, I would like to talk about Yin Yang 陰陽. In my previous letter, I said, "Yin Yang refers to heart". Why do I have this conclusion? All diseases influence the heart, and we can measure the heart function by taking pulse and, with that, know the situation of the disease and choose proper treatment. The ancient doctors knew that Zhang Zhongjing 張仲景 borrowed the concept of Yin Yang to explain six conformations and summarize all diseases. Zhang 張 believed he could detect the origin of disease by relying on pulse-taking for diagnosis. Actually, his methodology was based on heart.

In Native medicine, doctors say, "*Shang Han* 傷寒 summarises the diseases of six conformations, which comprises all diseases." In the preface of *Shang Han Lun* 傷寒論, Zhang Zhongjing 張仲景 said "I am not able to cure all diseases, but I am able to know their origin, so doctors who follow my theories can know at least half of the story, which is the disease origin." All febrile diseases manifesting symptoms such as headache, stiff neck, dizziness, dry throat, delirious speech, thirst, etc., are classified as Three Yang 三陽, and these are always accompanied by increase of pulse intensity or count. All other non-febrile diseases manifesting with symptoms such as diarrhea, vomiting, abdominal pain, vertigo, dyspnea, sweating are classified as Three Yin 三陰, and these are usually accompanied by decrease of pulse intensity or count, or even by a weak pulse that cannot be detected. Therefore it is certain that Yang 陽 is closely related to the heart excitement, while Yin 陰 is closely related with heart weakness.

Zhongjing 仲景 thought that Yang Ming 陽明 was the most important one among the Three Yang 三陽, so he started explaining it with floating pulse. He thought that Shao Yin 少陰 was the most important one among the Three Yin 三陰, so he started explaining it with faint pulse. Besides, he called all syndromes of six Conformations, "syndromes of pulse Mai Zheng 脈證". It is, therefore, reasonable to deduce that fever with diarrhea is considered Yang 陽, because heart doesn't weaken due to diarrhea, instead it excites due to fever. It is just like what *Tai Yang chapter* 太陽篇 is saying:

> If a doctor treats Tai Yang disease with purging, then it will lead to persistent diarrhea and rapid pulse, because the exterior syndrome hasn't been relieved. Use Ge Gen Huang Qin Huang Lian Tang 葛根黃芩黃連湯 to treat it if there is cough and sweating.

However, it is also reasonable that fever with diarrhea is considered Yin 陰, when heart doesn't excite from fever, but instead weakens due to diarrhea. It is just like *Shao Yin chapter* 少陰篇 says:

> Use Tong Mai Si Ni Tang 通脈四逆湯 to treat Shao Yin 少陰 disease manifested as watery diarrhea with undigested food, cold in the interior and heat at the exterior, cold limbs, faint pulse, no chills, reddish complexion, either having abdominal pain, or dry vomiting, or sore throat, or unrecovered pulse after the diarrhea stopped.

Jue Yin chapter 厥陰篇 says:

> Patient that has dyspeptic diarrhea, deep and slow pulse, reddish complexion, and slight fever must be weak and faint, because he has cold syndrome due to deficiency in the lower part of the body and pseudo-heat symptoms in the upper part of the body.

We can see that there are differences in the attribute of Yin Yang 陰陽 for cases of same syndrome having different pulses. It is quite clear that ancient doctors used Yin

Yang 陰陽 to represent the heart strength. The heart will fall into paralysis if being excessively excited, so excitement and weakness are not absolute. Take rapid pulse as an example: Zhang Zhongjing 張仲景 thought that rapid pulse was a manifestation of Yang diseases 陽病, while other doctors thought it was a dangerous case of Yin diseases 陰病. From the above discussions, we know the possibility of mutual transformation between Yin and Yang 陰陽傳變.

As for treatment, *Shao Yin chapter* 少陰篇 says:

> Ma Huang Fu Zi Xi Xin Tang 麻黃附子細辛湯 is used for early stage Shao Yin diseases 少陰病 that have fever and deep pulse.

Why are Ma Huang 麻黃 and Fu Zi 附子 necessary in this case? Native medicine doctors think that these two herbs can merge in harmony Yin and Yang 交和陰陽 (coming from the book *Chen Xiuyuan's Concise Annotation* 陳修園淺注). The new medicine doctors think that Ma Huang 麻黃 can reduce fever and Fu Zi 附子 can strengthen heart. The pulse is deep and therefore it is necessary to strengthen the heart. Tai Yang chapter 太陽篇 says:

> Use Gui Zhi Qu Shao Yao Tang 桂枝去芍藥湯 for Tai Yang diseases with rapid pulse and chest fullness after being purged. If the pulse is weak and the patient has aversion to cold then use a combination of Gui Zhi Qu Shao Yao Tang 桂枝去芍藥湯 plus Fu Zi Tang 附子湯.

What's the purpose of using Gui Zhi 桂枝 and Fu Zi 附子 here? Native medicine doctors think they are effective to treat the case of Yang deficiency and Yin excess. The new medicine doctors think that Gui Zhi 桂枝 can reduce fever, and Fu Zi 附子 is good at strengthening heart, because the pulse is weak and therefore it is necessary to strengthen the heart in this case. It is certain that treatments based on Yin Yang 陰陽 in Native medicine are equivalent to treatments based on heart function in Western medicine.

Tai Yang 太陽 diseases have a strong tendency to transform into Yin 陰, while Yang Ming 陽明 never transforms into Yin 陰, why? This is related to treatment. Tai Yang 太陽 diseases usually have mild fever without delirious speech, so it is acceptable to use prescriptions to strengthen the heart when it is weak. That's why Tai Yang 太陽 diseases easily transform into Yin 陰. *Tai Yang chapter* 太陽篇 says:

> If a patient has fever, headache, deep pulse, and body aches, use Si Ni Tang 四逆湯 to rescue the internal deficiency-cold.

Chen Xiuyuan 陳修園 explained that the deep pulse shows Yin 陰 hiding in the interior. On the contrary, Yang Ming 陽明 diseases usually have steaming fever and delirious speech, body temperature is quite high, and there are mind disorders. In this case one cannot use strengthening heart prescriptions indiscriminately even when the heart is weak, because heart weakness in this case is due to internal heat. This is why Zhang Zhongjing 張仲景 thought that Yang Ming 陽明 never transforms into Yin 陰. *Yang Ming chapter* 陽明篇 recorded:

> Patient with a weak pulse will survive, while with an unsmooth pulse will die…

Zhang Zhongjing 張仲景 didn't follow the method of rescuing pulse in Tai Yang 太陽. He refused to use Si Ni Tang 四逆湯 to strengthen the heart and recover pulse, because there was high fever and delirious speech. Therefore, transforming or not into Yin 陰 is just speculation, while being able to strengthen the heart or not is the key point, and this is why I say it is related to the treatment. What's more, among all prescriptions of Zhang Zhongjing 張仲景, Tong Mai Si Ni Tang 通脈四逆湯 is the most effective one that can support Yang and restrain Yin 扶陽抑陰. Tong Mai 通脈 [299] means supporting Yang, and supporting Yang can restrain Yin, so it is certain that Yin Yang 陰陽 refers to heart. It is absurd to say Yin and Yang 陰陽 are intangibles, or Qi activities, or mysterious opposites. These fallacies don't deserve to be discussed anymore.

Thirdly, I would like to discuss Wind Feng 風. In my previous letter, I said that "Feng 風 refers to brain." How do I get to this conclusion? Disease diagnosis is quite complicated; however, we are able to get a general overview of its causal relationship after prolonged observation. For example, there are causal relationships between head disorders and sensation and movement disorders of the whole body. Native medicine doctors didn't know the concept of brain, so they just used Feng 風 to replace it. In *Jin Gui* 金匱 chapter *Zhong Feng* 中風篇 section *Fang Ji Di Huang Tang* 防己地黃湯, Zhang Zhongjing 張仲景 recorded:

> The patient is manic, moves around with delirious speech.

[299] Here, "Tong Mai" means unobstruct blood vessel which—for Tan—implies the connection to the heart.

The symptoms are quite similar to epilepsy, which is a cerebral cortex disorder. *Feng Ying Tang* section 風引湯節 recorded:

> Adults have Feng Yin 風引, children have convulsion. It happens several times per day.

The symptoms are quite similar to convulsion, which is closely related with midbrain. The next section recorded "deviation of the eye and mouth", which is closely related with oculomotor nerves and facial nerves. "Speech difficulty, saliva drooling" are caused by impairment of hypoglossal nerves, or trigeminal nerves, which are related to medulla oblongata. Besides, all people know that stroke Zhong Feng 中風 belongs to cerebral haemorrhage. The first section of *Zhong Feng chapter* 中風篇 recorded:

> Diseases related to Feng 風 must have hemiplegia or paralysis of arms.

The second section said: "skin numbness, unconsciousness". All of these symptoms are almost the same as ones caused by cerebral haemorrhage. Chen Xiuyuan 陳修園 cited *Zhong Feng chapter* 中風篇 and said "unconsciousness, cataplexy, lockjaw, red complexion." These symptoms can also accompany cerebral haemorrhage. In a word, *Zhong Feng chapter* 中風篇 of *Jin Gui* 金匮 can prove that Feng 風 refers to brain. Besides, *Tai Yang chapter* 太陽篇 of *Shang Han Lun* 傷寒論 also says:

> After adoption of emetic or purgative, a Shang Han 傷寒 patient will have epigastric fullness, upward adverse flow of Qi to the chest, dizziness when getting up, floating and tense pulse. If a diaphoretic is adopted then nourishment of Channels and Collaterals will be exhausted, thus causing trembling and shaking of the body. Fu Ling Gui Zhi Bai Zhu Gan Cao Tang 茯苓桂枝白朮甘草湯 should be used for this case.

Chen Xiuyuan 陳修園 thought it was wind-wood shaking 風木動搖 but I think it is cerebral ischemia, since the patient feels dizziness when getting up. For Shao Yang disease in *Shang Han Lun* 傷寒論, its main symptom is alternating cold and heat, while its outline is "bitter taste of mouth, dry throat, and dizziness". Chen Xiuyuan 陳修園 cited the contents from *Nei Jing* 內經 and explained that dizziness was caused by stirring wind due to Liver-Yin deficiency. I think that this dizziness is caused by cephalemia, because the patient most probably has fever with high blood pressure.

Actually, Native medicine doctors use Feng 風 to explain symptoms of brain diseases. Furthermore, I have researched all causes of dizziness, and found out that besides cerebral haemorrhage, cephalemia and cerebral ischemia, there are still other complicated factors. However, most of them are closely related to blood circulation disorder. *Nei Jing* 內經 said "all Feng 風 diseases cause tremor and dizziness", so it is quite certain that Feng 風 diseases in Native medicine refer to cerebral diseases. The *Jing Bing* 痙病 chapter of *Jin Gui* 金匱 can also prove my conclusion. It says:

> A patient has fever throughout his body with cold feet, rigid neck, aversion to cold, fever in head, reddish complexion, red eyes, shaking of head, sudden lockjaw, and opisthotonos. It is called as Jing Bing 痙病.

It also says:

> Da Cheng Qi Tang 大承氣湯 can be prescribed for a Jing Bing 痙病 when the following symptoms and signs are observed: fullness in chest, lockjaw, opisthotonos that prevent the patient from lying flat on bed, leg spasm and grinding of teeth.

So symptoms of Jing Bing 痙病 and myeloencephalitis are exactly the same. Chen Xiuyuan 陳修園 always attributed Jing Bing 痙病 to Feng 風. *Nei Jing* 內經 also said "All sudden muscular spasm and rigidity are ascribed to Feng 風". Jue Yin 厥陰 is a channel of Feng 風 and Mu 木 wood. *Jue Yin* 厥陰 chapter of *Shang Han Lun* 傷寒論 recorded headache; it says:

> Wu Zhu Yu Tang 吳茱萸湯 can be prescribed to treat nausea with copious salivation and headache.

In a word, Feng 風 undoubtedly refers to brain. The herbs for Feng 風 in Chinese medicine are extremely complicated. For example, herbs that can relieve exterior and reduce fever are classified as herbs of dispersing exterior to expel Feng 風, such as Radix Saposhnikoviae Fang Feng 防風, Rhizoma et Radix Notopterygii Qiang Huo 羌活, Rhizoma Chuanxiong Chuan Xiong 川芎 and Radix Angelicae Dahuricae Bai Zhi 白芷. Herbs that have excitant action are classified as warm herbs to expel Feng 風, such as Radix Aconiti Lateralis Preparata Fu Zi 附子, Rhizoma Zingiberis Gan Jiang 乾薑, and Fructus Evodiae Wu Zhu Yu 吳茱萸.

Herbs that act on blood are classified as nourishing blood herbs to expel Feng 風, such as Radix Rehmanniae Di Huang 地黃, Herba Taxilli Sang Ji Sheng 桑寄生, Rhizoma Cyperi Xiang Fu 香附, and Radix Angelicae Sinensis Dang Gui 當歸.

Herbs with sticky substances are classified as moistening herbs to extinguish Feng 風, such as Radix Ophiopogonis Mai Dong 麥冬, Colla Corii Asini E Jiao 阿膠, Carapax et Plastrum Testudinis Gui Ban 龜板, and Carapax Trionycis Bie Jia 鱉甲. There are also other ordinary herbs that can expel Feng 風, such as Ramulus Uncariae cum Uncis Gou Teng 鉤藤, Bombyx Batryticatus Qiang Can 羌蠶, and Periostracum Cicadae Chan Tui 蟬蛻. Feng 風 herbs in Native medicine are quite complicated; in my opinion, it is because Native medicine doctors don't know the treatment for brain diseases. Terms such as evil wind Xie Feng 邪風, thief wind Zei Feng 賊風, transmit to center Chuan Zhong 傳中, and directly hitting center 直中 are completely imaginary.

Fourthly, I would like to discuss dampness Shi 濕. In my previous letter, I wrote "Shi 濕 refers to stomach and intestines". Why do I have this conclusion? As we know, Shi 濕 is closely related to Tai Yin 太陰. The *Tai Yin Yang Ming Lun* 太陰陽明論 of *Su Wen* 素問 firstly stated that Tai Yin 太陰 is a channel of damp earth Shi Tu 濕土. The *Tian Yuan Ji Da Lun* 天元紀大論 says "Tai Yin 太陰 is governed by Shi Qi 濕氣." The *Zhi Zhen Yao Da Lun* 至真要大論 also says "Tai Yin 太陰 is responsible for transferring the climate Shi 濕." These views have been accepted without any objection for thousands of years. Zhang Zhongjing 張仲景 created a chapter called *Tai Yin* 太陰 in *Shang Han Lun* 傷寒論, and the annotators explained this chapter based on Shi Tu 濕土 theory. So Tai Yin 太陰 disease is another name of Shi 濕 disease. In *Tai Yin* 太陰 chapter of *Shang Han Lun* 傷寒論, Zhang Zhongjing 張仲景 outlined:

> Patients suffering Tai Yin 太陰 diseases usually have abdominal fullness, vomiting, loss of appetite, severe diarrhea, and occasional abdominal pain. The upper abdomen will have a feeling of fullness and rigidity if using purgative.

All these symptoms are inextricably related to Stomach and Intestines. The Spleen is considered as the Zang 臟 organ of Tai Yin Shi Tu 太陰濕土. In Native medicine, Spleen and Stomach are linked to each other. *Su Wen Tai Yin Yang Ming Lun* 素問太陰陽明論 says, "The Spleen provides the essence to Stomach." And *Zang Qi Fa Shi Lun* 臟器法時論 says, "Spleen locates at the side of stomach." As for function, Native medicine doctors think Stomach is mainly responsible for receiving foods, while Spleen for digesting foods. *Zang Qi Fa Shi Lun* 臟器法時論 says, "Spleen helps Stomach Qi to digest water and grain." It also discusses Spleen deficiency: "Spleen deficiency causes abdominal fullness, borborygmus, diarrhea with undigested foods." *Su Wen Qi Jiao Bian Da Lun* 素問氣交變大論 says, "If the Spleen is invaded by pathogens then the patient will have diarrhea with undigested foods, loss of appetite, heavy sensation in the body, restlessness, borborygmus, and abdominal fullness."

Spleen deficiency is exact equivalent to indigestion. So the Spleen in Native medicine is equivalent to the pancreas, which produces substances helping the body digest food. Pancreas is an organ affiliated with Stomach and Intestines. That's why the Spleen in Native medicine is considered as the Zang of Shi 濕. Besides, pancreas, Liver and Gallbladder are also members of the digestive system. In Native medicine, jaundice is considered as a disease of Shi 濕. The chapter of *Tai Yin* 太陰篇 says "Tai Yin 太陰 patients usually have yellowish pigmentation of the skin."

In pathology, jaundice is caused by bile duct impairment due to gastritis and duodenitis. On the other hand, diseases of Liver and Gallbladder can also cause disorders of Stomach and Intestines. So there are causal relationships between them. I have discussed and proved that Feng 風 belongs to Liver-wood 肝木, but actually refers to brain, Shi 濕 belongs to Spleen-Earth 脾土, but actually refers to Stomach and Intestines. So the theories of Liver subjugating Spleen or Wood restricting Earth actually refer to neurogenic gastritis or gastric neurasthenia neuropathy. From the above examples, we know clearly that the relationships between Tai Yin Shi 太陰濕 diseases and other organs are actually the relationships between Stomach and Intestines diseases and other organs.

Next, I am going to prove my views related to treatment. In *Tai Yin chapter* 太陰, Zhang Zhongjing 張仲景 classifies all prescriptions of Shi 濕 as Si Ni Bei group 四逆輩, which includes Si Ni Tang 四逆湯, Li Zhong Tang 理中湯, Zhen Wu Tang 真武湯, Wu Zhu Yu Tang 吳茱萸湯 according to annotators' opinions. Actually, they are the main prescriptions for vomiting and diarrhea caused by Stomach and Intestines diseases of Three Yin 三陰 (Taiyin 太陰, Jue Yin 厥陰 and Shao Yin 少陰). There are some ancient prescriptions that include the Stomach character Wei 胃 in their name, such as Ping Wei San 平胃散, Wei Ling Tang 胃苓湯, etc. Later generations prescribed them broadly as effective treatments for Shi 濕 diseases. It strongly proves that Shi 濕 refers to Stomach and Intestines.

Furthermore, we can also find evidence in specific herbs. For example, Ding Xiang 丁香, Hui Xiang 茴香, Gui Zhi 桂枝, Dou Kou 豆蔻, Rou Kou 肉蔻, Gan Jiang 乾薑, Liang Jiang 良薑 etc., are used as aromatic and pungent herbs to invigorating the Stomach in Western medicine. Native medicine classifies them as drying Zao 燥 herbs that eliminate dampness Shi 濕. Though these herbs are used in different situations, they actually have similar functions in both Western and Native medicines. It proves that Shi 濕 refers to Stomach and Intestines.

Yin Chen Hao 茵陳蒿 can eliminate dampness Shi 濕. It is mild in nature and therefore prescribed in large dosage. It is an essential herb for treatment of jaundice, which was mentioned in *Shen Nong Ben Cao Jing* 神農本草經. Yin Chen Hao Tang 茵陳蒿湯 of *Shang Han Lun* 傷寒論 and Yin Chen Wu Ling San 茵陳五苓散 of *Jin Gui Yao Lüe* 金貴要略 regarded Yin Chen Hao 茵陳蒿 as a prominent herb for jaundice. According to pharmacological research, Yin Chen Hao 茵陳蒿 may have substances that can promote bile secretion, so it is also considered as an essential herb for digestive diseases. I would like to stop discussing dampness Shi 濕 here. The Shi 濕 in the terms wind damp Feng Shi 風濕 and damp warmth Shi Wen 濕溫 are completely different from the one I discussed above. The doctors of today don't follow the original meaning, rather, according to their opinion, almost all diseases can be titled as dampness Shi 濕 diseases and treated by eliminating dampness Shi 濕. It is all fabricated theories, simply pointing at a donkey and saying that it is a horse.

Fifthly, I would like to discuss water Shui 水. In my previous letter, I said "Shui 水 refers to body fluid". Why do I have this conclusion? Water Shui 水 is an inorganic matter, which occupies two thirds of the body weight. It is an element of life, which has been discussed in physiology textbooks in great detail. Native medicine regards water Shui 水 as the foundation for life, there is no place that it cannot be seen. However, secretion of glands, blood, digestive juice, urine, sweat, and tissue fluid are mixtures containing water Shui 水, these should be called body fluid rather than water Shui 水. Therefore water Shui 水 in Native medicine actually refers to body fluid.

The chapter of *Ni Tiao Lun* 逆調論篇 in *Su Wen* 素問 says "water Shui 水 flows together with body fluids." The body needs a certain amount of water Shui 水. If there are some factors that cause excess or deficiency of water Shui 水, the body will fall into a pathological state. I would like to firstly discuss nourishing water Zi Shui 滋水, which is usually called nourishing Yin Zi Yin 滋陰 in Native medicine. A severe deficiency of water Shui 水 can lead to death, so it is necessary to nourish water Zi Shui 滋水.

Zhang Zhongjing 張仲景 said "When a patient is thirsty, serve him water little by little. Then he will recover soon." It is simply a method for recovery after illness. Though the ancient doctors knew the importance of water Shui 水, they didn't know how to infuse a large dose of fluid into the body, i.e. they were only able to nourish water Zi Shui 滋水 through the absorption ability of Stomach and Intestines. Native medicine doctors normally use sticky herbs to nourish water Zi Shui 滋水, except for water loss due to vomiting and diarrhea, because these herbs are difficult to digest.

For treating difficult urination, E Jiao 阿膠 in Zhu Ling Tang 豬苓湯 or Di Huang 地黃 in Jin Gui Shen Qi Wan 金貴腎氣丸 are used. For upward adverse flow of Lung Qi, Mai Dong 麥冬 in Mai Men Dong Tang 麥門冬湯 is used. For palpitation with a slow-uneven and intermittent pulse, Di Huang 地黃 in Fu Mai Tang 復脈湯 is used. For insomnia, E Jiao 阿膠 in Huang Lian E Jiao Tang 阿膠黃連湯 is used. For fever, Zhi Mu 知母 in Bai Hu Tang 白虎湯 or Bie Jia 鱉甲 in Qing Gu Tang 清骨湯 is used. The prescriptions of nourishing water Zi Shui 滋水 are suitable for all patients having fluid deficiency accompanied by the following symptoms: dry tongue, thirst, dry cough without phlegm, constipation, oliguria with reddish urine. However, these prescriptions can only be used when the functions of Stomach and Intestines are not impaired. A proper use can promote production of fluids. These herbs are mild in nature and that's why they are also called restraining fire herbs 制火. These prescriptions have quite rarely side effects. However, on the other hand, they are not that efficacious and are usually used as a supplementary treatment. Though prescriptions of nourishing water Zi Shui 滋水 can produce some fluid, they are less effective compared to Western medicine methods. Some doctors advocate the theory of treating root 治本之說 and say that it is not necessary to remove fire if the body is in deficiency of water Shui 水. They suggest strengthening water in order to suppress Yang hyperactivity. In other words, they suggest to use prescriptions of nourishing water Zi Shui 滋水, but oppose using any prescriptions that remove fire. Though doctors may have individual style of using herbs, the above approach is rather superficial. For more details about fire and its remedy, see the next section of this article.

Secondly, I would like to talk about eliminating water Qu Shui 祛水. Chapter *Shui Qi* 水氣 in *Jin Gui Yao Lüe* 金贵要略 says, "Edema patient caused by Heart illness has heavy sensation of body, shortness of breath, and swollen genitalia." According to the symptoms, it is edema caused by heart valve disorders. It also says, "Edema patient caused by Liver illness has enlarged abdomen, difficulty in moving his body, hypochondrium pain, but the bowel movement is not obstructed." According to these symptoms, it equals to edema caused by hepatopathy of Western medicine. Chapter *Shui Qi* 水氣 also says, "Edema patient caused by Kidney disease has lumbago, dysuria." It fits the symptoms of edema caused by nephrosis. The section of wind edema Feng Shui 風水 says, "Wind edema patient has a swollen face, fever, puffiness of the eyelids resembling a dormant silkworm coming awake, visible pulse of neck vessels, frequent cough." I know wind edema Feng Shui 風水 refers to Kidney edema based on my research of *Nei Jing* 內經. *Shui Re Xue Lun* 水熱穴論 of *Su Wen* 素問 recorded:

> Huang Di asked "Why does the Kidney accumulate water and cause diseases?" Qi Bo answered "The Kidney is a Yin organ, it produces water and fluid. If water and fluid are neither able to sink deeper into the five Zang organs, nor able to get out through the skin, it will move within the skin, eventually causing edema. Edema caused by Kidney disorders is called wind edema Feng Shui 風水".

So wind edema Feng Shui 風水 is actually a synonym for Kidney edema.

Finally, I would like to discuss specific methods of eliminating water Shui 水. The chapter of *Shui Qi* 水氣 in *Jin Gui* 金匱 says "Edema syndrome below the waist, then adopt inducing urination; edema above the waist, then adopt inducing sweat." It also says "Purgative can be adopted to eliminate water." Honestly, these methods are quite similar to scientific methods. Water from edema is exuded from the blood, and prescriptions of eliminating water Shui 水 are actually aiming at promoting water to be absorbed by blood. However, some Shui Qi 水氣 discussed by Zhang Zhongjing 張仲景 are quite different, such as Shui Qi 水氣 in the epigastrium, Shui Qi 水氣 in the intestines and hypochondrium, etc. Water Shui 水 in the term Tai Yang Cold Water Han Shui 太陽寒水, and water Shui 水 in five elements, are purely imaginary.

Sixthly, I would like to discuss fire Huo 火. I said in my previous letter that "fire refers to the symptoms caused by stimulation". Why do I have this point of view? As we all know, every disease has a cause. Symptoms are closely related to the cause. Different causes will have different symptoms. However, symptoms may still exist even if the cause has been removed. All of them can be summarized as pathological stimulation, which is the same as fire Huo 火 in Native medicine. *Zhi Zhen Yao Da Lun*

至真要大論 in *Su Wen* 素問 says "all states of agitation and mania are ascribed to fire", which is the evidence for my statement.

The patient will have choking cough if the Lung is stimulated by pathogens; it is called fire Qi tormenting metal Huo Qi Xing Jin 火氣邢金, which is just like the chapter *Fei Wei Fei Yong Ke Sou Shang Qi* 肺痿肺癰咳嗽上氣篇 in *Jin Gui* 金匱 that says, "dyspnoea due to ascending pathogenic fire, uncomfortable feeling in throat". It should be treated by stopping fire and descending Qi. Chen Xiuyuan 陳修園 also explained this case with a theory of deficiency fire melting metal Xu Huo Shuo Jin 虛火爍金.

A patient will have bitter taste in mouth and dry throat if Stomach is stimulated by pathogens. This case is called "excessive fire in the stomach" in Native medicine. It is just like the *Shao Yang chapter* 少陽篇 of *Shang Han Lun* 傷寒論 which says "diseases of Shao Yang 少陽病 will cause bitter taste in mouth, dry throat, and dizziness." Chen Xiuyuan 陳修園 explained this case by quoting theories from *Nei Jing* 內經, such as "minister fire governs Shao Yang 少陽" and "bitter taste transforms from fire and when fire prevails dryness follows".

A patient will have insomnia if the brain is stimulated by pathogens. This case is called "hyperactivity of heart fire". It is just like the *Shao Yin chapter* 少陰篇 that says, "After suffering from Shao Yin disease for more than two or three days, the patient will have restlessness and insomnia." Chen Xiuyuan 陳修園 ascribed this case to the emperor fire of upper Jiao converting into heat. Besides, he thought the palpitations recorded in chapter *Jing Ji Tu Nu Xia Xue Xiong Man Yu Xue* 驚悸吐衄下血胸滿瘀血篇 were caused by hyperactivity of fire due to blood deficiency of pericardium.

He ascribed the yellowish eyes and continuous nosebleed discussed in the same chapter to upward disturbance of Liver and Kidney fire. The same chapter recorded "a patient with spitting blood and nosebleed should be treated by draining heart". Chen Xiuyuan 陳修園 explained that bitter and cold herbs were able to lessen fire and remove stasis.

However, there are many pathological stimulations that ancient doctors were not able to know the cause for, so they just called them fire Huo 火. There are many examples in ancient medical books that can prove my point of view. Native medicine divides fire into two types; real fire Zhen Huo 真火 and pseudo fire Jia Huo 假火. Taking reddish complexion and thirst as an example, if it is caused by fever, fire will be real fire due to Yang Ming Dry Metal 陽明燥金. If it is caused by diarrhea, fire will be pseudo fire caused by deficiency of Shao Yin 少陰. So we know that stimulation causes may be different even when symptoms are the same.

Next, I will discuss treatment. There is no anaesthetic in Native medicine, so doctors can only use cold prescriptions to moderate stimulation and reduce excitement. Cold prescriptions can be categorized into three groups; bitter-cold, sweet-cold, and sweet-moist. All of them can slightly moderate stimulation, so they are also called "prescriptions of lessening fire". Sweet-moist prescriptions can nourish water, so they are also called "prescriptions nourishing Yin". On the other hand, prescriptions supplementing fire can be categorized into two groups; tonics and stimulants. The stimulants usually contain Fu Zi 附子, Gan Jiang 乾薑, etc. Tonics usually have Ren Shen 人參, Huang Qi 黃芪, Dang Gui 當歸, Bai Zhu 白朮, Bu Gu Zhi 補骨脂, Rou Gui 肉桂, etc. If there is no fire, it is not suitable to eliminate water; instead, it is only suitable to replenish fire in order to treat Yin asthenia. In other words, it opposes the use of sweating, purging, or promoting urination, and it advocates using tonics and stimulants. Native medicine regards fire as the basis of life. Fire is just like the body temperature. People will die if they don't have a body temperature. However, fire in five elements theory and matching relationships of fire to tastes, colors and organs, are completely imaginary.

Seventhly, I would like to discuss deficiency and excess Xu Shi 虛實. In the previous letter, I said "deficiency and excess is the criterion for treatment". Why do I have this conclusion? A treatment for a similar symptom should vary according to the disease nature and individual differences. One should tonify to treat a deficiency, and sedate to treat excess. It is improper to treat deficiency with methods leading to further deficiency, or treat excess with methods leading to more excess. We must decide a treatment based on the patient's condition. Some doctors strongly advocate for adapting treatment to changing conditions. This principle is good for both Native medicine as well as Western medicine. If a specific treatment for a disease is available then it's better to use it. If there is no specific treatment available then it is better to decide treatment according to conditions, i.e. tonify deficiency and drain excess. The best doctors of both Chinese and Western medicines follow the above principle, however, unskilled doctors often tonify a patient who should not be tonified, or sedate a patient who should not be sedated. Therefore, we must use diaphoretic or purgative when it is required.

Tai Yang chapter 太陽篇 of *Shang Han Lun* 傷寒論 says, "A dose of purgative is given when diaphoretic is required, this is a wrong treatment. It is correct if a diaphoretic is first served. On the contrary, a dose of diaphoretic is the wrong treatment when a purgative is required. It is correct if a purgative is given." If one needs to strengthen brain urgently in order to stop dizziness then strengthening the brain should be used. *Tai Yang chapter* 太陽篇 says "Tai Yang syndrome: After the adoption of a diaphoretic, the patient perspires but the syndrome is not gone. He still suffers from fever, palpitation, vertigo, muscle spasms, and trembling and shivering which are likely to cause him to fall down. Zhen Wu Tang 真武湯 should be used for treatment." For rescuing a patient with exhausted pulse, strengthen the heart when it is necessary. Shao Yin chapter 少陰篇 says "Shao Yin disease with deep pulse should be treated by strong warming prescription, Si Ni Tang is suitable for it."

Doctors of both Chinese and Western medicines should apply treatment according to deficiency and excess. Native medicine doctors say, "For six Fu organs consider purgatives as tonics." Excretion of the old can generate the new. Therefore, treating diarrhea with purgatives can also be called using purgatives as tonics. *Shao Yin chapter* 少陰篇 of *Shang Han Lun* 傷寒論 says "A Shao Yin 少陰 patient with greenish watery stool, epigastric pain and dry mouth can be treated with purgatives, Da Cheng Qi Tang 大承氣湯 is suitable for this case." Chapter *Ou Tu Yue Xia Li* 嘔吐噦下利篇 in *Jin Gui* 金匱 says "If a patient has diarrhea with moderate pulse at Cun, Guan, and Chi, a hard mass is felt in the epigastrium. Purgative should be adopted urgently. Da Cheng Qi Tang 大承氣湯 is suitable for treatment. If the patient has diarrhea with slippery pulse, there is something in the interior that must be eliminated. The patient will recover after using purgative. Da Cheng Qi Tang 大承氣湯 should be used for treatment. Diarrhea with delirious speech indicates the existence of dry stool. Xiao Cheng Qi Tang 小承氣湯 should be used for treatment." In *Zhong Jiao chapter* 中焦篇 of *Wen Bing Tiao Bian* 溫病條辨, Wu Jutong 吳鞠通 said "In warm diseases of Yang Ming 陽明, if a patient has watery stool without solid waste matter, this condition is called heat retention with watery discharge Re Jie Pang Liu 熱結旁流. Tiao Wei Cheng Qi Tang 調胃承氣湯 should be used as treatment." The Native medicine diarrhea is quite similar to diarrhea caused by gastrointestinal dyspepsia, acute enteritis, or stimulation of stubborn stool to the intestinal canal. For Western medicine it is also urgent to eliminate toxic substances in the intestines.

Another method is taking tonics that serve as sedatives 以補為瀉. This method is actually strengthening healthy Qi to suppress pathogens. Zhen Wu Tang 真武湯 is an example of this method. Fu Zi 附子 and Gan Jiang 乾薑 are tonics, which can treat dizziness and palpitation. However, fever will also be reduced after using these tonics. This is exactly the method called "taking tonics as sedatives 以補為瀉". It is quite similar to Western medicine's use of camphor in heart failure caused by heat. There is a method in Native medicine called "simultaneous application of tonifying and sedating Bu Xie Jian Shi 補瀉兼施", which adds aromatic and spicy pungent herbs or tonic herbs to a sedating formula. Da Huang Fu Zi Xi Xin Tang 大黃附子細辛湯 from chapter *Fu Man Han Shan Su Shi* 腹滿寒疝宿食 of *Jin Gui* 金匱 is an example for this method. Western medicine has a similar method as well. Pulse condition is the most important aspect for differentiation of deficiency and excess. *Miu Ci Lun* chapter 繆刺論 of *Su Wen* 素問 says "check the channels, feel the pulse, and then treat according to differentiation of deficiency and excess." Therefore, we have to examine the pulse condition first before using tonifying or sedating method. In Western medicine, many diseases cannot be treated with purgatives, for example, intestinal typhoid with small pulse, cecitis with irregular minute pulse, and acute generalized peritonitis with frequent pulse. These few pulse conditions should be considered as deficiency, and may not be treated with purgatives. Deficiency should be treated with tonics. However, there are some cases of deficiency that cannot be treated with tonics, similar to excess that cannot be treated with sedatives. In *Qi Shi Jiu Nan* 七十九難, Bian Que 扁鵲 said "deficiency and excess are barely discernible in some cases." In a word, in the process of diagnosis and treatment, it is not proper to discuss deficiency and excess without considering the scientific cause and pathology.

Eighthly, I would like to discuss exterior and interior Biao Li 表裡. In my previous letter, I said "exterior and interior Biao Li 表裡 refers to the disease being deep or superficial". How can I get this conclusion? There are systemic diseases and localized diseases, however, a systemic disease may influence a local area of the body, and a localized disease may influence the entire body. This is the general meaning of exterior and interior Biao Li 表裡 in Native medicine. For example, fever, aversion to cold, alternating cold and heat, hectic fever, and aversion to heat, are systemic symptoms. However, fever will cause abnormal blood circulation, which may lead to continuous diarrhea, a localized symptom in the intestines. Native medicine calls it "the exterior problem of Three Yang transmits to the interior of Three Yin"; there are many examples of diarrhea Xia Li 下利 in the Three Yin chapters 三陰篇.[300] Another example: headache, fever, sweating and aversion to wind are considered as

[300] *Tai Yin*, *Shao Yin* and *Jue Yin* chapters of the *Shang Han Lun*.

systemic symptoms. Fever may increase and finally cause some localized symptoms of the brain, such as delirious speech. It is called "the exterior problem of Tai Yang transmits to the interior of Yang Ming". *Chapter Yang Ming* 陽明篇 recorded this case "After the symptoms of Tai Yang are relieved, the patient may have hectic fever, slight perspiration over hands and feet, constipation, and delirious speech." Headache, fever, and aversion to wind are systemic symptoms. Back muscles may be invaded and then a localized symptom will appear, such as spasm. Native medicine regards this case as "Tai Yang exterior skin problem transmits to Tai Yang exterior channel". The sections of Ge Gen Tang 葛根湯節 and Gui Zhi Jia Ge Gen Tang 桂枝加葛根湯節 are examples for this case. Common cold and other acute infectious diseases may lead to cystitis, and finally cause bloody urine. Native medicine calls this case "heat accumulation in bladder Re Jie Pang Guang 熱結膀胱". Fever and headache appear firstly, so it is considered as "problem at the exterior of Tai Yang transmits to the interior of Tai Yang". The *Re Jie Pang Liu section* 熱結旁流節 of *Tai Yang chapter* 太陽篇 discussed this case. The above are examples of systemic disease influencing a local area of the body. The above discussions on exterior and interior are completely based on the *Shang Han Lun* 傷寒論. Actually, Zhang Zhongjing's 張仲景 discussions are based on *Nei Jing* 內經. But I don't want to cite the original texts of *Nei Jing* 內經 here, because there are too many details.

Transmitting from interior to exterior is just the opposite. *Shao Yin chapter* 少陰篇 says, "A patient with Shao Yin disease has vomiting and diarrhea. If his limbs are not cold, to the contrary there is a fever, then he will not die." The following needs to be considered. A localized gastroenteritis leads to a systemic fever, which is called in Native medicine "the interior Shao Yin transmits to the exterior Tai Yang". There are some specific cases; for example, a patient with diarrhea may suddenly have deep and weak pulse accompanied by sweating and cold limbs. This may be seen by Native medicine as a type of inward transmission, transmitting from common organs to vital organs, for example, transmission from Tai Yin to Shao Yin or Jue Jin. However, a patient who has suffered diarrhea for several days may get worse due to complications or weak constitution. Native medicine may mistake this situation as inward transmission. What's more, there are many imaginary terms in Native medicine, such as transmitting to Liver, transmitting to Kidney, the upper and middle Jiao transmitting to lower Jiao by Wu Jutong 吴鞠通 etc examples.

Actually, though there are many meanings for exterior and interior, in my opinion, a transmission that makes the patient get better can be called "from interior to exterior"

出表, while a transmission that makes the patient condition worse can be called "from exterior to interior" 入裏. That's why I say that exterior and interior Biao Li 表裡 refer to the seriousness of disease.[301] Some doctors may suspect one example I brought above, which discusses diarrhea with fever. It seems that the patient's condition becomes worse and therefore not proper to call this case a "transmission from interior to exterior". However, diarrhea may cause weakness of heart, yet fever can excite the heart; that's why Zhang Zhongjing 張仲景 said "to the contrary there is fever 反發熱". It seems like a worsened situation but in reality it is better. There is no conflict with my conclusion, transmitting from interior to exterior indicates a better situation, while transmitting from exterior to interior indicates a worsened situation. However, in order to know clearly the pathology, it is necessary to examine the disease characteristics in detail.

Next, I am going to discuss the emergency of exterior and interior. *Zang Fu Jing Luo Xian Hou chapter* 臟腑經絡先後篇 of *Jin Gui* 金匱 says "There are some cases where exterior syndromes should be given a priority and others where interior syndromes should be given a priority. Why? When a purgative is adopted and the patient suffers continuous diarrhea containing undigested food and overall pain, in such cases, the interior syndrome should be considered urgent. When a patient has normal stool with overall pain, the exterior syndrome should be treated urgently." *Tai Yang chapter* 太陽篇 of *Shang Han Lun* 傷寒論 also says, "After adopting a purgative, the cold injury patient has continuous diarrhea with undigested food and suffers from overall pain. In such cases, the interior syndrome should be considered urgent. Si Ni Tang 四逆湯 should be used to rescue the interior syndrome. When the patient has normal stool with overall pain, the exterior syndrome should be treated urgently. Gui Zhi Tang 桂枝湯 should be used to dispel the exterior syndrome." It also recorded, "When a patient suffers fever and headache with deep pulse, if he doesn't recover, and feels overall pain then Si Ni Tang 四逆湯 should be prescribed to rescue the interior syndrome." The above examples are consistent with the disease seriousness. In Native medicine there is a method of relieving both exterior and interior Biao Li Jian Jie 表裡兼解, which usually combines herbs for reducing fever with ones that stop diarrhea. *Tai Yang chapter* 太陽篇 says, "In Tai Yang diseases, the exterior syndrome hasn't been dispelled, but the purgatives have been used for several times, which leads to repeated diarrhea and epigastric fullness. This is because both exterior and

[301] Seriousness of the disease 病情之深淺 also translates as "disease being shallow or deep".

interior syndromes did not resolve. Gui Zhi Ren Shen Tang 桂枝人參湯 should be prescribed for treatment."

Ninthly, I would like to discuss seven emotions and six Qi Qing Liu Qi 七情六氣. They are a remote or secondary cause of the disease. Wherefrom do I have this conclusion? There are two causes for a disease: internal and external. However, Native medicine only considers six Qi as external causes, and seven emotions as internal causes. That's why I say six Qi and seven emotions are a remote or secondary cause for a disease. I would like to discuss seven emotions first. Seven emotions include joy Xi 喜, anger Nu 怒, sadness Ai 哀, fear Ju 懼, love Ai 愛, hate Wu 惡 and desire Yu 欲. I am not able to find details about the seven emotions in the ancient medical literature, so I follow the common sense of *Classic of Rites Li Jing* 禮經. In my opinion, the emotions are closely related to physiology and the injury of emotions can indeed cause pathological changes. However, I think that seven emotions are not able to represent all the spiritual and emotional spectrum. Fen 忿[302] usually causes headache, so it belongs to anger Nu 怒. Bei Tong 悲慟 usually causes dizziness, so it belongs to sadness Ai 哀. Jiao Si 焦思 usually causes obstructed craziness Ma Bi Kuang 麻痺狂, so it belongs to desire Yu 欲. Lian Ai 戀愛 can cause hysteria, so it belongs to love Ai 愛. Jing E 驚愕 usually causes abortion, so I attach it to fear Ju 懼. Yet there are some cases that I really don't know to which one of the seven emotions they belong, such as epilepsy of a newly-married woman, tuberculosis due to melancholy, and neurasthenia due to nervousness or fatigue. It seems that joy and hate will not cause diseases. The ancients mistook seven emotions as internal causes of diseases. The above are some examples for that.

Next, I will discuss the six Qi, which include wind Feng 風, cold Han 寒, summer-heat Shu 暑, dampness Shi 濕, dryness Zao 燥, and fire Huo 火. There are two versions of six Qi in Nei Jing 內經, summer-heat Shu 暑 is replaced by heat in the other one. I don't want to discuss here what exactly dryness Zao 燥 and fire Huo 火 mean. However, all six Qi refer to the climate's temperature or humidity, which are indeed closely related to diseases. For example, common cold usually appears in the alternating progression of cold and warm. Sunstroke usually appears in the hot season. Digestive diseases usually happen in summer. Respiratory diseases usually happen in winter. Cholera is often seen at the end of spring and beginning of summer. Dengue fever is always seen in midsummer. Elevated grounds are not good for tuberculosis.

[302] In English, different Chinese terms may translate similarly so, to avoid phrases such as "anger belongs to anger", we keep the Chinese terms.

Rheumatism is often seen in low and damp area. The theory of spring-warm, summer-heat, autumn-dryness, winter-cold in Native medicine assumes that climate influences disease. This theory, nowadays, becomes more and more popular. Restraining the heaven Dao is hard but human's Dao is easy. One can convince people about it but can't convince heaven. This is not something that Native medicine should claim as climbing high and galloping far. There are many treatment methods for six Qi. There are prescriptions for dispelling wind, removing summer-heat, and expelling cold, which are quite similar to antipyretics. Prescriptions for eliminating dampness are equivalent to stomachics, which I mentioned in the previous section. Prescriptions for moistening dryness and suppressing fire are equivalent to cold and cool prescriptions; check the book *A Summary of Chinese Herbs Categorizations and Characteristics Zhong Yao Xing Lei Gai Shuo* 中藥性類概說 for more details. As for seven emotions' treatment, Native medicine thinks Chai Hu 柴胡 is the most important herb to relieve depression, which is similar to calming the brain. Bai Shao 白芍 can activate blood and Dan Cao 胆草 is bitter-cold. *Nature of Herbs Chapter Yao Xing Pian* 藥性篇 discusses these in detail. There is no need to repeat here.

Tenthly, I will discuss cold damage Shanghan 傷寒 and warmth diseases Wenbing 溫病. Both cold damage and warmth diseases are febrile diseases Re Xing Bing 熱性病; I will prove this by using the ancient classics. *Su Wen Re Bing* 素問熱病 says "all external-contraction febrile diseases are called Shang Han 伤寒." It also says "people who are injured by cold will develop febrile diseases." Wang Shuhe 王叔和, who rearranged the *Shang Han Lun* 傷寒論, quoted these views from *Su Wen Re Bing* 素問熱病 in his preface. So it is evident that Shang Han 伤寒 refers to febrile diseases. Warmth diseases are one kind of Shang Han 伤寒, so they are also febrile diseases.

Firstly, I will prove this with symptoms. There are records of warmth diseases in *Shang Han Lun* 傷寒論. Zhang Zhongjing 張仲景 said Shang Han 伤寒 must have aversion to cold, while warmth diseases must have no aversion to cold. Some scholars misused this quote for identifying diseases. Yang Ming 陽明 also doesn't have aversion to cold and so some scholars treated Yang Ming 陽明 as if it were warmth disease, and criticised others for separately creating the study of warmth diseases.

Secondly, I will discuss this from etiology point of view. *Su Wen Yin Yang Ying Xiang Da Lun* 素問陰陽應象大論 says, "People who are injured by cold in winter will have warmth disease in Spring." *Re Bing Lun* 熱病論 says, "Warmth diseases caused by cold injury Shang Han 伤寒 are called Bing Wen 病溫 if they occur before summer solstice, and Bing Shu 病暑 if they appear thereafter." Based on these views, warmth diseases develop from cold injury Shang Han 伤寒. Cold injuries Shang Han 伤寒 are febrile diseases, and therefore warmth diseases are also febrile diseases. Actually, both of them are acute infectious diseases in Western medicine.[303] *Shang Han Lun* 傷寒論 discussed mainly influenza, malaria, acute bronchitis, acute infectious intestinal catarrh, hemato-diarrhea, cholera, dengue,[304] rheumatism and epidemic cerebrospinal meningitis. *Wen Bing Tiao Bian* 溫病條辨 discussed mainly croupous pneumonia, febrile diseases with eruptions, typhoid fever, scarlet fever, diphtheria, malignant intermittent fever, septicaemia and epidemic parotitis. All of these were called "Fever" in Western medicine before modern bacteriology appeared. It is same with cold injury and warmth diseases in Native medicine. Besides, clinical identifications in modern science, such as typhoid fever and paratyphoid fever, influenza and dengue, red dysentery and local red dysentery, and cholera and bilious cholera, also appeared quite late. Ancient Native medicine was not able to identify diseases just like Western medicine, and it is understandable since instruments were not well-developed yet.

Some scholars suspect that Zhang Zhongjing 張仲景 used cardiotonic herbs like Fu Zi 附子 and Qiang Huo 羌活 to treat high fever. Actually, Zhang Zhongjing 張仲景 didn't do that. The heart may become weak when there is high fever and this should be treated by tonifying the heart or reducing fever. However, cardiotonic herbs are not suitable for high fever. Yang Ming 陽明 heat might be accompanied by large pulse or weak pulse. That's because heart action may be sthenic at the beginning and than become weak after hyperactivity. Zhang Zhongjing 張仲景 didn't apply any prescription, because he thought that cardiotonic herbs were not suitable for Yang Ming 陽明 heat. So it is obvious that Zhongjing 仲景 didn't use cardiotonic herbs to treat high fever. Now, when the pulse is quite weak, it is not suitable to use antipyretic herbs. So actually, Zhang Zhongjing 張仲景 didn't apply any prescription. I will use Tai Yang 太陽 to prove this. *Tai Yang chapter* 太陽篇 says "Use Gan Jiang Fu Zi Tang 乾薑附子湯 to treat patients who have restlessness in daytime, but are quiet at night, no vomiting, no desire to drink, deep and weak pulse, and no high fever." From the three words, "no high fever", we know that Zhang Zhongjing 張仲景 didn't use cardiotonic prescription to treat high fever. His treatment was correct. Later *Wen Bing* 溫病 scholars, unable to master Zhang Zhongjing's 張仲景 ideas, suspected that his treatment was improper. Wu Jutong 吳鞠通 even used prescriptions of nourishing

[303] In this article we translate the term "science" (Ke Xue 科學) as "Western medicine", simply to allow an easier read. For Tan, in this discussion, "science" means modern Western medicine.
[304] This word appears in English in the text.

Yin, such as Da Ding Feng Zhu 大定风珠 and San Jia Fu Mai Tang 三甲復脈湯 to replace Zhang Zhongjing's 張仲景 treatment for heart failure in febrile diseases. This was completely wrong. Actually, these two prescriptions are quite similar to Zhang Zhongjing's 張仲景 Zhi Gan Cao Tang 炙甘草湯. So the fight between cold and warmth schools was meaningless, it is better now to use scientific methods to deal with that, such as taking temperature.

The above are regarded as Native medicine's fundamental theories and methods. Cold and heat cover a wide range of topics, which should be discussed in a separate monograph. These theories and methods are based on experience. They are neither miraculous nor mystical. It is also not suitable to say that Native medicine is a scientific method. Native medicine is complicated and not systematic. It is without value to establish an independent medical system for Native medicine. Today, there are many things that still cannot be explained by science, however, this is not a reason to oppose science. I believe, as time goes by, modern science will explain more and more things. The Bureau for Native medicine should use science to reform the Native medicine, and combine both Native and Western medicines to form a unified medical system.

Author Remarks:

There is a saying that medicine is principle and principle there is only one. Native medicine is largely wrong about anatomy and physiology yet its accumulated clinical experience is vast. In pathology, Native and Western medicines are complementary and often arrive at similar conclusions and this is what I described in this article. So who said that it is not possible for them to merge with each other? Oppressive Qi is nerves, spleen is pancreas, six Qi is the origin of disease, liver controls spleen and wood controls earth is basically neurological stomach disease. My views are based on Yu Yunxiu's 余雲岫, and I just confirm them with evidence. Try and look at *Imperial Chinese Medicine* (Kokan Igaku 皇漢醫學), which was written by Yumoto Kyushin 湯本; the theories of Yin Yang Biao Li 陰陽表裡 have no scientific evidence to them. How can one try to convince someone like this? The Bureau for Native medicine didn't give any reply to my first proposal, so I wrote this one to present my suggestions again. Since the last one was not replied to, therefore I merged the new one with the previous one to make it clearer.

A proposal to the Academy:[305] Discussion on the importance of experience in herb research

By Tan Cizhong

Pages 46–93

This proposal aims to solve arguments between Chinese medicine[306] and Western medicine. Actually, I had presented a proposal asking the Academy to research Chinese medicine, to study Chinese herbs and to think highly of the accumulated experience in order to drastically stop arguments between Chinese and Western medicine. The office of the Academy replied "The proposal you presented on March 27th has been approved by president Feng 奉院長. Your proposal listed several advantages and disadvantages of Chinese medicine, which are with great insight. Our Institute of Chemistry has started studying some herbs and has published their research results. Due to financial difficulties, it is not possible to carry out a large scale research on herbs. We will forward your proposal to the Institute of Chemistry for reference." I appreciate this reply, which promises to bring many benefits for Chinese medicine development. But I still want to make a new proposal to further discuss the importance of experience[307] in the herb research.

Experience cannot be ignored during herb research. Without experience, we are not able to know the real situation and routine methods of Chinese medicine. What is the real situation of Chinese medicine? Though it knows a little about disease cause, it is quite good at symptoms. For example, blood and Qi, Yin and Yang, deficiency and excess, exterior and interior, principal and subordinate, dryness and dampness, wind and phlegm, etc. are related to symptoms; they are not metaphysical concepts. Exogenous six Qi, internal damage by excessive seven emotions, recurrence with improper food intake, recurrence caused by overexertion, recurrence caused by excessive sexual intercourse, coital transmission of febrile disease, etc., are not the real causes but rather inducements. Chinese medicine symptoms are not local but

[305] Zhong Yang Yan Jiu Yuan 中央研究院 The Central Research Academy of Sciences, established in 1928 in Nanjing, was the highest institute of the land for the research and development of modern science.

[306] Changing from the previous article, the author uses Chinese medicine 中醫 instead of Native medicine 國醫. We have changed the translation accordingly.

[307] Here and in the remaining article, "experience" has the meaning of practical experience accumulated over centuries of using Chinese herbs.

universal, such as vomiting, diarrhea, cough, warm in spring, heat in summer, dry in autumn, cold in winter, etc. Chinese medicine doesn't have detailed and clear records of diseases caused by specific factors, such as malaria, dysentery, measles, smallpox, lung abscess, intestinal abscess, tuberculosis, rheumatism, convulsive diseases, gout, etc. Though Chinese medicine is not able to know the exact cause of a disease, the therapeutic methods are still worthwhile. The four diagnostic methods (look, listen, question and pulse-taking) cannot possibly grasp all disease factors. However, Chinese medicine basic theories are quite helpful to herb research. For example, Radix Astragali Mongolici Huang Qi 黃芪 can treat wind diseases. We know wind may cause hemiplegia, arm paralysis, body numbness, leg atrophy etc., where body loses sensation and motoric ability, which may obstruct nourishment of the body. Based on this, we know that Huang Qi 黃芪 is able to treat nerve diseases. Nonetheless, we have to research it and make things clear, such as which aspect can it treat, neuritis or nerve palsy? Peripheral or central?

Radix Aconiti Lateralis Preparata Fu Zi 附子 can rescue Yang exhaustion, which manifests as vertigo, sweat, coldness in the extremities, faint pulse, collapse. Based on this, we know that Fu Zi 附子 is an essential herb for treatment of collapse. But we still have to research why it has this effect. Herba Ephedrae Minutae Ma Huang 麻黃 and Ramulus Cinnamomi Gui Zhi 桂枝 are able to treat winter cold, Flos Lonicerae Yin Hua 銀花 and Fructus Forsythiae Suspensae Lian Qiao 連翹 are able to treat spring warmth, Herba Moslae Chinensis Xiang Ru 香薷 is able to treat summer heat. Fever is the common symptom of cold, warmth and heat. The effect is considered good if the fever is reduced. So we know that Ma Huang 麻黃, Gui Zhi 桂枝, Yin Hua 銀花, Lian Qiao 連翹 and Xiang Ru 香薷 have a reducing fever effect. Other herbs similar to Ma Huang 麻黃, Gui Zhi 桂枝 and Xiang Ru 香薷 like Fang Feng 防風, Jing Jie 荊芥, Qiang Huo 羌活, Du Huo 獨活, Xiong Qiong 芎藭, Bai Zhi 白芷, Zi Su 紫蘇, Hao Ben 好本, Man Jing Zi 蔓京子 and Bo He 薄荷 can also induce sweat and help reduce fever. Do they have an effect on the adjusting temperature mechanism in the central nervous system? This still remains to be explored. Other herbs resembling Yin Hua 銀花 and Lian Qiao 連翹, like Chai Hu 柴胡, Qian Hu 前胡, Gou Teng 勾藤, Zhi Zi 梔子, Di Gu 地骨, Yin Hu 銀胡, Fu Ping 浮萍 and Shi Hu 石斛, don't induce sweat but still may reduce fever. Do they possibly affect material metabolism? This should also be explored.

Also, dryness can remove dampness and we can find these herbs in drying prescriptions. The herbs in Ping Wei San 平胃散, Hou Po 厚朴, Fa Xia 法夏, Cang Zhu 蒼朮, Bai Zhu 白朮, Chen Pi 陳皮, etc., have drying effect and belong to this type. What we call "Damp Disease" is described in Tai Yin Shi Tu 太陰濕土 outline sentence "abdominal distension and fullness, vomiting, food doesn't come down, chronic diarrhea and, at times, abdominal pain." From this, one knows that Damp Disease is actually stomach and intestines disease. Therefore, in Chinese medicine, drying prescriptions are prescriptions for stomach and intestines. Like this, understanding the entirety of Chinese medicine becomes the basis for researching herbs; without it, where could one start?

What are the Chinese medicine routine methods? Cold-hot method is one of them. It is a specific method of using herbs in Chinese medicine. There are mainly three kinds of prescriptions, specialty prescriptions, symptomatic prescriptions, and cold-hot prescriptions. Specialty prescription is a prescription that must be used for a certain disease. Using herbs which can eliminate phlegm to treat lung diseases and using digestive herbs to treat stomach diseases—these are symptomatic prescriptions. There is no obvious difference between Western and Chinese medicines with specialty prescriptions and symptomatic prescriptions.

However, the concept of cold-hot prescriptions is different. Compared to using symptomatic prescriptions alone, differentiating further cold prescriptions to treat excitatory diseases and hot prescriptions to treat inhibitory diseases yields much better efficacy. It is a principle of "within targeting the symptom there is further differentiation". The efficacy of cold-hot prescriptions is influenced by the nature and taste of herbs, dosage and composition. This knowledge is unique to Chinese medicine, and should also be the foundation for herb research. Hot prescriptions usually use herbs with pungent taste to achieve an exciting action, while cold prescriptions usually use herbs with bitter taste to achieve sedative action. So actually, hot herbs in Chinese medicine are quite similar to stimulants in Western medicine, and cold herbs are quite similar to anesthetics. Since, in the past, there were hardly any exciting formulas, they called them hot herbs and that's it. Likewise there were no sedatives and anesthetics, so they called them cold herbs and that's it. However, the objective of cold-hot prescriptions is diseases treatment, not increase or decrease of excitement. Therefore cold-hot prescriptions may treat many diseases, such as vomiting, diarrhea, cough, asthma, fever, vertigo, pain, etc. They can be used to regulate menstruation, prevent miscarriage, stop bleeding, relieve distention and fullness, stop hiccup, etc. The nature and taste of herbs impacts the entire body, not only the stomach, that's why cold-hot prescriptions are suitable to treat almost all diseases.

Dosage is a factor that may influence efficacy. Take Huang Lian 黃連 and Dan Cao 胆草 as examples. They are used only as stomachic in Western medicine. Yet in Chinese medicine Huang Lian 黃連 is used for sleep disorders, and Dan Cao 胆草 for eye diseases. This is because, in Chinese medicine, a large dose of these two herbs can reduce excitement. Small dose of Da Huang 大黄 has a reinforcing action, while a large dose has a sedative action. Generally speaking, in Western medicine dose will be less than half a gram, while in Chinese medicine more than 10 grams. Likewise, there are some anesthetics that have increasing excitement action in small dosage and anesthetic action in large dosage. So how come Western medicine doesn't pay attention to the dose being small or large? This problem is seen with the above example.

At the same time, the dosage is also influenced by the compatibility of herbs. For example, when a Western drug is combined with Gan Jiang 乾薑 and alcohol, it will have no side effects from the pungent sharpness only if dosage is below half gram. But if it is used, according to Chinese medicine, together with Gan Cao 甘草, there are no side effects even above 18 grams. Therefore, how to combine herbs is different from the substances that can modify taste in Western medicine and it is quite important for Chinese medicine herb research.

Without knowing the set rules of Chinese medicine well, it will not be possible to do proper herb research. In order to get achievements in herb research and prove clinical experience, we have to examine all related discussions in Chinese medicine and pay attention to their special points. Scholars usually research herbs only based on *Ben Cao* 本草. In other words, they are not able to research herbs based on a full view of Chinese medicine, including the connotation of cold and hot. Mistakes, therefore, are unavoidable in many aspects, for example, knowing which herbs treat which channels, or which herbs are attributed to which organs. Moreover, there are discrepancies between different schools, which causes confusion and misuse, for example, the mix up of Cao Wu 草烏 and Wu Tou 烏頭, the wrong use of Ren Shen 人參, the misunderstanding of Shi Gao 石膏. Likewise, *Ben Cao* 本草 is not infallible in herb research. In addition, there are some herbs that haven't been recorded by *Ben Cao* 本草 and we can only hear about them from some people living in seclusion. These herbs are difficult to discover, or looked down upon by doctors, but often they have miraculous effect. For any herb, it is rather difficult to first research its pharmacology and then prove it with clinical practice. It will be easier if we first research its clinical applications and then prove them with pharmacology.

I hope the Academy will conduct herb research starting with the easy ways first. Experience is quite important in Chinese medicine. It will not be possible to achieve great success with herb research without the help of experience. It is exactly like not knowing anatomy and physiology, and therefore unable to know pathology. Science is based on experiments and statistics. Both experiments and statistics are related to experience. As there are many herbs in Chinese medicine, it's better to divide them according to specific departments. The surgery and eye departments have many diseases only treated with surgery. We have to promote herb research based on experience for these departments. It will be rather easy to achieve success if we carry forward the advantages of Chinese medicine. In other words, we cannot just follow science. If there will be gain or loss largely depends on the choices the Academy takes.

A reply letter from the Central Academy for Sciences stated:

> On June 24th we have received your second letter on how to resolve the arguments in the medical field and that experience must be considered. We have forwarded it to our Institute of Chemistry to be considered together with your first proposal. We are hereby sending an acknowledgement letter to Mr. Tan Cizhong.

Reply to the Director of Shanghai Society Medical Gazette, Mr. Yu Yunxiu 余雲岫

By Tan Cizhong

Dear Mr. Yu Yunxiu,

I am pleased to hear from you. There are many wise thoughts in your feedback. Recently, my article was published in Shanghai Society Medical Gazette with your comments, which gives me plenty of praise and encouragement. Both of us are of the same opinion that the medical system should be reformed. However, there are a couple of divergent opinions on plans and procedures I would like to discuss with you in this letter. The fact is that Chinese herbs are effective, and people in our country are used to them and trust them, and this is something that cannot be easily changed. On the other hand, science wins more and more support and obtains great development. I think that your academic efforts are making significant contributions to the development of science. I am one who is greatly influenced by your theories. I therefore believe that it is better to reform medicine through academic efforts. Administrative strategy alone cannot possibly change the people's belief in Chinese medicine. To the contrary, it may lead to a stronger opposition to our medical revolution. What has happened in recent months proves it. In sum, administrative strategy is ineffective or even harmful to the reform of medicine.

You suggest that medical schools should assume responsibility for researching the effective herbs of Chinese medicine. However, scientific research of all herbs cannot be completed in a short period, and the establishment of medical schools is coming up within the foreseeable future. It is not realistic to simply stop using the effective Chinese herbs that haven't been proven by science just yet. In my opinion, it's better to first organize the historical experience of using herbs, and then move on to scientific research of these herbs guided by experience. Only in this way will we be able to achieve fast success with scientific reform of Chinese medicine. Long ago I already made a decision to organize the experience of Chinese medicine, and I have also followed some of your theories. I think you should better consider pledging a large-scale research on Chinese herbs. Since you are a famous doctor, both Western and Chinese doctors will support your reform of our medicine.

I hope you can carry out the proposition of establishing medical schools, which will bring enormous benefits for all Chinese people. I take liberty in making the above suggestions. I will feel honored if you could consider them.

Attachment: Reply letter from Yu Yunxiu 余雲岫

Dear Mr. Tan Cizhong 譚次仲,

I really don't deserve so many praises from you. Your propositions about the modern reform of Chinese medicine, conforming to mine, are quite practical. You suggest doing herb experiments based on experience. It is, actually, the gist of all medical reform, and also the thing that, it seems today, cannot be discussed by Chinese medicine doctors. Our sole divergence is the procedure of modern reform, yet our aim is exactly the same. I think that your measure of a transitional period is not thorough. I am going to list doubts below, please think them over.

In my opinion, you emphasize experience too much. I think that it's better to say experience should not be completely ignored. We have to deal with different experience in different ways. For example, the experience of scientists should be considered as science, but the experience of ordinary people should be treated as unreliable. Disease recovery is not only influenced by herbs, there are many other factors. Without scientific research and reliable statistics, can we say that an herb is effective just based on "having much experience"? Of course not. Da Huang 大黃 can remove excess, Dang Gui 當歸 may relieve pain and such experience should not be ignored. In my opinion, the experience accumulated after Song and Yuan Dynasties is not credible, because of the Confucianism influence. Dan Xi 丹溪 and Jing Yue 景岳 experience is even more questionable. Nonetheless, experience of ordinary doctors should be considered as research data. Now, if effective herbs from ancient legends prove to be "not scientifically viable" then we should just give them up.

You mention as well that experience may be invisible and complicated. I agree with your conclusion. We have to use scientific methods to prove them, make invisible things become visible and complicated things simple. A master craftsman is able to tell people the rules, but he is not able to transform a person into a master craftsman. Everyone can follow rules, yet people need a special talent to become a master craftsman. At the same time, without rules, nobody can become a master craftsman. Before we apply this "previously accumulated experience", we have to find out the scientific principle behind this experience. You think that it is not possible to get the core points without following the "previously accumulated experience". In my opinion, this is just a strategy to oppose science and refuse experiments. It is not possible to take all patients as test animals for the purpose of an experiment. Many medical accidents occur by just relying on personal experience, which is far away from a scientific principle.

Above are the points on which we differ. I am not able to discuss with you the "cold-hot", because your words describing it are not clear enough. It is not possible to do chemical experiments without a well-equipped laboratory. Shanghai Central Health Laboratory has the best equipment. The director of this laboratory is my friend, so I can do experiments there. Also, I can buy additional equipment that this laboratory doesn't have. If you trust me, you can send me some herbs with your understanding of their clinical efficacy. I will try to prove their efficacy and find out the contributing chemical ingredients. I will make chemically-constructed products, based on my research, then send them to many doctors for clinical trials, and try to get their feedback. I will also publish my research results in medical journals, in order to let domestic and foreign doctors know the newest in research of Chinese medicine and herbs. Such research will also bring benefits and fame to the researchers. So we have to keep it secret during the research process, in order to forgo the risk of discoveries being stolen by others.

I have skimmed your book, I will read it again more carefully when I am free, and then discuss with you the contents. It is not possible to express all my opinions in this letter, hope we can discuss more in following letters. Best wishes!

Yours,
Yu Yunxiu

Reply to the Editor of Hongkong Native Medicine Magazine, He Peiyu 何佩瑜[308]

By Tan Cizhong

Dear Mr. Peiyu,

I have received the magazine issue, in which is printed my article, A *Proposal to the Bureau for Native Medicine Guo Yi Guan* 國醫館*: How to Arrange the Nation's Medicine by First Establishing a Standard*. Thanks for your comment at the end of my article. In the comment, you wrote, "I am touched that you have totally expressed your opinions. You are a doctor who has read lots of ancient and modern medical books. You want to make a positive contribution to medicine by combining Chinese and Western medicine. I admire you enormously. However, it is a pity that your thoughts are unsystematic, which makes it impossible to guide practice."

After reading the full text of the comment, I feel your thoughts are disconnected and inconsistent, so I think you are not qualified to discuss the combination of Chinese and Western medicine.

Firstly, you agree to my opinion that anatomy and physiology are quite important, but on the other hand, you uphold ancient traditions, and believe in things without scientific grounds. So your thoughts are not consistent.

Secondly, I praise Chinese herbs for their efficacy in treating pestilence and bone fracture, yet you think they are non-scientific. Why do so many doctors prefer to use Chinese herbs for these diseases? You have many wrong assumptions in pathology and pharmacology, and you are also not able to completely explain your points in detail.

Thirdly, you believe that Zhang Zhongjing 張仲景 might also have made some mistakes, but you oppose my criticisms to his book without giving satisfactory explanation.

Fourthly, the main symptoms that Da Cheng Qi Tang 大承氣湯 can treat are delirious speech, hectic fever and sweating of hands and feet. Chen Xiuyuan 陳修園 thought that Da Cheng Qi Tang 大承氣湯 was suitable for treatment of other things besides abdominal fullness and dry stool. Yet you think that Da Cheng Qi Tang 大承氣湯 can treat only abdominal fullness and dry stool. It does show your ignorance of the classics.

---

308 The text has the name as He Yupei 何瑜佩, we have corrected the error.

Fifthly, science is based on evidence, but you only worship Huang Di 黃帝 and Zhang Zhongjing 張仲景.

Sixthly, you also think it is necessary to reorganize Chinese medicine, but you haven't provided any further opinions, such as which methods to use, which principles to follow, etc.

Actually, you don't understand what I am after in my article and proposal to the Bureau of Native Medicine. I think that medicine is not suitable to be divided as different medical principles, because humans all over the world are the same. Medicine should be a science based on experiments. Scientific experiments revolve around tangible physical reality. But in your comment to my article, you say Chinese medicine has its own science which is based on intangible formless things and Qi transformation. I have to tell you that Chinese medicine is not a science at all. If some parts of Chinese medicine are scientific, they should be based on tangible physical things. I would like to ask what exactly are these intangible formless things and Qi transformation? Do they refer to Yin and Yang 陰陽? I have written an article proving that Yin and Yang 陰陽, Blood and Qi 血氣, Wind, Dampness, Water, Fire, Deficiency and Excess, Exterior and Interior, Seven Emotions and Six Qi, Cold Damage and Warm Diseases are all tangible physical things that can be assessed with scientific methods. I invested great effort to break fallacies. I will send you a copy of this article and I hope you would read it carefully.

Science based on experiments is becoming more and more powerful and prosperous. Medicine, likewise, should develop based on scientific methods. Yet your words and actions are opposite to this trend. I resolved my heart to reform Chinese medicine through science and experiments and bring it to tangible physical reality, though I haven't figured out detailed implementation programs.

I have written a book, the first three chapters of which I have finished, containing circa 50,000 words, and it is called *My Opinion on Scientification of Chinese Medicine Zhong Yi Ke Xue Hua Zhi Wo Jian* 中醫科學化之我見, which includes my letters to the Research Academy and Yu Yunxiu 余雲岫. Shanghai Society Medical Gazette published all of my articles with Yu Yunxiu's 余雲岫 comments. Other newspapers, like Guangzhou Yue Hua Newspaper 廣州越華日報, in its medicine and public health column, reprinted them and added comments. Other newspapers, from Xia Men 廈門 to the capitol, too many to count, reprinted them and added comments. Their comments were humble and peaceful, clever, upright and valuable, many of which I accepted with great respect. As expected, there were also plenty of other deceitful comments such as "the yellow bell is ruined and abandoned" and "there is one crane in the flock of chickens".[309] Even though shamed, I did not deserve that. All my articles expound on the Chinese medicine principle. Alas, trying to convince the enemy in such a way, this will be judged at the end by public opinion and in every person's heart. (Now since every newspaper covered both opinions). My book is done but not printed yet. After it is printed I will offer respectfully to you one copy. The plan for the entire book is laid out and in the process of unfolding. After about five or six years it will be complete. The money will be paid for carving of the printing blocks, and five or six years after that I hope that we can achieve the following objectives:

1) There will be no barriers between Chinese and Western medicine; 2) Chinese medicine doctors will be able to communicate with Western medicine doctors; 3) Both Chinese and Western medicines will become essential for the research of Chinese herbs; 4) "Qi means nerves, Yin Yang means heart, Wind means brain, Dampness means stomach and intestines" will become the maxim of Chinese medicine; 5) There will be no Chinese versus foreign, ancient versus modern. Chinese and Japanese branches will merge into one river. One swipe will erase all differences, like a dragon rising with fire in the bright sky.

All above describes my belief in unifying Chinese and Western medicines. Isn't this "melting them together", what you claim as wrong? It seems that what the opponent tries to ascend I get rid of. Why is it obscure that learning has no national borders and is it really so that I am helping the flames of the opposition? Restraining me truly will be a curse, wouldn't the close ones have difficulty becoming good doctors and the far ones will not know their unworthiness?

Attaining nothingness is called the extraordinary origin, it is what the masses fear. When the fool hears of Dao he laughs at it with loud voice! [Replying here to the line "arousing laughter" circulating in the medical community.] My heart feels pity. I do not over-estimate myself. I sincerely want to mend their foolishness and confront the disorderly. I also heard "wearing a pot on your head and looking to heaven"[310] and "sitting inside a well and looking at the sun".[311] Now, the way you make yourself grand is not something the ancients approved of.

Respectfully yours,
Tan Cizhong

[309] One person that feels himself aloof above the others.
[310] Your action and objective are opposite to each other.
[311] Having a narrow minded view.

An additional reply to Yu Yunxiu 余雲岫 discussing ancient prescriptions

By Tan Cizhong

Yaron: Tan, in his reply letter, demonstrates a practical diagnosis of symptoms and treatment. This strategy, in my opinion, served later on as a foundation for TCM's "differentiating syndromes and applying treatment" (Bian Zheng Lun Zhi 辨證論治). When we practice TCM today, diagnosis involves finding a group of symptoms and naming them as a syndrome, for example, Liver Qi stagnation or Stomach Yin deficiency. The treatment that then follows entails selecting from a group of herbs appropriate for this syndrome.

This is how the originators of TCM designed Chinese medicine to be: practical; easy to diagnose; and easy to treat. Categorization of herbs to different groups was done by experiments. For example, thirst means Stomach Yin deficiency. If one drinks Mai Men Dong tea and feels less thirsty, then this means that Mai Men Dong cures Stomach Yin deficiency. Therefore, any time that a patient presents a syndrome, or group of symptoms, which includes thirst, this means that there is Stomach Yin deficiency and Mai Men Dong can be used—on its own or with other herbs, depending on symptoms present.

Differentiation of syndromes and application of treatment according to symptoms, even though it existed before, certainly became dominant in the early years of TCM's formation, from the end of the Republic until today. This is how Tan envisioned the way Chinese medicine should be practiced and it belongs to the group we defined before as "Tan Cizhong trend" (eliminating the old theory and using the accumulated experience of herbs).

Dear Mr. Yunxiu,

I have received your letter commenting on my article, *A Proposal to the Academy: Discussion on the Importance of Experience in Herb Research*, specifically the section talking about prescriptions. I sincerely respect your words. However, it is only about the previously-tried methods and that's it. Even though tried methods cannot always be followed blindly, ancient prescriptions stand out. I wish to discuss with you why ancient prescriptions are rather important for later generations. Ancient prescriptions include prescriptions from *Shang Han* 傷寒 and *Jin Gui* 金匱, and because *Qian*

Jin 千金 and *Wai Tai* 外臺 have close relationships with *Shang Han* 傷寒 and *Jin Gui* 金匱, the prescriptions from them can also be looked at as ancient prescriptions. The excellent efficacy of Zhang Zhongjing's 張仲景 prescriptions are based on following six factors: the individual herbs within; how to combine them; dosage; the physical form of the remedy; the application; and differentiation of cold and hot. Allow me to explain these points.

Most herbs used by Zhang Zhongjing 張仲景 are quite effective, such as Huang Qin 黃芩, Huang Lian 黃連, Zhi Mu 知母, Huang Bai 黃柏, Fu Zi 附子, Gan Jiang 乾薑, Zhi Shi 枳實, Hou Po 厚朴, Ma Huang 麻黃, Gui Zhi 桂枝, Chai Hu 柴胡, Bai Zhu 白朮, Huang Qi 黃芪, Dang Gui 當歸, E Jiao 阿膠, Tao Ren 桃仁, Di Huang 地黃, Dan Pi 丹皮, Shi Gao 石膏, Zhi Zi 梔子, Da Huang 大黃, Pu Xiao 朴硝, Yuan Hua 芫花, Gan Sui 甘遂, Da Ji 大戟, etc. All these herbs have excellent effect of being warming, clearing, purging or tonifying. This is the first factor allowing excellent clinical efficacy for Zhongjing's 張仲景 prescriptions. It is the individual herbs.

Zhang Zhongjing 張仲景 was good at combining herbs; for example, Ma Huang 麻黃 with Gui Zhi 桂枝, Chai Hu 柴胡 with Huang Qin 黃芩, Fu Zi 附子 with Gan Jiang 乾薑, Shi Gao 石膏 with Zhi Mu 知母, E Jiao 阿膠 with Huang Lian 黃連, Da Huang 大黃 with Pu Xiao 朴硝. These combinations increase the herbs' actions. If they are combined with Gan Cao 甘草, Shao Yao 芍藥, Fu Ling 茯苓, Ren Shen 人參, Da Zao 大棗, Chi Shi Zhi 赤石脂, Yi Tang 飴糖 or Jing Mi 粳米 then prescriptions' side effects decrease. In this fashion, Zhongjing's 張仲景 prescriptions are neatly organized. It is the second factor allowing excellent clinical efficacy of his prescriptions. It is herbs' compatibility.

There are many prescriptions that have the same individual herbs, but they have different actions because of the dosage used. For example, Gui Zhi Tang 桂枝湯 and Gui Zhi Jia Shao Yao Tang 桂枝加芍藥湯 have the same five herbs. The dosage of Gui Zhi 桂枝 is equal to Shao Yao 芍藥 in Gui Zhi Tang 桂枝湯 so it mainly treats headache, fever, sweating and aversion to cold. The dosage of Shao Yao 芍藥 is twice Gui Zhi 桂枝 in Gui Zhi Jia Shao Yao Tang 桂枝加芍藥湯 so it mainly treats abdominal pain. Si Ni Tang 四逆湯 and Tong Mai Si Ni Tang 通脈四逆湯 are composed with the same herbs. The dosage ratio of Zhi Gan Cao 炙甘草 and Gan Jiang 乾薑 in Si Ni Tang 四逆湯 is 4:3, but 3:4 in Tong Mai Si Ni Tang 通脈四逆湯. Zhi Gan Cao 炙甘草 can moderate Gan Jiang's 乾薑 pungent nature and so Tong Mai Si Ni Tang 通脈四逆湯 is suitable to treat more urgent syndromes than Si Ni Tang 四逆

湯. It is the third factor allowing excellent clinical efficacy for Zhang Zhongjing's 張仲景 prescriptions. It is herbs' dosage.

Decoction is easily absorbed by the body and can take effect quickly. Pills impact the body more slowly, so they are more suitable for diseases that require slow treatment. Zhang Zhongjing 張仲景 therefore created Cheng Qi Tang 承氣湯 and Pi Yue Wan 脾約丸, Da Xian Xiong Tang 大陷胸湯 and Xian Xiong Wan 陷胸丸. He also created Wu Mei Wan 烏梅丸 to treat ascariasis, because a pill allows herbs to pass the intestines slowly. The strength of powder is somewhere between decoctions and pills. It is good for treating stomach diseases, because it can slowly distribute the herb efficacy to the stomach. For example, Gua Di San 瓜蒂散 can promote vomiting, Wu Ling San 五苓散 and Wen Ge San 文蛤散 can quench thirst. That's the fourth factor allowing excellent clinical efficacy for Zhang Zhongjing's 張仲景 prescriptions. It is the physical form of the remedy.

Zhang Zhongjing 張仲景 preferred to treat diseases according to the symptoms, and he always used specific prescriptions to treat specific symptoms. For example, Gui Zhi Tang 桂枝湯 is specific for specific symptoms collectively called Gui Zhi Tang syndrome 桂枝湯證 and Chai Hu Tang 柴胡湯 is specific for some specific symptoms collectively called Chai Hu Tang syndrome 柴胡湯證. Which means that when symptoms of Gui Zhi tang syndrome are present, then it is proper to use Gui Zhi Tang and when symptoms of Chai Hu Tang syndrome are present, then it is proper to use Chai Hu Tang. The entire *Shang Han Lun* 傷寒論 is like this—when there are certain symptoms present then there are certain prescriptions to address it. The prescriptions have strict applications and prohibitions. For example, for Tai Yang disease 太陽症 having general symptoms such as headache, fever, and aversion to cold, if accompanied by sweating than use Gui Zhi 桂枝, if there is no sweating than use Ma Huang 麻黃. Even for the use of Ma Huang 麻黃 there are many options. To treat no sweating with asthma it is combined with Xing Ren 杏仁 to form Ma Huang Tang 麻黃湯. To treat no sweating with restlessness it is combined with Shi Gao 石膏 to form Da Qing Long Tang 大青龍湯. To treat no sweating with spasm of neck and back it is combined with Ge Gen 葛根 to form Ge Gen Tang 葛根湯. For Yang Ming syndrome 陽明證 with constipation, if there is delirious speech, hectic fever, sweating of palms and soles, use Da Cheng Qi Tang 大承氣湯; if there are only two of the above three symptoms, use Xiao Cheng Qi Tang 小承氣湯; if there are only one of the above three symptoms, use Tiao Wei Cheng Qi Tang 調胃承氣湯. It is the fifth factor allowing excellent clinical efficacy for Zhang Zhongjing's 張仲景 prescriptions. It is the application.

Differentiating cold and hot is the most difficult thing in Chinese medicine. In *Shang Han Lun* 傷寒論, both Xiao Qing Long Tang 小青龍湯 and Ma Huang Xing Zi Gan Cao Shi Gao Tang 麻黃杏子甘草石膏湯 are used to treat asthma, both Bai Tong Tang 白通湯 and Ge Gen Huang Qin Huang Lian Gan Cao Tang 葛根黃芩黃連甘草汤 are used to treat diarrhea, both Gan Jiang Fu Zi Tang 乾薑附子湯 and Huang Lian E Jiao Tang 黃連阿膠湯 are used to treat insomnia. In *Jin Gui* 金匱, both Bai Ye Tang 柏葉湯 and Xie Xin Tang 瀉心湯 are used to treat hematemesis. However, though they are used for the same disease, they have a significant difference: one is specific for cold type; and the other for hot type. This is the sixth factor allowing excellent clinical efficacy for Zhang Zhongjing's 張仲景 prescriptions. It is the differentiation of cold and hot.

Even though the above six factors are not entirely scientific, in my opinion, starting from these and reaching to science will not be that difficult. These are called "tried methods Cheng Fa 成法" in Chinese medicine. Tried methods honestly could be changed, yet originally they helped people establish rules. It prevented people from doing anything deceitful. Likewise, the artisan Gong Shu Zi 公輸子[312] could not have accomplished his crafts without the rules of circle and square. Now, to your esteemed opinion that one cannot stick to a fixed prescription, it will probably be that only the very clever ones can do it. Other than that, ones that deviate from orthodoxy and ones that follow the ancient ways religiously both will carry an equal offense. Both are actually not following the ancients' intent for these "tried methods".

Moreover, Dang Gui 當歸 is an essential herb for gynecological diseases according to *Jin Gui* 金匱 and it led to the invention of a new drug called Wu Lu Tuo 烏路托 in gynecology. So you see, the ancient experience is often consistent with modern science. Furthermore, in your article, *The Chinese Medicine Reform: Destruction and Reconstruction Zhong Guo Yi Xue Ge Ming Zhi Po Huai Yu Jian She* 中國醫學革命之破壞與建設, you wrote, "Western medicine found out that Ma Huang 麻黃 can treat asthma only after thirty years' research. Actually, the ancient prescriptions, such as Qing Long Tang 青龙汤 and Yue Pi Tang 越婢汤, have already used this action of Ma Huang 麻黃 and so ancient prescriptions should not be ignored." Therefore, experi-

[312] An artisan from the state of Chu 楚國 and contemporary of the philosopher Mo Zi 墨子. For the entire story of Gong Shu Zi 公輸子 see Mo Zi chapter 13.

ence is quite helpful for the experiments, and the routines should not be ignored. One person's claim is not equal a public claim by everyone. How can one ignore tried methods?

In Western medicine, there are also some tried methods that shouldn't be changed randomly by doctors. Like knowing about morphine and its wide distribution; it is first seen in the adrenal glands. Like Bismuth combined with soda, hydrochloric acid with pepsin, Liao Si De 了斯的 with iron, the efficacy is always increased with these combinations. Like opium and camphor combined with alcohol, "Mr. Tuo Fei Er Powder", all kinds of spirits and powders, all kinds of mixture drugs, mixed injections, they all have a fixed prescription, and each prescription must have specific ingredients and specific doses. The doctor certainly doesn't have any wiggle room with adding or subtracting ingredients in the drug. If one understands why drugs should not be changed like this, then he should have an easy time understanding why the "tried methods" should not be changed. If one departs from the ancients' tried methods then knowing the properties of herbs and how to apply them is impossible.

For example, the different claims that Shi Gao 石膏 induces sweat or arrests sweat. In *Shang Han Lun* 傷寒論, there are many lines using Shi Gao 石膏 for the treatment of diseases with sweating and not a few lines about using it without sweating. For example, if we look at its application together with Ma Huang 麻黃: Da Qing Long Tang 大青龍湯 is specific for diseases without sweating, while Ma Huang Xing Zi Gan Cao Shi Gao Tang 麻黃杏子甘草石膏湯 is for diseases with sweating. Knowing this, we therefore realize that, for the ancients, using Shi Gao 石膏 is not related to sweating or not sweating. In the *last chapter of Tai Yang* 太陽末篇, Zhang Zhongjing 張仲景 said, "diseases without sweating shouldn't be treated with Bai Hu Tang 白虎湯"—can we deduce then that Shi Gao 石膏 is able to stop sweating? In the *first chapter of Tai Yang* 太陽首篇, he said "diseases without sweating shouldn't be treated with Gui Zhi Tang 桂枝湯"—can we deduce that Gui Zhi 桂枝 is able to stop sweating?

I think Da Huang 大黃 and Shi Gao 石膏 are essential herbs for Yang Ming diseases. Da Huang 大黃 aims to relax the bowels, while Shi Gao 石膏 eliminates heat. Sweat is the product of heat; it will stop after heat has been reduced. That's why Shi Gao 石膏 is often mistaken for a herb that can stop sweating. Yang Ming 陽明 diseases usually have large pulse, and Shi Gao 石膏 has the action of regulating heartbeat. So misusing Shi Gao 石膏 will lead to profuse sweating and collapse. That's why Shi Gao 石膏 is often mistaken for a herb that can promote sweating. So stopping sweating and promoting sweating are not the direct action of Shi Gao 石膏. However, this view is based on experience and it should be proven by experiments.

You have said that Shi Gao 石膏 has calcium in it; I think this must be a result of an experiment. However, herbs that have the same chemical structure may have totally different actions, so it's necessary to do animal experiments and clinical trials. Finally, statistical methods to analyze data collected by experiments and trials should be used. Only in this way are we able to know the actions of any single herb. Therefore, we have to research further Shi Gao 石膏, and then we will know exactly whether it is suitable to use as a medicinal and also how to use it. In a word, it is feasible and valuable to communicate theories and facts. I send you this letter to discuss the above issues, hoping you can give me some suggestions.

Yours,
Tan Cizhong

Attached: Yu Yunxiu's 余雲岫 reply letter

Yaron: Following Tan's idea of making Chinese medicine practical and using herbs for specific symptoms, Yu Yunxiu advances his position that if one knows the application of a single herb for a single symptom, then he may actually understand the original intent of an old prescription.

Such is the case with Shi Gao, claims Yu: since we now know that Shi Gao restrains sweating, we therefore understand Zhang Zhongjing's original intent in the formula Qing Long Tang to restrain the diaphoretic action of Ma Huang. Building on this assumption, Yu furthers his theory saying that, based on this new understanding of the herb's action, we can substitute Shi Gao with other herbs having a similar action and reach the exact same clinical result. Such development of logic based on physiological reactions to herbs served as a foundation for TCM and "differentiating syndromes and deciding the treatment (Bian Zheng Lun Zhi 辨證論治)". We can contemplate together the following reply letter.

Mr. Cizhong,

I read your letter to the Academy. I think there are some things that need to be deliberated. I know that doctors of the "reviving ancient" type always prefer to use classic prescriptions without any modifications; they believe that classic prescriptions are perfectly effective and even miraculous. To the extreme, in recent times, some stray doctors even claim: "only pay attention to the prescription without considering single herbs." This is caused by a superstition that ancient people had super powers.

The famous doctors of Jin 晉 and Tang 唐 Dynasties normally didn't follow Zhang Zhongjing's dosage when they used his prescriptions. In *Qian Jin Fang* 千金方 and *Qian Jin Yi Fang* 千金翼方, there are many prescriptions that have the same name and indications, but with different herbs' dosage. So it is certain that prescriptions are not fixed and that we have to change the herbs as necessary. It is not possible to use fixed prescriptions to treat changeable diseases. The ancient prescriptions are not suitable for today's diseases.

Take Shi Gao 石膏 as an example, Haizang 海藏 and Danxi 丹溪 thought it can promote sweating. This view is based on the composition of the ancient prescriptions. In *Ben Cao Si Bian Lu* 本草思辨錄, Zhou Bodu 周伯度 said it can stop sweating, and explained that Zhang Zhongjing 張仲景 wanted to reduce Ma Huang's 麻黃 action of promoting sweating through the combination of Shi Gao 石膏 with Ma Huang 麻黃. We now know that Shi Gao 石膏 is calcium sulfate and it can stop sweating, so Zhou Bodu's 周伯度 view is right, he was a person who understood Zhang Zhongjing's 張仲景 original intention of compatibility between Shi Gao 石膏 and Ma Huang 麻黃. Haizang 海藏 and Danxi 丹溪 misunderstood Zhang Zhongjing's 張仲景 original intent. However, Zhou Bodu 周伯度 didn't know the chemical composition of Shi Gao 石膏, so he was not able to know why it can stop sweating. If we don't have the proper knowledge about the herbs' actions, we are not able to understand why prescriptions can treat diseases. We have to avoid such uncertainties. Ma Huang 麻黃 is able to promote sweating; Shi Gao 石膏 is able to stop sweating. If there is a disease that must be treated by Ma Huang 麻黃, and there is also a worry about the excessive sweating, then we can use it together with Shi Gao 石膏 to reduce its sweating action. Actually, other herbs that are able to stop sweating can be used to replace Shi Gao 石膏. They can also be used together with Ma Huang 麻黃 to achieve the same effect. It is really not necessary to strictly follow the ancient prescriptions, such as Qing Long Tang 青龍湯 and Yue Pi Tang 越婢湯.

In addition, from Danxi's 丹溪 view of Shi Gao 石膏, we can deduce that all his prescriptions including Shi Gao 石膏 are not reliable. Therefore knowing well the herbs can not only help us understand the original meaning of ancient prescriptions, but also help us know the misuse of herbs by other ancient doctors. In my opinion, only Xu Lingtai 徐靈胎 understood this point. It is really never possible to know how an ancient prescription works without knowing the single herbs within. Having efficacy or not, when to apply it and when not, without knowing the single herbs, where is there a point to talk about "tried methods"? While establishing the rules, if there is no proper measure, then what is the point of saying "this is the core"?

Now, you talked about statistics. The statistical method is a shortcut for herb research. However, herb efficacy statistics being accurate or not depends entirely on the diagnosis being accurate or not, which then allows one to know how to use the herb accurately. In my opinion, it is best to build a big hospital and to accept many patients, diagnose them with Western medicine and treat them with Chinese herbs. A nurse will be assigned for daily recordings of the patient's progress. Five or ten years later, we will get statistical results, knowing exactly which diseases can be treated by which herb, which herbs can treat which diseases. The efficacy rate can be reported with accurate numbers to the entire world. Then one will have a proper path to answer the questions: "is the native herbal production useful or not?"; and "should the ancient 'tried methods' be preserved or discarded?" I really don't know whether there are other shortcuts for herb research. I have read and thought about your letter to the Academy again and again, and wrote this letter based on yours. Unfortunately, I am not able to find your letter anymore, I think you may have a copy, please send it to me again, thanks.

Yours,
Yu Yunxiu

A Letter to Lu Yunlei 陸淵雷, the Member of Academic Committee of Chinese Medicine Administration

By Tan Cizhong

Yaron: The following letter is an example for the obvious push to modernize Chinese herbs, from planting principles to production and processing. It is the time when modern scientific versions of herbal products emerged—extracted, purified and modified. Today, in Chinese medicine, it is common practice to use pre-manufactured herbal patent pills. This is the time period where the idea developed, leading to fully-fledged mass-production during the Communist era.

Dear Mr. Lu Yunlei 陸淵雷,

I have read your letter to Yu Yunxiu 余雲岫, which was published in Shanghai Society Medical gazette 上海社會醫報 the 157th issue in the communication column. In this letter, you mentioned my articles and praised me a lot. Thanks for your encouragement. I have researched how to reform Chinese medicine for a long time. In my opinion, there are four main points to consider: the issue of standard, steps to be taken, the planning and execution, and the topic's research. I have discussed the first two points in my letters to the Bureau of Native Medicine and the Academy of Sciences. And I have contemplated the latter two for a long time, but it's a pity that I was not able to find a suitable person to discuss it with. I have read your article today in the *Shanghai Society Medical Gazette* on the reform outline for Chinese medicine, and I discovered that our opinions are quite similar. I therefore believe that you are the best person for me to correspond with. Having said that, there are some textual errors in your article that require deliberation, I will attach them at the end of this letter. First, I would like to discuss with you the reform methods for Chinese medicine. Indeed, you have discussed a few methods in your own article; I simply wish to discuss further.

As for planning and execution, there are three main points. The first point is Native medical textbooks. We have to edit and publish Native medicine textbooks according to modern standards. We can collect all kinds of effective herbs and methods based on clinical practice, and explain them with modern science. We must examine books that were written in recent years, and restrict the ancient medical books. In the past, Chinese medicine books were not systematized and did not have a standard. We have to reorganize these books, adopt their good points and avoid their shortcomings. The second point is doctors. We have to encourage Chinese Native [medicine] doctors to study scientific knowledge. The young and excellent doctors should be supported by studying medicine abroad or in good domestic medical schools. These are doctors who will greatly promote the Chinese medicine reform.

The third point is medical affairs. We have to reform Chinese medicine affairs in a scientific way, such as creating hospitals and schools, including science in medical textbooks and appointing proper teachers who conform to science and the scientific spirit. I am of the opinion that medicine should be self-sufficient; in other words, Native medicine should use only Chinese herbs and no Western drugs, and consequently explore all secret folk prescriptions and make them popular for the people's benefit. This, day by day, will perfect the efficacy of Native herbal medicine. In addition, we have to change the doctors' qualifications standard, as well as adjust procedures for planting, sales, and preparation of herbs. The reform will bring Native medicine closer to science. However, if a modern herbal pharmaceutical industry is not developed with this reform, then its future will be in danger. The Bureau for Native medicine should pay more attention to that.

As for topic research, there are also three focal points. The first point is to add internship in medical education. Medicine is a study combining theory and practice. It is not possible to get medical skills just from books. Therefore, it is necessary that students act as interns—learning, for example, how to apply acupuncture, the ways to prepare and administer herbal formulas or the way to combine Native and Western medicines in cases such as trauma and eye diseases.

The second point is about soliciting opinions. Native medicine is rather complicated and confusing. In it there are many things that should be rearranged and this cannot be accomplished with a small number of people. Therefore, we have to solicit opinions from many doctors in the entire country. For example, we have to collect opinions about questions concerning theories, such as: what exactly Yin and Yang refer to and how do they transform into each other; why Tai Yang is easily transformed into Yin diseases, but Yangming not; and what are the definitions of the terms "exterior", "interior", "deficiency", "excess", "blood", "Qi", "water", "fire", "principal", "subordinate", "healthy Qi", "pathogen", "wind", "dampness", "warm", "cold", etc.—how are they connected to the therapeutic effect of Native medicine and do they have scientific value? (See my *Proposal to the Bureau of Native Medicine*).

Regarding herbs, we need to collect opinions about specific issues, such as Fu Zi 附子 having toxicity or not, Chai Hu 柴胡 being able to disperse or not. We should also collect opinions about the actions, dosages, side effects, production areas, preparations, compatibility of herbs, and research them all.

The third point relates to scientific experiments. All aspects of Chinese medicine theory and herbs should be tested and proven by scientific experiments. Chinese medicine has developed for thousands of years, with abounding divergences between different schools. However, there is not one single theory of any particular school that can be totally trusted, because these theories haven't been proven by scientific experiments. In my opinion, the Bureau for Native Medicine has to launch a large laboratory, which imitates foreign medical and pharmaceutical laboratories, however, with slight modifications in order to conform to Native medicine needs. We should use experiments to solve all doubts regarding pathology, pharmacology, acupuncture, folk prescriptions and therapeutic methods. Only like this will we help Chinese medicine spread all over the world. Native medicine treatment relies on natural products and its application is quite simple and time-consuming, such as with cooking decoctions, so it is not suitable for emergency care that is needed in a rush. Native methods have rarely changed during the long history of medicine Medicine. Because of this, Native medicine was not able to compete with the world's medicine. We have to reform it in order to be more competitive. Otherwise, our medicine will never be able to catch up to the world's medicine. If the Bureau for Native medicine does not take care of this situation, then our medicine will have no option but demise. I am of the opinion not to use Western drugs, but in that case, we must advance a reform with Chinese herbs.

In order to promote Native medicine reform, the Bureau for Native medicine has to recruit excellent doctors and scholars from both Native and Scientific medicines, and try to get more financial support, because as a professional subject, Native medicine needs to combine both ancient and modern theories, which is rather complicated. In addition, we have to establish the needed facilities. Talent and financial support are essential issues, yet the authorities haven't paid enough attention to them. I have made efforts to help Native medicine reform for more than ten years. I have presented several proposals to the Bureau for Native medicine, but none of them was replied to. I am not sure why there was no feedback. Maybe the staff doesn't agree with my opinions, or maybe they have other difficulties or troubles to deal with, which are hard to disclose. Some people in the Bureau complain that my behavior and attitude are like attacks on Native medicine, but I also want to complain about behavior and attitude of some in the Native Medicine Bureau. Actually, I am the one being wronged. If a person is making a mistake that may lead to a dangerous situation, his relatives or friends may adopt unpleasant words or behavior to dissuade him. I am like the relatives and friends. In the past year, I worked hard on Native medicine and published some articles that have been reprinted by many medical magazines and newspapers from the capitol to Shanghai 上海 and Hangzhou 杭州 to Xia Men 廈門 and many other places. I simply expressed my opinions to the public. I really did not intend to attack Native medicine, and so I don't know why these people complain about my behavior and attitude. Some people, considering themselves Native medicine enthusiasts, like to praise the long history and great efficacy of Native medicine. I think such words are worthless for the research of medicine.

It seems that you don't agree with those wrongful opinions about Native medicine reform, and that you present your arguments supporting the reform. I appreciate your hard work and great sagacity. I present my opinions in this letter with great courage, hope you can read and think them over. Thanks.

Yours,
Tan Cizhong 譚次仲

Attachment: Corrections to the Draft Outline by Lu Yuanlei 陸淵雷, Member of the "Arranging of the Medicine Committee", Bureau of Native Medicine.

Yaron: The situation of teaching materials in Native medicine schools and the expectations from the Bureau for Native Medicine and medical reform. Lu Yuanlei was a student of Yun Tieqiao; however, this point in time is almost a decade after Yun has passed away. Chinese medicine's reality at that time, since the founding of the Bureau for Native Medicine, was different from a decade prior. Calls for Chinese medicine scientification and reform are stronger and louder.

Between Lu and Tan there is no discussion about keeping a unique theory for Chinese medicine, as was the case with Yu Yunxiu and Yun Tieqiao but, rather, it revolves around the scope of practice for Native medicine.

Tan strives to narrow the scope of Native medicine practice, while Lu hopes for equal status between Native and modern medicines: Native medicine should be valued for its accumulated practical experience, while modern medicine for its scientific understanding of nature.

Debates in the 1930s about Chinese medicine scientification shift away from its theory to its practical aspects. Lu claims that Chinese medicine theory needs to change a lot, whereas the accumulated experience just slightly arranged. Tan challenges this attitude; slight arrangement of the treatment method is not enough.

Note by Author Tan Cizhong 譚次仲: this draft outline is quite similar to my opinion; however, there are some text errors that should be corrected. I will list them with my corrections in the following article, so that all wise people can check and research them. Nonetheless, I have to declare that my article here focuses on the textual errors and hardly discusses the medical theories.

The first line to discuss is "As for academic studies[313] being right or wrong, we cannot have prejudice of being Chinese or Western, new or old 學術有是非，不可有中

[313] In academic studies Xue Shu 學術, "Xue 學" means the theoretical, while "Shu 術" the practical aspects of study.

西新舊之見." I think it's better to add the two words "good (or) bad 得失" in this sentence because Native medicine has more value with its practical aspect, and less value with its theoretical aspect. In other words, the good content of Native medicine related to practical therapeutics is nine out of ten. In the theory side, if we get rid of the mysterious, then out of ten there are only two or three left to consider. Therefore, theories can be right or wrong, while practical skills can be good or bad. So I think the two words "good or bad 得失" should be added, in order to avoid the loss of some important meaning.

The second line to discuss is "One thing has only one correct definition; all others are wrong 一事物之理解只有一個真是，容有若干之說俱非." I think "thing 事物" is too broad. Medicine is a science of nature, it researches entities based on experiment. In your article, you think medicine is quite different from social custom and laws. But "thing 事物" can refer to everything in the world, including social custom and law. That's why I think "thing 事物" is too broad. If you use this term it could mean "anything". For example, if you use it talking about a country and its type of government it could mean a federal system, unitary system, constitutional monarchy or democratic republic. If you use this term for the way it governs it could be national sovereignty, civil rights, presidential system, internal control system, centralization of authority, decentralization. So you see, each thing can be interpreted in several different ways, and every single item can have two meanings or more. Therefore, the term "thing 事物" is too broad.

Medicine should be defined as a science subject. Natural phenomena are explained by experiments. Anatomical knowledge obtained by experiments is evidential. This knowledge can be used all over the world and it does not change. Therefore we have to use scientific methods to research all things. Things that have been proven to be correct by science must be right, and things that have been proven to be wrong by science must be wrong. Things that have been explained clearly by science can be taken as a standard, while things that haven't been explained by science should be researched by scientific methods in the future. It is not allowable to use unreal theories to explain things. There are many things that cannot be explained by science in the interim, so it is quite important to specify that we must wait until science is able to explain them.

The third line to discuss is "Medicine is able to save lives and relieve sufferings. It is not related to preserving the quintessence of Chinese culture and preventing the spillover of national interest 醫藥所以救夭扎，已疾苦，不能與保存國粹杜塞漏卮諸主義相提並論.” I think this sentence is not good enough. Medicine is indeed able to save lives and relieve sufferings. I am of the opinion that herbs and theories that can save lives should be regarded as the quintessence of Chinese culture. Certainly, the ones that cannot save lives are not suitable to be regarded as the quintessence of Chinese culture. In other words, we have to preserve things that accord to different situations.

The national economy and people's livelihood are quite difficult nowadays. The spillover of national interest is one of the most important reasons for this situation. It is really necessary to prevent the spillover of national interest in all fields, including both Chinese medicine and Western medicine. Many drugs that Western medicine uses are imported from foreign countries, what's more, there are also many herbs used in Chinese medicine which are imported from foreign countries, just as you say in your article. Regardless whether Chinese or Western medicine, all doctors should work hard to prevent the spillover of national interest. However, we have to select methods of preventing spillover of national interest according to academic methods used by Chinese medicine. The Chinese medicine reform should not be negatively influenced by using "preventing spillover of national interest" as an excuse. It is rather feasible and necessary to make a balance between them and then hope that authorities invest efforts to keep this balance. In short, Chinese medicine reform is closely related to preserving the quintessence of Chinese culture and preventing spillover of national interest.

The fourth line to discuss is "arranging Chinese medicine means using scientific methods to improve Chinese medicine. It does not mean sacrificing Chinese medicine to science 今之整理，與醫藥利用科學，非以醫藥供科學之犧牲." The word "sacrifice 犧牲" is not proper. I guess it refers to the preservation versus abolishment of Chinese medicine (preservation and abolishment are not absolute terms). I think we should preserve the things in Chinese medicine that are consistent with science, and abolish the things that are contradicting science. This is the meaning of the word "arrangement". In other words, it means the scientification of Chinese medicine. This is the first "sacrifice 犧牲". Even between things which are consistent with science there are many differences. We have to select the ones containing refined theories, effective methods and detailed explanations and we must abolish the ones containing rough theories, ineffective methods and simple explanations. That's the second "sacrifice 犧牲". Theories and methods, which are now considered refined and effective, may be replaced by newer ones, so that we will use the newer ones and abandon the old ones. This is a third "sacrifice 犧牲". In the process of the new ones replacing the old ones, Chinese medicine will become gradually more and more similar to Western medicine. Therefore, Chinese medicine has to abolish the things that should be abolished first, and then it has an opportunity to preserve the things that should be preserved. That's the fourth "sacrifice 犧牲". Actually, there are many "sacrifices 犧牲". Everybody knows that new construction is usually accompanied by destruction, and that progress is usually achieved in the process of reform. Destruction and reform will certainly require sacrifice. In other words, "sacrifice 犧牲" is unavoidable in the reform of Chinese medicine. In the scientific developmental process, in order to get better achievement, later generations had to sacrifice the contributions of earlier generations. So "sacrifice 犧牲" is also unavoidable in the modern science development. In ancient Chinese medicine there were many schools that attacked each other on academic issues, in other words, they wanted to sacrifice others' academic opinions. Nowadays, people have to sacrifice their own values to convert to science. If Native medicine doctors are not willing to sacrifice anything, then the people's health will be sacrificed. In that case, Native medicine will never be able to make progress. I am really worried about its future if it refuses to reform and "sacrifice 犧牲".

In this section you also refute the views of Ke Sida 柯斯達, but I don't agree with your opinion. Diagnosis is an essential method to identify the exact cause of a disease in Chinese medicine, while treatment is the purpose. Both of them deserve careful consideration. Ke Sida 柯斯達 values diagnosis and neglects treatment, it is certainly not a fair attitude. But you value treatment and neglect diagnosis, it is also incorrect. Scientists always emphasize rational treatment; they don't value randomly effective experience. In addition, in the modern medicine schools, foundation courses, such as physiology, pathology etc. occupy 80%–90% out of all courses in the curriculum, and they are usually taught at the beginning. Courses concerned with treatment only occupy 10%–20% of the same curriculum, and usually are taught at the end. How can diagnosis take place without these foundation courses? And how can treatment reach any effect without diagnosis? It will be like a mistaken identity, even if the method is good and the intentions beautiful, it is all just empty talk. Without an accurate diagnosis one cannot speak of treatment. If there is accurate diagnosis then treatment is surely rational. If scientists don't value this then how come Mr. Lu 陸 is advocating scientification as valuable?

The fifth line discusses the theories and methods in Chinese medicine. You suggest that the methods are good enough and should not be changed, but the theories should be changed a lot. This discussion is incomplete because it separates theories from methods and it ignores the relationship between them. In such a case, theories and methods cannot form a coherent academic system. It is just like the teaching materials available today in Chinese medicine schools, the anatomy, physiology, and bacteriology are considered as one part, while *Shang Han* 傷寒, *Wen Bing* 溫病, *Liu Jing* 六經 transmission and *San Jiao* 三焦 entering and exiting are considered as a separate part, as if the two have no connection between them.

There are many conflicting aspects between them, which is the worst thing causing confusion and misleading students. How is this going to work? This is called perplexing. If, as Mr. Lu 陸 suggests, there are still some ignorant and near sighted people in the gully, who mock it as being a horse and not a donkey, how can this be excused? Experience is valuable, but experience based solely on clinical efficacy is not something that I find satisfactory. From the content of this item, I know you are satisfied with experience obtained only from the clinical efficacy, and rather not pursue further research based on experiments. It demonstrates that you lack scientific attitude. In my opinion, experience only shows the "how" but not the "why". If there is efficacy, one does not know why it worked. If there is no efficacy, one does not know the reason behind the failure. In that case, how can such experience spread all over the world? I will go so far as to say that this was not the government's intent when it established the Bureau for Native Medicine, and not the hope that everyone had for it; if the Bureau does it like this, isn't it even further from science?

As for Native medicine, where is the difficulty? It is difficult to understand it if it is explained via mysterious theories, but it is graspable if it is explored with science, when the methods and theories are merged together as one system. The famous theories of Chinese medicine such as Yin Yang 陰陽, blood and Qi 血氣, water and fire 水火, deficiency and excess 虛實, exterior interior 表里, cold and heat 寒熱, dampness 濕, wind 風, etc. I have already discussed and explained in my Proposal to the Bureau of Native Medicine.

Regarding therapeutic methods, I would like to make further discussion based on Mr. Lu's 陸 view of Chai Hu 柴胡, i.e. Chai Hu 柴胡 can treat discomfort and fullness in chest and hypochondrium. Fullness basically means that this area feels uncomfortable. In my opinion, discomfort and fullness in chest and hypochondrium is a side symptom of fever, which takes place all over the body. In addition, it is often seen in heart, lung, stomach and pleura diseases and in depression. Chai Hu 柴胡 can treat them because it is able to lower fever and calm the Stomach and brain. I have explained in detail these three actions of Chai Hu 柴胡 in my book *A Summary of Chinese Herbs Categorizations and Characteristics Zhong Yao Xing Lei Gai Shuo* 中藥性類概說. However, I bring here a few examples to briefly discuss them.

Xiao Chai Hu Tang 小柴胡湯 is able to treat alternating chills and fever with discomfort and fullness in chest and hypochondrium, this is Chai Hu's 柴胡 ability to lower fever. Da Chai Hu Tang 大柴胡湯 is able to treat constant nausea with discomfort and fullness in chest and hypochondrium, this is Chai Hu's 柴胡 ability to calm Stomach. Xiao Yao San 逍遙散 is used to treat headache, dizziness, bitter taste of mouth, lassitude, excessive thirst, depression, and discomfort and fullness in chest and hypochondrium, this is Chai Hu's 柴胡 ability to calm the brain. However, Chai Hu 柴胡 is not able to treat other types of discomfort and fullness in chest and hypochondrium. Even in the above three types, Chai Hu 柴胡 may not show efficacy in some stubborn situations. You believe that this symptom will be relieved in most cases after using Chai Hu 柴胡; honestly, I think your view is exaggerated and unrealistic. Otherwise, why doesn't Zhang Zhongjing 張仲景 use Chai Hu 柴胡 for all cases with discomfort and fullness in chest and hypochondrium?

For example, he uses Da Cheng Qi Tang 大承氣湯 to treat fever and chest fullness of convulsive diseases in *Jin Gui Yao Lüe* 金匱要略 and he uses Fu Zi Jing Mi Tang 附子粳米湯 to treat fullness in chest and hypochondrium with vomiting in the chapter of *Chest Fullness, Cold Hernia, and Indigestion*. Chai Hu 柴胡 seems to be applicable in the two above cases, because one is related to fever and the other to stomach. Yet, Zhang Zhongjing 張仲景 doesn't use Chai Hu 柴胡 in these two cases. There are many causes for chest fullness and some cases are not suitable for Chai Hu 柴胡. For example, Zhang Zhongjing 張仲景 uses Gui Zhi Qu Shao Yao Jia Fu Zi Tang 桂枝去芍藥加附子湯 to treat rapid pulse with chest fullness in the *Taiyang chapter* of *Shang Han Lun* 傷寒論. It is a method to treat heart weakness. In the *Phlegm and Cough chapter* of *Jin Gui Yao Lüe* 金匱要略, he uses Gui Ling Zhu Gan Tang 桂苓朮甘湯 to treat thoracic fluid retention with chest fullness. It is a treatment method for chronic lung diseases. In the chapter of *Chest Impediment, Heart Pain, and Shortness of Breath*, he uses Gua Lou Xie Bai Gui Zhi Tang 栝蔞薤白桂枝湯 to treat chest fullness. It is a method treating pleural diseases. These three cases of chest fullness are not related to fever, stomach disease or brain-related blood circulation impediment and therefore Chai Hu 柴胡 cannot treat them. So you see, if one liberally uses the ancient methods but doesn't seek the "why", rarely will he be able to reach the crux of it. What use is there for exaggerated talk?

The most important sentence in the draft is "Native medicine has many strong points, and they all conform to scientific methods". In my opinion, you should provide specific materials and examples to support your view. This will allow your views to convince people in modern-day and future generations. It will make the rearrangement of the medicine not an empty talk. Yet unexpectedly, you actually advocate abolishing ancient Chinese medicine theories such as five elements theory. It is completely opposite to your own view.

Above are textual errors that should be corrected. In addition, there are also many errors about medical theories, which I don't want to go into in this article. This article is based on the five items of the Draft Outline. I always hear that there are three important aspects for a good article, which are: the idea 義理, proof 考證 and wording 辞章. I hope that you and the other Committee members will respect all three points.

Remarks: The five main items in the draft proposed by Lu Yuanlei 陸淵雷:

The first item: Academic knowledge (including theory and practical skills) may be right or wrong, we should not have prejudice about Chinese or Western, new or old.

The second item: One thing has only one correct definition. It is not acceptable to have two correct definitions for a single thing. If there are multiple definitions for a single thing, we have to decide which one is correct, and the others should be considered as wrong. If there are some terms with the same name but with different definitions, or with different names but with the same definition, we have to first carefully check them and then decide which is correct and which are wrong.

The third item: Medicine is able to save lives and relieve suffering. It is not related to preserving the quintessence of Chinese culture and preventing the spillover of national interest. Therefore, the process of reforming Native medicine by scientific methods will not be considered as destroying the quintessence of Chinese culture and if doctors use foreign drugs it will not be viewed as spillover of national interest.

The fourth item: There are many natural phenomena that cannot be explained clearly by today's science. There are also some Native medicine methods that have been proven effective by clinical practice but without any scientific evidence. Therefore, the reform of Native medicine means using scientific methods to improve it. It is not the sacrifice of Native medicine to science. We can use all methods that have proven efficacy, regardless if they came from folk medicine or other sources.

The fifth item: Medicine can be separated into two aspects: theories and methods. In the process of reforming Native medicine, the theories should be changed a lot, while the methods only need to be sorted out which ones are more effective and rapid, and we also have to list the symptoms that these methods are able to treat.

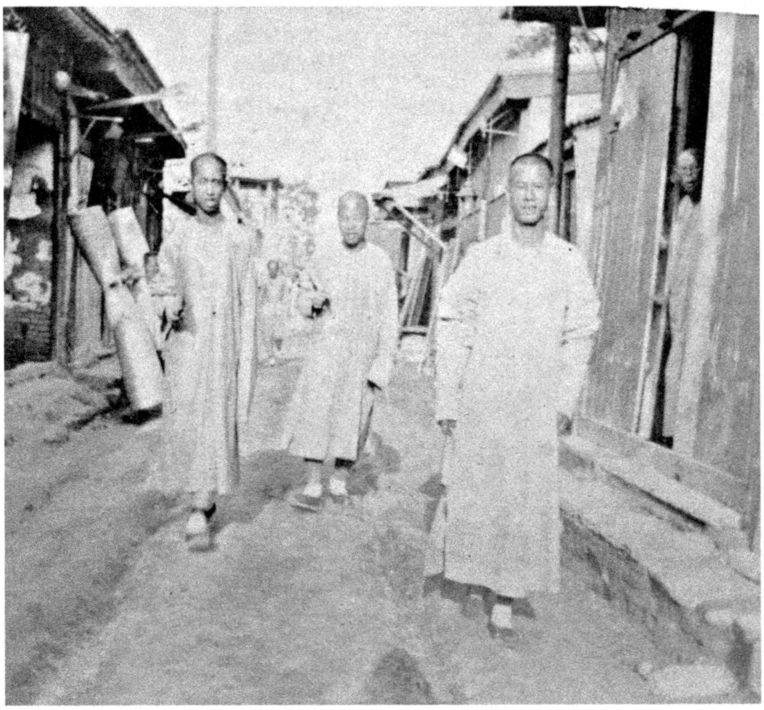

Photo by Mr P. Goux in early 1900s. "A street in Pao Ting Fu"

A letter from Guo Ruoding 郭若定[314]

Dear Mr. Tan Cizhong 譚次仲,

I have read your excellent book *A Summary of Chinese Herbs Categorizations and Characteristics Zhong Yao Xing Lei Gai Shuo* 中藥性類概說 in *Shanghai Society Medical Gazette*. I admire your achievements, you are a top expert. I have intended to write you a letter for long time, but it failed because I didn't have your address. Fortunately, I got your address from Mr. Wang Yaoliang 王藥兩. I hear that your other excellent book *Chinese Medicine and Science Zhong Yi Yu Ke Xue* 中醫與科學 will be published soon. I will buy it and it will be my pleasure to read it.

I am working on the categories of Chinese herbs. I wrote a book called *A New Chinese Herbs' Perception Xin Han Yao Jue* 新漢藥覺, in which I desire to explain herbs' clinical efficacy through scientific theories. I was not confident with my book, so I have published it in many medical journals in order to get instructions from the public. I don't know whether you have read it or not. I will send you a copy of *Shan Xi Medical Journal* 山西醫誌, which has one category of herbs from my book. I will be grateful if you can offer me some instructions to help me improve.

Yours,

Guo Ruoding 郭若定 from Zhejiang, Jiang Sheng county, Shifei 浙江江嵊縣石飛

[314] Guo Ruoding 郭若定 (1912–1946) a person of Zhejiang, Shengzhou county, Shifu township 浙江嵊州石砩. In 1928 he entered the tenth class of Shanghai Chinese Medicine Specialized School 上海中醫專門學校 and graduated in 1930. After graduation he returned home to practice medicine. Aside from the book mentioned in his letter, he also published a book titled *Measles Pathology Ma Zhen Bing Xue* 麻疹病 學. With his friends he has published several magazines including *The Voice of Medicine Yi Sheng* 醫聲 and *Tomorrow's Medicine Ming Ri Yi Yao* 明日醫藥, which was widely circulating and highly influential at that time. In order to help the profession, in Beijing in May 1937, *Ming Ri Yi Yao* magazine published the first part of his book *Han Yao Xin Jue* 漢藥新覺 as "Part 1", with an intention to publish the rest of it later on. However, since the war with Japan broke out soon thereafter, the magazine ceased publication and in 1946 Guo passed at an early age. In March 1947 *Ming Yi Ri Yao* started printing again in Shanghai and in the first issue they published writings left by Guo: *Han Yao Xin Jue Jie Re Yao Lei Yi* 漢藥新覺解熱藥類一. In 2010 , "Part 1" was reprinted by Shanghai Ke Xue Ji Shu Wen Xiang Chu Ban She 上海科学技术文献出版社; sadly, the article from March 1947 magazine has not been recovered.

A reply to Guo Ruoding 郭若定 on the book *Xin Han Yao Jue* 新漢藥覺

By Tan Cizhong

Dear Mr. Guo Ruoding 郭若定,

Thanks for your letter. You give me too much praise. I feel quite honored that you like my books. I admire your modest attitude, because you were able to lower yourself and ask for public advice. There are many categories of herbs in your excellent book; it's a pity that I am only able to read the second category, which is called blood-regulating herbs. What's more, I am not able to read the preface of this book, so I don't think it's possible to give you helpful instructions. However, since you directly ask for my opinion in your letter, I must give my humble opinion for you to check. From the category you sent me, I find out that there are many excellent views.

Firstly, you don't follow slavishly the theory of Qi Transformation 氣化. Secondly, you make innovations on ancient things. Thirdly, you try to unify medicine by scientific ways. You really make deep research and discussion. However, I think that the blood stasis theory is not proper. It is easy to find evidence in ancient classics that blood-regulating herbs can promote metabolism and improve blood irregularities. There is no need to import the blood stasis theory, especially the *Discussion of Blood Stasis* by Mr. Yumoto,[315] a Japanese doctor. Yumoto's *Imperial Chinese Medicine* 湯本皇漢醫學 is ridiculously exaggerated and unreasonable and has been strongly criticized by scholars for a long time. Your book quotes Yumoto's *Imperial Chinese Medicine* 湯本皇漢醫學, saying that "Blood stasis means dirty blood, i.e. abnormal blood. It is different from natural blood and it is rather a toxic substance that should be eliminated immediately." These words are really based on supposition. In pathology, there are only two factors that can cause blood diseases, one is poisoning, while the other blood irregularities. Stasis is not a factor in blood diseases at all. There are two types of blood poisoning; one is poisoning caused by foreign substances, while the other is endogenous poisoning.

Amongst poisoning caused by foreign substances, bacterial poisoning is the most common. For example, pus-forming bacteria in the body will cause sepsis, tubercle

[315] Yumoto Kyushin 湯本求真 1876–1941. Yumoto emphasized in his book that *Shang Han Lun* was experience-based. It was very influential in China after its publication in 1927.

bacillus will cause miliary tuberculosis, etc. In addition, there is also blood poisoning that occurs during experiments, vaccinations, diagnosis or treatment. There is some blood poisoning caused by chemical substances, such as acute or chronic mercurialism, arsenic poisoning, morphinism, ergotism, alcoholism, etc. In these, chemical substances invade blood circulation and damage cells. If a certain organ is sensitive to a chemical substance, then the symptoms of this organ will become apparent. Most deaths are caused by poisoning involving the central nervous system. Certain strong chemical agents such as acids, alkalis, heavy metals etc., may cause local corrosion or even death. Another type is called endogenous poisoning, such as secondary acidosis in diabetics, ammonia poisoning in uremia patients. All the above are called blood poisoning.

Blood irregularities contain three meanings: abnormal blood volume; abnormal blood timing; and abnormal blood location. Abnormal blood volume often manifests as blood loss, such as trauma, uterine bleeding and rupture of aneurysms and when there is high blood loss it is very dangerous. Abnormal blood volume can also manifest as insufficient blood supply; for example, the lower limbs will not be able to get enough blood supply if there is peripheral neuritis, arthritis, tuberculosis of joint, chilblain, etc., and it may eventually lead to gangrene. Abnormal blood volume also includes changes in blood constituents, such as hemophilia caused by low platelets, anemia caused by a lack of hemoglobin, leukemia caused by an abnormal increase in the number of white blood cells etc.

There are numerous examples for abnormal blood timing. For example, it is normal that hyperemia of liver and gastric mucosa appear after eating foods, whereas other types of hyperemia in liver and gastric mucosa will be considered as abnormal. Another example is irregular menstrual cycle.

There are also some examples for abnormal blood location. For example, normally, blood circulates inside vessels. If blood spills out of vessels it will cause hematemesis, hemoptysis, hematochezia, hematuria. In a word, blood appears in incorrect places. If the lower limbs are constricted then blood cannot provide nutrients to them, and eventually it turns into necrosis. In short, blood didn't appear in places it should have appeared. Another example is vicarious menstruation. All the above are examples of blood irregularities.

Blood poisoning and blood irregularities refer to all abnormal blood conditions. It is obvious that there is no such thing as "stasis".

Yumoto's *Imperial Chinese Medicine* 湯本皇漢醫學 says, "With females, if there is obstruction to blood flow or the flow completely stops then the toxins created will not only cause disease but they will also decrease the blood immunity to bacteria. It becomes the breeding ground for bacteria." From this statement, we know Yumoto 湯本 regarded menstruation as related to blood stasis. In reality, menstruation is a normal bodily function of discharging blood. It is an expression of the female reproductive function. Obstructed blood flow during menstruation is a result of certain diseases or life style influences. It cannot be compared to a bodily metabolic action at all. Menstrual flow is a part of the entire body blood system; if it does not flow this is not related to the moon accumulating blood in the uterus or in any other location. These are detailed wordings of Native gynecology that, without caution, give superfluous statements, they twist words beyond the good censure of the page. Menstruation cannot be a pathogenic factor of any disease. One cannot find any proven example that menstruation can cause diseases. Some people may say that vicarious menstruation is a disease caused by menstruation. Actually, vicarious menstruation is caused by the reflex of nerves. So it is really not related to blood stasis. Amenorrhea can be caused by long time lactation, hyperliposis, changes in life style, phantom pregnancy, etc. Blood stasis is not a cause of amenorrhea. Even if menstruation is a cause of diseases, what exactly are the causal relationships between menstruation and these diseases? How can we know the ultimate cause to be "blood stasis"? Is menstruation equal to blood stasis? Is blood stasis a substance of menstruation? What is the result of a chemical analysis? What is the result of pathology tests? How can menstruation turn to blood stasis? How can blood stasis cause diseases? If Yumoto 湯本 wanted to create a new theory for blood stasis, he would have to answer all the above questions and provide experimental evidence. Otherwise, his new theory on blood stasis is not reliable. It is just like Qi transformation theory, which is immaterial and intangible.

While his theory does not conform to modern science, furthermore, there is nothing in ancient literature to directly support Yumoto's 湯本 "blood stasis theory". In *Tai Yang chapter* 太陽篇 of *Shang Han Lun* 傷寒論, Zhang Zhongjing 張仲景 discusses Tao Ren Cheng Qi Tang 桃仁承氣湯 and Di Dang Tang 抵擋湯 and states that "Heat stagnates in the interior of the body 瘀熱在裏, which is manifested by sudden fever and hematuria". What Zhang Zhongjing discusses is acute cystitis, or liver and gallbladder diseases, which have no relationship with blood and menstruation. In *Yang Ming chapter* 陽明篇, there are a total of three "stasis Yu 瘀": one in the section of

Di Dang Tang 抵擋湯 referring to gastric ulcer and the other two referring to jaundice. There are many lines mentioning "Yu 瘀" in *Jin Gui Yao Lüe* 金匱要略. For example, in chapter *Blood Impediment and Consumption* 血痹虛癆篇, Zhang Zhongjing 張仲景 discusses abdominal fullness and dry blood Gan Xue 干血, which was paraphrased as blood stasis Yu Xue 瘀血 by You Zaijing 尤在涇 but actually, Yu Xue 瘀血 means here tuberculous peritonitis. In chapter *Puerperal Disease* 婦人產後篇, Zhang Zhongjing 張仲景 says, "...abdominal pain, and there is Yu Xue 瘀血 below the umbilicus...", this Yu Xue 瘀血 should be considered as placenta remnants. In addition, I really don't know what's the meaning of "Yu Xue 瘀血" in two sections describing it in chapter *Palpitation, Vomiting, Diarrhea, Chest Fullness, Yu Xue* 驚悸吐下血胸滿瘀血篇. For more details, please check the section of *Blood-Regulating and Anti-inflammatory Herbs* in my book *A Summary of Chinese Herbs Categorizations and Characteristics Zhong Yao Xing Lei Gai Shuo* 中藥性類概說. In a word, the "Yu Xue 瘀血" mentioned in ancient classics is completely different theory from Yumoto's 湯本 theory.

Yumoto 湯本 thinks that blood stasis Yu 瘀 is the pathogenic factor of all blood diseases. This is really a false view. He also thinks that the absence of menstruation is the cause for blood stasis Yu 瘀. I think that this view is even more false. These two statements cannot get any support from science or ancient classics. You advocate to reform Chinese medicine through science so you should oppose these views. I really don't know why you support them. I, too, appreciate blood-regulating herbs, and I have many opinions similar to yours, however, I don't dare to follow unscientific views. I suggest you replace blood stasis Yu Xue 瘀血 with blood blockage Xue Sai 血塞 or thrombus Xue Shuan 血栓, which are usually seen in cardiovascular diseases and trauma. For more detail, you can check the pathology books. It is fairly reasonable to use blood-regulating herbs for trauma, but it's a pity that you borrow the blood stasis theory from Yumoto 湯本 to discuss them.

Above are my personal opinions. Many of them are still in need of deliberation. I hope we can have the opportunity to further discuss. Besides, I also hope you can send me the full version of your book, I am certain it will enlighten me. Eagerly looking forward to it.

Yours,

Tan Cizhong 譚次仲

A sincere advice for scientification and uniting the entire Chinese medicine community

By Tan Cizhong

Yaron: Tan divides Chinese medicine practitioners into two groups: intelligent and unintelligent. In the intelligent group, the majority actively pursues scientification and a minority wants scientification but simply doesn't know it well. The unintelligent group is made up of people stubbornly opposing scientification.

In comparison, earlier on Yun Tieqiao claimed that most Native medicine practitioners are uneducated charlatans, whereas a minority are truly educated with Chinese medicine literature. Here, Tan's division includes street charlatans and traditional scholars of Chinese medicine in one unintelligent group. Such was the growing pressure for Chinese medicine scientification where one, regardless of his traditional scholarly achievement, is viewed as unintelligent.

Gradually, the idea of scientification became accepted in the Chinese medicine community. Whereas in 1917 Yu debated the contents of *Su Wen* and *Ling Shu* and later the *Shang Han Lun*, in the 1930s there was not much debate about theory left. There was less need to debate Chinese medicine ancient theories—if you believed in them, you were simply unintelligent.

In this article, point 'a' defines Chinese medicine scientification as a simple process: one learns modern medicine anatomy and pathology and when the situation is "serious" refers the patient to a modern medicine doctor. Point 'b' explains that a truly safe diagnosis and treatment can only be done with scientific diagnostic knowledge. Chinese medicine diagnosis, on its own, is not able to tell safety from danger when diagnosing a disease. Point 'c' explains that herbs can be used like drugs to remedy specific symptoms. Point 'd' explains that, without knowing physiology and anatomy and knowing the physical nature of a disease, one cannot treat it without mistakes.

In sum, making Chinese medicine scientific means making it physical and, in fact, making it follow and abide by modern scientific medicine. Alas, herbs need to be used like drugs for their known efficacy and this, too, only until modern drugs have been developed and no use for crude herbs remains. So for Tan, scientification of Chinese medicine meant assimilation into modern medicine and a gradual diminishing until there is only one modern medicine left.

Pages 94–112

In today's intelligent and broad-minded Chinese medicine circles, most people advocate the scientification of Chinese medicine. However, there are still a few who don't know scientification. There are also those who are not willing, or don't dare, to say "scientification". The crux of their problem is threefold: One, it is because they didn't investigate it thoroughly. Sometimes they just dream about it, and dreaming doesn't reach to the word "science". They imagine what kind of thing is science and, because of that, they don't understand the idea behind scientification.

Second, they don't know that Chinese medicine and science have a possibility for common root, middle ground and a thoroughfare that can be in agreement. They think that as soon as Chinese medicine goes through scientification, the theories of Yin Yang and Five Phases will be chopped away and that, with this, Chinese medicine will lack footing and, with indifference, be eradicated.

Third, while misunderstanding what medicine is, they think that they only need to reach a cure and this is it. They say, "Chinese medicine doesn't need science; when treating disease, it often leads to improvement, while Western medicine often talks about science, but when treating disease it is not always successful." In addition, with conviction, they claim that Chinese medicine is a method coming down from the ancient sages and that it is miraculous. The doctor himself feels his experience is great, so what is the need for having science? And so, they feel already satisfied.

These three stray attitudes indeed don't know what science is. So looking to these few in Chinese medicine circles, who are yet to investigate science further, they should more so urgently investigate anatomy and physiology. If they don't understand a little anatomy and physiology, I fear that my brethren—despite having many words and arguments and even if they remonstrate with good intention—simply can't participate in the conversation with everybody else. Even those fellows investigating the old doctrines of Chinese medicine, as soon as they open their mouth to say something they strike a pose, the kind without middle ground, that can't resolve the issue at hand.

And so with these three kinds, the first kind who doesn't know science is the worst problem. If the first problem can be removed then the other two can be addressed as well. However, everyone who wishes to research science must work hard at it and not just have a chat with today's brethren. As for the second group of brethren, there is already a book explaining Chinese medicine and science. It explains clearly the topic so there is no need to explain further here. As for the third group, who previously held the most absurd opinion, which seems to be unbreakable, who truly have suspicion that cannot be remedied, we just need to use words to try and inspire them.

In medicine, trying to assess whether doctors heal people adequately or less than adequately is a most difficult and complicated problem. One must use the "scientific experiment" principle and only then can he understand what truly happens within. What we call here "scientific experiment" means physiology, mathematics, physics and chemistry. The content of physiology, mathematics, physics and chemistry is vast. The procedure is complex but, simply put, if we talk about clinical experience, at the minimum one needs to carry out statistical calculations. So to say a million patients got curative result and it needs to be averaged to see the median good or bad success rate. Then one can expect a relatively true report of the efficacy rate. If one relies entirely on the doctor's opinion or the patient's subjective report, then over time it becomes a popular hearsay. Then the mistake becomes so perverse that logic can't fix it anymore. Simply put, it is not a true discrimination between right and wrong.

So let's take science as it is today and pick out several issues to present to the readership:

When we talk about science treating a disease, not necessarily it is all good. This is, of course, a fact. I even dare say that a thousand or ten thousand years later, when the level of science will reach to a peak in heaven, still they will not be able to cure all diseases and become kind of a sagely medicine that can cure all. But this kind of talk cannot become a theory reflecting on science. The reason we emphasize scientification is that even with low limits, they can still recognize a disease and they address it properly. This is the first and unsurpassed positive aspect of science. For example, if you come across a patient and you see that he has sudden fever then you know that it is acute contagious disease. If you see that he has cough and gasping then you know that it is in the respiratory system. If you see that he has endless vomiting and diarrhea then you know that it is a disease of the digestive tract. If you see in his head changes and that he has motor abnormality then you know that it is neurological. On and on with other systems like circulation, urination, motor diseases, they all can be differentiated very clearly.

If we talk about acute infectious diseases they can also be differentiated clearly that this one is in the intestines while the other is in the lungs. Talking about digestive diseases, one can be in the liver, while another in the stomach, they all can be diagnosed and then known. The analysis of diseases such as in the lungs, stomach, liver and intestines is difficult, yet even so you don't stray far from the truth. Because one uses pathology that follows the physiology of the person in order to diagnose then there is an understanding of the evidence. Therefore when they say that "all humans are built the same" it is different from relying on individual theories, where each holds different views, being confused and uninformed. This is another positive aspect of science in recognizing a disease. A disease must be known first and then everybody uniformly can apply the appropriate measure. Talking about the measure being proper or not is the most crucial!

Let's give now four examples that everyone can calmly discuss:

a. Let's take the example of tumor 腫瘤 (what Chinese medicine calls "a mass 癥瘕" more or less refers to this condition). If it grows outside, it is easy to see but if it grows inside, it is hard to know. If it is the external type, one does not have to be a doctor in order to see and know it. Now, regardless of the many names and types of tumors, their toxicity etc, if a tumor grows inside the body and not outside, let's assume even that they are all the same, and neither Western drugs nor Chinese herbs can scatter and remedy it, if you don't make abdominal surgery to remove it, there are no survival prospects for the patient. Let's take one example of uterine tumor, something that is often seen with female patients. At initial stages there are no symptoms whatsoever, but after long time when the tumor grows and presses anteriorly or posteriorly, then urination and bowel movement become pressing and there is a bloated feeling. These symptoms are sure to happen. When it gets to a stage where pathological fluids and material accumulate and symptoms such as exhaustion and endocrine gland swelling appear, then it is already at an advanced disease stage. Therefore tumors require early diagnosis and early surgical removal. However, if you don't rely on scientific imaging of the uterus, and only use physical examination, you can't diagnose this disease to be a tumor. More than that, you can't tell that this tumor is inside the uterus.

Hopelessly, one has to be indecisive and suspect Qi swelling, blood swelling, water swelling, parasite swelling, jaundice damp swelling, food accumulation swelling, etc—guessing. Then treatment follows as: scatter Qi; unobstruct stasis; eliminate water; expel parasites; remedy jaundice kind of unobstructing formulas. Often, only after having no efficacy for a long time, one gets a sense that the condition is grave and the patient is collapsing and weak, at which time the option of surgery is already not viable. Therefore Chinese medicine must undergo scientification. In addition, the process of this scientification is not difficult at all. One needs only to understand a bit of physiology and the pathology of tumors. And so when he encounters a condition that resembles this situation, he cannot be muddle-headed and give herbs; he must send the patient to get screened with scientific methods. This we can define as scientification of Chinese medicine.

b. Let's take typhoid fever as an example (also called "cold injury", but it is not the same "cold injury" from *Shang Han Lun* which is like catching a cold). At onset there is fever and headache; it looks exactly like any other febrile onset. Through bacteriological examination, one can know the cause. However, one can make a diagnosis also by relying on what science says the symptoms are. If the disease is caused by Bacillus bacteria, this bacterium resides in the gut and the age of affected people is normally younger than thirty. Running the three-week course of the disease, the heart is already exhausted and very often it ends up in intestinal bleeding or perforation. And so the patient's life being on the line is exactly at this time. In modern times, there is still no drug for treatment of this disease. There is also no benefit to reduce the fever early on in this disease. Therefore, any formula to reduce fever should not be used—in order to prevent further exhaustion. Any solidifying herbs should also not be used, in order to prevent further irritation of the intestines. During the disease, one must keep in full rest; purging formulas are even more prohibited so as to prevent hyperactivity of the intestines. Hyperactivity might spread the bacteria and increase the likelihood of perforation. This is the point of view of modern science according to what science can understand of this disease at this time. This is how they address it best. Because of this, they often can transform danger into safety. Treating the disease is not perfect; however, when following science, one can prevent mixing this disease with other febrile diseases. One has the ability to see the difference between this and the common cold and then can attempt to heal febrile diseases and cold injuries in a safe manner. Formulas to reduce fever and purging formulas are, of course, indispensible in the treatment of febrile diseases and cold injuries. However, with this disease one can instigate peril, taking safety and transforming it into danger. Now, one need only to know the intestine physiology and the pathology of this Typhoid disease, and with the four diagnostic methods—seeing, hearing, smelling and palpating—one can diagnose this disease. Chinese medicine has its own formulas for reducing fever but they should not be used in this case. Chinese medicine has its own purging formulas but in this disease they should not be used. By doing this, one can count it already as scientification, so how easy is that?

c. Another example is Stomach disease. Within the scope of stomach diseases there are cases that are easy to treat, no doubt about it. But as for the difficult cases of stomach disease that act up intermittently and irregularly, Chinese and Western medicine both don't have a grasp of the root cause. Sometimes when administering medicine it has no efficacy whatever. For example, acid reflux, hiccups, bloating after eating, heart burn, or reaching to a situation where one has no hunger the whole day, or has hunger but doesn't want to eat, or eats but lacks digestion, to an extreme even throwing up, or has heart pains radiating to the back, or back pains radiating to the heart, which can happen irregularly once every several months, or several times within one month, or to an extreme has a symptom like the above constantly without a break. So what is the critical point at this time? Take note of the following two sentences: if the patient eats, he dies of fullness; if he doesn't eat, he dies of starvation. What does it mean here? Since the stomach disease is severe, when food comes down, the stomach cannot do any labor and therefore the food stops there, stagnating untransformed. This must result in aggravated vomiting. When a bloated feeling reaches an extreme then every day it remains like this. This clearly shows that the patient gradually dies from fullness. However, if the patient does not eat, then he loses weight and becomes wasted. He doesn't get nourishment and this pathology transforms into what Chinese medicine calls "lack of Stomach Qi leads to death". Therefore, at this time, the appropriate thing is to use modern science nutrition therapy, using liquids that are rich in nutrients and are easy to digest (at times there are ones who don't care for liquid diets; one can also select a few appropriate solids, ones the patient likes, and give it to him). During this treatment the quantity has to be strictly regulated, every time during a feeding session one must confirm that there are no leftovers as to ensure that he gets his nutrients. He should eat small portions and let the stomach rest, until such time where the cause for the stomach symptoms subsides and then the patient gradually recovers. If one ignores this method then he may bring the patient's demise. At the least, it will delay the patient's recovery period or increase the occurrence frequency. In modern understanding of stomach physiology and pathology, sometimes there are no medications to treat it; in such cases, it is better to use hygienic preventative methods to help it. One advises the patient on food and drink modifications in order to help the situation. This is already scientification. Formulas and herbs in Chinese medicine like Mai Ya 麥芽, Ding Xiang 丁香, Bo Kou 波蔻, Gan Jiang 干姜, Huang Lian 黃連, Chen Pi 陳皮, Dan Cao 膽草 etc. are similar to stomach drugs in scientific medicine. Other herbs like Fa Ban Xia 法半夏, Hou Po 厚朴, Huo Xiang 藿香, Bai Zhu 白術, Cang Zhu 蒼術 kind of herbs, even though not part of the scientific medicine pharmacy, are all with similar effects to modern drugs. If one wants to practice scientification then I feel that there is no problem whatever.

d. Detailing one disease after the other is not possible on these pages, but to summarize what we have said already: taking abdominal fullness as an example, if we don't rely on scientific anatomy and physiology, then it is difficult to differentiate clearly the disease location being in the intestine or in the peritoneum. Likewise, if we don't use scientific methods then it is impossible to tell if there is inflammation or water retention in the peritoneum. Even if we only speak of water retention in the peritoneum, if we don't use scientific physiology and pathology we cannot tell if the water retention originates in the peritoneum or in the liver, heart or kidneys. If we can't differentiate clearly, how can the measure applied to it be appropriate? How can the herbs used be proper? Or, for example, cardiac arrhythmia hyperfunction due to Neurasthenia (in Chinese medicine it is called Zheng Chong and Xin Ji 怔忡心悸 palpitations). One may use appropriate exercises for palpitation, but with cardiac valve disease with this kind of palpitation hyper function, these exercises cannot be used. Another example is intestine disease; when constipated, a purging formula can be used but with appendicitis-related constipation, the same cannot be used. Also like a patient using opium formulation for pains, this cannot be used for stomach pains resulting from opium-related toxicity reaction. Like with fainting and dizziness during cerebral hemorrhage one should elevate the head, but in cases of fainting and dizziness due to anemia this should not be done. Or with cases of poisoning one can use drugs to induce vomiting, just with drugs that have corrosion of alkali and acid characteristics they should not be used. Or heart failure using heart-strengthening drugs, when there is high fever with weakened heart these cannot be used. Or with indigestion, after food one should pace around, but with cases of stomach prolapse leading to indigestion this is not the case. As you can see with these examples, cases might be similar but the measures used can be completely opposite. It requires one to first recognize scientifically the disease, only then can he speak of the appropriate measure and remedy. This kind of analysis extends to all diseases.

Summarizing the above four points:

a. An appropriate measure is early diagnosis and detection; operation should be used when needed and not herbs or drugs.

b. A proper measure is to assess the negative factors and not fix the eyes on the positive factor.

c. An appropriate measure is to use preventative methods and not solely rely on herbs and drugs.

d. A proper measure is to know what can be treated with herbs and what can't.

In summary, the four points above explain that one must first recognize the disease. Like this, even if modern science can't always treat and cure everything, at least it can recognize the appropriate measure that needs to be taken. Because of these appropriate measures, oftentimes health can be preserved. If we don't use scientific methods, despite having occasional efficacy, then not recognizing the disease often leads to missing what is appropriate and this mistake, I am afraid, does not benefit the patient. Chinese medicine has to go through scientification for this reason.

Science not only can recognize a disease, but it can also clarify the characteristics, application and efficacy of herbs. When science is used, one knows how to use the medicinal substance: why is this preparation reducing fever; why is it helping digestion; how is it removing phlegm; how is it benefiting urination; how is it purging;

how is it strengthening; or how is it stimulating (look for reference in my book: *A Summary of Chinese Herbs' Categorizations and Characteristics)*. One can differentiate these aspects clearly only by using science. Therefore, when a doctor sees a patient it is like an archer that has a target, like a boat that has a direction, the rules have their marking line; if it is not right on it is not far from it. This is the second good and unsurpassable aspect of science.

I bring forth a few examples to explain this to the readership:

a. For example, aconite Fu Zi 附子: Fu Zi in Chinese medicine is a stimulant. Because Fu Zi can treat dizziness, sweating, cold and weak extremities and fainting pulse kind of collapse disease, it thus has a stimulating effect on the heart and brain with no doubt. And so, in the old way of saying things, they would say that it goes to twelve meridians and can recover original Yang that was already scattered and lost. Or, for example, Shi Gao 石膏. Shi Gao is used in Chinese medicine to reduce heat because in the *Shang Han Lun* 傷寒論 *Yang Ming* 陽明 section it is used to treat surging heat (also means high fever), surging pulse (also can be seen as heart excitement) etc diseases. Therefore, one knows that its effect is of reducing heat. And while it can also suppress the heart force, it is said to be strongly slippery and moistening and can restrain Yang Ming dry metal. I am afraid that there is no way to prove that while theories seem to freely come about. Investigating what actually original Yang and Dry Metal are, it appears that in mythology, the legendary Pan Gu 盤古 and God, when creating humans, have inserted these two things into the human body. If one claims that original Yang and Dry Metal are Qi transformation, the eye can't see it, the ear can't hear it, the skin, tongue and nose can't feel, smell or taste it, then how do you know what it does and what to do about it? All herbs characteristics that rely on Qi transformation theories can be disqualified in the same way. If you don't use science to research herbs and their application, then you cannot escape the two realms of superstition and superstitious thought. As for the superstition of the ancients, it is displayed by their superstitious thinking, transmitted down for thousands of years, circling about without end. Therefore, there is no other way outside of science to pursue the true characteristics of herbs and their application. Now, with a scientific approach, one may discover why Fu Zi is stimulating and why Shi Gao is suppressing fever; other herbs may likewise be measured.

b. Going even a step further, when the ancients described herbs they didn't spare exaggeration of their efficacy and it was always like this, from Shennong 神農 onwards. They say that it makes the body light and not age, it benefits longevity and lengthens the years. It is allegedly in perfect superiority, but as soon as you turn the cup down finished drinking and lie down, with one dose you already know that it is not the case. How about after two doses? They say it cultivates Yang 陽 and benefits Yin 陰, tonifies Qi 氣 and blood, expels wind and removes fire, scatters heat and dissipates evil and the page is full of these words. They take herbs and present them as some sort of miraculous cure. In ancient times, this kind of exaggerated and flagrant wording was common-place but in modern day and for modern people, who use and are enlightened by science, this cannot be. In our modern environment, using the ancients' erroneous views, how is this not laughable? In reality, when using science to determine application and efficacy of herbs, we can use three categories. The first: An herb that must be used for a certain symptom must show absolute efficacy. It can cure seven or eight out of ten. In addition, it can resolve the problem from its root and this we can call special effect remedy. For example, Wang Fangan 汪訪庵 from the Qing dynasty in his book *Essentials of Materia Medica Ben Cao Bei Yao* 本草備要, says that Ji Na Shuang 雞納霜 can treat malaria, or like in the Republic's earlier years the Chinese medicine elder Mr Li Miliu 黎秘留 explained that Sheng Ma 升麻 can treat bubonic plague. This can also be categorized as special effect remedy (See *A Summary of Chinese Herbs Categorizations and Characteristics*). This kind of Ji Na Shuang can kill the malaria-causing bacteria, and so it can be categorized as special effect remedy. Sheng Ma being able to cure bubonic plague is also because it can eradicate bacteria causing it. (As far as I know, Chinese medicine has only one or two special effect remedies. However, these are still based on experience in clinic. It is unfortunate that they cannot be proven in experiments). Now, the medical establishment recognizes that there are maybe only five or six herbs from the entire world categorized as special effect remedies. This kind of special effect remedies should not be so rare and hard to attain like the scales of phoenix and unicorn horns. Only if there is a sufficient quantity of a certain herb that is applied directly to a disease and has efficacy, and when contraindications are known, or if it is specifically known not to cure the disease's root, but instead applies to certain symptoms of a disease, then it can be called a remedy targeting the disease. The remedy examples I described above for lowering fever, eliminating, expelling phlegm etc. are exactly that kind of treatment targeting a symptom. Now let's talk about fever in an infectious disease. What causes fever in an infectious disease? Most often it is because weather is not optimal during the four seasons and therefore bacteria grow and enter the body. When bacteria enter the body very often the body will contract the common cold, and therefore this bacterium is the disease cause. The weather is a secondary factor. Fever is a symptom. However, as soon as the disease develops, the secondary cause, namely the weather, has already no relationship to the body and there is no need to talk about it anymore. Therefore, when Chinese medicine describes herbs that can resolve winter cold, spring warmth, summer heat and fall dryness, like Ma Huang 麻黃, Gui Zhi 桂枝, Yin Hua 銀花, Huo Xiang 藿香 etc, they are actually a type of lowering-fever remedy. In other words, they lower the fever caused by different kinds of bacteria. They absolutely cannot eradicate bacteria that enter the body and reside in the blood; therefore they are called a remedy targeting the symptom. Symptom-targeting remedies have only relative efficacy. In simple words, relating to space, the term "relative efficacy" means that if a disease is easy then there is efficacy but if the disease is severe then there is none. Relating to time, "relative efficacy" means that at the disease's tail end there is efficacy but at the disease's head there is none.[316] In summary, without specifically considering time and space, all remedies, after entering the body, need to have an effect of resisting a disease. They need to reach a certain action restraining the disease's evil to an appropriate degree. A symptom-targeting remedy has its distinctive efficacy. The majority of herbs belong to this type. Amongst the remedies of both Chinese and Western origin, this kind constitutes at least 90% or more of all remedies. Some herbs, however, have little efficacy and yet they have startled the ancients who forcefully transmitted them down. Later generations learned them without questioning, and therefore believed them to be effective. They used them as if with pre-destiny. Alas, within the stray act of blindly using prescriptions with pre-fixed ingredients without questioning it, Chinese medicine can't recognize which herb does the main action and which one has a secondary action. It is like Han Xin 韓信 commanding the

[316] This means that at the beginning of the disease these remedies can't locate the problem, only when the disease is fully developed later on that they can target the visible symptoms.

troops,[317] the more you have of it the more important it seems, the bunks pile up in the room,[318] and this kind of error kept on accumulating. Because of this, herbs with no efficacy were oftentimes mixed in and there was no way to separate them. For example, Lian Zi 蓮子, Huai Shan 淮山, Yi Ren 苡仁, Nan Dou 南豆, Chi Dou 赤豆, Shou Wu 首烏 and the kind occupy a huge percentage in herbal stores. If one exclaims that there are many kinds of existing diseases that cannot rely on medicinals for a cure, then we can likewise say that no matter the number of herbs in existence, they are all ineffective. This is the reason why medicinal substances are considered ineffective. The scope of medicinal efficacy does not fall outside of this.[319] With modern science, one can expose and dismantle the ancients' exaggeration of herbs' efficacy.

c. Another level to consider: whenever a herb has a good side it also has a bad side. Beforehand, we explained only the good aspects of herbs. Now, we also want to speak about the unfavorable aspects thereof. Science defines this negative aspect as side effects. For example, if a patient takes the herbal prescription and then feels unwell then we, the doctors, have to examine our hearts fearful. We ask our heart, have we established diagnosis properly, did we use the proper prescription and within the prescription were the herbs and dosages proper according to the rules and, if so, why did the patient feel unwell? If we did everything according to the rules then these are the herbs' side effects. If an herb's potency is great then the side effects are also great. In addition, there are people with sensitivities to certain herbs that create particular reactions. These kinds of side effects are numerous; sometimes it seems to alternate, for example administering remedy to reduce fever but the fever, to the contrary, aggravates. Or administering a cough remedy and, instead, the cough aggravates. Any doctor, no matter how good he is, cannot prevent this scenario. It's just that when the disease is not clear, then the prescription and herbs within it are incorrect according to the rules, and then one can never use the term "side effects" to cover up his mistakes. As for herbs' side effects, these can also be determined by science. Amongst our na-

---

[317] Han Xin 韓信 was the general of Liu Bang 劉邦, the founder of the Han dynasty. This idiom means: on the surface, it seems that the more the better but in reality, there is something else more important. As legend goes, Liu Bang asked Han Xin, his general: "how many soldiers do you think I can command?" Han Xin replied: "about 100,000." Liu asked: "How many can you command?" Han said: "The more the better." Liu Bang laughed: "So if you can command so many, why do you subject yourself to me?" Han answered: "Your highness' ability to command regular troops is limited; however, your ability to command high ranking generals is unsurpassable."

[318] The idiom means excessive and repetitious.

[319] That is, if they can cure the symptom or not.

tion's Native doctors, the ones who study Zhongjing 仲景 emphasize ginger Jiang 姜 and cinnamon Gui 桂 and are afraid of Mai Dong 麥冬 and Shu Di 熟地. The ones who study Wu Jutong 吳鞠通 hate Huang Qi 黃耆 and Fu Zi 附子 and love Huang Qin 黃芩 and Huang Lian 黃蓮—an academic sectarianism. The ones who hold fast to warm tonification know that cold cool herbs can kill, but they don't know that warm tonification can kill as well. The same holds true for the opposite group that hold fast to cold and cool herbs. In reality, how will you know the adverse effects of herbs, if not through science?

Summary of the last three points:

a. Explanation needs to be scientific—the characteristics and application of herbs and then their categories.

b. Explanation needs to be scientific—the force of the herbs being strong or weak.

c. Explanation needs to be scientific—the adverse reactions and positive actions of herbs. The good side and bad side should both be discovered.

If we get to this level of research, is it not goodness that will come out of Chinese pharmacology scientification? Thus, basing Chinese pharmacology on science makes it transparent. When pharmacology knowledge is transparent, then there is no place for the ancients' toxic theories, taking herbs and making them inconceivably mysterious and letting imagination run riot. There is no place for applying herbs' invisible actions to a patient and when it doesn't work, then not understand which supposed action of the herb did not work.

When one knows the herbs' actions in a transparent pharmacological way, then he can master the herbs' application. He can discern clearly what will be the outcome, big or small, of administering these herbs before he even administered them to the patient. He can forecast ahead of time what will be the possible side effects. Like this, he doesn't get into a situation where herbs exacerbate the disease. He doesn't get into a situation where several prescriptions were ineffective and yet he switches again to another prescription, where these few herbs were ineffective so he tried those other few herbs. Lastly, he views herbs as the courtroom of experience and he makes an attempt with human life. Like this, what do you think, is science useful or not? Is scientification of Chinese pharmacology crucial or not?

My dear colleagues of the Chinese medicine community! May I ask: amongst the doctors of my generation, who doesn't hope for bringing herbal medicine back to life? Who doesn't hope that as soon as you use herbs they bring a cure? That, over time, we have destiny to have many medical friends, and receive both gain and fame? There is no way of doing this with such a herb that when you use it first it has an amazing efficacy, but when you use it the second time, it doesn't perform well. Likewise, for the same disease, using medicine from my hands it works, but the same medicine from another doctor's hands doesn't work. Getting to the bottom of it, does this herb cure this disease or not? Using this prescription for this symptom—is it effective or not? Sometimes it gets so baffled that, as a result, one cannot master it until the end of life.

Isn't there a common saying by the elder Chinese medicine doctors: "at first, after three years of study, one does not know heaven but, after another three years, he doesn't even dare to speak"? We can only tackle the errors of Chinese pharmacology through science, otherwise the research will be tottering, and by the patient's bedside it will seem as very difficult. My brethren, I am also a Chinese medicine doctor, I researched books and practiced in clinic for twenty years. As for the deficiencies of Chinese medicine and pharmacology that I have highlighted—truly, I have fully tasted the flavor, and only after that I began researching science and therefrom found a way out. This is where my great resolve for Chinese medicine scientification is coming from. It is my great aspiration for Chinese pharmacology scientification (the first is easier to achieve; the latter very difficult).[320] Today, I don't dare to achieve this goodness by myself; I hope that all you gentlemen will share this goodness with me. The mistrustful gentlemen who don't have resolve for this goodness, I hope they have courage to advance toward it. Looking amongst my brethren there is no such a person.

How do I know that there is no such person? Because men, no matter how stubborn they are, cannot oppose "becoming better". Dear gentlemen! You should know that scientification means becoming better. Men, no matter how conservative they are, cannot oppose advancement. Dear gentlemen! You should know that scientification is advancement. In addition, if Chinese medicine departs from science then it has no hope for becoming better and more advanced.

[320] The first means Chinese pharmacology, while the latter means scientification.

What is the proof here? Generally speaking, the historical changes in China's medicine took a big turn in the Song 宋 and Yuan 元 dynasties. Before Song and Yuan, everybody followed the path of Zhang Zhongjing 張仲景. After the Song and Yuan, the medicine started dividing into different schools, which were not in agreement with each other. Later generations, when studying medicine, either followed the old way or the modern way, each with its peculiarities. The ones who followed the old ways naturally revered Zhongjing, while the ones who followed the modern way opposed Zhongjing. Even the Japanese Kampo 漢醫 medicine followed the same pattern I described. May I ask, was this an improvement or not? Was this an advancement or regression? If we say that it is an improvement and advancement then this means that later generations were winning. I am not willing to acknowledge that the scholars of Song and Yuan were better than Zhongjing. As far as I can tell, most of my colleagues will not acknowledge this as well. Because, in today's Chinese medical circles, when we call ourselves Confucian scholar-doctors Ru Yi 儒醫, we still revere the old and look lightly at the modern. The value of Zhongjing's voice still surrounds the great sage who was the first teacher to lead the way. In later generations, there was not one who dared turn their back on him. Judging by this, where was the point for improvement and advancement?

Taking a broader look at modern scientific medicine, is it the same kind of nonsense? In recent years, it soared high and forcefully advanced. It charioted ten thousand miles towards the south and it went straight up to the blue sky. It is unlike the theory of evolution that exclaims a spiral object forms by the thread repeating itself. Thus, in this theory, whatever is supposed to advance, advances while repeating itself over and over and, like this, excellent benefits the excellent and it grows. In reality, after numerous years, this only becomes a relic, not to mention that after hundreds or even thousands of years this can only become an exhibit in the library or an antique in the museum. Alas, if you let those who only contemplate the ancients take charge and do textual research of scientific materials, they lack youthful vigor. Dignified, they stand there and, after advancing, style themselves as kings, feeling lofty and honorable. Instead, bring about those who are happy to follow the world, the ones who are highly knowledgeable about Zhongjing 仲景, yet not necessarily know things at birth[321] nor are supposedly able in all directions. It is not possible that before Zhongjing 仲景 there were no brilliant ancients and that after him there will be no

[321] To know things at birth is a Confucian saying from the Analects that the one who knows at birth, or knows naturally, has the best knowledge. Here the author points out that these "know-it-all" doctors are unsuitable or have the wrong attitude needed to pursue science.

other brilliant scholars. In summary, later generations didn't know how to research medicine and pharmacology in a scientific way and so there was a change, but not for the better. They took steps without advancing. This statement, nonetheless, is a general overview of the situation. If we were to take article after article of the ancient doctors' writings and analyze them then we will easily see that without a scientific process in medicine and pharmacology, the statement "lack of change for the better and no advancement" cannot be refuted. Allow medicine to go through scientification first and then allow pharmacology to become scientific as well.

Gentlemen, you should know that, for a disease, there is no division between Chinese and Western medicine. For example, fever of contagious disease: Western medicine calls it acute infectious disease; the ones who study the *Shang Han Lun* 傷寒論 call it Cold Injury; while the ones who study *Wen Bing* 溫病 texts call it Febrile Disease—but, in reality, it is not different kinds of diseases. Even though our terminology is different from Western medicine's term, "acute infectious disease", I ask those of us following the Shang Han Lun school—which was transmitted down for thousands of years—what is the deal with "six conformations transmitting to each other; root, manifestation and Qi seen in center; opening, closing and pivot"? Or, those of us following the Wen Bing school, which was also transmitted for thousands of years—what is the deal with "in winter doesn't store essence then in spring there will be febrile disease, before summer solstice the disease is warm while after summer solstice the disease is hot"? May I ask, having researched these theories through such a long history and many generations, at the end, what was the achievement? What kind of positive aspects did it make transparent? In reality, it only had contending schools fighting against each other with erroneous explanations and baffled statements. They wanted to reach high, but correct explanations didn't form.

Now, contagious diseases all have bacteria that cause them (also called microorganisms) and along with this knowledge came disinfection which can sever the transmission of bacteria. It became clear how to use toxic material and vaccinate against bacteria, which allows the human body to develop resistance to these bacteria. Because of this, a great advancement ensued in the prevention of infectious diseases. The production of bacteria serum was possible, like diphtheria serum, tetanus serum—a real lifesaving accomplishment. This is enough to startle a person. These two kinds of serum are considered in the entire world as special effect remedies. Think about this accomplishment—because of this, the treatment of these infectious diseases attained an astounding accomplishment. Isn't it proof that medicine using science has reached a better place, an advancement?

Now, when you look back at our own preventative methods for infectious diseases, like in the *Su Wen* 素問, posthumous writing of *Ci Fa Lun* 刺法論 chapter, stating: the five Qi guard the body etc nonsense. There is no need to further explain. Or in *Ci Fa Lun* 刺法論 the formula Xiao Jin Dan Fang 小金丹方 is using what kind of red yellow cinnabar to make pills? Bury it in the ground for seven days, remove from the ground and swallow, then there will be no epidemics etc. (Only bubonic plague, during the spread of an outbreak, can be prevented by using two three Qian of Sheng Ma in rice congee. My experience shows that it can serve as a preventative measure. Therefore Sheng Ma is Chinese medicine's special herb for bubonic plague). The reason I say these things is not in order to make everyone laugh and have convulsions of the abdomen's skin, so this is enough.

When it comes to treatment, even though there are different kinds of fever-reducing remedies in Chinese medicine, there is only one remedy or half a remedy that can be called "special effect remedy". These remedies, however, are experience-based and not related to heat-cold theories kind of research, because, in reality, this epidemic disease is caused by bacteria and not by heaven Qi being hot or cold. It is a fundamental mistake and, naturally, anything coming out of it is devoid of essence. If, in theory or practice, there is no real accomplishment to describe, then where can there be a discussion about changing for the better? Where can there be a discussion about advancing? Medicine is like this, pharmacology likewise is like this.

For example, Camphore Zhang Nao 樟腦, the one used by science and the one used by us in Chinese medicine materia medica, is one and the same. However, what use do we have for it? We say that Zhang Nao can stir fire to come out of water, unobstruct and benefit the orifices. I have never seen what becomes unobstructed. Only those people who used scientific research immediately knew that this drug can strengthen the heart. Even though at initial stages, its smell and flavor being too strong, it bothered the stomach and therefore reached no accomplishment. However, later on, scientists changed it to intravenous injection, bypassing the obstruction caused by intestines and stomach, and allowed it direct entry into the blood. Like this, Zhang Nao demonstrated 120% efficacy. It became, in the entire world, the first or second best drug for strengthening the heart and reviving people from the dead.

Another example is arsenic Xin Shi 信石, the common name is Pi Shuang 砒霜. In Chinese pharmacology, it doesn't have any outstanding function. However, going through scientific research, it was composed into 606 and 914, two different drug compounds. They became the liberator of syphilis. This is a fact that everybody knows in the Chinese medicine community. Or like Chaulmoogratree Seed Da Feng Zi 大楓子. Even though it has a common use in Chinese medicine, after it went through scientific extraction of its volatile oils and made into intravenous injection, it became the most essential drug for leprosy. Its efficacy is considered top notch. What do you think, isn't this a proof that using science in pharmacology is a great advancement? And so when we look back and observe the time when our nation did not know how to use science to research pharmacology, truly the more they wanted to do, the more it was nonsense.

Take the materia medica that narrates absurdities. Let's take something relatively practical and explain it. Aconite Fu Zi 附子: does it or does it not have toxicity? The ancient books say different things, according to beliefs of different doctors. They all can't agree on it. Is Chai Hu 柴胡 scattering or not scattering? The ancients' theories were all in a sorry plight. The modern man even more so has no unified opinion to follow. Sheng Ma 升麻 has a characteristic to go to the head, Di Long 地龍 has characteristic to go to the foot—is it true or false? What is the proof? Or let's take Shou Wu 首烏 that can make the hair black—until today some still try to use it. Cao Ma Zi 草麻子 applied externally has an absorbing action, whatever people want to say they say, but one can see that the pharmacological actions are not conforming to science. The efficacy can never be verified. It is difficult because forever there is no hope to resolve this inadequacy. Wherefrom should one claim change for the better and advancement? According to this narrative, the crux for advancement or regression is established. Medicine is like this and pharmacology is also like this. If it uses scientific methods then it may reach this grand accomplishment. If it doesn't use scientific methods then it cannot reach even minor undertakings. These examples clarify for everyone, already to an extreme, the proper measure needed.

Alas! The words are long and I am afraid that with you, gentlemen, the ears detest it. To conclude, Chinese medicine must go through scientification (this includes Chinese pharmacology). If it is for medicine itself, if it is for the people's sake, all are eagerly looking forward to it. Brethren, if you have a concrete plan toward this affair then lay it out. I wrote this article as a concluding sermon for advocating Chinese medicine scientification. I have started a task of bringing about the scientification methods. I sum up with two sentences the work that needs to be performed in the future: science is the foundation; pharmacology is the application. In other words, we use Chinese herbs according to science. This, my brethren, is the first step for Chinese medicine scientification.

Humans are all alike, so can knowledge really be different from one to another? He is a doctor and I am a doctor. He can advance with science; how come I cannot advance with science? Gentlemen, read about the history of medicine in Europe. The ancient medicine was practiced by monks and priests; it has the same origin as our shaman doctors. Thereafter, they used wind, fire, earth and water and magnetism to explain medicine's principle. It is like our nation's Yin Yang and five elements in the recent several hundred years. Even though through great difficulties and winding paths, at the end they established an experimentation system through dissecting, on which basis the Dao of scientific glory came about. Isn't this for us the best mirror to borrow? Gentlemen! Why be discouraged? Why lose confidence? Even if they already went ahead and we follow behind, nonetheless, the rules and measures are established and readily available. If Chinese medicine will turn scientific then easily it will become many folds better than Western medicine. It only requires you gentlemen to use great resolve and great courage, and with that early success will soon be seen.

In modern day's communication level, like sandals at the entrance hall of a house, all affairs cannot tolerate proclaiming oneself in ancient manners. From a big perspective, it includes the country and the people; from a small perspective, it includes every single technique and art. In the middle of all this, what survives or perishes, what rises or falls, is determined by it fitting the tidal current of the entire world. If one wishes to be outside of this progress then he brings his own demise. Looking at medicine of all countries, is there one which does not follow the common path of science?

When I look at our nation's medicine, it is still occupied with the two Qi, five phases, seven directions, ten key formulas, seven emotions, six Qi, three regions, nine domains, four phenomena, eight trigrams, twelve branches and stems. It is still occupied with all kinds of uninvestigated obscure words, superstitious assumptions and absurd theories. Look at all those who are hazed by resisting science; is it laughable? Isn't it pitiful? Alas! Gentlemen, you know the philosophy of an empty structure. It does not surpass the experiments of science. These kinds of old tricks in Europe, already in the seventeenth and eighteenth centuries didn't have a platform to dance on. Performed already so many times, how come it is not already realized over here as well? I hope that all gentlemen will soon self-reflect and prepare to discharge forward toward science.

What should the new skill be like? Seek out the logic of Zhongjing 仲景, the experience and the methods, but believe not the uninvestigated mysterious words of the *Neijing* 內經 and Song Yuan 宋元 later scholars. Use not herbs and formulas blindly but instead differentiate diseases first. Follow not a certain doctor's claim for fame and persistently keep on following his incorrect thoughts. Hope not that each herb will come back to life and instead seek what follows the principles. This is, gentlemen, the golden needle remedy for all patients. It is also my sincere therapeutic advice for all brethren. Gentlemen, if you have the resolve and courage for scientification then you should seek these four points of preparation. Enlightenment is not far off, in this ascent there is light, I cannot express all I wish to say, but I hope that all you gentlemen can imagine it.

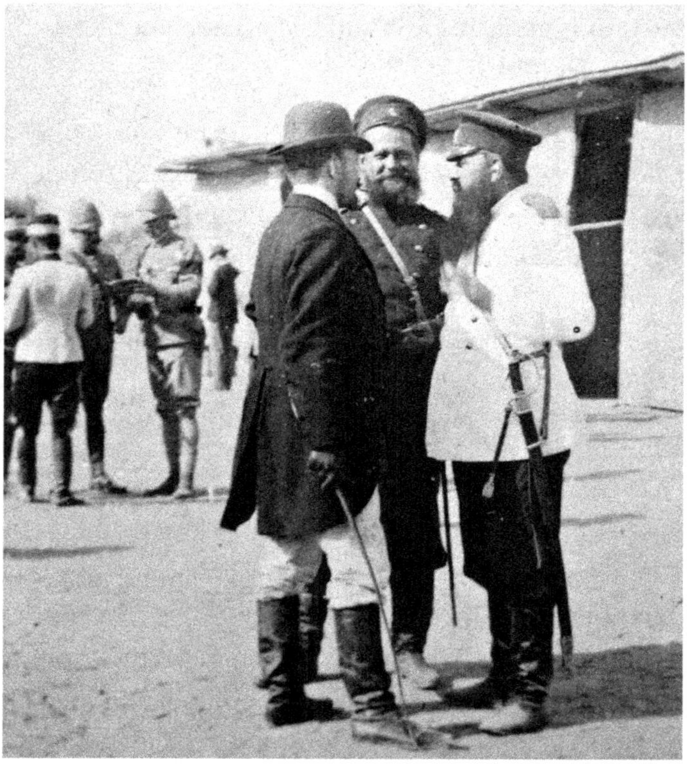

Photo by Mr P. Goux in early 1900s. "Russian officers".

Admonitions to Western medicine

By Tan Cizhong

Yaron: Tan's sincere appeal to the medical community simply asks Chinese medicine to become better. For him, there is no other way but science.

Pages 113-118

Western medicine is a branch of science. Since we advocate to reform Chinese medicine by science, naturally we have to absorb the advantages of Western medicine. There is an old saying: "people who give us fair criticism can be our teachers, and people who give us unfair criticism can be our friends". So Western medicine doctors can be our teachers and friends. Nevertheless, it is still quite necessary to learn from each other by exchanging views. I have often heard from some prominent people in science that science itself has some things not yet good enough. Science develops gradually over many generations, so it is not proper to despise the work of the ancients. However, it is also not right to have blind faith in ancient theories. Nowadays, Chinese medicine doctors are quite passive, yet many foreign people play progressively more significant roles in the research of acupuncture and herbs. Being too content is not good for the progress of science; however, abandoning Chinese medicine is not virtue of a Chinese sage. This is the first exhortation.

Science is related to knowledge but not to politics. However, reforming the current medical policy is an issue. A scientific doctor, on the basis of medicine, talks about science and, on the basis of science, talks about medicine. A real scientist doesn't have time to talk about all kinds of things outside of science. In the old medicine there are many mysterious things, but there are also many reasonable things. So it's better for Chinese medicine to evolve naturally and sort it out by itself. If one is trying to abolish Chinese medicine by external force it will not succeed, but instead the medicine of China will simply regress. The contempt for Chinese medicine will divert many talented people away from Chinese medicine. Therefore, Chinese medicine will be monopolized by rogues, and will become more and more mysterious and deceitful. The quintessence of Chinese culture will be destroyed, and people's life will be in danger. Unexpectedly, the interests of our country and people both will be damaged, and the result of Chinese medicine reform will be just the opposite of what we have wished for. This is the second exhortation.

No matter how many times we repeat it, it's better to make overall reform plans and take all factors into consideration. Only in this way can plans be systematic and realizable. A doctrine will be more valuable if it can fit the demands of current times. Nowadays, the majority of people hope that doctors can develop the rich treasure of Chinese medicine through scientific methods. If one simply wants to attack the mysterious doctrines and, with this attack, correct the old medicine, then a second-year junior high school student, who knows a little bit about anatomy and physiology, is able to do it. If he argues with my brethren, who have very little modern knowledge, he does not need a butcher's knife to chop a little chicken.

To sum up my aspiration for the medicine, I hope that from negative it will turn into more positive, that people will give words a rest and start taking actions, that they will have a spirit wanting to purely benefit the art, that via academics the progress will be benefiting the people, that the development of the nation's art and herbs will be the objective. In other words, for the people's welfare, Chinese medicine doctors have to work hard to promote Chinese medicine development. Only in this way, Chinese medicine can act worthily of the country and people, and doctors will not feel guilty for what they are practicing. From that time on, Chinese medicine doctors will equal Western medicine doctors, and gain well-deserved reputation.

There are many issues that I want to talk about, but I have discussed them in letters to the Academy of Science and Mr. Yu Yunxiu 余雲岫, so I am not going to repeat them here. For more details, please refer to those letters.

Honestly, I am not familiar with science and it seems I am not qualified to discuss it, so I sent letters to the Academy of Science to express my opinions about it. However, science has developed quite well and gained many embracers, so it doesn't really need more flattering words. There is an old Chinese saying: "one person's fair criticism is more valuable than the praises from thousands of people". So I choose to criticize science instead of praising it; I hope scientists will like to hear my criticism.

Gentlemen in both Chinese and Western medicine communities, the aim of science today is the same for everyone. One should not leave for the other what he should do himself when it comes to a grand mission such as Chinese medicine scientification. There is an equal responsibility for both sides. I would like to ask all of you to bring out scientification in a real way so everybody can see it. Science aims to standardize everything; it only allows one correct explanation, and this will greatly reduce the dispute.

Finally, I would like to warn people and myself with this current slang:

> *The sound of science is filling our ears,*
> *What does it reform? There is nothing dishonest,*
> *What the pen writes and the mouth speaks are like weapons,*
> *Western medicine is a spear, while Chinese medicine is a shield.*

Gentlemen, doctors of Chinese and Western medicines, do you resonate these words?

Discussion of the necessity of Chinese medicine scientification

By Tan Cizhong

The problem of medicine in our country has been discussed openly for many years. Both Chinese and Western medicine doctors agree that Chinese medicine has many advantages, and that it also has many disadvantages. Most doctors advocate Chinese medicine reform by scientific methods, i.e. the scientification of Chinese medicine. Both Chinese and Western medicine doctors have a responsibility to reform Chinese medicine. However, I am only going to discuss the most basic issues, such as what science is and what the benefits of Chinese medicine scientification are etc.

What is science? Firstly, scientific knowledge can be obtained not only by ancients, but also by modern people. There are many old stories about the superior efficacy of Chinese medicine such as bringing people back from the dead, but none of today's doctors can repeat them and achieve similar results. They say that the transmission for such skill was lost—but what is the use for such talk? Such things cannot be regarded as scientific.

Secondly, the scientific phenomenon should have concordant theory. It is not allowed to have different theories for one phenomenon. In Chinese medicine, it is quite common that a son learns medicine from his father or an apprentice from his master. Such ways produce many different theories among them. They argue with each other based on their personal theories. These things in Chinese medicine are not scientific.

Thirdly, the scientific phenomenon should be based on evidence. The aspect of Chinese medicine that exists without evidence cannot be regarded as scientific. Bring out the evidence and let us see it. All the big empty talk, even though it sounds good to the ears, has no evidence to rely on. It does not conform to science.

Actually, the above three points are the main disadvantages of Chinese medicine. However, Chinese medicine has many advantages—it has shown efficacy in treating diseases for thousands of years. The efficacy of Chinese medicine is based on herbs and people's experience using them. However, experience is not reliable because it cannot explain the true origin of a disease. We should know that many diseases cannot be treated with herbs and that many herbs also cannot produce instant results.

The most important thing is for doctors to understand the diseases correctly. Doctors may achieve great efficacy in treatment if they understand the disease correctly and apply herbs based on that. Otherwise, it is not possible to achieve good efficacy even if the herbs are good. The improper use of herbs will influence the herbs' effect. Therefore, it is not reliable to use herbs based only on experience. Besides, there are many quack doctors that still insist on false theories like Yin Yang 陰陽 and five phases 五行. They are unable to understand exactly what these theories mean so, most often, they cannot cure the patient even with the most efficacious herbs. I am really worried that good herbs become poison because of improper use. If we improve Chinese medicine with science then we are able to understand diseases based on anatomical experiments and not just experience.

When there is malpractice it can be attributed to the doctor's personal fault. Since science will standardize Chinese medicine, a situation where different doctors make different diagnoses will become rare. Moreover, we will know herbs better through scientific experiments, such as channel entry, indications, side effects etc. Herbal knowledge will be based on evidence so it will be possible to avoid subjective opinions. The scientification will make Chinese medicine more reliable and accurate and people who love Chinese medicine will not need to worry about its future. Furthermore, the progress of Chinese medicine will promote the welfare of all people.

I am a Chinese physiology teacher in a middle school. Actually, I haven't made deep research on both Chinese and Western medicines so I'm not partial to any of them. Due to academic principles, my conscience and the conditions of both the country and people, I firmly believe that Chinese medicine should be reformed through science. I have researched Chinese medicine scientification for many years. In my opinion, in order to achieve this goal, Chinese doctors should cooperate with Western doctors. Therefore, I have written four letters presenting my opinion on Chinese medicine scientification. Two were presented to the Bureau of Native Medicine and the other two to the Academy of Sciences.

I think medicine should not be divided into Chinese and Western and its most important point should be whether it is effective or not. As a doctor, academic research is more important than words. It is quite rare to have people who love Chinese medicine and at the same time understand its disadvantages and the need to reform them through science. Yet these people are the ones who truly love Chinese medicine. Medical specialists should create standards deciding the advantages and disadvantages of Chinese medicine and, accordingly, make procedures reforming the disadvantages. It is really necessary to make such standards and procedures; otherwise, people will not know how to reform Chinese medicine. I hope that both Chinese and Western doctors can remove prejudice and misunderstanding, making efforts to develop an effective medicine.

Complete impartiality is quite important for academic research. Science is seen as Truth because it is always impartial. Furthermore, science is based on facts that can be proven, so even ordinary people can easily understand it. However, Chinese medicine uses theories of Yin Yang 陰陽 and five phases 五行 to explain all things in the world and so even the smartest doctors have difficulties understanding them. Some doctors deceive ordinary people based on such theories. So actually, these theories are neither common-sense nor scientific at all. In a word, Chinese medicine scientification aims to reform it and make it more common-sense. It is really not a fanciful issue.

End of Tan Cizhong book excerpts

What is Western medicine?

1925 by Yang Ji Shi 楊濟時

Source: *Chinesische Zeitschrift fur die Gesamte Medizin (Chinese Journal for the Entire Medicine) (Min Guo Yi Xue Za Zhi)*, June 1925 民國醫學雜誌 第三卷第六號

Yaron: A good example for the social pressure felt by Western medicine doctors. It was a situation where a compromise with Native medicine would mean a complete obstruction of modern medical science in China. It is also the backdrop for the *Native Medicine Abolition* proposal by Yu Yunxiu.

Pages 281–287

1. What is Western medicine?

What is the method of Western medicine? What is the foothold of Western medicine? What is China's role in Western medicine? What is Western medicine's mission to improve society? What makes the native intelligentsia misunderstand Western medicine? What are the new medical trends?

These are very important questions, which I can hardly answer, so I hope to get some advice with the following discussion.

2. The evolution process of medicine

Western medicine comprises many theories but none of them are imagination without foundation; its process of historical evolution is worth learning. Without knowing the historical background, we cannot understand the Western medicine spirit as well as the scope of Chinese medicine. Unfortunately, there is no good book about the history of Chinese medicine. As for the history of Western medicine, it can be divided into four eras: Spirits; Observation; Obscurity; and Experiments. Generally speaking, the evolution of Western medicine followed these four stages.

In the Spirits stage, illness was seen as connected to spirits and ghosts, so people needed to please them in order to cure disease. Nowadays, the aborigines of some undeveloped areas, such as Africa and America, are still at this stage.

Observation era began with Hippocrates from Greece, who wrote many books using precise words to describe what he saw with diseases—from an objective angle. As the ancestor of Western medicine, he laid the foundation for the scientific method of Western medicine. One representative of the Observation era was Galen, whose theory was rather complicated. He adopted four elements theory: Fire; Air; Water; and Earth. Fire is primarily hot and secondarily dry. Air is primarily wet and secondarily hot. Water is primarily cold and secondarily wet. Earth is primarily dry and secondarily cold. His theory also adopted the four humors theory which says that the human body is filled with four basic substances called humors, being in balance when a person is healthy. The four humors are: black bile; yellow bile; phlegm; and blood. Galen developed his own tripartite soul theory following the idea of Plato.

In the Obscurity stage, Western medicine was mysterious, practiced only through experience and did not significantly progress until the fifteenth century.

During the Renaissance era, it developed key wisdom and became more scientific than imaginary, indicating the beginning of Experiments era. Vesalius is the ancestor of this stage. As the founder of modern human anatomy, he carried out dissection as the primary teaching tool and suggested hands-on direct observation as the only reliable resource. In the seventeenth century, Harvey discovered systemic circulation. In modern times, there was some research of biochemistry and biophysics and the improvement of nutrition and endocrinology.

3. Western medical treatment

In English, the word "medicine", which may mean "medical treatment" or "medical drugs", is mentioned in Walpse's book, *Medical Sociology,* as being unfortunate. Medical treatment is not exactly equivalent to medical drugs, and medical drugs are not the only way to treat. For example: heliotherapy for tuberculosis; radiation therapy for cancer; electrotherapy, massage and exercise for muscle weakness; blood injection for anemia; appropriate food for diabetes; fish oil for rickets; and so on. There are so many diseases that medical drugs can't cure. Only a handful of diseases can be cured with chemical drugs, such as quinine for malaria, arsphenamine for syphilis, etc. It is a worldwide superstition to regard medical drugs as the only way to treat disease.

In addition to medical drugs, there are many ways to cure or improve disease or halt its course. Western medicine has five principles to cure disease (or five battle strategies to fight disease). The first is to save life, second is to figure out the cause and weed it out, third is to eliminate the patient's pain, fourth is to emphasize nutrition and hygiene and fifth is to prevent other diseases from forming. If the doctor's responsibility was to only prescribe drugs, then this would not be the meaning of "cure disease". Unfortunately, people often think that ingesting drugs equals curing disease and so they believe that doctors should give out a prescription in every case. If a doctor only mentions lifestyle modifications without prescribing any drugs, then he/ she will certainly be regarded as a quack who underestimates the patient's wealth.

Some people think that Western medicine is liquid drugs; some see it as a pill medicine. The first one is intravenous infusion of normal saline, which costs 6 or 7 dollars. Some people feel more comfortable afterwards and believe that the injection is effective and, as a result, they think that the doctor is great. The annual fee collected for those pills, liquids and injections totals a tremendous sum. Some people think that Western medicine is improper; even the "water pillow", widely used in other countries and proven effective to cool down fever and make the patient feel better, is still not accepted in China—even if the patient loses consciousness from high fever. It is as if those who refuse water pillows are willing to suffer.

If we want to cure the disease from the root then we need to know the cause of the disease—this is called diagnosis—and then we can prescribe the appropriate medicine. It is very difficult to correctly diagnose if information is limited to pulse and tongue. This is why we need to record patient history in detail and include every change of symptoms since the disease onset, everyday life and family history, and the patient's recollection of events. In addition, the patient needs to undergo detailed physical examination, including laboratory tests. Most disease causes are found following the above steps. One should understand that these exams and procedures are part of disease treatment and, as discussed before, not only drugs are responsible for treatment.

Whoflen once said to his students, "Nature is reflected in the doctor's healing of disease. The doctor's job is nothing more than nature's work. You [doctors] need caution to not leave any permanent harm". This illustrates the capacity of medicine and drugs to be harmful sometimes. We, doctors, know more about physiological and pathological changes and, therefore, should do more than merely prescribe drugs. If one has money and he desires to have those colorful medical powders and liquids, that's his choice. However, we should avoid dispensing medicine excessively. Otherwise, even if it has strong efficacy, it will gradually become less effective. Our body belongs to nature. It has a natural ability to resist poisonous invasion and fix the damaged part. The doctor's job is to assist nature.

4. The status of Chinese medicine

I did not research Chinese medicine so I am unable to comment on it. However, regardless of what we research, we should look at it objectively. Chinese medicine has many topics in need of research. For example, it has no correct understanding of the human body, its physiology and anatomy. There are only random details, so we hope that some graduate students can research these topics further. At the least, we should compile the history of Chinese medicine and then try to assess its value. Chinese medicine has not yet arrived at the Experiments era, nor is it still in the Spirits stage. Some claim that Chinese medicine is our country's essence and that it does not follow the same evolutionary path as Western medicine. If these people are happy about Chinese medicine's current situation, then my words are all in vain. If, however, we recognize that there is not enough understanding of basic modern medicine in Chinese medicine then we will want to get rid of the rubbish part, such as Yin-Yang and five elements theories. We will keep the part worth preserving and save the less worthy parts in museums. Then it will be possible to rearrange Chinese medicine.

5. The strategy of organizing Chinese medicine

First of all, we need to analyze Chinese medicine from an objective angle and not be influenced by its title as if it is the embodiment of China. Medicine is a valuable thing, regardless of national borders and religions. The difference we make here between Chinese medicine and Western medicine is to emphasize that Chinese medicine is not based on science. In order to organize Chinese medicine, we need to destroy many useless parts and save the worthwhile parts, which then can be devoted to science as a great treasure. Next, we need to destroy Yin-Yang and five elements theory, leave the explanation of climate and weather to astronomers and leave the philosophy lines to university professors. Then we can do research into things worth studying in a scientific way. Chinese medicine, overall, includes very little anatomy, chemistry and physiology. However, some people disagree. They find some farfetched explanations in Chinese medicine books pretending that there is no lack of this knowledge. Those ones just lose themselves and abandon the pursuit of progress. My friends often say that Chinese medicine is based on accumulated experience passing down for thousands of years and instructing us how to cure disease. The correctness of this statement we can discuss later. Nonetheless, we should figure out a standard that explains how to assess this experience and which way we should head towards.

6. The comparison between Western and Chinese medicine

Advocates of Chinese herbal medicine claim that the secret is with the herbs' application. If herbs can cure disease, then many people will not have to die, especially Chinese people. However, if we were to cure diseases only with drugs, then ten times more people will die. These words make a lot of sense to people who study modern medicine—even to common people, after they think about it carefully.

Even though there are diseases that seem to be cured with Chinese medicine, if we have no scientific proof that Chinese medicine causes any physiological change, then how can we claim that it can cure disease? It is equivalent to declaring war on science and betraying the truth. If Chinese medicine has no scientific proof then it is not true that Chinese medicine can cure what Western medicine can't.

First, we can consider that the mortality rate in China is three times higher than in other countries. In China, the mortality rate is more than 30 out of 1000 (according to hygienists' speculation), 23.7 in Beijing, 10.6 in UK and Ireland (1923), and 10.6 in USA (1923). There are many factors causing the high mortality rate and we cannot attribute the factors solely to Chinese medicine; however, it should take partial blame. Second, many people recover without taking any medicine. Third, we only see those odd cases that support Chinese medicine, but we never examine the failed examples. It is blind, arbitrary and illogical to advocate Chinese medicine just because it cures several people and, at the same time, not mention the deaths it causes.

7. The relationship between medicine and society

Since we recognize science as truth, then medicine based on a scientific principle is also truth. Although Chinese medicine has popular support while Western medicine attracts suspicion, Chinese medicine has no leg to stand on during this scientific era. Western medicine will not lose the truth, regardless how uninvited it is in China. Despite all those negative words aiming at our extermination, we—the enlightened intelligentsia—should be aware of the situation of science in China. We should not cover our ears and eyes in blind support for Chinese medicine, uttering "preserve the national essence" and "Chinese medicine is good", while ignoring the hardships that befall the people. Deaths caused by it are more than all wars and natural disasters combined. All you gentlemen who promote Chinese medicine, do you carry the responsibility for all those who have died in vain?

This Chinese medicine problem is directly connected to our lives. However, this problem does not receive much attention because there are old ethical codes, warlords and scholar-tyrants in our country. There are still people who promote Chinese medicine and others who follow it. Maybe it is due to our large population that, even with this high death rate for hundreds of years, Chinese people still survive. The fact that both airplane and donkey-drawn cart exist side by side in the best areas of our country is indicative of the essential chaos in China. No wonder some Chinese medicine advocates also support the scientific method.

Some have already noticed how serious the problem is but thought, "Why do we compete with Chinese medicine? It will die anyway." I thought so before, too. However, instead, Chinese medicine trends become more and more popular, which turns into not only a medical problem but also a negative influence on our culture. Western medicine is a study involving scientific principles about the human body, and its connection to biology is obvious. It also relates to physics. For example, the element radium can be used in medicine, where changing its characteristic is done through chemistry and knowing its beam emission through physics. Knowing the occurring change after the beam was emitted into a cell is through biology. Many diseases are congenital, so here medicine is connected to genetics. Knowing geography and climate are related to disease distribution, where different kinds of diseases happen in different communities. The Western medicine point of view, therefore, includes principles from all scientific fields, which results in knowing the scientific interaction between different activities inside a human body. To be suspicious of Western medicine implies having no belief in science or scientific methods and to support Chinese medicine means to deny science indirectly. Western medicine started in Japan no earlier than in China and I hope that Chinese medicine advocates can see the progress that Japanese people have made in Western medicine. Dr. Kitasato discovered the pathology of bubonic plague and tetanus, Dr. Noguchi discovered the pathology of yellow fever, and Dr. Katsurada discovered the pathogenesis of Japanese schistosoma. These are the most important discoveries in the entire world. Compared to us, there are many famous Japanese medical scientists whilst there are almost none in our country.

8. The medical trend in Europe and USA

In recent decades, medicine has improved in preventive medicine (or "Public health"). If one sees a doctor after he already fell sick, the question remains if he will recover or die. Even if one has recovered, it remains unanswered if he had compromised himself for the disease. When sick, one not only impacts himself and his family, but also the community and the country. In Japan, the national annual budget for the hygiene industry is, on average, one hundred million Yen. In New York City, where hygiene equipment is considered the best in the entire world, the budget for the hygiene industry is fifty-one million six hundred seventy-eight thousand three hundred fifty-two USD. It shows how popular the trends are in Europe and USA.

Most importantly, the UK established the Ministry of Health in 1918 as being on the same level as Ministry of Foreign Affairs and Ministry of National Defense, proving that the UK emphasizes development of preventive medicine. Although the USA and Japan haven't gone this far, they are almost there. Preventive medicine has made big progress causing the mortality rate to drop by more than half in UK and USA.

Practicing preventive medicine means to record causes of death in the entire country, the reproduction rate and the occurrence of infectious diseases, and find a solution to correct causes of death. Any and all foodstuffs, drugs and drinking water in markets, factories and houses need to be examined. Women and children in factories should be protected by healthcare regulations. All doctors need to pass a licensing exam in order to practice medicine. Children in schools should get regular physical exams practiced by professional personnel and, if sick, should not go to school but, rather, seek a doctor. Now, our Ministry of Health also disseminates information on how to prevent diseases by lectures and stripfilms, showing that modern medical trends have been accepted by people in all other countries. Recently, some good medical schools in other countries have adopted preventive medicine into the medical science curriculum.

In our current directionless Chinese society, Western medicine is positioned at the same level as Chinese medicine. Western medicine's fate will only be decided by the people's feelings. If we reject Western medicine, it will be reluctant to stay and will be eradicated by this ill and old country. It will spread its goodness only in countries that welcome and treasure it. Then intelligentsia leaders will have to assume partial responsibility for the intelligentsia's lack of understanding towards Western medicine. However, the reason people don't challenge Chinese medicine is not only because of its alleged embodiment of China's essence and metaphysics, but also because the intelligentsia don't understand fully and believe in science. They attain knowledge about philosophy and astronomy, but know nothing about protecting and nurturing their own bodies and there is even no sex education in schools. Like this, they create more people who do not understand—and have no interest in—Western medicine. When people don't understand Western medicine, not only does it impact life and death, but it also strengthens the erroneous belief in Chinese medicine. Please let me repeat once more, Western medicine is a science closely connected to human life and it is not useless mysterious metaphysics. It directly results in people's happiness rather than merely curing diseases. It ambitiously seeks health and follows every rule of human survival. One cannot blindly advocate Chinese medicine if he had understood what I just said above.

9. The principle of the new medicine

From the Spirits stage to the Experiments era, in the evolution of medicine, the progress represents how far and successful people were with science. The meaning of "Experiments era" is not only numbers in labs, but also practising all truths found by scientists and using them to improve people's life. In short, the goal of the new medicine is medical sociology. What is medical sociology? In old times, medicine only helped individual sick people. Now, the new medicine treats the entire society. It utilizes its knowledge to help the entire society grow healthier. Varied topics such as parenting, population, labor hygiene, municipal hygiene, schools, prostitution, races, prevention of infectious diseases and hygiene education are all part of it. The purpose of medical sociology is to make medicine the crux of all social activities. Medicine should benefit the community by improving people's health across the board. Medicine should be owned by the society as a whole and not be secretly possessed by a selected group of doctors. I am of the opinion that medical sociology is the main element showing progress with human evolution.

10. Conclusion

Western medicine is the crystallization of all life sciences; the way it treats disease is all based on scientific truth. There are three kinds of danger in supporting Chinese medicine:
1. It blocks the development of Western medicine in China;
2. It stops the improvement of all kinds of science; and
3. It causes death indirectly.

It is absurd to advocate Chinese medicine because of the following reasons:
1. Many diseases recover on their own;
2. If people do not know the exact effects of drugs then they cannot claim the drugs are working;
3. Chinese medicine supporters only bring success examples and not the numbers of deaths; and
4. The death rate in China is higher than any other country.

The intelligentsia should not have zero understanding of Western medicine because of these:
1. The leader is supported blindly;
2. People don't understand scientific truth; and
3. There is no physiology in the curriculum of schools.

To organize Chinese medicine we need to:
1. Break the preconceived notion of "Chinese essence";
2. Eliminate Yin-Yang and five elements theories; and
3. Seek the truth by scientific means.

We cannot totally depend on medical drugs; that they can cure disease doesn't mean that it's the only way to treat disease.

Preventive medicine has been practiced in Western countries and Japan. However, people in our country even haven't unveiled the real faces of Chinese and Western medicines. The principle of new medicine is to medicalize the community, which is medical sociology.

Article end

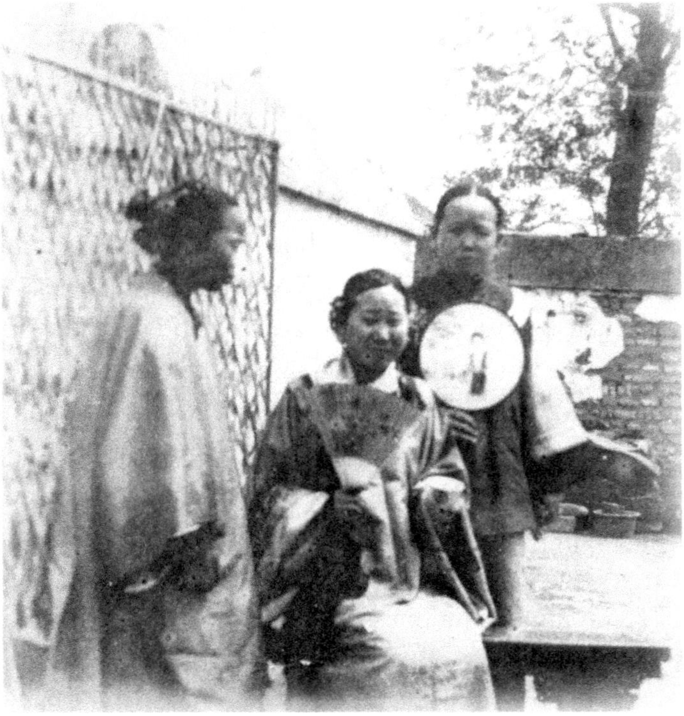

Photo by Mr P. Goux in early 1900s. "Chinese women".

The similarities and differences between Chinese and Western medicine 論中西學說之異同

1926 Composed by Longshan old man Dizhenzi Mr. Guo Jingtang 龍山老人諦真子郭金堂撰

Copied by junior scholar from Jing Nan Mr. Zhou Yuxi 後學涇南周禹錫抄錄

Source: *San San Medical Gazette,* 3rd scroll 3rd issue, published in Hang Zhou by San San Medical Society 1926 三三醫報 第三卷第三期 杭州三三醫社

Yaron: During the Republic, some wanted to believe that Chinese medicine and Western medicine were actually similar to each other. It was a convenient escape route: an idea that modern scientific medicine and ancient Chinese medicine pointed to the same things with different points of view and terminology that could easily be reconciled. In such an ideal situation, there was no need to get rid of old theories or despise modern medicine. It was a small trend having little chance to succeed; neither defenders of old nor proponents of new subscribed to such a notion.

1. About Shen 神

The difference between Chinese and Western medicines is the concept of Spirit Shen 神.[322] In Chinese medicine, heart stores Spirit Shen 神, so heart is the monarch amongst the officials, where spirit appears.[323] So people attribute Spirit-Shen to heart. In Western medicine, Shen only exists in the brain; therefore, in physiology and psychology, the most important chapter is about the nervous system 神經篇.[324] This is the biggest difference between Chinese and Western medicines. Shen existing in the brain has material fact. It has been proven and accepted by the entire world, including China. However, it is not totally absurd to say that heart stores Shen from Chinese medical point of view. Why is that? It is a fact that Shen is from the brain. When we observe the brain structure, we can see that it is definitely coming from there. However, nutrients carried to the brain, aren't they carried by the blood? If this supply declines then nerves Shen Jing decline. There is no difference between Chinese and Western medicine in regards to heart governing blood. When there's blood deficiency, it will result in a brain illness that begins with the heart. In addition, in Western medicine, the pneumogastric nerve largely distributes to the chest and abdomen and it is also called an involuntary nerve. The heart itself has a nerve, so what they both feel[325] is consistent. In addition, heart is fundamental for the building-up of brain. It is, therefore, very reasonable to claim that heart stores Shen.

Out of my personal experience, I can say that when a person uses his heart too much,[326] then heart Shen is restless and, truly, this is felt in the physical heart, with symptoms such as heart palpitations and blood-deficiency heart-pounding. If it lasts long, a mental disease Shen Jing Bing 神經病[327] will ensue. Ancient people said, "If a person does not sleep at the third night watch, then blood does not return to heart and the person's Shen naturally declines." This shows that Shen is in the heart and everyone can experience this themselves. This is the evidence in Chinese medicine showing that Shen belongs to heart.

Nowadays, some people who know a tiny bit of Western medicine slander the ancient theories badly, without doing any research. That is why Chinese academic

---

[322] There is difficulty in this article to translate Shen as it contains several meanings, but mostly refers to spirit, mental faculties and mind. It also means a spirit such as in spirits and Gods. In this article, we keep it untranslated as Shen 神 to allow readers a visual indication of how often this term is being used for multiple meanings.

[323] A quote from chapter 8 of the *Su Wen*.

[324] Note that the word "Nerve" Shen Jing 神經 in Chinese includes the word Shen 神.

[325] Heart and the nerves serving it.

[326] Thinks too much.

[327] Mental disease in Chinese is "Nerves Disease" Shen Jing Bing 神經病.

knowledge is retrogressing and the quintessence of Chinese culture becomes less popular. At the beginning, Western medicine was inclining to thoughts and assumptions more than reality, which was similar to Chinese medicine. They have researched further and finally it became science. Although ancient people were smart, first with developing Chinese medicine theories, this knowledge, nonetheless, cannot be perfectly accurate. If we don't continue researching it, then this will be our mistake that we hand down to later generations. No matter if it is Chinese or Western medicines, each may have an attainment. Regardless of what some people say and that they look down at the ancient sages, a sincere person knows no limits and we should all encourage each other.

2. About Qi 氣

There are many theories about Qi in China. The main idea is Yin-Yang and five elements, especially what master Zhuzi 朱子 said, "Heaven gives birth to myriad things via Yin-Yang and five elements, Qi makes them into a physical shape," is a very accurate explanation. And so, when doctors talk about all kinds of Qi, such as heart Qi, liver Qi, spleen Qi, lung Qi, kidney Qi, upright Qi and evil Qi, it is based on Zhu's remarks.

In Western medicine, since they discovered the concept of air, they think that human body's Qi gets in and out from the mouth and nose. The air is inhaled from the nose and goes to the lungs and then in the veins and blood exchanges the old with the new, and then it is exhaled with carbon from the mouth or nose. They think that the Qi of the human body is like this and that's it. If a person gets his mouth and nose blocked for twenty minutes then he can't live. This can be examined by experiment. Thus the idea of supplementing Qi in Chinese medicine they see as totally made up and not trustworthy. However, patients with short Qi,[328] often feel better after taking Chinese herbs to supplement Qi. Why is that?

I've been researching this twice and trice and saw that it applies to all things in the world. I found out that, in addition to air Qi, everything has its own origin Qi, such as fragrant Qi of fruit, pungent Qi of peppers and cinnamon, which are obvious examples. Isn't it a good proof that everything has its own origin Qi? In addition, when fruit is rotten due to air exposure, it has foul odor, thus how can we say there's no other Qi except for the air? It is just that we, human beings, can't sense every kind of Qi.

[328] Shortness of breath.

Origin Qi is the Qi of Yin-Yang and five elements. Furthermore, the method of supplementing Qi in Chinese medicine is not only supplementing Qi but also facilitating functions of organs. For example, lungs are an important organ carrying air, so when there is lung deficiency or atrophic lung disease, then lungs can't carry air properly. We, therefore, use herbs to tonify lungs which results in lungs recovering their function just as before. In addition, air gets in and out through the mouth and nose but origin Qi doesn't. For example, Qi of magnetic electricity doesn't need an orifice to get in or out of an object. Recently, Western people invented x-ray, which penetrates every organic object. They figured out that in the air there is another kind of origin Qi. Their philosophers call it Ether "Tai 太" which, until today, cannot be explained thoroughly. Believing firmly that there is origin Qi in between heaven and earth is something which was held fast in China since antiquity. This kind of academic knowledge, Chinese and Western medicine should examine both without a bias, where each believes theirs is true. There is much transformation within heaven and earth and many things that haven't been discovered, even for those leaning toward and believing only in Western science. I therefore think that we should merge our efforts and seek a middle road. It is the right thing to do.

3. About Jing 精

The Jing 精 essence[329] of the human body comes from the Jing of things. In Zuo Zhuan 左傳 it is said that much comes from the Jing of things, the principle of which is extremely accurate. Even Western medicine cannot escape this principle. Only that Chinese medicine says Jing comes out of kidneys, while Western medicine says that the testicles are the manufacturing organ. It is a minor difference. I've tried to figure out the differences between Chinese and Western medicines through different theories and experience, and discovered that both of them are indispensable. People indulging in sexual activity usually suffer from lower back pain, which is the main sign for kidney deficiency in Chinese medicine. This is the evidence of Chinese medicine.

Western medicine's point of view is that the testicle function is to produce semen. Testicles are the "pair of kidney seeds", which makes Chinese medicine then hardly different. I also think that although kidney is said to be the residence of Jing fluid, this Jing fluid belongs to blood and not to semen, whereas semen and sperm are stored in testicles. All these can be verified through dissection and anatomical experiments. When excessive sexual intercourse becomes intensive, the patient will have

[329] Jing 精 may contain different meanings like essence, sperm, pure extract, so we keep it untranslated.

hematuria, because testicles are too damaged to function properly and so the body excretes the original building block of semen from the kidneys, which is blood.

Another example is "Yang collapse", of which nine out of ten die. It is caused by deficient kidneys and tendons becoming lax and weak resulting from a serious disease. The restriction control is lost and so, during action, the semen building block in kidneys and semen in testicles all come out together with the origin Qi in torrents. This is then called loss of origin Qi. Some might not die from this disease because they still have some origin Qi left in their kidneys, even if they lost all semen. To treat this kind of patient effectively, we need to supplement their origin Qi by having another person connecting his mouth to the patient's mouth to continue the patient's breath. This method started from theory and became practice in China and it could also be proven by experience. There's no similar concept in Western medical theories and therefore they didn't come up with this idea. Now, Jing in both Chinese and Western medicines has great similarity with only minor differences. Both of them have advantages, so how can we emphasize only one of them?

4. About blood

Human blood circulates all over the body. There are big and small blood vessels, arteries and veins. The theories are generally the same in Chinese and Western medicines. The only difference is that in Chinese medicine there are also twelve meridians and fifteen main collaterals plus eight extra meridians as an aggregation path for blood. About pulse taking, it is divided into three parts as Cun, Guan, Chi 寸關尺, which Western people totally disagree with. In Western medicine blood circulation goes from heart to lungs via artery and from lungs back to heart via the vein. Both circulate endlessly all around the body, which has been checked several times through anatomic experiments. Every one who practices medicine can get the rough idea that pulse may feel floating or sunken, rapid or slow; however, how can one divide the pulse into three and see organs' particular conditions? It seems that the meridians and other theories were all false.

I did textual scrutiny and found out that Huangdi 黃帝 made Linglun 伶倫[330] use bamboo to make the yellow bell harmony tubes Huangzhong Lüguan 黃鐘律管[331] to measure the solar terms Jie Qi 節氣[332] and made Qibo use Qikou 氣口[333] to establish

[330] The text writes Linglun name as Lingpian 伶偏; we have corrected it.

[331] To establish pitches, 12 bamboo pipes, closed at one end, were cut into graduated lengths. When blown across their open ends, they produced the 12 Lü, or fundamental pitches.

[332] Jie Qi are 24 seasonal division points.

pulse-taking method in order to measure people's moving Qi. The human body is a micro heaven and earth. Since yellow bell Huang Zhong 黃鐘[334] harmonic tones can detect the preexisting omens of the solar terms Jie Qi 節氣, we can therefore measure the pulse Qi based on the harmony tubes Lüguan 律管. It makes a lot of sense that heaven, earth and human Qi are connected to each other. Many profound theories are concealed within the diagnostic methods of pulse-taking in the book *Nanjing* 難經 written by Qin Yueren 秦越人. These theories were discovered by enlightened people and are not something commoners are able to guess. Wang Shuhe 王叔和 composed his book, *Pulse Classic Maijing* 脈經, based on those theories and not on empty talk. However, when it comes to blood vessels and collaterals the ancient people only described this concept in general. They did not imagine stuff like later generations did. These theories have been practiced for over four thousand years by all the famous doctors through all dynasties always carrying good effects, so we shouldn't regard them as useless or nonsense.

On the other hand, Westerners only do dissection anatomic experiments to research medicine, which can teach us a lot; however, blood vessels often spoil after people die, so when they do the anatomic experiments on dead people, how can the result not be lacking? I actually think it's not correct to regard all ancient theories as nonsense and get rid of them, and it is also not correct to stick to ancient theories and regard them as error-free. Although Wang Mang 王莽 ordered his doctors and butchers to dissect a living person and investigate within, their report of meridians beginning and end points matching the ancient theories, I am afraid, must have been fabricated. Anyway, blood vessels are very fine; both Western and ancient theories have not discovered it fully. This draft, for the time being, just raises doubts. I hope that, in the future, someone wise can discover the answer.

The four points I mentioned above are the big similarities and small differences comparing Chinese and Western medical theories. The reason I talked about it first is that Shen, Qi, Jing and blood are the fundamental functions of the human body. As for the similarities and differences, I only mentioned a general idea. There are more I can introduce on another day. Composed by Longshan old man Dizhenzi Guo Jintang 龍山老人諦真子郭金堂 in San Li Literary Society 三立學社 in Hengyin 恒陰 County.

---

333 Radial pulse

334 Huang Zhong is also the name of the first of the twelve harmonic tones.

Yuxi 禹錫 followed the categories of Shen, Qi, Jing and blood and merged into it some Western medical theories and, like this, discovered some new medical knowledge.

This article was published in the first book of *Shi Quan Shou Shi Xue* 十全壽世學 as its first article. Yuxi saw that his friend had it so he ask where to get one, then the friend replied that it was from an old vendor in Beijing, and that he only got this one book out of the whole series. There was no address in the book, only "Published by Heng Yin county San Li Xue She" and "Procuration for every kinds of books 各處代理流通者善社藥店書莊" printed on the book. So I copied this down to publish it in the newspaper and hope anyone who knows the address can publish it in the newspaper or mail it to me, Mr. Zhou Yuxi 周禹錫, and the address is: Chinese and Western Medicine Society, inside little south gate, Wan County, Sichuan Province 四川萬縣小南門內中西醫藥社. I'll pay proper amount for a medical book as reward but it's necessary to give clear indication where the mail is from to prevent my mailing it to a wrong address. Written by Junior scholar from south of Jing River Zhou Yuxi on April 8th.

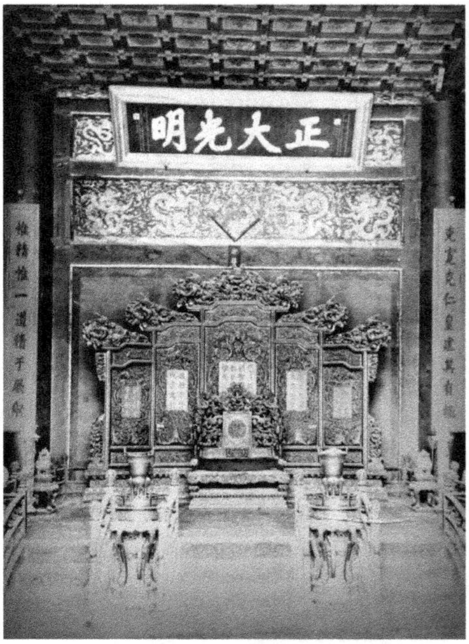

Photo by Mr P. Goux in early 1900s. "Imperial throne".

One of Shanghai's things: Chinese medicine

By Du He 獨鶴

Source: *Compilation of Discussions about Chinese Medical Education* 中醫教育討論集

Yaron: A personal account of the problems associated with medical practice during the Republic years.

Pages 494–498

Doctors and medicine take the two most important roles for the wellbeing of everyone and this is why they have such a high status in our society. There are countless doctors, hospitals and drug stores, which appear to outsiders as trustworthy and life preserving. However, there are just too many hidden maladies to write about. The number of people who have died from medical malpractice in Shanghai may actually be bigger than that of those who have died without adequate medicine (or proper treatment) in remote areas. I live here and know much about medical malpractice. I am not blaming anyone but I truly hope that they would realize how much responsibility they are shouldering and try to mend their ways.

It is reasonable for doctors in Shanghai to charge more than those who work elsewhere, considering the high standard of living here. Medicine is a profession and the role of doctor is an occupation. Doctors should be paid just like any other occupation.

What doctors should receive as a consultation fee should be measured by their right to charge and their duty to provide treatment. In these years, the amount of money that doctors charge has risen so rapidly that it is getting away from acceptable standards. Even those who are not so famous, and with affordable outpatient charges, cannot be called out without five or six Yuan, not to mention doctors of Western medicine and those famous Chinese medicine practitioners. As the saying goes, the poor in Shanghai better not get sick. Not only the poor but also middle class families are not be able to afford medical fees. There are often sad incidents where people with serious illnesses are unable to afford medical treatment and end up as fatal cases. (There are some doctors advertising doing call outs regardless if patients are poor or not. This is actually a way for beginners to attract customers. After one year or so when they manage to improve their skills and have a better reputation, it is almost certain that they will no longer care for poor patients.)

On the other hand, not only individual doctors but also the community as a whole is responsible for the high consultation fees. People in Shanghai are used to a luxurious lifestyle and they tend to appreciate things according to their monetary values. Take ticket sales at theaters as an example; the more expensive the tickets are, the more popular the movies will be and the more tickets will sell. Also, in the market, the goods with higher prices often have greater popularity than those cheaper. People tend to weigh everything according to how much it costs. Gradually people become convinced that the best doctors charge the most, and the opposite holds true as well. This is why doctors have to ask for more, just to go with the tide and avoid being looked down upon.

There is another malpractice by doctors in Shanghai—they are never punctual with call-outs. It may sound reasonable for experienced doctors who have a high reputation and lots of call-outs to be a little bit late. Nevertheless, there are lots of ridiculous cases in which odious doctors will not get to their patients' place before dusk, even though they are not really busy. Moreover, these doctors do not start with taking care of their patients when they arrive. Instead, they make polite noises to explain their being late, such as they were so busy out there taking care of so many patients. These doctors want to become famous through showing off, putting their patients in second place. In Shanghai, most people prefer outpatient services to home visits due to the high consultation fees. For those who need a home visit, it is very likely that the patient is in a more severe situation, being unable to visit the doctor. So this is the situation, those doctors are late for the appointment only to put a show that they are busy and popular, while their suffering patients need them so badly. What's more, how can doctors be liable for being late if they are called for urgent cases? What if the patient dies while waiting for them?

The doctors' rebuttal is that patients may have early callouts (the call out service before the outpatient service hour). Of course, it is much more expensive. Everything is about money. In recent years, doctors in the city are becoming much more ostentatious. Most of them travel by car and carriage, while only a few take the rickshaw. As for their dress code, most Western medicine doctors are in suits while Chinese medicine doctors are also fairly well dressed. Theoretically, dressing up does not improve the doctor's healing skills. However, people in Shanghai look down at doctors who don't wear fancy clothes. My friend Lu Zhiping 陆治平 has been a doctor for many years and there were times he has cured my family. He may not have miraculous healing skills but he is definitely better than many of those so called famous doctors. However, he does not advocate fancy clothes and his career suffers, maybe because of this.

A doctor showing off by wearing fancy clothes does not do harm to his patients. Nevertheless, doctors put on airs from time to time, forgetting their duty as a doctor. They may not notice that it creates difficulties for their patients, which is unforgivable. Eight years ago my brother's newborn son became sick and they sent for a doctor. It was around eight in the evening, which is not that late. However, the famous pediatrician refused to offer a call-out service arguing safety reasons. He claimed to be concerned about public security and afraid of being blackmailed by those who pretend to be patients and call him out, so he never goes to patients' homes after sunset. My brother had no choice but to continue asking him for help, however, it was useless. Finally, we invited the pediatrician in by writing him an invitation letter, signed by me and stamped by a newspaper office, just to prove that we are not going to blackmail him. After a visual examination, the pediatrician insisted that it was only a mild bellyache and the child would feel well after taking his medicine. He prescribed the medicine and left in a hurry. A few hours later, the child's limbs began to twitch and we asked the same pediatrician for help in the morning. However, what we heard in the morning was totally different from that in the last evening—the child was going to die soon and there was no need for medication. My brother was so shocked about the great change in only hours. We asked the pediatrician why the situation worsened so rapidly but he was turning a deaf ear to our questions. He tried to calm my brother by telling him that the child would become a hierarch in the other world after his death and then left without prescribing anything for the child. The consultation fee for the two call-outs was more than 30 Yuan.

My first son also died by the hand of a so-called famous pediatrician at the age of one. He had a cough, which was not a severe case. My son coughed for a long time so we visited a lot of pediatricians. The child improved with medication but he was never cured completely. One day he coughed out sputum with a little bit of blood in it. I was not at home then, but my wife panicked and took our son to a famous pediatrician recommended by a relative. The famous pediatrician had a room full of visitors. After waiting for the whole morning, my wife got a prescription for our son. However, the situation changed enormously. The child's chest was like a kurgan and had opisthotonos.[335] We sought help from another doctor and the doctor prescribed a "cool" tonic medicine after having a look at the original prescription by the famous pediatrician. My son died eventually. From then on, I have tended to be more leery of those doctors with high reputations and lots and lots of patients, especially the pediatricians. (Among all the pediatricians, Mr. Yun Tieqiao 惲鐵樵 is a good one, with good diagnosing skills and not an air on him like a "famous doctor".)

Some doctors can have over a hundred patients in a day. Due to limited outpatient service hours, they have to have their apprentices write down the prescriptions in order to save time. However, no matter how fast the apprentices write, it is never going to be as fast as the diagnosis making process by those doctors. As a consequence, it is common for a doctor to utter the last patient's prescription for the apprentice to write down while the doctor himself is already taking the pulse of the next patient. Sometimes they can be so busy that there are three to four prescriptions still being recorded for prior patients while the current one is being diagnosed. Outsiders may think that those doctors have excellent memory and diagnosing skills. Actually, there is no doubt that those doctors make mistakes in that way. I heard that there is a trick among some doctors. They prescribe light dose prescriptions to the patients who come to visit them because, so they think, if patients can come by themselves they cannot be suffering from severe illnesses. Moreover, the light dose medicine will never have strong side effects (even though the light dose medicine will not have adequate healing effects as well).

Without a doubt, a doctor having too many patients doesn't do any good for the patients. There is somehow another kind of doctor who sets limits on the total number of appointments he books. These normally charge even more compared to the general Shanghai standard. Moreover, patients must make the booking one night in advance. To all appearances, they are taking their time to see every patient in great length, but they are actually just trying to do something different and make use of that to advertise. In fact, the number of visiting patients may not reach the doctor's limit by the end of the working hour. Nevertheless, they always show the board as "fully booked" or "no appointment available" and refuse any other walk-in patients after the so-called working hours. All I can comment about this kind of doctors is: why do they have to do this?

[335] A tetanic spasm in which the body arches backwards and stiffens

There is another vital drawback for Chinese medicine doctors (which Western medicine doctors do not have)—they don't sterilize their instruments. It is no big deal for normal diseases, but can do great harm with acute infectious diseases, for example, if a Chinese medicine doctor uses a tongue depressor in two patients without proper disinfection. With the conceivable amount of dirt and bacteria remaining on it, it is undoubtedly likely for patients to contract a much more serious disease even though they have visited the doctor just for a mild sore throat. My nephew once had a sore throat and a doctor, famous for his strength in throat related diseases, was invited. That doctor had previously cured my younger brother's sore throat with a single treatment. I really appreciated him as a result. My nephew was getting better with the doctor's medication. Then one night after a visit to his clinic, my nephew started to have a fever with extreme sore throat, which was irreversible. After a lot of consideration, I think that my nephew has contracted the disease from the tongue depressor which was reused without disinfection.

My speculations are not over-sensitive. (There are always a lot of people inside a Chinese medicine clinic. This can be really dangerous if someone with flu or other infectious disease is in the crowd. While the same scenario may take place in a Western medicine clinic, they have better disinfected instruments than those used by Chinese medicine doctors.)

Article end

General situation of Chinese medicine doctors in Shanghai

By Jin Yin Hua 金銀花

Source: *Compilation of Discussions about Chinese Medical Education* 中醫教育討論集

Yaron: Corruption in Chinese medicine politics started early on.

Pages 498–503

At the first Health Conference in the 18th year of the Republic (1929), the entire Chinese medicine community stretched up their eyebrows like having a very sour and spicy soup. After all, Shanghai is a place with so many talented people. Some petty men were calling on people in the fields of Chinese medicine and Chinese herbal medicine under the guise of "facts", which they made up out of the blue. Outside Shanghai, people in the two fields[336] responded with great vigor, resulting in the formation of the so-called National Union for Societies of Chinese Medicine 全國醫藥團體聯合會. At that time, Chinese medicine leadership fell into the hands of Shanghai Chinese medicine circles and, as of today, it remains the same.

It is a pity that while transportation is being improved and communications increasingly convenient, people in this field are still sleeping. Dear Chinese medicine doctors! Please do not laugh at or be angry with me. I am not chewing on my own tongue. I will absolutely provide the evidence. Just wait, I will make it all very clear in a special publication about Chinese medicine history. Please wake up, Chinese medicine doctors! Since everyone thinks that Shanghai Chinese medicine doctors represent the entire nation, I would like to present here the actual situation of the field in Shanghai.

1. About doctors

    i. Doctors specializing in providing profit-based medical services to the general public: These are the majority and the most complicated. Amongst them are so-called "multi generation scholar doctors" San Shi Ru Yi 三世儒醫 as well as quacks Jiang Hu Pai 江湖派. Now, because of the materialistic lifestyle in Shanghai, their minds are filled with ideas of fake legal tender, house calls

[336] Chinese medicine and Chinese herbalism

and early calls 早拔.[337] As for their way of doing business, it is not within the scope of this article, thus I will write another one to discuss it.

ii. Doctors working for charity 善堂派: Shanghai is a city of kindness and the significant number of charities provides the best proof. Generally, medical services are included in charity work, with a pre-registration fee of 0.2 Yuan. I have heard that all Chinese herbs used in those clinics are provided by drugstores, with any daily dosage at the price of 0.1 Yuan. Doctors, who receive a monthly salary of around 20 Yuan, would never be able to work there if they did not know the charity chairperson or another influential person. Some doctors in the clinic are not paid at all, but they still need to be introduced to the charity by some tycoons. What kind of medicine they sell in this melting pot, only God knows.[338]

iii. Doctors who work as professors: The field of Chinese medicine seems to be even more energetic after having the sour and chili soup. There have been a whole lot of Chinese medicine specialty schools Zhong Yi Zhuan Xiao 中醫專校, Native Medicine Colleges Guo Yi Xue Yuan 國醫學院 and Research Institutes for Native Medicine 國醫研究院. Those doctors, who cannot take care of patients, change direction and become lifelong teachers who educate students.

iv. Doctors in medical associations Yi Hui 醫會: They look to the future of Chinese medicine. Prime Minister Sun's idea to educate the general public gave birth to Native medical associations Guo Yi Gong Hui 國醫工會. In their lifetime, these doctors draw people in and earn loads of money every day. When they die, they have lots of obituaries and titles. As a consequence, the associations are filled with politics and intrigue where they write to newspapers daily to speak ill of each other. Here is an article as evidence. I will not put up all their articles here, as I respect Mr. Li Zi's 力子 request not to waste too much paper.

Article excerpt end

[337] The service which is more expensive

[338] The idiom used is "Jesus has its own logic".

A Request from Shanghai Native Medicine Association 上海國醫公會 to all members to deny those despicable behaviors

To whom it may concern,

The latest elections were full of fraud and malpractice unlike ever before. The place was an absolute mess. Some were even physically fighting with each other, which was witnessed by many including myself. The association used to have a high reputation amongst us so it was beyond our dreams that this election would be rigged by those ambitious people cheating any way they can, completely ignoring all members. Here are some of their misdeeds:

1) Just one day before the election meeting, every member received a letter from Jiang Wenfang 蔣文芳. It pointed out that there are a few ambitious individuals. I was not planning to attend the meeting. However, someone came to my place claiming that I must attend the meeting and there would be medicine (about 6–7 Yuan at cost) to be given away for free. Before leaving, the person repeated more than twice that during the election on the next day, I should vote for the candidates who proposed the "Suggestion of membership fee deduction", all of them. I knew what that meant in an election and was not fooled.

2) The 20th was Election Day. I accepted the invitation and went to the meeting. There really was a leaflet promoting the "Suggestion of membership fee deduction" for every single member entering the meeting room. On the leaflet it clearly listed 21 names of those who proposed the deduction of membership fees. And 21 is also the number of executive committee members to be elected. There were even some "helpers" who were distributing pencils and telling people where to copy from. I saw a lot of members copying from the leaflets according to their instructions without any hesitation. Obviously they were not aware of what they were copying and supported candidates they don't really support.

3) I talked to some others in the meeting. In fact, countless "agents" went to meet with all members to collect meeting invitations. With every meeting in-

vitation paper, they could have one more voting sheet. That was why we saw many members having some TEN voting sheets in their hands.

4) According to observation, there are two groups of people controlling the election and they are competing for executive positions. Shame on them.

5) Before the vote-counting session, I wanted to observe the counting process as a third party. It was obvious that the two parties are just about the same size. Party A had their supporters copy the 21 names of the candidates from the leaflet mentioned previously. And there were more than 200 votes with those 21 names in exactly the same order. And more than 100 votes with the 21 names without the same order. Party B had another set of candidate names with about 300 votes. In both parties, some people of high status are used to winning the election. This kind of election is a total failure.

We seek the following:

1) Check the name list mentioned previously in the leaflet promoting "suggestion of membership fee deduction". Those who vote for the exact 21 candidates in the same order should also be investigated.

2) Action should be taken against those who tried to fix the election result behind the scenes and were liable for the mess of this election.

3) The elected candidates should not be approved.

4) This election should be declared invalid. There should be another real election at another date for members to vote freely.

   i. Doctors who serve as officials: the Bureau for Native Medicine **國醫館** is definitely an academic organization. However, those who work there receive subsidies of 5000 Yuan from the government every month. Therefore they are all officials.

1. About hospitals

The so-called Chinese medicine hospitals mostly refer to charitable organizations which are part of the charity industry. There may be only one or two doctors, or as many as ten or more in each clinic. Working hours are generally from 9:00AM till noon. During these three hours, the doctors see as many as one hundred patients or even more. These doctors' working efficiency must be incredible. With hundreds of patients inside a single room, some of the patients simply cannot afford to wait. What they normally do is pay another 0.2 or 0.4 Yuan directly to the doctors so that they can skip the queue. Otherwise they might as well wait until 5 minutes to noon. As for the herbs, all clinics have their own so-called herbs department. Every prescription contains more than ten types of herbs. From time to time, there are newcomer doctors who are not experienced enough and so they forget to write the word "separated" on the prescription next to expensive herbs. (Other doctors will not do this as the herbs department can make more money by providing the expensive herbs separately.) As for the sick rooms, patients enjoy so-called caring service. I have no idea what kind of service is provided. The first- and second-class rooms cost 3–4 Yuan. Without rules as in Western medicine hospitals, the sick rooms are actually quite popular.

2. About schools

In Shanghai, we have a lot of specialized schools and institutes teaching subjects like *Huang Di Nei Jing* 黃帝內經, *Nan Jing* 難經, *Jin Gui Yao Lüe* 金匱要略, *Shang Han Lun* 傷寒論, Physiology, pathology, diagnosis… some of them even offer the *Three Character Classic of Medicine* 醫學三字經 and general education of Western medicine. They mix Chinese and Western medicines together. As for their students, they are mostly graduates or undergrads from high school or primary school. Some of them came from traditional private schools 私塾 and had never attended public schools. Some students are second generation of some medicine store owner or a famous Chinese medicine doctor. I once saw the enrollment sheet and noticed that high school graduates are only 2% of the enrollees. Successfully graduating from these medical schools are just about 99%. Professors in these schools have either learned from someone famous in classical studies or have graduated from a similar Chinese medicine school and then become famous. The only teaching materials in these schools are *Bu Ji Huang Quan Wu Xiang Jian* 不及黃泉毋相見 and *Xi Nu Ai Le Kong Bei Jing* 喜怒愛樂恐悲驚.[339]

3. About Medicine Society

The meaning of having this medicine society is to keep in touch with friends and get more membership fees from more members. Currently the field of Chinese medicine is separated from other sectors and the concept of qualifications as in other sectors does not exist. People just want to grab a title in the society as an attraction, since the people who make a good living must have fame. Since the approval of the government for this organization, it has become a hidden battlefield for power. Chinese medicine's influential figures and politicians use this place as a meeting point. In the Central Bureau for Native Medicine, any senior or junior participant is a politician and they have an air on them. In Shanghai, naturally, there is a branch. Even though the Central Bureau for Native Medicine receives a monthly subsidy of 5,000 Yuan, the Shanghai branch, being honest and exemplary, arranged that any and all uses of that money will be controlled by the branch director.

Article end

[339] Superstitious books about topics that the eye can't see and emotions.

Research on Chinese Medicine and the view of scientific evidence: Report delivered at National Member Congress of Chinese Medical Association etc.

1956 by Russian Professor B.T Vadim Gabrielevich Vogralik 華格拉立克

Source: *The New Chinese Medicine Magazine*, August 1956 新中醫藥第七卷第八期

Yaron: Here we switch to the Communist era. It is a contrast to scientification debates during the Republic; now, debates become scarce. Noteworthy is the reintroduction of Yin Yang and five elements theories justified by dialectical materialism—a completely new factor not previously seen during the Republic. This piece is written by an influential Russian professor, dispatched to China as part of a larger team, helping China find a proper path toward building a new socialist nation. Reconstructing Chinese medicine became a part of the larger reconstruction of new China.

Pages 339–341

Chinese culture is one of the oldest cultures. Mao Zedong has said, "China is the earliest civilized country in the entire world. China has had written history for almost four thousand years." (From *Selected Works of Mao Tse-tung* Volume two p.593). The description above fits Chinese medicine well. For centuries, Chinese medicine has accumulated evidence and improved upon therapeutic experience curing people. Now, it's time to do scientific research on this great treasure of wisdom.

In my opinion, in order to accomplish proper development of Chinese medicine, one requires four basic conditions shown below:

1) Correct thoughts at work
2) Correct working method
3) Correct working organization
4) Sincere and ambitious cooperation between Chinese and Western medicines

These conditions need to be assured in every phase and every aspect of Chinese medicine research. I think this research can be divided into several parts as follows:

1) Research about Chinese medicine history
2) Research about Chinese medical theory
3) Research about Chinese medical diagnostic method
4) Research about Chinese medical treatment

It is an important mission for Western medicine doctors to learn Chinese medicine so they can become the next generation of Chinese medicine doctors.

It is indisputable that the ideological foundation for this research is the most advanced, suitable to develop, and the only scientific philosophy needed—the philosophy of dialectical materialism.

It is also indisputable that, in order to research the abovementioned Chinese medicine topics, we should use the most modern, complete and accurate methods and not just clinical observations. Instead, we should also perform animal and clinical experiments.

Chinese medicine research needs organized institutions and a leading institution. I believe that there should be, in every Chinese medicine research institution, a leader who is skillful and experienced in scientific fields. This position should be reserved for professors from modern medical colleges or from science and technology institutes.

Next, I'm going to explain some issues about Chinese medicine research.

A. Research about Chinese medicine history

Researching Chinese medicine history gives us access to facts that are worthy of learning and knowing. We may be able to discover multiple inventions in ancient medicine.

Researching Chinese medicine history allows us to understand many famous Chinese doctors and scientists, their personalities and activities as well as their living and working environment. Through this information, we may understand their devotion to Chinese medicine and to worldwide medicine. Inspired by their achievement in the masses health-work, we can learn from them.

Thus far, in Chinese medicine academia, research has gone deep into Chinese medicine history, however, this Chinese medicine history research should be even more. History of any science or industry is closely related to economical, political, and cultural developments of a country, and it is also related to the masses. However, due to social environment there is often one outstanding person among the people.

When this person has some special traits, he can affect the masses. Nonetheless, people's personal lives and working conditions cannot capture the entire history of Chinese medicine.

Researching Chinese medicine history in a thorough way requires multiple aspects, of which the main parts are:

1) Deep, scientific and real analysis is necessary for unraveling the development of Chinese medicine history.
2) Division into stages of scientific development in Chinese medicine history is necessary, which should be based on socioeconomic changes rather than dynastic changes.
3) Historical materials need to be deeply analyzed. We should assess the continuous Chinese medicine history based on this and, through this, mark both people's personal impact and Chinese medicine overall impact in history.
4) We need to focus more on historical materials from recent eras in Chinese medicine history.

No doubt that the accomplishment of this research is going to facilitate the correct development of Chinese medicine history.

B. Research about Chinese Medical Theory

Chinese medical experience has proven that its basic theory is correct already since centuries ago. The theories of Yin-Yang and five elements describe the basic idea of a relationship between viscera and treatment principle. All these academic thoughts, as proven by lengthy research, include correct and advanced ideas and totally conform to the principle of dialectical materialism.

Nonetheless, it should be pointed out that these theories were recorded in ancient Chinese words, which are not easily accepted by Western medicine doctors. Even some Chinese medicine doctors treat diseases based on symptoms alone, while disregarding these theories.

Therefore, I believe that from Chinese medical theory point of view, the following basic points should be noted:

1) Chinese medical theory should be expressed with modern language in an explicit, clear and approachable way.

2) Chinese medicine ancient realizations should be explained with a modern perspective, especially the theories of Yin-Yang and five elements.

3) We should verify these theories through science and seek truth from facts. Factors changed with time and customs should be considered so we can adjust Chinese medical theory according to our time as well.

4) It is necessary to explore the classification of organs, syndromes and diseases. We should keep a fair attitude, value good ones and criticize bad ones and create new ways to develop these theories in such a way that the essence will be preserved while also fitting modern science. For example, Chinese medicine concept of an organ is not only a physical unit but also a functional unit, which is in an advanced cognition state. Furthermore, while we develop these theories, one needs to pay attention to preserving the principle of disease classification.

In short, I believe we should research Chinese medical theory more than we did in the past.

C. Research about Chinese medicine diagnostics

Everyone knows that the main diagnostic methods are as follows:

1) Question the patient about disease onset, speculated cause, initial symptoms, previous treatments and disease development.
2) Inspect patient and sometimes palpate patient's abdomen and extremities.
3) Inspect carefully patient's tongue.
4) Examine patient odor and for some cases examine patient's excrement.
5) Auscultate patient's voice and breath.
6) Take the pulse on patient's two wrists.

Taking pulse is the most meaningful among the diagnostic methods above; the other ones are just lending support.

Facts show that Chinese medicine solves diagnostic problems by using these examinations, so this diagnosis becomes the foundation for preventive treatment.

Within diagnosis there are several points warranting further attention:

1) Chinese medicine diagnostic methods require more scientific verification than before, especially the important methods such as inspection, ausculta-tion, olfaction and pulse-taking, which are often more advanced than the modern equivalents.

2) People should research the theory behind these diagnostic methods and veri-fy their correctness in practice.

3) People should enrich Chinese medicine with modern diagnostic methods and use Chinese medicine diagnostic methods in Western medical practice.

D. Research about Chinese medicine treatment

In *Huangdi Neijing* 黃帝內經 and other ancient books, some basic principles of Chinese medical treatment were already mentioned:

1) Do not use artificial things for treatment; instead use natural products.

2) All substances in nature—such as minerals, plants and animals—have curing effects. It is also effective to change the patient's lifestyle.

3) Treatment is always individualized and it should vary according to patient's specific condition.

4) Treatment should be based on disease syndrome and characteristic of symp-toms, and especially the patient's constitution. We should follow Chinese medicine treatment theory to formulate treatment. Since every syndrome and symptom has its mechanism, we therefore know that the treatment men-tioned above is the most specialized for an individual patient.

5) All treatments should be general for the entire body but also focus on specific diseases.

6) Correct treatments should not only attack disease but also strengthen the body so as to resist disease, except for some particular situations.

7) Help the patient believe in his recovery, which is very meaningful during treatment and shouldn't be overlooked.

I believe that we can establish reasonable and modern principles for Chinese medi-cal practice. These principles should serve as foundation for Chinese medicine treatment and development.

Chinese medicine treatment is currently being studied and verified scientifically in many medical institutes and special research institutes around the country. Yet their attitude and research needs to be improved. I'll provide my opinions in this aspect as follows:

1) Research should be based on modern physiology, while considering that Chinese medicine also treats through lifestyle, physical activity and diet.

2) Research done in a modern scientific way to test the physiological difference between massage, local herbal application and acupuncture by both experiments and clinical practice should determine the best condition to gain an appropriate physiological reaction.

3) All herbs within different formulas should be investigated and so should the formulas themselves with their synergetic action. Formulas should not be tested as a standard treatment for one disease, but rather with patients based on individual conditions.

4) While researching herbs' efficacy, people should not focus on a subjective clinical impression, but rather on physiological indicators.

5) People should research not only short-term effect but also long-term effect. Patient's lifestyle and labor intensity should be considered as well.

These are my opinions about Chinese medicine research and the methodology of scientific evidence; I hope they can be helpful for you.

(Translation from Russian to Chinese by Xu Wufeng 徐五鳳) (Originally published in *Jian Kang Bao* 健康報)

Article end

Chapter 4: Ideological, political and other influences shaping Chinese medicine

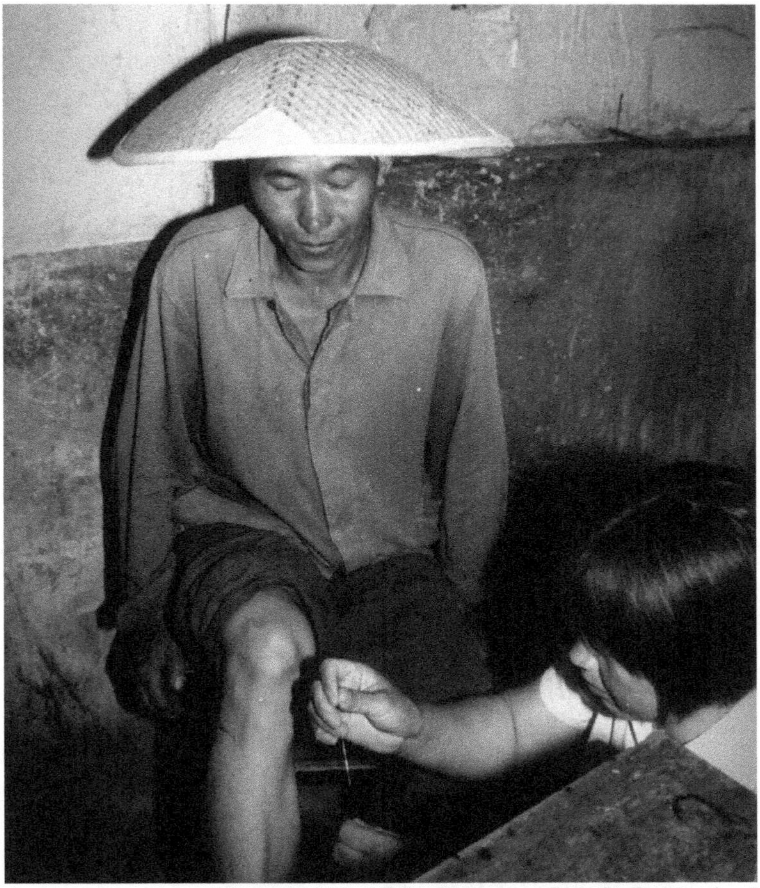

"Chinese barefoot doctor performing acupuncture" By World Health Organization, photo by D. Henrioud (http://ihm.nlm.nih.gov/images/A13744) [Attribution], via Wikimedia Commons

"We want to take the mentality and mindset of the old society and thoroughly transform it. We want to change the perceptual knowledge into rational knowledge, change secrecy into openness, eliminate the established rules, use it in an agile way, merge theory together with practice, come together with enthusiasm, resolutely struggle for it, undergo a revolution in Chinese medicine, study harder political affairs, elevate the technique level, undertake the rebuilding of our health system, fulfill the task of defending the mother nation, study the Soviet Pavlov's love of his motherland, love mankind, love the spirit of science, magnify the vision, fight for incorporating China's medicine into the world's medicine and serve the masses of the entire world."[340]

[340] *Chinese Medicine of the new China must militarize its thinking process; only then can it travel toward scientification.* 1952 by Zhao Yuqing

Work Guidance: Inspecting a few issues with one's mindset

1946 by Qi Zhonghuan 齊仲桓

Source: *The Medical Journal of Central China* (Kunmintang controlled areas)

Published on June 1st, 1946

Published By: The New Fourth Army Central China Military Region Health Department

華中醫務雜誌 第三期 新四軍華中軍區衛生部出版 一九四六年六月一號

Yaron: 1940s China is engulfed in war. First was the resistance war against Japan and then, after the end of the Second World War, came China's civil war: the Kunmintang[341] nationalists, who had just lost the support of foreign nations, fighting the Communists, who were vigorously supported by the Russians.

During that time, other than minor discussions about Western medicine merging with Chinese medicine in Yan'an or the north-west "liberated areas", the struggle between Chinese medicine and Western medicine became overshadowed by warfare. We bring the following article simply to highlight this point.

Pages 1–2

The Kunmintang diehards amassed a million soldiers encircling China's central liberated[342] area but, even after the truce, scattered attacks continued without end. The entire country is in civil war and so they are all mobilized for Jiang Kai-shek.[343] In order to resist the civil war—in order to win the civil war—we must use our hands to prepare for this war.

Since Communist policies are not the same as ours and class nature is also not the same, if Kunmintang diehards falter one day then the civil war disaster cannot be avoided for one day. Therefore, war preparation work must be calculated for the long run.

---

341 國民黨 Guo Min Dang is the modern Chinese Pinyin (Romanized letters); however, in this book we keep the old rendering as Kunmintang or KMT, the translation of which is "the nationalist party".

342 Here, "liberated" refers to liberation from the Japanese occupation, which is different from the Communists' use of the same term "liberation". The latter often refers to liberation from the Kunmintang and the foreign powers that assisted the Kunmintang.

343 We use old rendering for the Kunmintang leader's name. In modern Chinese Pinyin rendering: Jiang Jieshi 蔣介石.

We went through a long war; from the beginning of the civil war until now we had a campaign against encirclement and suppression, we repulsed the enemy's "mopping-up" campaign, we got rid of bandits from the countryside, we attacked and eradicated the enemy, we had guerilla warfare, positional warfare and mobile warfare. This gave us many health solutions that we have acquired out of experience during the war. This has also created many heroic rescuers and heroic nurses who did model work. In reality, the war taught us how to serve the fighting organizations with special techniques. In reality, the war fostered and strengthened our class consciousness and allowed us, with resolute heart, to pursue the truth. We say that the civil war broke out and because the civil war broke out we have to give even greater service. Therefore, we cannot afford to be unfamiliar with any comrade or have thoughts of avoiding personal difficulties. With a calm and cheerful manner we should welcome the task of fighting the civil war.

Specific tasks were already distributed in all sorts of meetings and assemblies; we shouldn't elaborate on them again. Here, we raise a few issues with one's mindset that need self-criticism. Inspecting for a moment the one-sidedness of medical comrades' thoughts, we see that, in each level of medical institution, there are issues to be addressed requiring further education in order to correct this one-sidedness and in order to strengthen the work. Strengthening the work of fighting the civil war, it strengthens the long-term work of social revolution.

Here, we present four not-very-honest mindsets: one is interest discussion; second is learning discussion; third is returning home discussion; and fourth the big screw discussion.

Interest discussion

For interest there are two types: one is lifestyle interest, the other is work interest. Lifestyle interest means desire to eat sour or desire to eat sweet, wear something long or something short kind of things that the person likes. Lifestyle interest must trail behind work interest. For example, participants in the resistance war were very happy with plain clothes and vegetarian diet; the ones who enter deep into the rural peasant areas were happy with the peasant lifestyle. There were many bourgeoisie and petty bourgeoisie who have participated in the liberation work, and their old and decayed lifestyle desires naturally were replaced with new lifestyle desires. To an extreme, even international friends like Norman Bethune and Andrei Orlov,[344] when they participated in China's liberation work, did not feel hardship because there was no milk and bread; to the contrary, they climbed mountains and traversed rivers, they slept in rice fields and ate coarse cereal. Contrary to the norm, they felt content because their work desire took precedence over their lifestyle desires.

Work interest can also be divided into two: small interest and big interest. Small interest is like desiring literature over martial things. Big interest is like giving one's life for the revolution. Big interest, may we say, is for the large view of life.

The small interest must follow the big interest. Often, there are people who give their life for the revolution and so they quit their jobs and their small interest. The ones who like to have a moving work do stillness work, the ones who like to be still start moving work, the ones who like the work in the front do the work in the rear, and the ones who like the work in the rear do the work in the front. Therefore, many comrades serve as small screws in the big machine, and their own interest is not important, this is because the interest of the entire machine is unified, and this matches their big interest.

There are some comrades who express their interests making an argument. They say: "my interest is like this and like that". Naturally, what they talk about is their small interests. They often raise it and it is not impossible to arrange consideration for it.

However, there are also comrades, after they put forth their small interests, they love to keep on pushing it, they talk about it to support it, they write letters to support it, they report about it to support it or even use some inappropriate negative methods to support it. Naturally, they feel indifferent to the big interest. The development of the small interest is derived from the vanishing of the big interest. It is built in the mindset of the person. The army commander Chen[345] said: "when one sacrifices his life for the revolution he undertakes to do a difficult job the best he can". This talks exactly about this point.

When the small interest conflicts with the big interest, what can we do then? Naturally, the small interest should lag behind the big interest. The big interest is to sacrifice one's life for the revolution, this one is certain. This is because our life view

[344] Two doctors that helped the Chinese during the resistance war against Japan.
[345] At the time of the resistance war against Japan, Chen Yi 陳毅 (1901–1972) was the commander of the new fourth army.

is to sacrifice our life in order to help the oppressed, in order to create a new society. Who can still doubt this? And so, these that we call small interest, we can completely give up. The personal interest of the people, if we persistently support them, they naturally influence the small part of the big job that a person is doing and so, for the revolution, if it is training soldiers, fighting the civil war or constructing the new society, this can only be detrimental. When the enemy stands in front of us, the only thing we need is a weapon in our hand. Be it a gun, a knife or a cannon, we should use all our might to tackle the enemy. We should not hesitate if we have a gun or a knife in our hands, because both knife and a gun can tackle the enemy. In our battlefield, knife and gun are both important.

Summary of the article's remaining 3 points:

1. Learning discussion talks about the need to learn hard in order to serve the revolution well.
2. Returning home discussion talks about soldiers not motivated to serve because they just think of going back home.
3. The big screw discussion talks about people hoping to do big tasks and they don't want to do little jobs. But it is important to do little jobs in order to accomplish the big task.

Article end

Yaron: The preceding article is printed by the military office of health, so naturally topics are war- and army-related. Nonetheless, it demonstrates the circumstances of the 1940s. This helps us transition through a decade-long period of chaos and into the Communist era. It is a decade when fighting between Western and Chinese medicines became utterly inappropriate and unpatriotic. Within Kunmintang and Communist controlled areas, first united against the Japanese and later fighting against each other, all doctors needed to work together to help war efforts. Following, we resume in 1952 and the Communist rule of China. Many articles in this section talk about forming TCM schools and a Chinese medicine education system, a topic similar to Chapter 2, however we include them here for their concentrated ideological influence.

Central Government of the People, Ministry of Health: About the stipulation of organizing Chinese medicine advanced studies schools and advanced classes

Source: *Beijing Chinese Medicine* (periodical), 1952 June 15th (1st volume 3rd publication), Published by Beijing Chinese Medicine Association Publication Committee
北京中醫一九五二年六月十五號 (第一卷第三期) 北京中醫學會出版委員會出版

Yaron: Below is a government directive on how to form Chinese medicine schools.

(Heading: Reprinted Articles. Glued on the page is a sticker with original date: First Announced on December 27th, 1951)

It has been a year since the scientification of Chinese medicine. Under the leadership of the Ministry of Health, local organizations all across the country, to date, include 17 Chinese medicine advanced studies schools 中醫進修學校 and, in 101 locations, advanced classes 中醫進修班 carrying different names. However, these schools and classes don't have a standard for a fixed curriculum. There are some locations where equipment does not match the content of Chinese medicine advanced studies. The graduation period is also not uniform. Some advanced studies school curricula are only 3 months long while the longest is 18 months. Amongst the advanced classes, the shortest curriculum is only a few weeks. In order to unify the standard of organization and curricula of different Chinese medicine advanced studies schools and advanced studies classes, this topic has made its way through the National Medical Labor Conference, State Administrative Council and State Culture and Education Committee. The following was decided:

Chinese medicine advanced studies schools and Chinese medicine classes should have the following differences:

1) Chinese medicine advanced studies schools should have the character of a proper school. It must meet a minimum standard for equipment, like a school building, laboratory facilities, practical teaching rooms, dissecting room etc. Students must finish the length of schooling and curriculum, which is 12 months, and then they can start practicing. Because of this, Chinese medicine advanced studies schools must merge with local, relatively large, hospitals or medical schools so they can utilize their equipment.

2) Chinese medicine advanced classes should be run by local people and subsidized by the state. Initially, teaching materials' requirement need not be very high. The class can mobilize the energy of the masses and gradually be supplemented with teaching materials. Schooling length should be fixed at 6 months and, according to necessity, shorter periods can also be used (3 months) for specialty classes. For example, preventive medicine class, acupuncture and moxibustion research class, first aid class can be divided into sections and studied separately. This will help bring these graduates to the graduation level of the Chinese medicine advanced studies schools.

The methods of organizing Chinese medicine advanced studies schools and advanced studies classes are as follows:

1) Forming an organic structure. A Chinese medicine advanced studies school should have its own organic structure. However, it is a pity that teachers are all qualified to teach in the regular medical schools. From equipment point of view, it is also a pity that they rely heavily on medical schools. It is best for its foundation studies department to gradually hold its own. Curriculum should include, as a rule, preventive medicine, foundations, clinical studies and social sciences. Study term should be divided into two semesters, each semester 6 months long (432 hours), with graduation taking place after 12 months. The curriculum's first part should focus on foundation studies, while the latter part should incorporate foundational studies with clinical studies, emphasizing especially practical measures. What we fixed above as a 12-month schooling term may agilely be adjusted according to each locality's necessity and need. In general, the objective of advanced studies is to end up as a Chinese medicine worker. It should accept all people selected and dispatched by local administrative regions to help them become doctors. Rules should be established for students' entry examination, registration, checking in, semester exam etc education administration management items. In order to accommodate the working life of Chinese medicine doctors, classes can take place on half days or during free time. In order to practice the new democracy, the students can form students' associations. In addition to the State-run organizations, Chinese medicine advanced classes should be organized by the masses of Chinese medicine doctors. Each region's Ministry of Health should lend full support and assistance in qualifying teachers for the job. The curriculum content (aside from preventive medicine and specialty classes)

should include foundation studies, clinical studies and social sciences. Schooling term can be divided into two terms, each term 3 months long (159 hours), with graduation taking place after 6 months. Preventive medicine class, acupuncture and moxibustion class and first aid class can all be set up as specialty classes, each lasting 3 months (87 hours).

2) Curriculum standard. The curriculum of Chinese medicine advanced studies schools includes the following four categories: foundational studies (includes dissection, physiology, pathology, history of medicine, pharmacology, bacteriology, parasitology); preventive medicine studies (includes public hygiene, infectious diseases); clinical diagnostic and treatment skills (includes internal and external medicine, first aid, acupuncture and moxibustion therapy, tissue therapy); and social studies (includes the historical development of society, the new democracy treatise, current affairs reports). These four categories can be combined and instructed in an agile way. The following three points need attention:

   a) First, a clear thinking process of "serving the people" must be established. While advancing the social sciences curriculum, one must carry out the policy of "preventative is the main thing" and thoroughly teach preventive medicine. At the same time, accompany the movement of "resisting America and helping Korea" and instruct in first aid and rescue studies. For guarding each locality's epidemics, one can insert relevant classes.

   b) The Chinese medicine cultural level is untidy, the ability to receive science is not uniform; therefore, teaching materials and instruction must follow a planned out and drafted teaching. Following the principle of making things popular and fitting to current reality.

   c) Curriculum and instruction must merge theory with reality, experiments and practical application. These need to be knitted tightly together in order to reach the objective of "study in order to apply".

Chinese medicine advanced classes curriculum will include the following three categories: foundational studies (includes dissection, physiology, pathology, bacteriology, pharmacology and diagnostics); clinical studies (includes internal and external medicine, pediatrics, ophthalmology etc specialized departments); and social studies (includes social development history).

Preventive medicine specialty classes will focus on infectious diseases and preventive inoculation methods.

Acupuncture and moxibustion research specialty classes will focus on the new acupuncture teachings and instruction, as well as simplified foundational studies (includes dissection, physiology, pathology, bacteriology and sterilization).

First aid classes will focus on rescue and first aid as well the study of simplified foundation (includes dissection and bacteriology).

The advanced studies classes and specialty classes should also pay attention to the three points (above) mentioned for advanced studies schools.

3) Instruction methods. Teaching of Chinese medicine should incorporate and criticize the experience of old Chinese medicine. Simultaneously, students should be encouraged to develop new points of view and new methods. Therefore, instruction should focus on foundational studies merged together with clinical diagnostics in order to adapt to current needs. In addition, after class is over and there is leisure time, concrete questions about Chinese medicine's old theories should bring about a discussion, in order to stimulate the enthusiasm for learning science.

Additionally, as for instruction methods, one hopes that theory can be implemented while merged together with physical reality (one may use graphs and tables, models, material objects demonstration or printed materials to supplement deficiencies) in order to accomplish hearing, seeing and doing all done together.

When explaining content, one should do one's best to be vivid in order to help listeners become clear about the objective of practicability. One should do one's best to talk only in technical terms (however, basic terminology should become clear to them).

Printed materials can tentatively be set as dictation notes, which may help the listeners' concentration. However, during each instruction, one can hand out the general outline.

The above instruction methods can be used by both Chinese medicine advanced studies schools and Chinese medicine advanced studies classes.

Article end

Central Government of the People, Ministry of Health: An instruction how to organize Chinese medicine associations

Source: *Beijing Chinese Medicine* (periodical), 1952 June 15th (1st volume 3rd publication)

Yaron: This government directive demonstrates how government influenced the shaping of Chinese medicine education and what people were allowed to teach and think. Most importantly it shows the close relationship between Chinese medicine professional activity and political education, without which one could not become qualified to practice.

(Glued on the paper is an updated date of "First Announced on December 27th, 1951")

In order to strengthen the merging of Chinese and Western medicines and advance the scientification of Chinese medicine, each locality should establish a Chinese medicine sciences group of the masses. For this, we have specially drafted "how to organize a Chinese medicine association" as follows:

1) Name and characteristics: Chinese medicine associations should form under the leadership of the People's Government Ministry of Health varied organizations, in order to advance merging of Chinese and Western medicines, organize advanced studies and elevate the level of Chinese medicine. An association should form in order to fit the needs of the people. They should organize in order to serve the people of each locality and the masses. Therefore, the association name should first reflect the locality name. Association members may be Western medicine doctors. They can also mobilize qualified members to take part in local Ministry of Health and health labor associations.

2) Tasks and objectives: The foremost task of Chinese medicine associations is to advance Chinese medicine scientification and closely integrate Chinese and Western medicines. Therefore, a Chinese medicine association should be a bridge closing the gap between Western and Chinese medicines. It should follow the Chinese medicine advanced studies leadership and organizations. Other than that, it should abide by the overall directives of the Ministry of Health and Labor, mobilizing its members to participate in our nation's

building of public health. In addition, it bears the responsibility to research and advance Chinese medicine sciences.

3) Organization style and methods: According to different circumstances in each locality, there may be the following three different organization styles:

   a) Under direct leadership of Ministry of Health local branch, organized as a Western and Chinese medicine unity, like Beijing Chinese Medicine Association.

   b) Merging together several groups originally having different Chinese medicine character, adopting and smoothing differences during the organization process, like Shanghai Chinese Medicine Association.

   c) First undergo extensive study of Chinese medicine political affairs, ferment preparations for relatively long period of time and then gradually organize, like Guangzhou Chinese Medicine Association.

The above three organization styles should conform to the leadership and, for optimum results, simultaneously study in advance the different styles. Other than that, according to each individual case, the following documents: *Draft of Chinese Medicine Association Statutes* and *Draft of Democratic Rights of the Association* should be approved by the Ministry of Civil Affairs and Ministry of Health local branches, then be mastered thoroughly, adopted and implemented.

Association members can be divided into two types: Proper member (one who has a local license to practice the profession of Chinese medicine); or expectant member (one who researched Chinese medicine for many years, but didn't attain yet the proper qualifications). Selecting people with outstanding character, who are treasured by the masses, is the backbone of the association. When accepting new members, newcomers should go through elementary study and careful observations and, at the same time, be persuaded against keeping secrets and suspicion of advancement. This will prevent the phenomenon of "being closed and guarded".

The association should take care of its members' study time and living conditions and should give additional help to its members, preparing them to improve their skills and their political affairs education level. This will, in turn, allow them to attain qualifications more easily.

Article end

Beijing Chinese Medicine Association campaign against the Three:[346] An inspiring report by the assistant director Zhang Wenqi 張文奇

1952 by Zhang Wenqi 張文奇

Source: *Beijing Chinese Medicine* (periodical), 1952 June 15th (1st volume 3rd publication)

Yaron: The government altered the doctors' thinking process, in line with socialism, and impacted the practice of medicine. Doctors could not practice what they thought was right, but only what was told to them is right. If, in the past, a Chinese medicine doctor had prescribed expensive herbs or large doses of herbs, from this point on he could no longer, at least not without risking public prosecution and humiliation.

Pages 5–6

Published on January 28th, 1952

Gentlemen, the campaign opposing corruption, waste and bureaucratism is unfolding everywhere enthusiastically! Some people understand this campaign well, but there are some people who don't understand it 100%. These people who don't understand it 100% think: "for people who practice medicine, where is there corruption?" They think: "the clinic is their own, it provides their own livelihood, what kind of waste is there?" They think: "myself, I am not an official, where is the need to talk about bureaucratism?" Therefore, the ones who think that the campaign opposing the Three has nothing to do with them, view it with ignorance.

The campaign opposing the Three is a grand affair which is very important. It is a grand affair closely connected to every single person. Who wants to view it ignorantly? Who wants to commit this offense of their understanding? Why do I say it? We must talk a bit about the campaign opposing the Three.

Why do we want to unfold a campaign opposing the Three?

After liberation, workers, peasants and soldiers became politically conscious and much improved. With current production equipment, they practice "increase production while economizing". They increased the production level, which was entirely possible.

[346] "The Three" refers to three evil things: corruption, waste and bureaucratism.

However, here we come to a problem. If one thinks of increasing production while economizing, he must first eradicate corruption, waste and bureaucratism. If you can't eradicate these three things, then you can't reach to an increased production while economizing. Instead, you can only harm China's industrialization.

We often hear: "we must make China a prosperous country." How can we make China prosperous? One very important work is to materialize our nation's industrialization. The result of China becoming industrialized is having our own machines, increasing our production—then the people's life will drastically improve. Our national defense will drastically strengthen. Only like this can we become a prosperous China.

Here, there is a precondition. If we want to industrialize our nation, we must first accumulate resources. Capitalist and imperialist nations use a method of exploiting the people in order to collect revenue. We oppose these methods. Therefore, these are methods that we ourselves cannot utilize. Socialist nations, like the Soviet Union, use economizing (saving) methods in order to accumulate revenue. We ourselves welcome these kinds of methods. Therefore we can practice them. As a result, only by vigorously practicing saving that leads to accumulated revenue, can we materialize the possibility of our nation industrializing. However, if corruption, waste and bureaucratism exist, it becomes an obstacle for economizing, which also becomes the enemy of our nation's industrialization. If we don't do away with corruption, waste and bureaucratism then China cannot become industrialized. Then there is no guarantee for the nation's prosperity. Like that, there will be the danger of "the Party vanishing and the nation losing its independence".

The idea of the campaign opposing the Three is so grand. Can it be that we, colleagues of the medical service circle, should fall outside of this campaign? I think that we should not. It would be a mistake.

When we practice medicine, can there be corruption, waste and bureaucratism? If we think it over carefully, not only do these exist, they exist abundantly. For example, if using immoral methods I take someone's property and make it my own. This is considered an act of corruption. So let's inspect it for a moment—is there this kind of action? According to my knowledge, some gave bribes to get licensure. Making fake certificates, this happened already. In order to profit more from the patient's money, treatment got prolonged and number of sessions increased, one sees these cases too. To an extreme, cheating the patient with fancy words, not caring about the patient getting well or not, so long as one pockets the money. These kinds of methods, cheating people out of their money—is it any different from an unscrupulous merchant fabricating receipts, bribing, seeking large profits or cutting corners in workmanship?

If, for example, we say, "what shouldn't be used is used,"[347] or "what should be used scarcely is used a lot," isn't this much wasting? If we can use Gypsum Shi Gao 石膏 to lower fever, then why use rhinoceros horn Xi Jiao 犀角[348] to eliminate fever? In herbal formulas, why is there a need to add some "precious" herbs? Why take the herb Che Qian Zi 車前子 and write in the prescription as Pie Yi 芣苡[349] and cause the patient to do extra leg work? Can it be that wasting money and time like this is not an expression of waste?

Now, when we talk about bureaucratism, it mainly talks about not caring for the masses. Of course, for doctors, "the masses" are mainly the patients. How is our level of caring for patients? Is it already 100% caring for them? This is worth self-reflection and criticism. Truly, there are ones who are impatient with their patients. Some dislike when patients talk a lot, some are sloppy and diagnose the patient incorrectly. Some find doctors who then shift responsibility on to them. This kind of shirking from responsibility, isn't this an expression of bureaucratism?

Therefore, it does not matter if the scope is of the entire nation or just in the medical circles—the campaign of opposing the Three needs to unfold. More so, it must unfold. How to unfold the campaign opposing the Three?

It is mainly by developing the mindset of doctors, improving their self-realization, and then tying it to current reality, allowing them to be courageous with eliminating their own mistake of corruption, waste and bureaucratism. At the same time, with great courage, they should report to authorities other peoples' mistake of corruption, waste and bureaucratism. One should take this campaign of opposing the Three and view it as an extremely serious war. He should participate in this campaign with great courage and determination. After going through the tests of this campaign, he should attack corruption, waste and bureaucratism in an unyielding fashion. Only like this can this campaign unfold in a positive way and yield good result.

I believe that after we, in the medical circles, will go through this campaign, we can form a new prevailing spirit. Everyone will elevate a level in their mindset. I wish all of you that with this campaign you will gain a great victory!

Article end

[347] Using herbs that are not needed, or using large doses instead of small.

[348] Using expensive herbs instead of cheap ones.

[349] Che Qian Zi 車前子 is seed of Asiatic Plantain; in the very ancient Book of Poetry (ca. 1000 BC), this herb is named Pie Yi 芣苡. The question posed here is why use ancient names nobody recognizes anymore, just causing the patient aggravation that they need to find out for themselves what the herb is.

A short introduction to Beijing Chinese medicine circles' campaign opposing the Three.

Source: *Beijing Chinese Medicine* (periodical), 1952 June 15th (1st volume 3rd publication)

Yaron: Beijing Chinese Medicine Association's response to the previous article, explaining in detail how exactly they implemented the campaign against the Three. Not only the few reported criminals mentioned in this article, but every single person felt threatened. What transpired then and how it influenced the minds of all Chinese medicine practitioners we should carefully contemplate.

Pages 6–7

Following Chairman Mao's call, Beijing Chinese medicine circles excitedly put forth the campaign opposing the Three. This unprecedented grand campaign caused every single person to elevate their thinking process one level. A brief introduction to how it was implemented is introduced here.

1) The steps and methods of implementing it.

   a) Members and inspiration. On January 28th, Beijing Chinese Medicine Association invited Beijing's office of public health assistant director Zhang Wenqi 張文奇. At Beijing's merged medicine hall, he gave an inspiring report (see the previous article). The focal point revolved around the importance of the campaign opposing the Three for medical workers. The members of 81 small groups (totaling more than one thousand members) immediately resolved to study the inspirational report, research and discuss it and, thereafter, put together all pertaining important articles and successively study them. These included Chairman Mao's treatise on opposing corruption and waste and Comrade Bo Yibo's[350] report on the campaign of opposing the Three. Political affairs study, normally required in every region by the Department of Health, should be carried out simultaneously by groups divided into Chinese medicine groups and Western medicine groups. This will allow comrades to elevate their understanding capacity to

[350] Bo Yibo 薄一波 was an important politician and member of the politburo during that time. He was later jailed for over a decade, charged for being a traitor during the Cultural Revolution, then later on reinstated to power by Deng Xiaoping. An influential politician during the 1980s and 1990s, he helped his son, Bo Xilai 薄熙來, rise to power and become the party secretary of Chongqing municipality (recently, in 2013, Xilai was accused of corruption and removed from power).

said magnitude of this grand campaign. Members who study or serve in advanced studies schools should likewise study it simultaneously.

a. Put forth examination of common problems. Chinese medicine association regulatory committee, starting with the committee head completing his own self-criticism, will draft explanatory outline for common problems, mainly within the scope of corruption, waste, bureaucratism, unlawful actions and exaggerated publicity. They should draft detailed rules and regulations, allowing the comrades, according to the spirit of the draft outline, easily to self-criticize. The outline should be as follows:

I. Corruption:

1. Herbal medicine shop kickbacks.
2. Increase in visit fees.
3. Accepting gifts from herbal shops.
4. Make up prescriptions for the patient in order to make money.
5. Make false report about free numbers.[351]
6. Any other improper ways of making money off of the patients' backs.

II. Waste:

1. Using unnecessary expensive herbs.
2. Writing prescriptions with alternative herbs' names.[352]
3. Prolonging treatment course.
4. Extravagantly wasting while attaching importance to external appearance.

III. Bureaucratism:

1. Unnecessary emergency treatment.
2. Shifting responsibility.

---

[351] When a patient comes to the clinic they take a number and wait their turn. When a patient gets a number, the clinic can report it for reimbursement unless the patient should receive free treatment. Here, the clinic reports free treatment as a reimbursable ticket.

[352] Which confuses the patient and causes him to do extra work to find out which herb it may be.

3. Not caring about the patient's time.
4. Not sympathizing with the patient's pains. Not inspecting carefully severe ailments.
5. Giving out a prescription without even seeing the patient.
6. Not recording carefully the patient's case.
7. Making oneself grand, attacking others in order to elevate oneself.

IV. Unlawful acts:

1. Use or sell drugs.
2. Broker.
3. Trade in gold.
4. Organize gambling or take a cut from gambling winning.
5. Unrestrained conduct regarding male-female affairs.
6. Induce abortions or teach how to induce abortions.
7. Forge certificates or credentials.
8. Sell fake certificates or credentials, certificates of injections, vaccination certificates.
9. Give bribe to get a certificate.

V. Others:

1. When buying herbs not issue and paste a receipt with a stamp (to avoid paying taxes).
2. Listen to the patient and write an increased sum of money (encourage corruption).
3. Ask the patient to make a public announcement thanking him, or hang leaflet announcing advertisement.
4. Post a sign outside guaranteeing a cure and ensuring recovery (exaggerated publicity).

b. Making confessions and reporting offenders. After the members were all inspired, they became clear about the policy. Integrated with current reality, they entered deep and examined. Self-confessions and reporting other offenders type of reports came in from small groups, one after the other, to the association regulatory committee. Some also brought them in by themselves. The regulatory committee, in compliance with the rules, inspected them all and categorized and numbered them, summarized them together and submitted a report to Beijing public health office. From beginning to end, the scope of this report included over 200 documents.

2) The benefits gained from the campaign.

   a) The issue of fake certificates, breaking the law and deceiving the government. The task of medical workers is to protect the people's health. However, in the past, there were those who didn't follow the law. Only caring about making money, they didn't care about the danger lurking for people's lives. They had the audacity to sell fake certificates. Through this learning process, they were all reported. The most notable example of these was from the prior[353] Beijing Native Medicine College 北京國醫學院, education administration director Kong Zhonghua 孔中華. After liberation, he has sold fake certificates, presumably of the old Beijing Native Medicine College, deceived the government and broke the law. Unfolding the campaign of opposing the Three and gathering reports of offenders by association members, after initial calculation, he has sold nearly 50 fake certificates. (Each certificate for circa 300,000 to 1 million cash). This kind of Chinese medicine doctor, scum of the community, invoked resentment of the entire Chinese medicine community. One after the other, asking the government to punish him severely according to the law. Kong Zhonghua also wrote a confession and even surrendered with it the counterfeit certificate mold, seal etc. And so the Chinese medicine association took all the reports of the offender about counterfeit certificates, confession statements, and also Kong Zhonghua's own confession statement, all the equipment and literature and surrendered it to the Office of Public Health to handle. At present and according to the law, Kong Zhonghua was arrested. The ones who purchased fake certificates were also individually investigated by the Public Security Bureau. At the same time, many association members reported offenders in Tianjin, forging certificates from the China Native Medicine[354] School 中國國醫學校 and

[353] Prior to Communist liberation.

[354] Chinese medicine was called "Native Medicine" Guo Yi 國醫 before the Communist takeover in 1949.

Tianjin Native Medicine College 天津國醫學院. These two kinds of fake certificates were sold relatively cheaply and their distribution was rather wide. Amongst them, there are fake disorderly introductory certificates made by swindlers and there are those which were fixed at a high price and sold by mail correspondence and even had the official seal of northern Liaoning province stamped on at the time of certification. All kinds of odd documents were collected from beginning to end and handed over to the Office of Public Health to act upon after ascertaining the facts. One document that was handed over was even an abstract sample with a form to fill in.

b) Commonly exposing poor quality style of work. About those whose style of work is of poor quality, it is like the idiom "ugly form appears in droves". They guarantee a cure and promise recovery. They hire a person to stand in the vicinity of the hospital and lure patients in. Some don't understand the principle of medicine, some are unlicensed, they combine herbs to make a sudden huge profit, turn a profit of over 900 folds over cost. Some who practice without a license extort patients, some perform abortions, some trade in gold. All the aforementioned cases were also handed over to the Bureau for handling.

c) Truly realize and correct the bureaucratic style of work. Average doctors—and especially those who were famous doctors—benefiting from special dignity in the past, allowed themselves ostentation and extravagance and, to an extreme, even put on airs. They really could not have the attitude of serving the people wholeheartedly. Now, through this education, they became clear about their past mistakes. They all did a profound and thorough self-criticism.

d) Other aspects. During this campaign, historical problems needed further explanation, even the most trivial corruption and waste. For example, receiving gifts, intentionally prescribing expensive herbs and causing the patient uncalled-for loss etc. They were all categorized and reported to the Bureau or kept on record by the association. The organized medical association became also an inspection organization. It is now in the process of inspecting all items.

In summary, our Chinese medicine community's "opposing the Three campaign" truly and earnestly brought about enlightenment. Each person sincerely handed over his self-confession and educated himself hard. The old famous doctors Xiao Longyou 蕭龍友, Luo Zhiyuan 羅止園, Zhu Weinian 諸位年, even though advanced in age, also enthusiastically participated in the small groups' self-criticism discussions. Emotions were rather high; famous doctors like Shi Jinmo 施今墨 etc also earnestly and thoroughly performed self-inspection, which then served as an example for others. We cannot but acknowledge that this was a special advancement. Through a struggle in every aspect, the foundation level was overall elevated. We must consolidate this victorious accomplishment and continue to develop further. We need to allow every single medical worker to go through this campaign. Eliminate the degenerate bourgeois mindset. Cast aside the heavy millstone around one's neck of stench dragging him down. Happy and relaxed, walk toward the pure and bright future of serving the people.

Article end

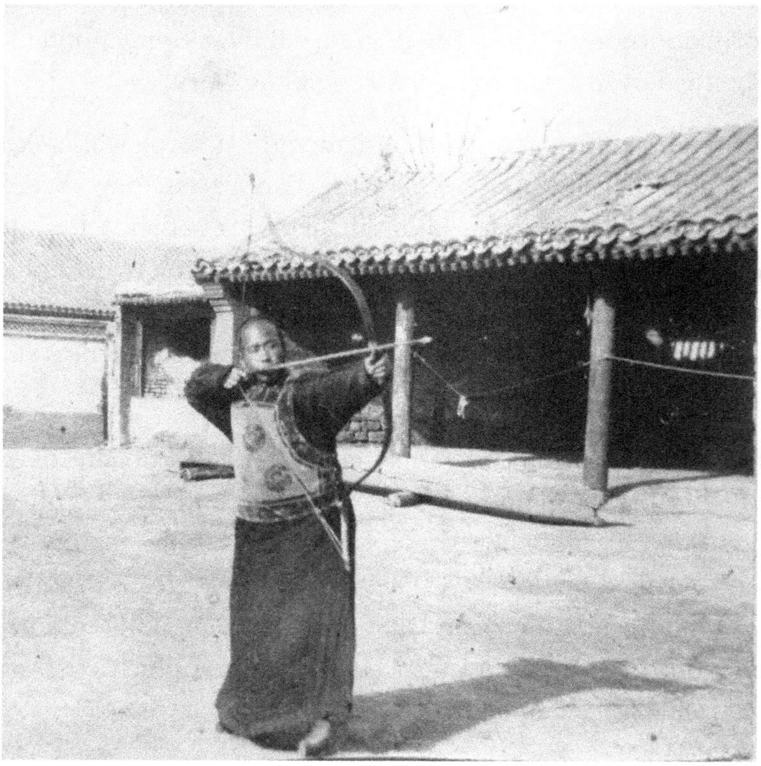

Photo by Mr P. Goux in early 1900s. "Chinese man shooting his bow".

Chinese Medicine of the new China must militarize its thinking process; only then can it travel toward scientification

1952 by Zhao Yuqing 趙玉青

Source: *Beijing Chinese Medicine* (periodical), 1952 June 15th (1st volume 3rd publication)

Yaron: This article, with point 3 carrying our book's title, is important. The uncertain times reveal a delicate balance between what is and isn't allowed for Chinese medicine as it transforms into TCM. Bouncing back and forth with uncertainty is in the hearts of all practitioners at that time. Western medicine belongs to imperialists, is it allowed? Chinese medicine belongs to the feudal society, can we use it? Should we change it? Should we keep it? This uncertainty and fear is at the root of forming TCM. There is no debate here, there is fear!

Pages 11–14

Chinese medicine scientification must start by altering the thinking process using Marxism, Leninism and Mao Zedong thinking to militarize our own thinking. Using dialectical materialism point of view to research, criticize and analyze the quintessence of our nation's medicine. Grouping together the ancients' experience of medicine and, in a systematic fashion, arranging it in an orderly way. What needs to be developed should be developed; what needs to be preserved should be preserved; what needs to be deleted and revised should be deleted and revised. Only the quintessence should be left, with all the dregs removed. The medical science of the past used all kinds of names and phrases and formulas; they should all be clarified. Turning it into a modernized medical science of China, following the principle of development. It must have a scientific view, a revolutionary spirit—only like this can it open up a very promising future.

We want to stand firm the position of the Chinese people, develop and correct the precious scientific heritage that our ancestors left for us and look out for our workers, peasants, soldiers and the masses. We oppose imperialism, feudalist influences, bureaucratic capitalism, merchant's class, and all others who are not good for the people. All remnants obstructing scientific studies, we should resolutely fight against them.

Medical science includes two kinds: preventive and treatment. It is an important art of preserving health. It is a kind belonging to natural sciences. Medical science coming from Western Europe is called "Western medicine"; our nation's own medical science is called "Chinese medicine". (Japanese medicine is called "Kampo"—Han Chinese style of medicine). No matter if it is Western medicine or Chinese medicine, they all are for the people wanting to guard against and treat disease. Their objective is one and the same. Why do some say that Chinese medicine is not scientific? I narrate the following few points to explain this:

1) Chinese medicine theory is not uniform

Chinese medicine of antiquity is shamanistic. Starting from the Qin and Han dynasties, Chinese medicine has Yin Yang and five phases. After the Song dynasty, Chinese medicine started incorporating natural sciences. And so, in the past, Chinese medicine came out of self-study, from examination for public service, from friend teachers, or from secret transmission, or study at home from the elders, or from reading books and self-realizing things, or from private people teaching others as students. There were no proper schools and teaching materials. No opportunity for a concentrated study. Everyone followed their own teacher within different schools of thought. They could not unify into one research and therefore could also not attain any real advancement. Some studied at very high level, while others studied at an inferior level. And so there were different designations like Confucian scholar-doctor, famous doctor, doctor of the time, city doctor, charlatan doctor. To an extreme, it became all spiritual-like; they took the true spirit of medical science and, in the void, lost it (this is my own impolite self-criticism). During the nationalist era, even though there was a small number of privately owned Chinese medicine schools and specialty classes schools, most were established in an uncontrolled fashion. They did not receive political help or unified teaching materials, and so the theory was still not uniform.

The outline of the six conformations in the *Shang Han Lun* 傷寒論 is a formulation of disease pathology. It takes pathology, diagnosis, pharmacology and prescriptions and mixes them all together. The principle is profound but the text is very mysterious because, at that time, there were no scientific instruments to help out and diagnosis explanation leaned towards Qi transformation. There was no way to do laboratory tests. There was no way to see pathogens and so Yin Yang took over describing a disease advancing or retreating. Hypothetically speaking, if Zhang Zhongjing 張仲景 had lived after the invention of the microscope, he would have developed much more and his contribution would have been even greater.

Chinese medicine principle is scientific. Chinese medicine of later generations had true accomplishment in reaching a certain standard of medical science. However, there were Chinese medicine doctors who didn't attain mastery, who passed something sham as real, who made up things as they went along. They were those who had the fame of Chinese doctors but not the substance. Not only could they not merge with the newer theories, they also didn't understand the quintessence of the old theories. Their technique and theory could not merge. And so now, everybody is saying that Chinese medicine is not scientific. However, people of antiquity and present are the same. If not scientific, how could they have solved problems? It is because they couldn't ascertain the real cause that people today say it is not scientific. Nonetheless, in treatment they had their strong points and they also had their shortcomings. If one says that a single doctor could resolve all diseases then this must be a false claim. These kinds of empty claims, such as one being a divine doctor or a divine acupuncturist, are uncalled for. However, the spirit of the entire thing is precious.

Zhu, the commander in chief,[355] said, "If it has an effect, it is scientific. Acupuncture and moxibustion have scientific value." Japanese scholars like Yumoto Kyūshin 湯本求真, Asada 淺田 and Hara Shimetarō 原志免太郎 etc[356] all researched our nation's medicine and pharmacology and made commentaries on the *Shang Han Lun*. They realized that Chinese medicine and pharmacology is great and worth researching. Their works were many and, at the same time, they established acupuncture and moxibustion schools and colleges and studied it seriously. French scholars also paid special attention to acupuncture and moxibustion therapy. They revered China's art of acupuncture and moxibustion. One can see that our nation's medicine has scientific value. It should be researched further, thoroughly arranged and its advancement sought.

2) Chinese medicine was under political pressure during the different dynasties

The earliest history of Chinese medicine was created by laboring people, trying to preserve their own health and fight against diseases. They created treatment methods like stone needles, acupuncture and moxibustion, massage, herbs and formulas etc, within which, imperceptibly, they incorporated natural laws and chemistry principles. One sees that China's earlier people were very clever. However, these

---

[355] Zhu De 朱德, the commander in chief of the Red Army in the resistance fighting against the Japanese.

[356] Yumoto Kyūshin (1876–1941) was considered the pioneer of current Kampo pharmacology in Japan during the Meiji and Taishou eras. Asada Souhaku (1815–1894) was a scholar of Kampo medicine during Meiji period and was the personal physician of the Tokugawa Shogun. Hara Shimetarō (1882–1991) was well known for his use of okyuu (moxibustion), especially its effect on the immune system. He used moxa on himself from the age of 40 for over 60 years. Also considered the "Sage of anti-aging." Footnote source: Jeffrey and Yumiko Zurawin.

kind of model laborers were covered up; throughout history there were very few records of them. What is the reason for that? It is because, following from earlier society, feudal influences exercised oppression. History belonged to the emperor's genealogy. Therefore, it is said, "Reading books should be sold to the emperor's family." It is, truly, why what the vast masses discovered was not transmitted down. Only the monarch, ministers and officials had alleged accomplishments. Only with these people was it taken into consideration and viewed with importance. For example, acupuncture and moxibustion were created by the working people but, intentionally, it was said that they were created by the Yellow Emperor and Qibo.[357] The people, however, started researching it because when the emperor and minister recommend it, then it has value. Only then can it be transmitted down. Here, one can consider the *Inner Canon*[358] documents.

One can tell that the Inner Canon was written by working people during the Qin and Han 秦漢 dynasties. This document does not have "unpronounceable words"; it contains exclusively language from the Qin and Han. Compared to the *Book of Historical Documents Shu Jing* 書經, it is much easier to read. This is a proof that this work was produced by the working people of the Qin and Han. So how can anyone say that it is a Yellow Emperor composition? Everybody knows China's cultural development. The Yellow Emperor is considered to be the originator and, because he attacked the mythological Chi You 蚩尤, discovered the compass and created cloths and caps, he held the spirit of research for medicine as well as abundant other things. But if one wants to claim that the Inner Canon was written by the Yellow Emperor, then it is a mistake.

So if it was not written by the Yellow Emperor, then who is the anonymous writer? Of course, it was the hard toil of the working people. Why don't they introduce themselves? It is because the words of the lowly carry no significance. Wanting to transmit their art, they needed to use the Yellow Emperor and Qibo, the monarch and the minister, in order to compete for the people's belief. They also wanted to commemorate the spirit of the Yellow Emperor and become the unknown heroes. Looking at the corpus of the *Neijing* 內經, it seems that it was compiled by various people. The content is complex and was certainly not the work of one single person. It was written by the accumulated experience of the working masses.

---

[357] One of the legendary ministers of the Yellow Emperor.

[358] *The Yellow Emperor Inner Canon Huang Di Neijing* 黃帝內經

According to Chinese medicine history, the end of the Zhou was the golden era of this art development. It is when the hundred scholars flourished. Every scientific society and natural science has its sprouting era. After medicine became ready and harmonious, there were great physicians appearing one after the other like Bian Que 扁鵲 and Cang Gong 倉公 etc famous doctors. Therefore, during the Han dynasty, medical sciences flourished. Zhang Ji, from the eastern Han, assembled medical science of his time and became a medical sage. He composed the *Shang Han Jin Gui* 傷寒金匱[359] books, which are of excellent standard up to present day. Hua Tuo's 華佗 surgery and ability to dissect may serve as a representative model. Therefore, with great courage, we can say that the *Neijing* is a work created during the Qin 秦 and Han 漢.

Ancient China emphasized medical politics and, less so, medical schooling. There was no medical school equipment but there was a medical official who served the nobility. He didn't serve the masses. The term "medical officials" is seen first in the book *The Rites of Zhou* 周禮. Transmitted down through dynasties, there were such designations as the imperial physician Taiyi 太醫, imperial physician assistant Taiyi Cheng 太醫丞, serving doctor Shiyi 侍醫, imperial court doctor Yuyi 御醫 and doctor literati Yishi 醫士. There was also the organization of an imperial college, all established to serve the nobility class, the capitalist class. They were not meant to serve the masses.

Qin Shihuang 秦始皇, the first emperor of Qin who burnt books and buried scholars, Emperor Wu 漢武帝 of the Han, revering Confucianism and banning other scholars, all restrained the people's minds and obstructed the art's advancement. Even though they always wanted to prolong their own life and rule the people forever and they sought alchemists and skilled doctors, yet they always placed the medical arts in a dark cave of superstition. They lost the scientific value and could never advance. Since medicine and natural sciences are very closely related, naturally if science falls back then how can medicine advance? What kind of equipment can it use? With what can it experiment? They could only rely on experience and the naked eye to formulate their diagnosis and treatment. Therefore, they extinguished the vigorous development that took place at the end of Zhou dynasty and exercised a policy of keeping the people ignorant. These two emperors carry the responsibility for this autocracy. Next to that, when Cao Cao 曹操 killed the physician Hua Tuo 華佗, it inflicted great damage on the medical circles. Because the person was killed, his

[359] *Cold Injuries Treatise* and *Summary Treatise of Golden Casket Shang Han Lun* 傷寒論 and *Jin Gui Yao Lüe* 金匱要略.

books burnt and his art lost, then Chinese medicine remained without a surgery department. What a great misfortune!

During Wei 魏 and Jin 晉 dynasties, even though there were works and annotations by Huang Fumi 黃甫謐, Tao Hongjing 陶弘景, Ge Hong 葛洪 etc explaining their own compilations, they still didn't break out from the same old stuff. After the invasion of China by northern nomads in the fifth century, medicine was transmitted in a secretive way.

Sun Simiao 孫思邈, of the Tang dynasty, followed the spirit of Nan Yang 南陽, and compiled the book *Essential Formulas for Emergencies [Worth] a Thousand Pieces of Gold Beiji Qian Jin Yao Fang* 備急千金要方. Tradition says that he attained the secret prescriptions of Long Gong 龍宮 dragon palace. The name Long 龍 dragon was not a superstitious dragon spirit kind of "Long" but, rather, the "Long" from a place name Wo Long Gang 臥龍崗 (where Zhongjing resided).[360] He attained secret recipes of Zhang Ji 張機,[361] which impacted the resurgence of medicine during the Tang dynasty. Wang Tao 王燾 also received medical science from abroad and compiled the book *Secret Measures as Written Outside the Ministry Wai Tai Mi Yao* 外台秘要. The materials within these were rich. It is a pity that, since the Tang, medicine was influenced by Buddhism and Daoism and the practicability of the theory became less and less. It became an empty cave of guesswork and lost its scientific meaning.

From the Song 宋 dynasty onward, Yin Yang 陰陽 and Five Phases 五行 theories were widespread. Medicine was influenced by Confucian philosophy. It accumulated speculative philosophical ox horns. It became close to illusory. It divided into different categories, which gave birth to different schools, each school having its own persons and theories. It took different forms, holding different opinions under the same roof, which caused people not to know which one to follow.

In the Ming dynasty, persons such as Li Shizhen 李時珍 and Yang Jizhou 楊繼洲 carried on the spirit of medicine. They compiled books and had their sayings and, for that, spent great toil. Yet they couldn't lead in a new direction nor revolutionize the new. Their contribution to medicine starts and ends with a compiling and arranging work.

The Manchus of the Qing 清 dynasty, who controlled China, encouraged literary inquisition. They restrained Chinese people's thoughts and freedom. Since the

[360] Wo Long Gang 臥龍崗 is in Nan Yang 南陽 city, Henan 河南 province.

[361] Zhang Ji 張機 was another name of Zhang Zhongjing 張仲景.

Opium war, foreign imperialists entered and influenced their policy. The entire population was under the oppression of a feudal society. The spirit of studies could hardly be developed. Even though there was one work, *Golden Mirror of Medicine Yi Zong Jin Jian* 醫宗金鑒, which emphasized textual research, even so, one cannot find a new direction within. Wang Qingren 王清任 compiled *Correcting Mistakes of the Medical Community Yi Lin Gai Cuo* 醫林改錯 and emphasized dissection studies. Despite his spirit to develop a new direction, and because he didn't have the right instruments, he couldn't succeed.

At that time, under conditions of poor and backward China, divided and ruled by joint sovereignty, the Chinese people were called the sick people of East Asia. Not only could they not raise their heads to resist the foreigners, but they also lost their self-trust. They took their own skill and sunk it a thousand measures. Our medicine—acupuncture, moxibustion, pharmacology—was streaming eastward to Japan. It was given importance by the Japanese who viewed it as a treasure and, with great vigor, carried it on. European wind and American rain[362] used the invasion power of capitalism and imperialism to expand and reach China. Their medicine, following the capitalist expansion, also developed. Their medicine advanced very quickly. When they came to China, it served as an invasion tool, enticing the masses' belief. Because of this, their medicine entered China first. At that time, the Chinese people were ruled by a numb and corrupted government. The people of China became valueless. How could have China's art raised its head!

After the 1911 revolution, Sun Zhongshan 孫中山 advocated developing the inherited arts. China's dying art of Chinese medicine became alive again. However, because the revolution was led by the bourgeoisie, it couldn't complete its revolution. After the death of Mr. Sun, the bandit Jiang 蔣[363] assumed great power in his hands and used anti-revolutionary measures to suppress the Chinese people. He used a nominal attention to play with Chinese medicine. He used, for his benefit, the entire group of Chinese medicine practitioners.

Our Chinese medicine fellows went around campaigning for our cause. They went on a struggle for our art and organized themselves as a group. Their proposed schools came and went, the schools would not go on record at the Education Department, their hospitals would not go on record with the Ministry of Health. What

---

[362] Western cultural influences.

[363] Jiang Jieshi 蔣介石, also known as Chiang Kai Shek, took over the leadership of the KMT (Guo Mindang 國民黨) after Sun Yatsen's 孫中山 passing, later becoming the president of the Republic until its overthrow by the Communists in 1949.

kind of oppression did Chinese medicine receive! Because of this, the 317 Chinese medicine movement formed.[364] The great traitor, Wang Jingwei 汪精衛,[365] not only wanted to sell the motherland but he also advocated extinguishing Chinese medicine. At this time, Chinese medicine was, truly, like an orphan without a mother. The state of the art[366] was precarious, and its standing was in no position to improve. Therefore, it became open to all kinds of occupation. Not to be pessimistic, just stating it from a professional point of view. The entire preceding historical narrative demonstrates the extent of oppression and destruction to which, over time, Chinese medicine was subjected.

During the anti-Japanese resistance days, many of China's big cities became Japanese colonies. Another part of China was used by the imperialists as a semi-colony and semi-feudal society, like in the southwest and northwest sections of the country. One section was our own resisting-the-Japanese base area, the liberated area. Most of this area harbored poor and out-of-the-way villages in the mountains. It was the masses of the Chinese people. They all needed us. Our existence was all due to the need of the people for us to exist. We are here for serving the masses of the people. We are closest to peoples' old-time sufferings and the fact is that we were always like this.

3) The liberation of Chinese medicine

After the establishment of the People's Republic of China, under the leadership of the brilliant leader chairman Mao, the three grand health policies were put forth: Chinese and Western medicine must unite; prevention is the focus; and gearing towards workers, peasants and soldiers.

Chinese medicine advanced studies schools and specialty advanced classes were established. These remolded Chinese medicine and cultivated Chinese medicine. Other Chinese medicine research organizations were also established. They researched Chinese medicine and, at last, Chinese medicine could free itself. It stripped itself from the feudal smelting and from the capitalist shackles. It strode towards the great path of a scientific new China, a scientific medicine.

We want to take the mentality and mindset of the old society and thoroughly transform it. We want to change the perceptual knowledge into rational knowledge,

[364] In February 27th 1929, a measure was offered during the First Health Workers Conference to abolish Chinese medicine altogether and replace it with modern medicine. On March 17th 1929, there was a fierce fight-back by Chinese medicine doctors and associations against this measure. 317 stands for March 17th.

[365] Wang was the president of the puppet government installed by the Japanese during their occupation of eastern China.

[366] The Chinese medicine art.

change secrecy into openness, eliminate the established rules, use it in an agile way, merge theory together with practice, come together with enthusiasm, resolutely struggle for it, undergo a revolution in Chinese medicine, study harder political affairs, elevate the technique level, undertake the rebuilding of our health system, fulfill the task of defending the mother nation, study the Soviet Pavlov's love of his motherland, love mankind, love the spirit of science, magnify the vision, fight for incorporating China's medicine into the world's medicine and serve the masses of the entire world.

4) Performing well the work of coming together

At present, everyone is after true principle; everything is done for the benefit of the people. Medicine is an art aiming to preserve people's health. It is not separated by country borders. Each emphasizes its strong aspect in order to serve the people. Everybody is enthusiastic about the same health objective. There should not be visible separate doorways for Chinese and Western—be it seeing, tapping, listening and feeling, or seeing, hearing asking and palpating,[367] scientific instruments, laboratory tests diagnosis—Chinese and Western medicine both should use it. Each brings forth its strong point. Whichever way has benefit for the people is the way to do it. The principle is "whatever fits the people's needs". Western medicine should adopt a "masses" character, a China character. Chinese medicine should become scientific and modern. Since Western medicine is the product of capitalist society, while Chinese medicine is the product of a feudal society, each has its deficiencies. The first and the latter both need be corrected and straightened up. They should help each other and collaborate. They are all part of the motherland, and together will build the new medicine of the new China. Pavlov[368] said, "Scientists are not divided by national borders, but they do have a motherland." Therefore, we must perform properly the merging of Chinese and Western medicines; only then will it be right for the people.

The people of the entire world are of the same heart; they walk the same path. Everybody forges ahead towards an accurate path. The work of medical service should learn the new materialism. Western medicine should not be divided into the

[367] The first four are Western diagnostics; the latter four are Chinese diagnostic methods.

[368] Ivan Petrovich Pavlov (1849–1936), a great Russian scientist, Nobel prize winner in 1904 for his research on the nervous system reflexes and the relationship of the cerebral cortex to the organism's environment. His discoveries led to great breakthroughs in modern medicine. An official document, signed by Lenin on January 24, 1921, stated: "The outstanding scientific services of Academician I.P. Pavlov, which are of enormous significance to the working class of the whole world".

American Anglo school or German school.[369] Chinese medicine, even more so, should not be divided into febrile disease school, cold and cool school, southern and northern schools, ancient and modern schools. The scientific principle is all-encompassing; it has no branches.

When it comes to unifying the theory of Chinese medicine, one must compile standardized teaching materials. This should be divided into foundational studies and clinical studies. Use textbooks to systemize it, treasuring the Chinese and consulting the Western. Be it in schools, self-study or examinations, this should be the standard for everyone. This will allow every single person studying Chinese medicine to not slave over the books. At the same time, they will not receive poisonous transmissions, where they attain no results and even harm the people's health. They should also, however, not forget their roots or lose their self-confidence. Standing foot with the motherland, they should not lose the essence of Chinese medicine.

This work is easily described with words but extremely difficult to do. It requires the revolutionary spirit in order to overcome these difficulties. The large wheel of social development is propelling forward. After China's victory of liberation and the upcoming success of establishing the new democracy, then socialism will come, communism will come. We have already leaped out of the darkness towards the light. We should ourselves become clear, teach ourselves, correct our thinking, study Marxism and Leninism and Mao Zedong thinking, arm our own mindset, vigorously study, not hold a purely technical point of view, not embrace businessism, not be impacted by foreign language restraints. We must enrich the theory, elevate the technique, participate in advanced studies, utilize scientific instruments, recognize pathogens,[370] focus on preventive medicine and promote "the highest doctor's approach is to treat the disease before it has formed". We should gear it towards the workers, peasants and soldiers. Not repeating the times of backwardness, instead we stand firm with the proletariat and eliminate the bourgeois mindset. We want to reform vigorously under the banner of Chairman Mao, undertake the revolutionary task and together build new China.

Article end

[369] In the first half of the 20th century, Western medicine physicians were divided according to the school they attended; more prominent were the German, English and Japanese schools. Their literature was in different foreign languages.

[370] Here referring to Western medicine pathogens like viruses and bacteria.

Introduction to initial steps of organizing Chinese and Western medicine United Clinics

1952 by Wei Longxiang 魏龍驤

Source: *Beijing Chinese Medicine* (periodical), 1952 June 15th (1st volume 3rd publication)

Yaron: Several articles about the United Clinics, where Western and Chinese medicines are forced together and optimal results are expected. Merging a scientific Chinese medicine and Western medicine for the masses created a hybrid, a foundation for TCM.

1) United Clinics are a newly-formed organization

In April 1951, in the Central Ministry of Health announcement during the national health conference titled *The decision about the relationship between the private and public medical and pharmacological healthcare*, the third item stated the following: "Medical organizations should give adequate support and guidance to an alliance with private doctors. They should mobilize all medical workers to arrange an alliance with hospitals or united clinics. They should become assistants of the public health organizations." In July of the same year, the People's Central Government State Administrative Council issued a directive supplementing national defense construction with help from health workers. It stated, "Because of the harsh reality, when it comes to private medical workers who cannot help the construction of national defense or participate in public health organizations, each local health organization, at their discretion, should assist them to participate in forming united medical organizations. Help them bring to play an even greater medical impact." The problems highlighted by the above two directives point to the current state of affairs around the country and, specifically, instruct the solution thereof.

Ever since the great campaign of "resisting America, helping Korea and defending the motherland" started, medical workers from the entire nation leaped with enthusiasm and participated in it. Especially after the State Administrative Council has issued the directive supplementing national defense construction with help from health workers, one branch of medical workers did participate in the construction of national defense. Another branch of Chinese and Western medicine medical workers, following the appeal of the government, began organizing Chinese and Western medicine United Clinics. This also fits the current needs for national production and defense construction. This is to say that United Clinics utilize current manpower and material resources and economically bring them together into play, with whatever else is viable to supplement it. They reinforce the "here and now" of healthcare organization work. From another perspective, they also highlight past weaknesses where every private health worker was on his own. Private health workers were like scattered sand. Weak and forceless, they could not serve well the workers, peasants and soldiers. Today, under the banner of Chairman Mao, we don't separate Chinese and Western medical doctors. Everybody is united together. From individualism going toward collectivism, with a face gazing toward the people, medical work of new China now assumes a new direction.

Following the appeal for making Chinese medicine scientific and Western medicine for the masses, and through the mutual learning between Chinese and Western medicines, everybody elevated their political enlightenment and technical skills. Especially after the mass style of learning Chinese medicine in the advanced studies classes, people refigured their own new path how to take this new practical medical knowledge of preventive and treatment work and put it into practice in a scientific way. This required initiatives advancing even more the merge with Western medicine. While studying and helping each other, they established a foundation for correcting each other and coming together. Because of this, Chinese and Western medicine United Clinics fit the people's needs. They relieve people's suffering and practically materialize coming together of Chinese and Western medicines. It is an organization that better serves the people in our new democratic society.

In recent years, in relatively developed areas like in the north eastern cities of Benxi 本溪, Harbin 哈爾濱, Shen Yang 沈陽 etc, because of the revolution's development, Chinese and Western medicines style United Clinics and hospitals sprang first. In addition, in northern China Tai Yuan 太原 city and in the center-south Wuhan 武漢 city there were first signs of United Clinics early on. But especially following the promulgation of the Central Ministry of Health directive, directing to organize United Clinics, and without even counting in the entire country all of them, in the spring of 1952 there were 1672 United Clinics, the majority of which were organized by Chinese medicine doctors.

In the capitol in the spring of 1951, under the direct guidance of the Central Ministry of Health, using the enthusiastic effort of fresh graduates from Beijing Chinese

Medicine Advanced Studies School, four Chinese and Western medicine United Clinics were established. After gaining experience and serving as a model for others, 21 United Clinics were created within one year. With such rapid development, they created the capitol's medical circle's new atmosphere. Medical doctors stemming out of China's 2000-year-old feudal society—and the last hundred years of half-feudal half-colonialized society, especially ones who followed the never-changing way of Chinese medicine secrecy—broke away from the old habits they previously immersed themselves in, and with vigor entered the new style of United Clinics. This abundantly demonstrated that the time for a grand transformation has come.

In the capitol, during the graduation ceremony of the Beijing Chinese Medicine Advanced Studies School, Chinese medicine doctors sang with high spirit the school's song "Wherever the People Need Us That Is Where We Shall Go". More than half of the students went to the outskirts to establish United Clinics. It was evident that they realized that only wholeheartedly serving the people is the highest honor. Since their political understanding increased, they resolutely followed the Government's calling, and so their one and only hope was to relieve the sufferings of the people. No wonder that, when comrade Li Qinghua 李慶華 from eastern China Ministry of Health, visited Beijing's United Clinics, he witnessed how passionately they serve. Western and Chinese medicine doctors seemed like members of one family congregating together. With distinct admiration he said, "It is no wonder that such a high level political product emerges right here at the feet of Chairman Mao."

Normally each United Clinic has its own progress; however, when compared to a private doctor's clinic, it has more equipment and more specialization and it concentrates more ability. In addition, since Western and Chinese medicine exchange their experience with diagnosis, it improves the art and changes the overall style of work. It reinforces the collectivity, merging together and creativity. More so, for assisting preventive work and local sanitation work, they are very useful. From medical treatment point of view, they relieve much pressure from public medical facilities. Since they gear towards workers and peasants and have established relationships with surrounding factories, they therefore offer a convenient treatment option for workers and farmers, establishing a foundation for a regional system of job responsibility.[371] This testifies to the correctness of the Government's calling and also increases trustworthiness of United Clinics. The United Clinics today, still in a sprout-

[371] Job responsibility means the workers need to be taken care of.

ing stage, are not 100% fully established and with still few deficiencies; after all, they are a new kind of organization. However, the people embrace them and the Government supports them. Now, since they practice it already in several localities then they should practice it everywhere around the country. Its guaranteed future, with no doubt, will follow the law of development. It will propagate daily and vigorously to become grand.

2) A few fundamental problems with one's recognition

Chinese and Western medicine United Clinics are a creation never seen before in history, breaking new ground. With its scarce experience fumbling around, it should match exactly reality requirements and attain anticipated result. Therefore, at its initial stages of organization, if the basic spirit is not mastered, then its posture will seemingly be such yet its substance will not. It will fundamentally take on a different form and the wrong turn. And so the following few points must be contemplated carefully:

a) The character problem: It should mainly express the collectivity force. It should divide work into specializations. It should supplement the physical condition by having more equipment in order to increase treatment efficacy. Because of this, it has a fundamentally different character from a traditional herbal store. For example, in Baoding 保定 city, as the United Clinic was organizing, local druggists immediately drew in local doctors in order to remonstrate with the local Ministry of Health office, attempting to sanction the establishment of a pharmacy.[372] They attempted an opposition. Since we, as well, are responding to the Government's calling, how is this not allowed? In addition, half-public local health clinics, run by the commune hospitals' administrations, which have cooperative style yet the masses have to pay for medicine, are all different from United Clinics. Because United Clinics, under the Government's guidance, have the doctors themselves raise funds and be self-sufficient. Their joint-venture medical organization is self-managed. So to say, this is one of the social welfare projects that are part of the new democracy economy. It is entirely different from the common profit-seeking commerce.

b) The task problem: First, one should be responsible for the people. When medical technology and equipment are inadequate, then patients must be referred out to state public health facilities. This gives patients a complete

[372] In the United Clinic.

guarantee. One must change the old attitude that even when not knowing, he must appear to be knowing and when he can't cure it, then he must refer to a famous doctor that can. The old style of doing things must be cast away. Only then can a United Clinic become an assistant to State public health facilities. In addition, treatment should be combined with preventive care. It breaks the norm of only using medicine for treatment. It takes the initiative to the masses; it guards the people's health within the locality. United Clinics should accept free numbers[373] and help the government promote preventive and sanitation work. They should establish a trusted medical relationship with collectivized factories and schools. They must gradually establish a foundation for a system of job responsibility for every area and sector.

c) The objective of this service and regional distribution: Since care is geared for workers and peasants, therefore concentration of doctors in the city center is not the objective of United Clinics. Under correct guidance and planning, and according to local needs, emphasis should be placed on distribution to areas where workers and peasants live and lack of medical care and drugs exists. For example, in Shanghai's new city district, there is a concentration of doctors and, therefore, the United Clinic there did not develop well. Its impact in that location was very small.

d) The problem of scientification: When Chinese doctors establish a United Clinic, in a locality that has good conditions, it is best that the core doctors will be graduates from advanced studies classes. Thereafter, they should also recruit other Chinese medicine doctors and seek Western doctors and midwives. For diagnosis, they should use thermometer and stethoscope. From testing point of view, they should perform blood and urine tests. If equipment is lacking, they should utilize State public health facilities to arrive at a scientific diagnosis. If they still use old-style Chinese medicine diagnosis, it is then inadequate scientification of Chinese medicine. Nor can one thoroughly have the spirit of preventive medicine. For example, in the north east district in a summary given by Tie Xi 鐵西 Chinese Medicine United Clinic, the Chinese medicine doctors exclaimed that their knowledge of science is inadequate.

[373] As mentioned in a prior footnote, patients get a ticket with a number on it and wait their turn for treatment. The clinic receives payment for the ticket from the patient or from the government. In this case they should give five tickets for free, without reimbursement, or basically provide free healthcare.

3) Undertake an effective mobilization work

The first work of leadership is mobilization work. Normally, other than masses' conferences, giving reports and inspiring, small group discussions etc mobilization strategies, which allow the masses to have a clear cut understanding of the United Clinics, the key for success or failure of mobilization lies with being able to get through to the people's minds and relieve their worries. From leadership standpoint, one first needs to supplement, in people's minds, what practicing medicine means. Then analyze it and put forth whatever problems exist. Thereafter, persuade and educate how the mobilization tackles those problems. Like this, it comes from the masses and goes back to the masses; like this, it chimes in easily. This kind of mobilization does not fail. In its progression path there are very few obstacles. From mindset point of view there are the following few situations:

a) Professional work and skill: Ones that are very professional and have high skill level can easily hesitate, worried that others in the United Clinic will benefit from being associated with them. They, themselves, will suffer as they share the clinic with inferior skill doctors, and together they will lose their own reputation. On the opposite end, ones who have low skill level are afraid to pale by comparison. In addition, there are those who have learned from their ancestors and are afraid that, in the United Clinic, they will have to reveal their secret recipes, which will break their metal bowl of rice. These issues should all be thoroughly explained, in order to remove all the different heroic postures of feeling oneself arrogant, explosive, renounced, inferior etc. selfish and narrow points of view.

b) Lifestyle issue: One is afraid that, when uniting in the clinic, his lifestyle will be restrained. He will not have the freedom as when he opens his own enterprise. A person has himself many expenses; what if, in the middle of it, the family will collapse—what should he do? The leadership needs to explain that, in collective organization, everybody is helping each other. The power to do this is great. The profession develops and the field of vision expands. Naturally, this inspires their courage.

c) Uniting Chinese and Western medicines: Normally, in the counties and villages surrounding the city, the concentration of Chinese medicine doctors is more than Western medicine doctors. Therefore, adopting an organization style of Chinese and Western merged medicine is the best. During mobilization, need to emphasize the impression that Chinese medicine is scientific and Western medicine is for the masses. This can only materialize when Chinese and Western medicines unite. In addition, if mobilizing Western medicine doctors, who do not partake in State public health facilities, they may participate in United Clinics half-days or full days. They can help Chinese medicine doctors with diagnosis and treatment.

d) Doctors leaving the city: Doctors from the city are used to life in the city and are unwilling to go to villages to organize United Clinics. The leadership needs to emphasize that, after the villages' land reform,[374] lifestyle level gradually increases and the future is bright. The cities' propertied class[375] declines with each passing day. It[376] is not the objective of modern day medical service. It is not worthy to keep on longing for. What a glory it is to take the skill and offer it to the workers, enlighten their political thinking process and self-recognition. In addition, one needs to show them real examples of United Clinics in villages that have already succeeded. Ones who still resist going to the villages will immediately change their minds and solidify their trust. For example, when establishing the first United Clinic in Beijing's suburbs, some of the Chinese medicine doctors said: we left the city and we were not doing good business anymore. We hurried to the desolate outskirts of the city, and suffered from cold and hunger. From morning to evening we walked hungry, but after several months the United Clinic prospered, then the others all struggled to reach first the Ministry of Health office and apply for registration. They got worried that later on they will have no spot left for them.

4) One must first resolve several factors

After mobilization has reached to the minds of people and got rid of old notions, a large number of activists will spring forth without difficulty. The leadership needs to seize upon the activists, weigh their motives, and select for them what to do first, allowing them to become pioneers. Through meetings, undertake preparatory work and further express the mass character of creativity and enthusiasm. The leadership

[374] During the first years after liberation, there was a massive land reform in the country side, seizing lands from landlords and distributing it to poor farmers. Decades later, it was revealed that these land reform campaigns were a destructive mobilization of the people to a class warfare and bloodshed. For more on this topic, see *The Tragedy of Liberation* by Frank Dikotter.

[375] Urban doctors.

[376] Being an urban doctor.

should assist and guide from the sidelines and, even better, if one cadre will personally participate, specifically offering solutions to the following few factors:

a) Human affairs factor: a United Clinic's organizing members, a very important factor, should have a personal and deep relationship with the personnel rallying together and developing; they should resolve and make good all personal matters. This mainly includes:

    1. Establish a foundation for everyone's wish to voluntarily unite and create an atmosphere for everyone's motivation to cooperate. This means that one must open the gate wide and not guard things that are only close to him. It should not be like a small coterie[377] that you can see outside. But it can also not be like push and pull crowding it, each with a different opinion. If you force its merging than it will lead to gradual breakup.

    2. Through a democratic process, a virtuous and talented leader should be elected. His authority should be clearly defined and he should have a clear understanding of the masses. In addition, duties should be assigned and medical treatment and administrative tasks allotted. Each should exhaust his ability in different ways in establishing the united clinic.

b) Capital factor: Strive for doctors who have accumulated a lot and can contribute a lot of capital. Like in Xuancheng city in southern Wan 皖南宣城,[378] the second district doctor, Jiang Jianwu 江健吾, voluntarily donated ten million Yuan. He resolved completely the problem of raising funds for that clinic. Most doctors, however, have medicine as their trade and what they accumulate is not much; the best is that each will invest according to shares. Average what you gather together and each needs to get at least one share. The ones who contribute more will get more shares. At the same time, to the maximum extent, do not recruit external shareholders in order to avoid working capital strife. In addition, herbs contributed can be evaluated in terms of money and acquire shares. If the economic viability is lacking, one can also ask for government aid. Like, for example, the United Clinic in Matou township in Huai Yin 淮陰碼頭鎮[379]—they received a government subsidy of two

[377] A small group of people that gather together to share their own common interest.
[378] Wan is another name for Anhui province.
[379] Jiangsu province.

million Yuan, while the county hospital sent 600,000 Yuan. In addition, Western doctors contributed Western drugs in exchange for shares. Its total funds raised reached four million Yuan.

c) The physical building factor: These clinics are geared towards workers' and peasants' areas. Because of being at the city outskirts and industrial areas, building or renting a building is difficult. This can be solved as follows:

    1. In a village. One can utilize a house or a public temple that was not confiscated and already redistributed during the land reform. This can be accomplished with the approval and help of the local government.

    2. While advancing propaganda to the masses about the United Clinic, it should be explained to them that this clinic is for serving the people and not for private profit. The masses can be relied upon to open up or rent out a space for this clinic.

    3. In addition, at times of renovation, one should be content with whatever is available. Try to save on every aspect and avoid extravagance and waste. At the same time, establish attitude towards labor; encourage, to the extreme possible, that everyone will partake in the work.

d) Herbs and drugs factor: In a big city there are many pharmaceutical factories, so large United Clinics like in the northeast in Shen Yang 沈陽 and Fu Shun 撫順 can have a large-scale joint venture with pharmaceutical dispensaries. However, in villages and suburban remote districts, pharmaceuticals are in short supply. Therefore, one needs to establish his own pharmacy. The solution used by Beijing United Clinic can be adopted:

    1. Promote collaboration with herbal shops. For example, the United Clinics of Yong Dingmen 永定們 and Guang Anmen 廣安門 set up a collaboration with the traditional herb shop Xi He Nian Tang 西鶴年堂. In the clinic they established a supply station, while the tax burden was carried by the herbal shop. This way a hope was given to farmers to get genuine medicine at a fair price. The United Clinic takes the pharmacy to the village and develops this trade there.

    2. Provide a small pharmacy for oneself: With herbals, there is no need to stock up a lot—just provide for common applications. Buy and sell for

low price so as to avoid exploitation of herbal trade and reduce the burden from the masses. For example, Beijing's Hai Dian 海甸 and De Shengmen 德勝門 United Clinics are like members of the same family. Since there were few doctors with prior experience in herbal dispensing, they took over this task. In addition, they recruited a pharmacist trainee and since they didn't sell outside prescriptions, their profit was adequate. They could also enjoy a tax-free status from the government.

3. Western drugs are expensive and purchasing them is difficult. The government can lend some drugs. Borrowing and returning drugs can help circulate capital.

e) The factor of medical equipment and instruments: From Chinese medicine perspective, there is not much problem; from Western medicine perspective, one can give shares to Western doctors and midwives in exchange for equipment evaluated for their cost. As for tables, chairs and furniture, everybody can use their own first and then gradually buy additional furniture and take back what they brought. This will help offset startup costs.

f) The name factor: Because United Clinics gradually establish a local system of job responsibility, the purpose of the name is unlike a few clinics in Wuhan city 武漢市 which named themselves "The Masses", "Benefiting the Masses" and "The Common People United Clinics". It fits the reality better to use names like that of Beijing clinics of Yong Dingmen, Hai Dian[380] etc.

Other than that, while going through the regular procedures of registering the clinic, setting up the proper connection with tax authorities etc issues, the leadership can lend a hand in solving all these problems and, thereupon, the operation of the clinic can commence.

5) The results of Beijing Chinese and Western medicine united clinics

Chinese and Western medicine United Clinics conform to the objective of making Chinese medicine scientific and making Western medicine for the masses. A relatively simple Chinese and Western medicine United Clinic has to meet the people's needs. The results of a Chinese and Western United Clinic are as follows:

[380] These are names of local districts in Beijing.

a) Chinese and Western medicine merge from work standpoint. In Chinese medicine in the past, there was constant mutual suspicion and jealousy. This has changed direction to become mutually beneficial as it gradually helps unifying differences within Chinese medicine theory of different schools. For example, Chinese medicine doctors from the United Clinics of Yong Dingmen, Hai Dian, Xi Zhimen 西直門 etc were, in the past, disciples of the so-called "great four doctors" but now they all write similar prescriptions, with no difference treating patients. Doing diagnosis from both Chinese and Western medicine can much more easily resolve the vast problem of treating people's diseases while randomly dispensing medicine. For example: rapid diagnosis and treatment of acute infectious diseases; acupuncture treatment of chronic diseases; surgery and sterilization for external injuries; and accurate diagnosis of internal diseases in a scientific way while using proven effective herbals for it. These methods can be measured by the true principle of science and their experience exchanged, their validity proven or disqualified and, like this, Chinese and Western medicine advance together toward treating diseases and saving people. It reaches the objective of preserving the people's health.

b) Becoming an assistant to the State public health medical facilities. When Chinese and Western medicine unite, they enrich the new diagnostic methods and they bring into play the old accumulated experience. Prevention and treatment merged together helps resolve the lacking of public health organizations not being able to handle the workload of patients.

c) Women and children get guaranteed care. Western medicine gynecology and midwifery can help Chinese medicine gynecology inaccuracies. Because of this, the safety of women and children is guaranteed. This avoids accidents during labor and child bearing.

d) Chinese herbals are improving. For a doctor to master herbs, not only should he simplify the formulas to fit reality, but also should change the old habit of prescribing many herbs, which is wasteful. He should also create effective pills and powders, like Fu Chengmen 阜城門 United Clinic, which took all the efficacious decoctions and reformulated powders out of them. San Jiadian 三家店 United Clinic used refined herbs of Xingqun 星群 brand and replaced their decoction of raw herbs in order to make it more convenient for patients. The quality of those herbs also increased a lot.

According to the four United Clinics in the suburbs of Beijing, the treatment statistical results of a single month are as follows:

Total patients	1,921	
Workers	295	or 15.41%
Peasants	266	or 13.85%
Soldiers, policemen and cadres	121	or 6.3%
Students	88	or 4.58%
Businessmen	152	or 7.91%
Children	458	or 23.84%
Together workers and peasants	540	or 28.11%

In the suburbs, United Clinics are close to industrial districts and so it is easy to create medical relationships with the workers. From an objective need of current reality, in order to benefit the farmers' economic situation, they offer free numbers[381] (the city's Ministry of Health office helps the free numbers by allowing 5 lb. rice each). They also give preferential treatment to workers and half-price off. Everybody can gain experience from that.

From the above statistics, one can see that Chinese and Western United Clinics are gearing towards the peasants and workers.

Chinese and Western medicine United Clinics also take the policy of "prevention comes first" and thoroughly put it into practice. Like Yong Dingmen United Clinic, during the summer months and in order to prevent an epidemic, divided the clinic's ten doctors into groups. One of the groups assisted the number 9 factory clinic to complete Yong Dingmen neighborhood vaccinations of 1200 people. Another group went to the outskirts of Liu Li, Chengshou temple 六里以外承壽寺 region, and assisted the southern district local sanitary clinic, completing vaccination of three elementary schools and six administrative villages, with a total 1700 people. The Hai Dian United Clinic vaccinated 850 people in the local township during the summer in their epidemic prevention efforts.

381 Free treatment.

Since they are geared towards workers and they receive lower fees, and since Chinese and Western medicine are in joint effort, they resolve many problems for the people. For example, De Shengmen United Clinic is viewed by the masses as a small hospital. Nan Yuan United Clinic 南苑聯合診所 successfully treated the wife of the village head and cured her long-unresolved menstrual problems; therefore, the village head wrote a letter to the Ministry of Health commending them. This kind of new organization gave to the masses a good impression for both Chinese and Western medicines. After the four United Clinics were established, the Central Ministry of Health came to visit and inspect. They listened to local Ministry of Health representatives, local government officials, and representatives on the street, women and children all praising the clinics. As one can see, they received the welcome of the people and, thereupon, their trade developed. Like in Beijing's Hai Dian, every day they get 50 to 80 patients and between eight and nine out-referrals. Their income, not including expenses, can reach a remuneration of 500 lb. rice for each doctor. At work, everyone is in high spirits. They certainly realized that it's only by serving the people that one can receive the great benefit of the people. Everybody can march together toward the reward.

Setting up this kind of an exemplary model inspires Chinese and Western medicine doctors, one after the other, to organize United Clinics. Talking specifically about Beijing, within less than one year, all in areas outside the city, there is not one without a new united clinic being established. To the farthest, it reaches more than 10 Li[382] outside of the city, to Ci Yun temple 慈雲寺, Nan Yuan 南苑, Qing He 清河, before and after Qing Long bridge 青龍橋 etc 13 small villages and towns where united clinics have organized. By the end of 1951, more than 21 united clinics have established already, with more than 230 members. According to initial calculations, patients seen in these clinics reached 72,820. In preventive measures, people receiving vaccinations have reached 28,000. This demonstrates that the United Clinic development in Beijing is flourishing and it also shows that the force of "coming together and unite" yields a new kind of achievement.

6) How to strengthen and develop

This new kind of organization, a "United Clinic", working in a strange area, how can it develop? How can it gain popular trust? How can it overcome difficulties?

[382] About 5 km.

How can it solve all these different problems? These relate directly to the strengthening and developing of a United Clinic. How to strengthen and develop? We put forth the following few points:

a) The first is lifestyle issue: Right at the founding of the clinic, for a period of time it is not easy to quickly have a large base of people. It is hard to have professional work develop immediately. Most of the organizing members use this establishment for their livelihood. A few doctors have accumulations but themselves need to support their families, which often wavers their conviction in the most basic glory (of serving the people). In Beijing there are two kinds of solutions that one can utilize:

    1. Doctors that have the masses' trust should be the core. This is a beneficial aspect for expediting the development process. For example, in Beijing Hai Dian United Clinic, the director Zhu Boquan 祝伯權 is a local famous doctor. On the first day that they opened for business, the patients all crammed to get in and the reception welcome was flawless. The reason is that all the villagers heard that Dr. Zhu had expanded his clinic, and that there are more doctors now. Because of this, each doctor's pay has reached 500 lb. of rice.[383] The doctors organizing the United Clinic in a distance of more than ten Li outside the city immediately had their livelihood needs met and so they could serve with a calm heart.

    2. Practice half-days at home seeing patients and half-days at the United Clinic. Like Beijing Yong Dingmen United Clinic, doctors see patients half-days at home in the city in order to support their livelihood, and half-days outside the city to serve. In addition, a few doctors with no familial obligations should be sought after and allowed to live in the Clinic. Give them livelihood subsidiary payments and so there will be attending doctors in the Clinic day and night. Like this, using half-days work and simultaneously caring for one's family and gradually pacing toward specialization, one can say that it may succeed in becoming a model example.

    The above two methods have their deficiencies. In the first solution above, when patients come to see the doctor, the ones who were busy before are now busier and the ones who were idle are now more idle. For the second so-

[383] During the initial years of the PRC, local currency had no value so people were paid with grains and other goods.

lution, if the distance is far between the United Clinic in the suburb and the private clinic inside the city, there is no professional conflict. But if it is in a small city and the distance is near, then it does not work. In Baoding 保定 city, the United Clinic is in the city center so they only use full days work; in addition, each doctor's private clinic had to stop operation.

b) The masses work: The United Clinic must merge together and integrate with the masses, allowing the masses to shift from knowing about it to believing in it. There should be propaganda all the time and frequent contact. For example, Beijing Hai Dian United Clinic, during the encephalitis epidemic, printed posters and pictures and hung them in the waiting room, advertising to the masses the way of eradicating mosquitos in order to eradicate the epidemic. Like this, the people commended "the United Clinic does not only treat disease quickly and the herbs are cheap, but they also explain to us the cause of things." When Yong Dingmen United Clinic traveled out of the city six or seven Li during the summer to give vaccinations, one old lady said, "The doctors of Chairman Mao are completely not the same like the old doctors. Not only do they treat disease, they also prevent it, and they also explain to us why they give us injections." And with this, the patients kept on coming one after the other.

When each of Beijing's United Clinics had its opening ceremony, cadres from the Central Ministry of Health and City Sanitation always came to participate. Prior to the event, local government, local police, small local public clinics, village heads and representatives on the street were all communicated to and kept informed. Like this, the masses not only knew that the Government is in support of this but also, during the opening ceremony, they helped spread the word.

In addition, they often participated in meetings with the village head, listened to opinions, welcomed criticism and gave house calls to very ill patients. The masses all realized the modest and enthusiastic approach of the United Clinic. The relationship with the masses became closer and closer.

c) The uniting together issue: Only when uniting together is there power. The separated individuals walk toward uniting together. The unity in the core is the most important link for becoming stronger. Uniting together must follow on the foothill of political studies. It must be grounded in the point of view of serving the patient. After undergoing improvement studies, one acquires the habit of collective living. One has belief in science. One follows the method of sharing the work and helping each other. He can peel off the selfish and profit-oriented mindset. If they all have energetic and responsible attitude towards work, then they can do well "uniting together". At the same time, from leadership point of view, they should give recommendations often—often encourage, educate, inspect and correct. Like this, it can reinforce the "uniting together".

d) The issue of Rules: most doctors are from a petty, bourgeois family line and they have the habit of being lax in discipline. One must establish a set of rules, drawing up a joint pledge with his colleagues. Everybody should inspect and keep each other within the set limits. For example, the pay of compensation, the dividing up of capital profit, should be fair and reasonable, assessed in a democratic way. Treatment should follow on the first-come first-served basis. There should be doctors in attendance day and night. From treatment point of view, it should be divided into departments. An average Chinese and Western medicine United Clinic has the following departments: internal medicine; external medicine; obstetrics; acupuncture and moxibustion etc. One needs to take careful patients' records. The specialist needs to carry responsibility and, at the end of the month, report the summary and statistics to the leadership.

e) Increasing study: this should be divided into professional studies and political studies. In professional studies, one researches the doctor consultation process, discusses methods, like Yong Dingmen United Clinic that has fixed a time to review and discuss patients' records. An enthusiastic Western medicine doctor, Dong Xuwu 董序五, stated, "not only that I help diagnose and treat, I took whatever techniques I know and taught it to the other doctors so they can practice it as well." In political studies, one should constantly study the policy content of serving the people and establish, with that, serving-the-people attitude. Study the work style of Norman Bethune "Everything for the sick and wounded". With vigor, one should merge his medical skill with the political policy, thoroughly embracing the spirit of the three great health policies.

f) One must scrutinize intensively the profession: Today, as for the United Clinics, it is spring sowing and not fall harvest. It is like a sprout not fully matured. It is a new product. It requires endless new and fresh things to cultivate itself. It should be the people's head, not the people's tail. No matter if it is the organization or the medical skill, it often needs to be self-criticized, summed up into experiences of successes and failures. Like the United Clinics committee which was organized by Beijing Chinese Medicine Association. They often hold meetings and discuss the common actual problems, how to overcome specific difficulties and how to strengthen and develop Beijing's United Clinics. In addition, there is an exchange of experiences between different regions. In the entire country, exchanges of thorough self-scrutiny take place, seeking new creativity with vigor. Only like this can there be something new every day.

With the principle "Chinese and Western medicines need to merge", the Chinese and Western medicine United Clinics organized. The medical and sanitation needs of China at present not only resolved, but at the same time the need to make Chinese medicine scientific and Western medicine for the masses was also resolved. The health problems of the people, as a result, also resolved. Amidst the string of solving all these difficulties, there have been many developments strung together: a development reaching to industrial areas; a development reaching to mining areas; a development of medical safety toward women and children; and a development reaching to several different levels of health care. These are the accomplishments of the United Clinics. If there are ten treatment beds then this can become a united hospital. In sum, this kind of United Clinic thoroughly captures—and is the concrete manifestation of—the entire health policy of China. Chinese and Western medicines unite and forge ahead into the bright future!

Article end

Reflections on how I participated in a United Clinic

1952 by Dong Xuwu 董序五

Source: *Beijing Chinese Medicine* (periodical), 1952 June 15th (1st volume 3rd publication)

Yaron: Testimonies of doctors participating in United Clinics. We bring partial articles since repetition of ideas and content is prevalent, a fact in itself reflecting the spirit of the time.

Pages 30–31

1) How did I partake in Yong Dingmen United Clinic

When I was young, I studied the *Acupuncture Great Compendium Zhenjiu Dacheng* 針灸大成. I also learned and memorized the *Shang Han Lun* 傷寒論. At that time, I had a fameless teacher instructing me and there was also no opportunity for practical studies. This mysterious and subtle medicine I knew, I only half understood and I couldn't apply it to reality. With courage, I sat and passed the examination and entered Hebei Medical University. Then I got my chance of understanding the scientific theory behind medicine. After school hours, my school fellow Li Xiangliang 李香亮 and I studied from Mr. Zhang Weiting 張魏庭, from the vocational school of agriculture, the Chinese medical arts. We spent two years of hard work at it. Just when Hebei Medical University reorganized to become a medical hospital, beginner students underwent a very shallow learning of clinical studies. It was against the rules to dispense Chinese medicine herbs and traditional prescriptions and so one would have no hope to enter deep into its research. After graduation, I stayed and worked in that hospital for more than ten years. I was saturated with European and American negative cultural and medical influences and the long-gone traditional Chinese medical arts were a thing of the past.

In the summer of 1950, the Chinese medicine advanced studies school was established. Under the leadership of school director Meng 孟校長, Chinese medicine gradually became scientific. Rejoiced at the good outcome, Chinese medicine was pacing towards a new revolutionary path, where science was its foundation. Based on thousands of years intuitive knowledge of herbal and prescription experience, now it added an appropriate scientific principle and style. This allowed the medicine of China to unfold something new. I think that, as long as Chinese medicine is under the leadership of the Communist Party, it can attain development and advancement.

In the summer of 1951, six districts opened classes for Chinese and Western medicine and political studies. Comrade Zhang Nianzhong 張念仲 was our leader. It advanced our knowledge of the policy and firmed our view of life of serving the people. During political studies, the call for merging Chinese and Western medicines gave us a bridge. It was a first step for Chinese medicine doctors to unite with us and for us to learn from Chinese medicine doctors how to have more of a mass character. Together we went to the outskirts and got close to workers and peasants.

2) The communist party has changed me; it firmed my new view of life

How many years did I receive imperialist oppression, feudal society and bureaucratic capitalism oppression? The medical work completely lost its direction and was in a state of chaos. Medical work completely lost the element of "gearing toward workers, peasants and soldiers". It became commercialized with a view point of selling procedures. Treating disease and saving people—the sublime virtue of medicine—was put in the rear in order to enjoy individually making money. They forgot that science is the crystallization of the masses' common effort. It became an enterprise of betraying the people's health.

At liberation, the people attained liberation. We, as well, attained liberation. The Communist Party led us accurately. Chairman Mao profoundly instructed us "for serving the people" and "gear toward workers, peasants and soldiers". And so we achieved new understanding, a correct direction, a correction for the work style of the past. It settled our position. Workers and peasants are the building force behind our national development. Soldiers are the fortress protecting our national safety. Gearing toward workers, peasants and soldiers and serving the people is the guiding principle of our medical work. Recalling the earlier days, our medical work was clearly cut off from the people. By myself, within a small circle of people, offering plain medical treatment, I was not able to see preventive work. Like on the eve of going into battle, I was facing the enemy and offering passive resistance. With no doubt putting the masses under the risk of contracting pathogenic bacteria. This is, for me, engaging in medical work, an absolute must-do self-criticism. Therefore, we medical workers, the combatants on the battle line, must sincerely come together and merge. We must work as a team, neatly organizing our steps and pace towards villages, factories and the army, taking bacteria and viruses that harm people's health and ruthlessly eradicating them. We should do propaganda with sanitary education, make it common knowledge for the masses, concentrating ever larger power. We are the spearhead—the masses serve as reinforcement—we should thoroughly eradicate all serious illnesses. We should make forceful, preventive attacks in order to guarantee people's health and serve as our lifelong mission.

Partial article end

The bright future of Chinese medicine: United Clinics

1952 by Luan Zhiren 欒志仁

Source: *Beijing Chinese Medicine* (periodical), 1952 June 15th (1st volume 3rd publication)

Pages 32–34

Chinese medicine scientification and serving the people are the objectives and obligations of every single Chinese medicine doctor. However, until today, how scientific did Chinese medicine become? How much more scientific should it become? Should it become Western medicine? When some people graduate from the advanced classes, is this a success? Or is it only after they can do experiments, tests, give injections or use Western drugs that it will be considered a success? As for serving the people, where should they go to serve the people? How should they serve? This article hopes to utilize some facts and explain these problems and their solutions.

1) About Chinese medicine scientification

   a) Beijing Chinese Medicine Advanced Studies School 北京中醫進修學校: In 1950, the Central Ministry of Health established the Beijing Chinese Medicine Advanced Studies School. To date, four classes have graduated. Originally it was six months to graduation but now it has changed into a one-year course. 90% of the instructors teaching the curriculum are hospital directors, professors and doctors from Beijing University Medical School 北京大學醫學院, Xie He medical school 協和醫學院, The Central People's Hospital 中央人民醫院 etc. Chinese medicine doctors who are practicing in Beijing city can partake in the advanced studies for free. After graduation, and according to their level of political understanding and aspirations, each can decide for himself on the path he wants to pursue going forward.

   b) Chinese Medicine Institute of the Central Ministry of Health Research Academy: The Chinese Medicine Research Institute 中醫研究院 was established over a year ago. Within it, there are units researching history of medicine, prescriptions, acupuncture and moxibustion, raw herbs etc. They invited specialists to take charge of these units. Lately they formed the Chinese Medicine Scientific Research Committee, using this pool of wisdom to strengthen the research efforts.

c) Cultivating specialists: Recently, the Central Ministry of Health decided to initiate specialization classes within Beijing University Medical Hospital. They enrolled in the school only Chinese medicine doctors who are younger than thirty years of age. After a five-year course, they will graduate and commence the task of Chinese medicine scientific research.

d) Assemble talented people: Zhu Yan 朱顏 was, originally, a practicing Chinese medicine doctor and he also graduated from a medical school. In 1951, he came to Beijing to assist teaching in Xie He 協和 Medical School. Not only does he have thorough foundations of Chinese medicine, but he also deeply investigated Western pharmaceuticals. Now he has transferred to Beijing Chinese Medicine Advanced Studies School, where he holds an important position.

From the above several points, the following can be clearly determined: Chinese medicine scientification, under the leadership of the Government's plan and organizations, gallops forward in its development. Chinese medicine is the creation and crystallization of our nation's thousands of years and millions upon millions of workers. It is part of our national culture. However many years ago it started to stagnate in the feudal society realm. More recently, by the mutual trampling-over of imperialism, remnants of feudalism and bureaucratic capitalism, it became a dying candle, having the posture of living precariously on morning dew. And so, like this—on the verge of death, like a person almost dying—one morning, liberation came. The people's Government sent for a doctor in many ways, in the open countryside in all directions. It summoned Chinese medicine to advance in science, and invited specialists to further research. Doctors who were versed in both Chinese and Western carried the heavy responsibility of drafting the plan. Chinese doctors in their prime were appointed to take full charge and diligently study and research it, to take this one that has still one breath left in it and bring it back to life, make it sturdy, enhancing it in order to benefit the people.

I have practiced medicine my whole life. When a disease comes about, even if there is a supreme drug for it, it also requires adequate rest and nourishment and gradually it becomes better. Step by step, health recovers. Chinese medicine scientification cannot be completed with one kick. You cannot finish it on a definite date, nor can a small group of people complete it. As testimony are all the histories, where social development has a rule of starting with a gradual change that leads to a total change. How can our Chinese medicine scientification escape this true principle?

In addition, this kind of mighty task has no precedence in history. Chinese medicine had no set rules and lacked indications. Like its impatient handling, as soon as it reached a fork in the road, one then had to reflect back and needed one hundred years to make a move. As a result, Chinese medicine not only could not become scientific, but also the people's loss of health was immeasurable.

Chinese medicine circles today are concerned about scientification and everyone has the same heart of seeking science. However, each person carries responsibility. They should consult the many ideas and materials offered by the government about scientification. The great leaders of the government and every fact mentioned before prove it; we can say without a doubt, "Chinese medicine scientification can be realized." If the entire Chinese medicine community works together as a team and thrusts forward with fierce development toward this upcoming scientific path, then success is within reach. One can be certain of this.

Science is now in the full swing of developing "scientific Chinese medicine". It runs parallel to the development of science itself. When we master science it is, then, "scientific medicine". Science does not distinguish between Chinese and Western. It is a tool that, likewise, serves all people. Chinese medicine advanced studies is the initial learning about science. Following this, science will advance. Beijing Chinese Medicine Advanced Studies School originally was six months to graduation and now it has changed into a one-year course. This explains that, as soon as we ourselves seek progress, the government will give you the opportunity to accomplish it. We, ourselves, if all we want is to serve the people, then the government will supplement and fulfill all conditions required for you to serve the people. Chinese medicine becoming scientific is in order to serve the people. Our people's government is a government allowing service for the people. In order to "serve the people", Chinese medicine becoming scientific means even better and even more serving the people.

Excerpt end

My motive for and reflection on participating in a United Clinic: Dong Zhimen United Clinic 東直門聯合診所

1952 by Jia Liangcai 賈亮采

Source: *Beijing Chinese Medicine* (periodical), 1952 June 15th (1st volume 3rd publication)

Page 37

1) My motive to participate in a United Clinic

My motive to participate in a United Clinic ties in together with my entry into the Chinese Medicine Advanced Studies School. The reason I entered the advanced studies school was that I thought to take my knowledge of Chinese medicine theory, thousands of years of Chinese medicine precious experience and clinically effective formulas, and use scientific methods to systemize, organize and analyze them. I wanted to incorporate Chairman Mao's recommendation to make Chinese medicine scientific and make Western medicine for the masses. I wanted to put this conviction into practice. Therefore, after I graduated, I thought about it twice and thrice… "engaging the trade individually is like the olden ways, will it not be the same like before my advanced studies?" I resolved then to partake in the government's undertaking. If it is not geared toward workers, peasants and soldiers, then it cannot attain the objectives of "preventive comes first", "Chinese and Western must unite" and "making the treatment for the masses". With this, I have struggled in my heart of hearts for many days until I resolved this problem. I have decided, with my co-student Jia Menglian 賈夢蓮,[384] to set up Dong Bianmen United Clinic 東便門聯合診所. Using a lengthy three months of hard toil, aside from taking up the matter with the government, we contacted our co-students, raised funds and arranged shares, looked at potential buildings, purchased equipment etc tasks. Without even noticing, three months of hard work have flown by. Because of building difficulties it was, all along, hard to set it up and so some co-students did not want to wait and therefore left our not-yet-established clinic. They started collaborating with other people. Menglian was very sad and seemed like wanting to quit. Alas, at last we mustered up some courage and firmed our determination. We again connected with a few comrades and, in the heat of summer, sweat dripping on our backs, we decisively overcame the building difficulty and all other problems. Our clinic was finally established

[384] Jia Menglian was later known as three needles Jia 贾三针 and, as a famous doctor in Beijing, he would occasionally give treatment to Chairman Mao and the premier Zhou Enlai 周恩来.

on October 14th of last year. My first step of reaching my heart's desire to be part of a United Clinic was fulfilled.

Article excerpt ends

A plenary meeting and exhibition of Native products of the South Central Region: Summary of clinical work

1952 by Xu Jianquan 徐鑑泉

Source: *Beijing Chinese Medicine* (periodical), 1952 June 15th (1st volume 3rd publication)

Yaron: There were arbitrary decisions about treatment modalities and medical practice. In addition, forcing together Chinese and Western medicines in this manner differs from an organic harmonious transformation. If we take seed, earth, fertilizer, compost, sun and water and force them abruptly together hoping to get a fast plant, then likely nothing will grow.

Article section pages 40–41

Within our work we should reach the objective of exchange and merge between Chinese and Western pharmaceuticals.

The doctors in our clinic's three units—Chinese, Western and acupuncture-moxibustion—all come from different backgrounds. In order to unify everyone's mindset toward serving the people and putting into practice the merging of Chinese and Western medicines, at the very beginning we divided the tasks. We have created a system of treatment divided between the different departments. According to what patients believe in, we decided which diseases will be treated by which departments. Give injections to the ones who need injections, give acupuncture and moxibustion to the ones who need acupuncture and moxibustion, give herbs to the ones who are supposed to get herbs, give special efficacy Western drugs to the ones who are supposed to get special efficacy Western drugs. Like this, we have avoided conflicts between the different departments.

After a prolonged period of time working in the above fashion, and going through the process of merging Chinese and Western theories, the first and the latter can now mix well in one room. Chinese and Western doctors have now respect for one another. They learn from each other now very well. For example, in Western medicine, there are not many advanced Western medicine doctors who have seen the miraculous effects of acupuncture therapy and now they expressed their willingness to study acupuncture. Chinese medicine doctors see how Western medicine doctors wear surgical masks as they do their diagnosis, wear medical uniform and take body temperature. In every aspect it is scientific and so they too wear white lab coats and use thermometers to take body temperature. They demonstrate a spirit of advancement.

But there are also some who belong to the "keeping secrets school". Even though they don't oppose what we do, they don't put effort in researching it (this includes Chinese and Western style doctors). In their hearts, they still harbor some sort of recalcitrant attitude. On some occasions they display it in an unfavorable way. Their lack of political studies is showing. They fundamentally don't understand the calling of Chairman Mao to merge Chinese and Western medicines. That it is for mutually learning, mutually improving, it is for strengthening the prevention of epidemics with the people. It is unifying the battlefield frontline of strengthening public health and sanitation work. If one only holds fast to his own school then he doesn't understand the government policy or the current level of the people's needs.

Because of this, in order to do well the integration of Chinese and Western medicines and exchange their techniques, we used our afternoon breaks to gather in meetings. Aside from learning the government's distributed documents relating to the merging of Chinese and Western medicines, we went a step further and frequently reviewed the positive and negative experiences of each comrade doctor as well as commenced their self-inspection and self-correction. All mistakes were promptly corrected, all accomplishments were praised. During this time each comrade's political understanding was elevated, which strengthened the merging between the two sides. It had reached a true state of working together and helping each other. Every comrade was able to express his opinion and contribute his own best ability, bringing forth high level of "serving" spirit. This work is unlike the usual stuff. Here, with this kind of great exchange in our clinic of Chinese and Western treatment modalities, we have reached to the first steps of the work "Chinese and Western medicines should unite".

The work cadres should be leading this work, and then this may harmonize better. The ones who don't understand the task at hand should learn it humbly. Chinese doctors should learn the strong points of Western medicine; Western style doctors should learn the strong points of Chinese medicine. This is the prerequisite to increase the level of medicine. The ideal doctor should be able to utilize ancient and modern, Chinese and foreign medicines in treating diseases and saving people. It is improper for him to impose restrictions on himself; rather, it should be what we call "study to old age". Study until one is old means that the process of learning is forever without a limit.

Article excerpt end

Beijing Chinese Medicine Association, acupuncture and moxibustion research class: A report about the work of the first class

Anonymous author

Yaron: The rise in popularity of acupuncture as an affordable treatment modality, its merge with science and its use as a political tool.

[Article section] The purpose of establishing the acupuncture research class

---

Page 44

The Beijing Chinese Medicine Association Acupuncture Committee's first acupuncture research class was established three months after the Beijing Chinese Medicine Association Acupuncture Committee was formed. Because it is one of the Committee's main tasks in following the call of Chairman Mao to "make Chinese medicine scientific" as well as the Central Ministry of Health policy of "preventive is the main thing; gear toward the workers, peasants and soldiers; and merge Chinese and Western medicines". It is a basic work in developing, improving and popularizing this excellent, simple and effective treatment modality.

In this work, the acupuncture research class needed, first and foremost, to correct the mindset of other practicing acupuncturists. Since liberation and the new style of new China, in our motherland every corner gives rise to buildings that surge high. Since liberation, there is also a wide struggle against, and criticism of, people with old society mindset, for not using the practical study of Marxism. In addition, following the path of the three great and most important policies of "resisting America and supporting Korea", "suppressing counterrevolutionaries" and "land reforms", advances a step further the knowledge of most acupuncturists who, at present, practice in their own private clinic. It encourages everyone's objective and subjective need to enthusiastically partake in political study. Most special is the study of government policy and line of thinking. It requires one to correct himself and establish a new revolutionary outlook on things. Then acupuncturists can advance a step in serving the people.

Acupuncture and moxibustion[385] treatment modality is one of our nation's precious inheritances of folklore experience. From economic and treatment efficacy perspectives, for thousands of years, this simple and powerful treatment of disease has helped resolve so many problems. From this perspective, it is precious and requires us to earnestly study and creatively develop it. However, being subjected to biased and destructive government powers of the different dynasties in history, the development of acupuncture theory and technique was scattered, not balanced and, in addition, many kept it a secret. In the past, under oppressive reactionary governments, acupuncturists did not stand a chance. They absolutely could not elevate their own level by inquiring into scientific knowledge. This is clearly demonstrated by the fact that, in the past, most acupuncturists would give no importance to sterilization when administering acupuncture. Likewise, one can see that acupuncturists in the past did not know scientific physiology, anatomy, pathology and diagnosis, as well as bacteriology, sterilization etc. This, of course, obstructed the development of acupuncture into becoming a science. Therefore, in order to promote responsibility toward the people and use greater effort to guarantee the health of the workers, there is no doubt: we must improve the acupuncturists' level of scientific knowledge.

Beijing Chinese Medicine Association Acupuncture Committee established the acupuncture research class in order to address the above problems, the purposes of which are the following three:

1) Based on the foundational policy of our nation's people's democracy, it will help practicing acupuncturists strengthen their political studies, correct

[385] Acupuncture and moxibustion 針灸 hereafter shortened to "acupuncture".

their own mindset, advance a step in understanding the meaning behind "serving the people", and thoroughly change their point of view of "service for the people".

2) It will strengthen their study of new scientific medicine knowledge and help them use a new scientific point of view. It will allow them to practically criticize the old medicine's secrecy and spirituality aspects, while expanding upon past experiences which may still be useful. It will break open the door of prejudice and, within no time, in a creative way, they will improve.

3) Under the principle of a centralized democracy, it will organize acupuncturists and bring them together. It will advance a systematic, planned and organized way of studying and working in order to harmonize together with local healthcare needs. In addition, it will firm up the merging of Chinese and Western medicines and all other aspects that are included in the merging together scheme.

Therefore, it will elevate the acupuncturists' political understanding (this includes also other practitioners of Chinese medicine who simultaneously use acupuncture). It will elevate their scientific skills and organization at work. Within a short period of time, they will master these aspects of knowledge and methods associated therein which, in turn, will increase their treatment efficacy. It will perfect all these different objective issues within their job and it conforms to the present urgent problem of responding to the masses' needs. In sum, this is the objective of establishing the acupuncture research class.

Other than that, it is a step further in making acupuncture modality popular, and cultivating new kind of work cadres able to respond to the mass of workers' (especially farmers') needs. The acupuncture committee has also drafted an initial plan for an "acupuncture study class", but this item's development must wait until all our city's acupuncturists have advanced their study and graduated from the current "acupuncture research class".

[Article section] Students' origin and content taught

Page 45

The first acupuncture research class admission criteria is "acupuncturists who hold acupuncture certificate and are Chinese medicine practitioners already practicing and using acupuncture treatment modality" (these are mainly members of the Beijing Chinese Medicine Association). In the first class there are 82 students, among them 76 are actual students while 6 more are Ministry of Health cadres just listening in. In total there are 82 fellows.

Sex of participants are 77 males and 6 females,[386] their ages range from 30 to 70 years of age, but the majority are 40 to 50 years of age.

The study course is 3 months; each week there are classes on 3 days (Mondays, Wednesdays and Fridays) and class duration is 2 hours. In order to protect the student's professional activities, classes are held in the evening from 7:00 to 9:00pm. Classes were held at the Central People's Government Ministry of Health Department Beijing Chinese Medicine Advanced Studies School.

The students, even though older folks, were studying in high spirits. There were very few absentees or tardy arrivals, except for a small number that were accident-related. There are many folks who, despite heavy rain, would come from a long distance away. For example, 65 year old Dr. Nuo Songshan 那松山, living in Beijing's suburb, close to Qinglong bridge 青龍橋 past Wan Shoushan 萬壽山. Even though he lives 10 kilometers away, everyday he risks the wind and rain and insists on not being absent. Every day he rides his bicycle even though he gets home very late at night. This kind of earnest studying spirit has already inspired all the fellow students in the class. In addition, in the classroom, the way the class is arranged is in small groups. There is an excellent atmosphere of observing the rules.

The acupuncture research class curriculum and time follows, in general, the Central Ministry of Health planned curriculum and time for such an acupuncture research class. It is physiology and anatomy 14 hours, pathology and diagnosis 14 hours, bacteriology and sterilization 6 hours, the new style of acupuncture 36 hours, political studies 14 hours and, according to the need, this can be a bit longer or shorter.

[386] This adds up to 83, we kept the mistake as in the article.

From teaching content point of view, because this is a new kind of setup, the teaching materials selected are simply seen as an initial attempt. Before we started the program we have summoned many meetings to discuss the teaching task, the result of which was our determination of a specific outline for each and every class (see attached list number 4).

Teaching style was mainly of personal demonstrations and, as needed, in every class we included real specimen, corpses, hanging charts, slide projector, microscope etc teaching materials. The students on the one hand were taking notes themselves and on the other also contemplating the class handouts and requested reading materials given by the teachers. In addition, they organized in small groups and developed discussions.

In the practical study of acupuncture, since the students themselves were practicing acupuncturists, and since the overall course was rather short, then only a short time of observation-style study was included. According to the number of students from each city district, we divided them up to small groups and dispatched them to an Acupuncture Treatment Laboratory 針灸療法實驗所 to observe. Because of work condition limitations, we have divided the class to small groups of 3 students each. Every morning, for 10 days, we dispatched 2 small groups. After observing and after the class ended, the small groups will organize to discuss their experience.

The class organization was according to a seating arrangement, where the entire class was divided into eight small study groups. Each group commonly selected one leader, who was responsible for leading the group in their study as well as attending to students' various other difficulties. The entire class also elected two main representatives to lead the entire class studies and submit an overall report.

In order to seriously address school security, the acupuncture committee selected a few members to be on duty daily, in order to help with security work.

After classes, most students, depending on their residence being far or close, have organized six after-hours small study groups, two in the eastern city area and two in the western and two in the southern. They also elected a member to be responsible for the group. They often held discussions about each one's methods and experience in treatment as well as the issue of sterilization. In one small group, because of their brotherly love and affection and in order to help the profession and advance a step in serving the people policy, they accepted local acupuncture practitioners into the groups that were not part of the class.

Page 47

About the new acupuncture curriculum, most of the students expressed satisfaction. Some, however, raised their opinion. For example, most felt that practical studies connecting theory to reality were too scarce. They hoped that next time it could increase a bit. Some were hoping for more exchange of each other's experiences while discussing it in small groups. This was a natural expression of everyone having elevated their own skill level. When it comes to the teaching of the course, everybody particularly welcomed director Zhu's 朱[387] teachings. Many old folks said: "Director Zhu put so much toil into developing our acupuncture. He truly took his own precious experience and made it public, sharing it with us. The people's government, for each and every one of us, is truly our government."

Attached list number 4

Page 49

Each class content and outline

1) Physiology and anatomy (total 8 classes, each class 2 hours)—This class has handouts. In these 8 classes cadavers, specimen, models and charts were used.

Class 1: The inner organs normal location part 1 (teacher Ma 馬)

Class 2: The inner organs normal location part 2 (Ma)

Class 3: Circulation and respiration (Ma)

Class 4: Anatomy and physiology of the digestive system (Ma)

Class 5: Urinary, reproductive and endocrine systems (Ma)

Class 6: The composition and classification of the nervous system (Ma)

Class 7: The distribution of peripheral nerves and regions (Ma)

Class 8: Neurological distribution and its connection to the location of acupuncture points.

[387] Zhu Yan 朱顏.

2) Pathology and diagnosis (total of 7 classes, each class 2 hours, but because the content was so much it became 13 classes and 26 hours)

Class 1: Physiology, pathology and diagnosis of the skin, muscles, tendons, pleura, peritoneum, bones tissue, joints (teacher Yin 殷)

Class 2: Physiology, pathology and diagnosis of the blood vessels and circulation (Yin)

Class 3: Physiology, pathology and diagnosis of the respiratory system (teacher Cai 蔡)

Class 4: Physiology, pathology and diagnosis of the digestive system (Yin)

Class 5: Physiology, pathology and diagnosis of the urinary and reproductive systems (Yin)

Class 6: Physiology, pathology and diagnosis of the nervous system (Yin)

Class 7: Physiology, pathology and diagnosis of the five sense organs (Cai)

3) Bacteriology and sterilization studies (total 3 classes each class 2 hours)—classes include handouts

Class 1: Understanding Bacteria (Yin)

Class 2: Understanding immunity (Yin)

Class 3: The importance of sterilization in acupuncture and the methods to implement it (Yin)

4) Political studies (total 8 classes, each class 2 hours)—mainly pointing out reading materials, no handouts.

Class 1: [missing]

Class 2: The resolutions of the first national health symposium (teacher Bao 鮑)

Class 3: The common program of the Chinese people political consultative conference (Gao 高)

Class 4: The common program of the Chinese people political consultative conference (Gao)

Class 5: The people's democratic dictatorship (Pan 潘)

Class 6: Practical discussions (Meng 孟)

Class 7: Practical discussions (Meng)

Class 8: Practical discussions (Meng)

5) The new acupuncture (total 12 classes, each class 2 hours. At the end since the practical study of acupuncture was done during the day, the remaining unused hours were used for pathology and diagnosis studies)—This class pointed to reading materials, mainly Zhu Lian's 朱璉 book "The New Acupuncture". No handouts.

Class 1: General introduction (teacher Zhu 朱)

Class 2: The issue of selecting and combining points (Zhu)

Class 3: How to know and cultivate political affairs for acupuncturists (teacher Wang 王)

Class 4: How to know and cultivate political affairs for acupuncturists (teacher Wang)

Class 5: Acupuncture technique of sterilization (Wang)

Class 6: Acupuncture technique of sterilization (Wang)

Class 7: [missing]

Class 8: The principle of action in the acupuncture treatment (Wang)

Class 9: The principle of action in the acupuncture treatment (Wang)

Class 10: On the different opinions of the acupuncture points' locations and a thorough discussion about the standardization of point location (Ma 馬)

Class 11: On the different opinions of the acupuncture points' locations and a thorough discussion about the standardization of point location (Ma)

Class 12: On the different opinions of the acupuncture points' locations and a thorough discussion about the standardization of point location (Ma)

Article end

Chinese medicine advanced studies organization and management: selected articles

1953 Selected by Yu Daoji 于道濟[388]

Distributed by Beijing Health Book Store 1953

中央人民政府衛生部北京中醫進修學校

中醫進修講義

中醫進修組織管理選輯

于道濟選

北京健康書店發行

Yaron: The following book, published in 1953, contains several articles from *Beijing Zhong Yi* magazine we have translated in the section from 1952. These appear here again as the government official position, so from being an opinion in a magazine it became a government-supported "Party line" that everyone must follow. Materials compiled into this book served as guidelines for newly-forming Chinese medicine organizations all over the country; a Chinese medicine mass mobilization on a national scale not seen in China since 1929.

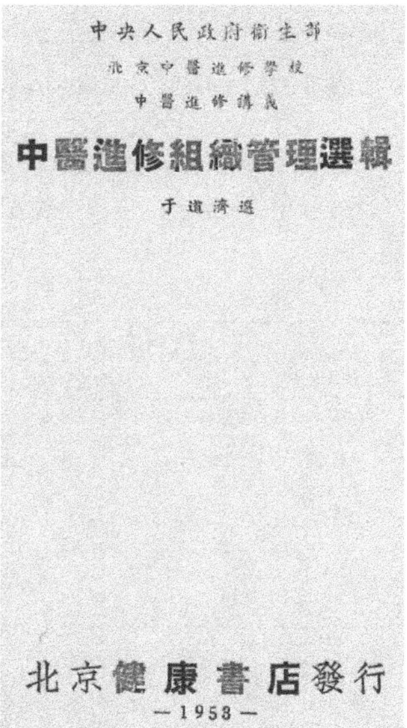

The book title format highlights its official nature:

Line 1: China Central People Government Ministry of Health

Line 2: Beijing Chinese Medicine Advanced Studies School

Line 3: Chinese Medicine Advanced Studies Teaching Material

[388] Yu Daoji studied medicine in 1927 in Tong Shan hospital in Shen Yang 沈陽同善醫院. In 1931 he started a private practice and was teaching Chinese medicine in Beijing. In 1949 he served as Academic Dean of Hua Bei Native Medicine Academy 華北國醫學院教務長 and in 1950 served as Academic Director of Beijing Chinese Medicine Advanced Studies School 北京中醫進修學校教育主任. In 1954 he served as director of general affairs of Beijing Chinese Medicine Research Institute attached clinic 中醫研究院門診部業務主任. In 1956 he served as education director of Beijing Chinese Medicine College as well as director of the college hospital 北京中醫學院教務長兼附屬醫院院長.

Foreword

In our school teachers' class, at the beginning we set up an additional Chinese medicine advanced studies organization and management course, total of six lectures and 18 hours. The reason for setting this up is that, after the teacher class graduates, the students will return to their original organizations. While partaking in the Chinese medicine advanced study work and studying in this school, in addition to political studies, we need also to supplement some government policy education, especially related to advanced studies of Chinese medicine. This education strengthens our thinking process and clears the capitalist old point of view from the medicine. It establishes a new road for medical work and it puts into practice the call of Chairman Mao for Chinese medicine scientification. It thoroughly realizes the "three great policies" and their associated struggles. It is the focal point of this course. We first selected and compiled the directives coming out of the First National Health Congress and the Central Ministry of Health director's report. We require students to discuss and study it carefully. We hope that, in your thinking process, you can reach great transformation and accurate proper knowledge. When going back to your work units, reach a state of serving the people with a complete heart and strong will.

Up until now, each provincial city health organization has set up a Chinese medicine advanced studies organization; many have inquired by letter regarding our school organization methods as well as teaching plan. We have also replied by letter with a general outline. From 1953 on, in each provincial city in the entire country, Chinese medicine advanced studies organizations will be set up; they will certainly require all sorts of reference material. Therefore, we take here our Chinese medicine advanced studies school, advanced studies class, preventive class, acupuncture and moxibustion class—all these advanced studies materials, we select and compile them, in order to serve as reference materials. When it comes to the Chinese Medicine Association it is a mass character Chinese medicine research organization. The Chinese medicine teachers' rules are rules respected by all Chinese medicine doctors and so they are selected as well to enter the curriculum. Recently, United Clinics were established; they respond to the peasants' needs—this is required all over the country. Participants in medical work of these United Clinics are, indeed, a true expression of "serving peasants and workers". Therefore, introducing the United Clinics is even more so a must. The materials for this course are mainly selected from *The Health Newspaper* and *Beijing Chinese Medicine Magazine*; however, because of time constraint, it is not meticulous. When time allows, we need to supplement and correct it.

Yu Daoji 于道濟 October 21st, 1952

Foreword end

A Report on the National Health Congress: (On September 8th, in the Central People Government, State Administrative Council at the 49th Government Affairs Meeting)

1953 by Central Ministry of Health director Li Dequan 李德全

Yaron: The restructuring of Chinese medicine from top to bottom, from government down to the people. Different from the Republic when Chinese medicine practitioners hoped to reform Chinese medicine in order to be included in the state organization, here the government willingly includes Chinese medicine practitioners in state organization, however this time dictating to them what needs to be done and how. Many practitioners, who struggled in the past to be included, now felt legitimized and accepted. It seemed a victory in the eyes of many.

Pages 1–5

The first National Health Congress was already planned from September into October last year by the military commission of the Chinese Communist Party Central Committee and the Ministry of Health during their Health Administration Congress. In that Congress, they decided that this year, during the summer, the Ministry of Health, together with the Military Committee Health Administration, convene this congress. (Therefore, last year's Health Administration Congress was the preparatory congress for this year's health congress). In that congress, the general policy target was preventive medicine, and that health work must guarantee production and national defense construction. One must gear towards peasants, workers and miners and rely upon the masses. Since these policies were already implemented in each administrative region, one could see that the policies were accurate. The purpose of the first National Health Congress was to exchange and summarize previous experiences, discuss and, even more so, reinforce the proper policy for our national health construction. In addition, it formulated concrete measures to implement the policy thoroughly.

During preparations for this congress and during the congress itself, we have discovered that even though China was under great oppression of imperialism, feudalism, bureaucratism and capitalism for so long, the reactionary Kunmintang government did not pay importance to the people's health undertaking. Health and medical institutions were simple and crude, their distribution not fair, while some of them even carried the name without having the substance. They were divided into factions between Chinese and Western medicines and even within Western medicine itself. They struggled amongst themselves and served only a few people. The majority of villages usually lacked medicine and drugs. Farmers could only look for spirits and Buddha for salvation. Contagious diseases were rampant and people were under the mercy of heaven. The number of sick people in our entire country has reached every year about 140 million, and mortality rate was well over 3%. Among them, more then half died of infectious diseases that could be avoided with preventive medicine, such as: bubonic plague, cholera, measles, smallpox, flu, dysentery, typhus, relapsing fever, etc aggressive diseases, as well as Kala Azar, Japanese schistosomiasis, malaria, venereal diseases that also impacted many people. Women in labor, most at the hands of midwives, have experienced, more or less, 40% infant mortality rate.

The congress began on August 7th and lasted 13 days (this included one day break to tour the Ministry of Health exposé), concluding on the 19th. In attendance were 421 participants; attending as non-voting delegates were 161 participants. Among the participants were delegates from all regional military health administrations, plus famous Chinese medicine and Western medicine doctors. During the congress and in accord with our nation's current health conditions and the main guiding policy of "preventive comes first", we have performed deep discussions. We strove to perfect and develop our nation's health organization within three to five years. In our discussions we were in agreement that, considering different factions' medical education point of view, we must talk some Western medicine doctors over their extreme opinion towards Chinese medicine. We need to remove their fear of Chinese medicine and have them reach an agreeable place. We have decided the following three main policies of "gear toward peasants and soldiers", "prevention is the main objective" and "merge together Chinese and Western medicines". We have also passed resolutions on the following issues: development of medical education, cultivating large numbers of health workers, building and developing a national basic health structure, adjusting within health departments the ratio between public and privately owned, uniting and reforming pharmaceutical enterprises and reorganizing hospitals. This demonstrates the congress's success and it also expresses the new appearance of health, medicine and pharmacology of the new China.

Next, I will summarize a few issues we discussed during the congress:

1) About the policy "prevention comes first"

Medicine and pharmacology is science of people struggling with disease and participating in this struggle are all the people. Medical profession is the spearhead of this struggle. It is the organization and leadership of this struggle. If health workers do not take this science, this struggling method, teach people and help them understand what to do, how by themselves they should act upon it instead of relying on a health workers minority, then this cannot solve the problem at hand. In the past, medical work was separated from the masses, and so it only included a treatment perspective. At present, we emphasize serving the people and the masses; it is not "wait for the people to get sick and then come look for us". It is us who need to take action and mobilize the people to preemptively struggle against disease. This mobilization to struggle against disease of course means prevention. Therefore, the policy of "prevention comes first" stems out of, and is in accord with, "when serving the people first serve the workers, peasants and soldiers". As for the health work itself, only when one has this prerequisite in mind and he stands for this position, that truly "prevention comes first" will be achieved.

2) About establishing a basic health structure

Establishing on different levels a national basic health structure in order to resolve the healthcare needs of the masses means to realize the healthcare profession service of the people. First, it must be a key service for workers, peasants and soldiers. If we want to resolve healthcare needs of workers, peasants and soldiers we must establish a basic healthcare structure. This work is extremely important; however, we must strive to accomplish this within three to five years. So to say, within this time frame, throughout most of the country, in each county there should be two to seven specialist doctors and one pharmacist or one drug personnel in a public health clinic organization. Gradually we should have, in each and every district, one to two doctors and one midwife in a local health clinic. In factories and mines and in each neighborhood there should be a health clinic. These personnel should come, on the one hand, from people cultivated in schools and, on the other hand, from medical workers out of the big cities. In summary, at least in the next few years, our healthcare construction should not be focused on big cities but, rather, on the medium-to-small sized cities as well as villages and factories, mines and military units.

3) About education

With old education standards in our nation in the past 40 years, there were not even twenty thousand proper doctors cultivated. With these kinds of medical standards, facing the current reality, one certainly cannot resolve the problem at hand. Therefore, first and foremost we need to establish new standards for medical education. This is in order to develop medical education and cultivate a large number of medical professionals. The new standard for medical education should be divided into three categories: high level, intermediate and lower levels. In the high level medical education one should create sub-specialties. The new medical education should spread and elevate the foundations. While improving it, the policy of spreading it should be implemented. So at present condition, in our entire nation, spreading it should be prioritized. As for teaching methods, they should combine theories and practicality into one.

4) About uniting and reforming the pharmacology world

Before liberation, the tasks of government health offices on all levels were arduous and glorified. Our nation's health workers, including Chinese and Western medicine doctors and pharmacology personnel, must unite and work hard together—only then can we elevate the task of the people's health. In the past, there was estrangement between Western and Chinese medicine doctors and pharmacologists and the battles between the factions were stern. Therefore, in the congress, while discussing the uniting and reforming of the pharmacological world, we required that Chinese and Western medicine doctors will unite under the same banner of "serving the people"—they should reform as well. Chinese and Western medicine doctors should increase their political and professional studies. We should charge the regional administrations' health institutions to truly reach to the level of "Chinese medicine scientification" and "Western medicine for the masses".

This year, at first is in each administrative region big cities then next year, gradually in every province and provincial city we should establish Chinese medicine advanced studies schools or Chinese medicine training classes or, with presently existing Chinese medicine schools and associations (The City Medical Circle Federation), establish an advanced studies school, training classes and part time schools. For private individuals who establish their own Chinese medicine schools (or take on disciples) we should not add restrictions; however, their curriculum must equally contain scientific medicine foundations and political studies. Their curriculum standards must be negotiated with the Central Ministry of Health. This is in order to reach a uniform level of scientific training for the entire country's Chinese medicine doctors. Then they can become villages' talented medical workers.

5) About restructuring a relationship between private and public medical and pharmacological enterprises

In general, this principle was pointed out as being advantageous to both public and private interests. In the medical and pharmacological world it should likewise be executed. Since the motherland economy still awaits recovery, the distribution of health workers and institutions still did not change enough to meet the needs of the masses. At present, China's public medical systems cannot immediately do the job; private health professionals are, today, still a need for our society. In the past, governmental health agencies had little experience with helping and managing private health care providers and they paid them little attention. Therefore, in many geographical areas, especially areas liberated a relative short period of time, they still don't have a close relationship to private healthcare providers. Private healthcare providers have a depressive appearance, and so this problem must be appropriately dealt with.

In order to resolve this problem, we must first better organize the private healthcare providers. Workload should be divided appropriately in relation to the Health Department healthcare mission. In regional districts, responsibility regulations for public health should assign distinct tasks to privately-held hospitals. As for resolving their difficulties, we should certainly supervise them and offer help. As for levying taxes on them, we should reduce the burden, especially for enterprises in villages and industrial and mining regions—they should be tax-exempt. Governmental health offices should regularly guide private healthcare professionals, help them change their attitude, reform their art and change their standards for the better. Of course we should restrain and punish the minority who act in crooked ways, for example the ones who cheat patients for profit. At the same time, healthcare personnel working in private enterprises should initiate a change of the old attitude. They should study current political affairs and build a "serving the people" mindset. They should mend and correct the mindset of "do things only for profit". Only like this, there is a future path of development.

6) About reorganizing the hospitals

At present, the current state of affairs with hospitals around the country has already improved, compared to before liberation. However, there are some workers' attitudes that still did not change enough. Their spirit of earnest responsibility is insufficient. Their techniques are not good and their secretive attitude is still severe. On top of this, their treatment standards are not being perfected and negligence accidents are plenty. In the past, we did not pay enough attention to this and so it needs a thorough discussion. Because organizing the hospitals is a need for everyone, it requires each and every hospital to investigate thoroughly three aspects: their mindset; their professional skills; and their rules. We should reorganize them as follows: First, improve their leadership, establishing a centralized democratic hospital administration committee. Then instruct the mindset of every hospital personnel, strengthening their political affairs studies. Establish a mindset of "everything for the sick and wounded". Next, perfect different kinds of rules and thoroughly implement them. When establishing rules, have in mind the patients' interest; simplify formalities, earnestly perform diagnostic work, nursing and increase professional skill. In addition to increasing professional studies, also establish patient cases summary meetings, research association for clinical studies, pay attention to sterilization and reduce complications.

7) About military health work

This congress was convened for both regional health work and military health work. Therefore we must discuss, as well, the military health work; gearing toward workers, peasants and soldiers. In our liberation army, health work for the past 20 years was always like this. The path our liberation army health work took in the past was correct. From now on, we should continue to follow this path. Not only, as completely agreed in this congress, the direction of the liberation army health work should be the direction of the entire country's health work, but also the experience of the liberation army health work from now on should be the development starting point for the entire country's health work. The liberation army health work, on the one hand, should initiate this glorious starting point and, on the other hand, recognize that this is only the starting point.

There is an even bigger affair we all must do. There are still many things we must learn with humble hearts. There are also other good experiences outside of the liberation army and we need to absorb them as well. The liberation army health workers should pace forward, hand in hand, together with the entire nation's health workers and take a beautiful tradition, propagate and glorify it. In deficient localities we should study harder and, other than that, we should especially increase the military health work in order to guard the fighters' health, making this a cardinal point for the military health work.

Article end

About the decision to merge and study from each other in the medical and pharmacological world: Extracts of four decisions reached in the National Health Congress about medicine and pharmacology education

1953 (anonymous)

Yaron: Chinese medicine throughout history was subjected to selection; from a vast and accumulated knowledge, people selected what seemed appropriate for their time. It was also the case during the Republic and during the Communist era. In this article we can see a valid selection process, valid for the time. Today, selection criteria must be different. In fact, highlighting a need for different selection criteria is the purpose of this book.

Pages 6–7

According to estimates, Western medicine doctors who have graduated from medical schools in the entire country add up to less than twenty thousand and Chinese medicine doctors some several hundred thousand. Since, in the past, the reactionary government had in mind to drive a wedge between different groups, Chinese medicine and Western medicine were estranged. To an extreme, they became two contending schools. Within themselves, Chinese and Western medicines were further divided into different schools of thought. This phenomenon must be corrected now. Regardless if it is between Chinese and Western medicines or internal conflicts, everybody should unite together under the banner "service for the people". They should all study together.

Chinese medicine has several thousand years' history and its accumulated experience is rich. Its medical treatment methods (such as acupuncture and moxibustion etc) and herbs are valuable. However, they lack scientific knowledge of physiology, anatomy and pathology. Therefore, Chinese medicine must labor hard to accept scientific medicine knowledge. It should reform its medical treatment methods. Within Western medicine, there is also a trend of being removed from the masses. It does not conform to deficiencies of current reality. It must, with great vigor, conform to current reality and gear toward workers, miners and the mass peasant workers. In summary, Chinese medicine should undergo scientification and Western medicine should transform toward the masses. From the practitioners' perspective of studying, researching and exchange of experience, they must break free from past division of factions. In order to strengthen the merging together, collaboration and mutual study of medical and pharmacological circles, the following decisions have been reached:

1) In order to improve efficacy of service, both Chinese medicine and Western medicine doctors must increase their study of political affairs and professional matters. Western medicine can offer, via their high or intermediate level schools, or through their Western medical associations and organizations, lectures and classes advancing after-hours education. Chinese medicine, in each administrative region and each city, should plan to gradually establish new Chinese medicine advanced studies schools and advanced studies classes or, through existing Chinese medicine schools and associations and city medical and herbal associations, arrange to add Chinese medicine advanced studies schools, training classes and evening after-hours schools etc. In these schools, they should teach basic scientific medicine and political studies; for example, foundations of modern medicine, preventive medicine, social science etc. Chinese medicine advanced studies schools' curricula will be determined by the Central Government Ministry of Health and Central Government Education Department. Each Chinese medicine advanced studies school and training class, according to local conditions, local contagious diseases situation etc, may add classes to the curriculum, allowing the "study" and "application" to be closely related, in order to answer the masses' needs in each locality.
2) The Central Government Ministry of Health will establish Chinese medicine and Chinese pharmacology research institutions. These will use scientific

methods to organize and research China's medical treatment methods and China's pharmacology. This work should unfold in unity with all local experienced and cultivated Chinese medicine doctors and herbal producers. They will collect from these persons all valuable medical methods, prescriptions and medical and herbal literature, as well as all sorts of secret recipes and folk efficacious remedies. They will research them, discriminate between them, propagate and develop the scientific part of Chinese medicine and pharmacology and discard the unscientific part.

3) Every local healthcare institution should mobilize all Chinese medicine doctors, who went through advanced studies and training, to participate in preventive medical work. Every county and smaller healthcare institution should accept Chinese medicine doctors, who have completed advanced studies and training, to partake in diagnostic and treatment work. This will allow Chinese and Western medicine doctors, in practice, to study from each other and supplement their deficiencies.

4) There will be no restraints on private Chinese medicine doctors to have their own Chinese medicine schools (or take on disciples); however, these schools need to add scientific foundation of medicine and pharmacology.

5) In order to strengthen the merging and collaboration of Chinese and Western medicines, every locality, according to their need and ability, will establish a medical and pharmacology federation or medical and pharmacology forum. This should be a Chinese and Western medicine doctors' joint organization. Previously existing societies or scholarly associations, with separate branches of Chinese and Western medicines, may remain. In addition, according to labor union laws, they should organize the health labor union.

6) Higher-than-provincial-level Ministry of Health administrative organs may establish and handle Chinese medicine professional institutions according to need. They should supervise Chinese medicine doctors' registration, merging activities, advanced studies, training etc appropriate activities.

7) These resolutions were petitioned by the Central Government Ministry of Health to the State Administrative Council for approval and then were announced and put into force.

Article end

The merging of Chinese and Western medicines and Chinese medicine advanced studies: He Cheng 賀誠 Vice-Minister's[389] speech at the Beijing Chinese Medicine Association opening ceremony

Yaron: The force and might of the Communist state was different from the Republican regime. With great vigor they succeeded in unifying the entire country from the top down, from the government down to the people. The last paragraph shows the new attitude: if Chinese medicine doctors' opinion conforms to what the government wants then the government will adopt it naturally. It was the basic premise for founding TCM.

Pages 8–10

In October last year, our Association convened in the National Health Administration Congress. In this Congress we received guidance from Chairman Mao, commander in chief Zhu 朱[390] and other leaders. They have asked us to unite Chinese medicine in the entire country and help it elevate its level. After the Congress we have immediately instructed each local Chinese medicine association to organize Chinese medicine study and research teams and perform well the work of merging Chinese and Western medicines. In some localities, they have already started doing it but it was not widespread. After the Central Ministry of Health was formed, it has already performed some Chinese-medicine-related work; for example, forums, committees and establishing Chinese medicine advanced studies schools. It collected Chinese medicine opinions from the entire country and performed Chinese-medicine-related surveys. Today, Beijing Chinese Medicine Association is formed. It is yet another circle within these many very important tasks.

According to estimates, every year five million people die in China and about 100 million people become sick from all sorts of minor as well as severe illnesses. Even with these kinds of large numbers, the previous reactionary government power of state has never adopted any effective measures to resolve it. A large percentage of these sick and dying people have never received any proper medical care. According to local surveys

[389] 賀誠 1901–1992 Was a lieutenant general in the liberation army, Vice-Minister of the Department of Health, later became the military Medicine And Science Academy Director 军事医学科学院院长 and from 1975–1982 became Vice Minister of the Logistics Department. He was prosecuted during the Cultural Revolution.

[390] Zhu De 朱德 (1886–1976)

in villages, 80% of the sick do not get any medical treatment. According to this calculation, every year there are four million people who die without being able to get proper medical care. From the sick, there are 80 million people who remain without medical care. Therefore, medical personnel carry a very heavy burden.

We should be responsible and use all our power to help solve this. You all know, in the Chinese People's Political Consultative Conference the 48th Common Program, it was already explained clearly "encourage the people's physical education; promote health, medicine and pharmacological professions; and pay attention to protect mothers', babies' and children's health". We should be conscious of solving this problem. If, in order to resolve this problem, we plan to only rely on the twenty thousand Western medicine doctors we have, then this will not satisfy the job. We have no way of carrying this burden alone. From another aspect, many illnesses are infectious. If we only rely on the "not yet advanced" Chinese medicine doctors to do preventive treatment work, from the perspective of scientific measures, this too is insufficient. Therefore, in order to accomplish the task just mentioned, we must take the twenty thousand Western medicine doctors and the several hundred thousand Chinese medicine doctors and merge them together, collaborating and helping each other. Only then can we solve this problem.

We should self-criticize the poor state Chinese and Western medicines were in the past; they had a gully between them. Western medicine felt itself to be scientific while Chinese medicine wasn't scientific—it considered itself to be better. From the Chinese medicine side, there were also many who looked down at Western medicine. They felt that China's medicine had several thousand years' history and felt that it surpassed Western medicine. Therefore they didn't want to get close to them. This is also wrong. This kind of phenomenon is detrimental to the common solution needed for this health problem. In the past, these two factions also didn't feel that their responsibility is significant, or maybe their feelings were not deep enough to realize that only joint effort can solve this problem. In the past, the reactionary government didn't pay importance to the people's health; instead, they manufactured fights and famines and crop failures, capitulating to imperialism and becoming the servant of imperialism and feudalism. These were conditions harmful to the people's health. Of course, even more so, they couldn't take care of organization, promotion and education of merging together Chinese and Western medicines. In reality, they actually didn't want people to merge together, because this would be detrimental to their power of state. In the past, Chinese and Western medicines did not have the objective of merging for the people's benefit. On rare occasion, there was a mention of this, but by very few people and, indeed, there was no appeal, instruction or organization. It was such that a small minority could not have had a big impact.

From now on, we must turn our back on this past situation; we must do well the merging of Chinese and Western medicines. We should take the entire nation's medical personnel and not divide them into factions. Under the call of "serving the people", we should systematically merge together. We should clearly tell all our medical workers to merge together under the call for "serving the people's health". As long as we want to serve the people, it means we want to gather together, and then we can merge together.

In China, there should be many undertakings for the people's health; for example, nutrition, dwelling, clothing, infectious diseases and prevention and treatment of all sorts of diseases. There are dozens or hundreds of different tasks that need to be done but since manpower is in short supply, we can only select, as an initial step, the most urgent ones posing the greatest risk to the people's health. As for the construction, the new motherland economy and national defense, the most harmful are infectious diseases, endemic diseases, occupational diseases, and amongst them infectious diseases constitutes the majority. Therefore, Chinese and Western medicines should emphasize research of infectious diseases treatment and prevention. Like this, we can decrease disease and mortality rate. On this point, Chinese medicine must increase its scientific knowledge and experience and only then can the task be completed. Because of this, we cannot but think of the next problem and this is the advanced study and improvement of Chinese medicine for prevention and treatment of infectious diseases. This requires equipment, laboratory, collection of Chinese and foreign literature, and only then can one undertake this research.

In the past, Chinese medicine did not have these conditions—and other elements helping Chinese medicine scientification were also scarce. Today we need to shoulder this new task; we must resolve the problem of advanced studies and improvement. Some may think Chinese medicine scientification may prove very difficult, while practitioners possibly would not be able to. In reality, it is not that they are unable to learn this. For example, we have arranged epidemic prevention training classes and within 2-3 weeks the majority was able to understand some epidemic prevention knowledge. Of course this is not thorough learning of the topic but, for example, with prevention of umbilical tetanus of neonates one can learn the topic within a few hours. Because these are often-seen problems, Chinese medicine advanced studies schools have infectious diseases courses and other courses allowing Chinese medicine scientification to take place. Chinese medicine doctors are able to learn this.

Another aspect: if one wants to learn a new art he must break down sectarian biases. One must study with a humble heart. From now on, as for the issue of improving the level, Chinese medicine may attain some good conditions, and so Chinese medicine should use very well these new conditions. Chinese medicine should build up its own experience and so it will be able to enrich itself. This is the future path of Chinese medicine. Developing the art of Chinese medicine conforms to the people's needs. Therefore, the Ministry of Health handles this affair as one of its tasks.

In this year's National Health Congress in July–August, a scheme was proposed and a discussion developed about the merging of Chinese and Western medicines, elevating it and together serving the people's health. This allowed the experience of both Chinese and Western medicine doctors to tackle these problems. Attending this Congress, as well, were Chinese medicine delegations hoping to put forth their opinion on how to help the people in order for the entire congress to research it together. As long as it was an opinion that benefited the people's health, everybody in the congress naturally adopted it.

Article end

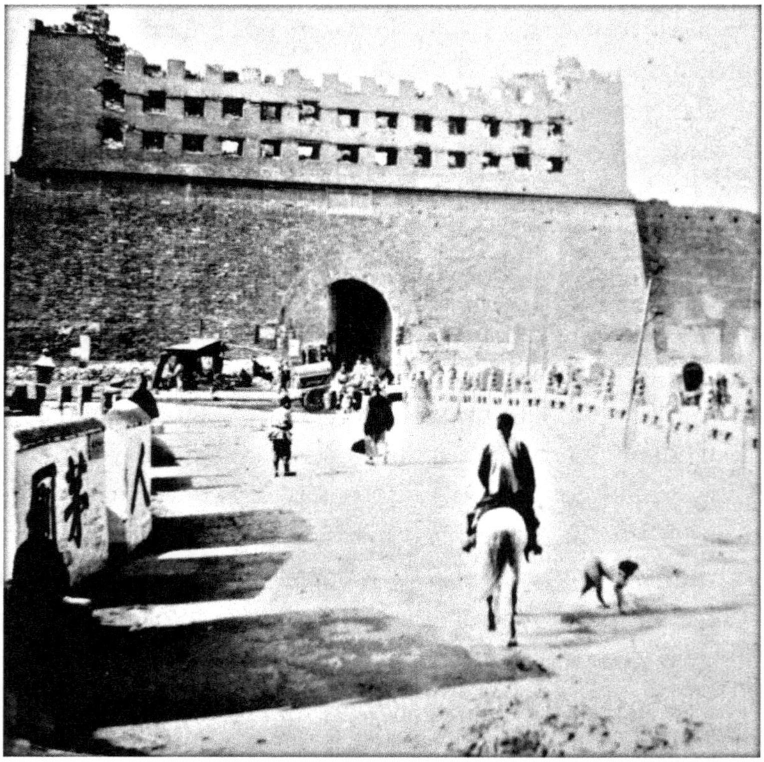

Photo by Mr P. Goux in early 1900s. "Entrance of the Inner City—Peking".

Why does Chinese medicine need to engage in advanced studies? Central Ministry of Health Medical Policy Office, Office Director

1953 by Bao Jinghuan 鮑敬桓

Yaron: Mobilizing Chinese medicine practitioners just like soldiers, in fairness, was needed during the early years of the Communist take over of China. They faced extreme conditions of poverty, lacked healthcare organization and had no viable economy to fund a healthcare system. However, as the situation today is different, so must be the selection process.

Pages 11–12

China's old medicine is one part of China's thousands-year-old culture. In recent years, even though natural sciences and social sciences advanced by leaps and bounds and Western medicine theory, treatment and techniques have sprung forward, yet Chinese medicine "100 years as if one day" did not change at all; it remained together with the masses, offering treatment to the masses. The masses having deep rooted belief in it, is something recognized by both Chinese and Western medicines.

In the 1944 Yan'an Culture and Education Plenary Meeting, the call for "Chinese medicine scientification" was put forth. It was pointed out that Chinese and Western medicines must merge together; Chinese and Western medicines must learn from each other. Western medicine carries the responsibility to help Chinese medicine acquire new medical knowledge in order to serve the people. Following on from that, in liberated regions, Chinese and Western medicines had great transformation. Chinese medicine attained knowledge and techniques from Western medicine, which enriched the Chinese medicine art greatly. Western medicine, likewise, learned from Chinese medicine and this helped greatly overcome the Western drugs shortage during the war. When we compare this situation of Chinese and Western medicines to regions that were not yet liberated, it was entirely different.

Now, the entire nation is liberated. The entire country should follow the example of the liberated areas just like following a teacher. They should merge and synchronize in production and construction. Under the leadership of the Central Ministry of Health they should advance the construction of health in the new China in order to guard the health of the working people. At the same time, the Central Ministry of Health, in accord with policy regulations as well as financial and cultural needs, has decided that the main direction for health work should be "prevention comes first".

In the past, Chinese medicine doctors (to an extreme even many Western medicine doctors) performed only treatment work. Their knowledge of preventive medicine was lacking; they couldn't do it, they had no idea where to start. If Chinese medicine doctors want to partake in the national health scheme, they must first learn the foundation of medical science. Only then can they shoulder the task of "prevention comes first".

Next to that, as everybody knows, Chinese medicine medical knowledge is still on the level of "experience-based"; it did not elevate yet to the theory level. In addition, it does not fully understand complex physiological structures and anatomical systems. It does not have any knowledge of pathology. When it comes to diagnosis and treatment methods and techniques, it still uses thousand-years-old rules. Even though there is some good experience, it varies from one person to another. They know that it is like this but they don't know why it is like this, and still it was transmitted down. When compared to modern medicine, it lacks greatly.

According to the aforementioned two points:

In order to perform "prevention comes first" health policy, Chinese medicine doctors must undergo advanced studies based on modern standards and only then can they perform the task.

We must cause China's medicine to expel the old and take in the new, being truly responsible for the health and life of the people. Chinese medicine also must follow the changing times and the evolving medical knowledge, urgently catch up and directly pursue it; it must learn the new theory in order to supplement and enrich the Chinese medicine knowledge. This is the only viable option to love and protect Chinese medicine.

Article end

Introducing several experience-based formulas

1954 by Qing Ye 青野

Source: *Beijing Chinese Medicine* (periodical), 1954 July (3rd volume 7th publication)
Published by Beijing Chinese Medicine Association Publication Committee
北京中醫
一九五四年七月號(第三卷第七期)
北京中醫學會出版委員會出版

Yaron: The new Chinese medicine uses experience-based formulas. Herb dosages are small, tying in with the "campaign against the Three" instructing doctors to be sparse with herbs in order to help the motherland, not being wasteful or corrupt. It also firms the TCM model of differentiating syndromes and selecting treatment accordingly (Bian Zheng Lun Zhi 辨证论治).

Page 29

Diarrhea: Chinese medicine guards against diarrhea. Even though, up to present, there is no (scientific) research or rather no special effect remedy that was discovered, yet many articles describe in clinic formulas that have efficacy. In addition, no matter what kind of formula it is, its efficacy strength first and foremost relies on the ability to recognize the disease. No matter the diagnostic used—seeing, hearing and smelling, asking or palpating, what we call the four diagnostic methods—if one is able to match the formula to the disease, then its special effect must come about. Otherwise, one may come to the wrong conclusion that experience-based formulas are ineffective. Next I introduce several experience based formulas I have translated from the Japanese periodical "Japan Medical Matters New Publication" published in 1954 in February and May issues. Is it truly effective? I can only ask my fellows to experience this in practice and further advance the investigation.

1) Ge Gen Tang 葛根湯: Ge Gen 葛根 8,[391] Ma Huang 麻黃 Da Zao 大棗 each 4, Gui Zhi 桂枝, Shao Yao 芍藥 each 3, Gan Cao 甘草 1, fresh Sheng Jiang 生薑 3. The disease that it fits: At initial onset pulse is floating tight, fever and aversion to cold, lower back pain, some have stomach pains with diarrhea, if above formula is given warm there is slight perspiration, it can decrease the symptoms, and it can shorten the length of the ailment.

[391] All dosages are in grams.

2) Gui Zhi add Shao Yao Da Huang Tang 桂枝加芍藥大黃湯: Gui Zhi 桂枝, Da Zao 大棗 each 4, Gan Cao 甘草 2, Shao Yao 芍藥 6, Da Huang 大黃 1, fresh Sheng Jiang 生薑 3. The disease that it fits: Light case of diarrhea and the like, the patient has no fever or slight fever, there is stomach pain with urgency and heavy feeling after evacuation, but there is no thirst, nausea, vomiting, fullness, knotted feeling in the stomach area, thick tongue coating etc symptoms. It is appropriate to use in light cases.

3) Da Chai Hu Tang 大柴胡湯: Chai Hu 柴胡 6, Ban Xia 半夏 4, Huang Qin 黃芩, Shao Yao 芍藥, Da Zao 大棗 each 3. Zhi Shi 枳實 2, Da Huang 大黃 1–3, fresh Sheng Jiang 生薑 4. The disease that it fits: After using Ge Gen Tang and inducing sweat, or after several days when the disease resolved and the body seems to have recovered (from the cold injury) but the pulse is deep, there is thirst, tongue coating is brown yellow and dry, there is a lump feeling in the stomach area, no appetite, or nausea, abdominal pain, diarrhea, urgency with a heavy feeling after evacuation, then this formula is appropriate.

4) Shao Yao Tang 芍藥湯: Shao Yao 芍藥 4, Huang Qin 黃芩, Dang Gui 當歸, Huang Lian 黃連 each 2, Gan Cao 甘草, Mu Xiang 木香, Zhi Shi 枳實, Da Huang 大黃, Bing Lang 檳榔 each 1. The disease that it fits: At initial onset or after few days, there is stomach pains and diarrhea, urgency and heavy feeling after evacuation is severe, and there is thick tongue coating and poor appetite, then this formula is appropriate.

5) Shen Gui Shao Yao Tang 參歸芍藥湯: Shao Yao 芍藥 4, Ren Shen 人參, Dang Gui 當歸, Fu Ling 茯苓, Shan Yao 山藥, Chen Pi 陳皮 each 3. Suo Sha Ren 縮砂仁 2, Gan Cao 甘草 1. The disease it fits: Even though the disease has subsided, yet the diarrhea didn't stop, in addition the body is weak, and so it is prohibited to use Da Huang kind of formulas. Then this formula is appropriate. Normally it will take three weeks to resolve the problem.

6) Zhen Wu Tang 真武湯: Fu Ling 茯苓, Shao Yao 芍藥 each 5, Bai Zhu 白術 3, Fu Zi 附子 1, Sheng Jiang 生薑 0.5. The disease it fits: Abdominal pains, diarrhea without end, hands and feet a bit cold, the pulse is small and weak then it is appropriate to use this formula. Or if the disease lasts very long and the lower limbs have edema then this formula is good as well.

The formulas above use grams as measuring units; for an adult, one should add 500ml water, boil and reduce to 300ml, remove the sediment, divide to three and administer three times per day.

Another disease is warts (this includes ordinary warts, adolescent warts and old age warts). Common warts and adolescent warts use Ma Xing Yi Gan Tang 麻杏苡甘湯 internally, administer for ten days to one month in order to resolve the problem. One can also use alone Yi Yi Ren 薏苡仁 and treat it. But the effect of the single herb is inferior to the formula above.

1) Ma Xing Yi Gan Tang 麻杏苡甘湯: Ma Huang 麻黃 4, Xing Ren 杏仁 3, Gan Cao 甘草 2, Yi Yi Ren 薏苡仁 12. Preparation method: For an adult for one day add 500ml water, boil and reduce to 300ml, remove sediment, divide into two or three doses and administer within the day twice or thrice. Patients younger than fifteen years old can still use the above dosage, ages 7-10 use half the dose, ages 4-6 use a quarter to a third of the dose.

2) Yi Yi Ren 薏苡仁 Decoction: Yi Yi Ren 薏苡仁 12 (it is most effective if the hard shell is removed). Use the prior cooking instruction and administration method.

Excerpt end

Section: Chinese medicine development in different regions

Source: *Beijing Chinese Medicine* (periodical), 1954 July (3rd volume 7th publication)
Published by Beijing Chinese Medicine Association Publication Committee
北京中醫
一九五四年七月號(第三卷第七期)
北京中醫學會出版委員會出版

Yaron: In the factory there is a blend of Chinese Western doctors, which meant Chinese medicine doctors who have learned basics of modern medicine.

Page 31

Report: Building Chinese medicine industry in Tai Yuan City 太原市: Energetic service (for the people)

Our society reports: In Shanxi 山西 province the Party and government give importance to Chinese medicine. At present in Tai Yuan city there are relatively many factories with medical facilities. Within them there are not a few that accepted Chinese medicine doctors for work; some have one practitioner, some two or three, and altogether they accepted more than fifty practitioners. Treatment efficacy is normally good, receiving the workers' praises. For example, in factory XXX there are twelve doctors; ten of them are Chinese and Western doctors (seven of whom are internal medicine, 3 external medicine) and two are Chinese-medicine-only doctors. In April, the internal medicine clinic saw 3727 patients, among which the combined Chinese and Western doctors diagnosed and treated 1324 patients, or about 35%. The Chinese-medicine-only doctors diagnosed and treated 2403 patients or 65%. For smaller factories lacking medical facilities or having poor facilities unable to handle medical care, the Tai Yuan city Department of Health plans to gather private doctors and concentrate them in six United Clinics around the factories, in order to overcome this deficiency. In addition, factories and construction sites have a relationship with nine United Clinics which, in April this year, have treated a total of 28,238 patients.

Tai Yuan city already gained experience and success last year laying down the foundation for workers' organizations connecting with private doctors. Today, they still use it to overcome workers' medical care deficiencies. Tai Yuan Trade Union Federation, in order to protect the workers' health, established two workers' medical facilities. Among the two, the second medical facility solely utilizes Chinese medicine and Chinese herbs for treatment. It contains 100 patient beds and, regarding treatment, it uses both acupuncture and herbs as a combined treatment method. Treatment efficacy is excellent and recovery phase is relatively short.

Report end

Report: Curriculum expansion and revision scope (Hebei 河北 Province Chinese Medicine Advanced Studies School)

Page 31

Our society reports: Hebei province Chinese Medicine Advanced Studies School, in accord with the local Ministry of Health directive, already revised the contents of the advanced studies curriculum, expanding the proportion of Chinese medicine. With the entire curriculum of 720 hours, political classes (including the Party general line, current affairs education and Ministry of Health policy) occupies 15%. Foundation of medicine's general knowledge (physiology, public sanitation and infectious diseases) occupies 15%. The remaining 70% is divided equally between Chinese medicine departments: acupuncture; internal medicine; gynecology; pediatrics; pharmacology (mainly Chinese herbs, but there are also new drugs commonly used as special effect remedies); diagnosis (this includes modern medicine diagnostics); exchange of experience; and practical study.

The arrangement of experience exchange in the school has two types. The first, inviting fourteen local famous doctors to form Chinese medicine research association, divided into four departments of acupuncture, internal medicine, gynecology and pediatrics. The selected study materials are then discussed by the group, annotated and the deficiencies supplemented. At the end they make a report and during this discussion the fellows raise different opinions and correction ideas. After that, it goes through the research organization's research and then it is corrected once more.

The second way of arranging fellows' experience exchange is taking the most efficacious experience from each one in regards to disease: diagnosis; handling; method of preparing; application; prohibitions; explanations; modifications according to symptoms; contraindications; and how to guard against the unexpected—and equally differentiate and explain every single one of them. If it is possible to use scientific explanation for the disease etiology and pharmacology, then they merge it. Otherwise they use factual phenomena in their experience in order to explain it. They do not use strained interpretation to explain it.

Report end

How did I come to learn and use acupuncture therapy?

1954 by Xiong Yi 雄毅

Source: *Beijing Chinese Medicine* (periodical), 1954 September (3rd volume 9th publication)
Published by Beijing Chinese Medicine Association Publication Committee
北京中醫
一九五四年九月號(第三卷第九期)
北京中醫學會出版委員會出版

Yaron: The author is a Western medicine trained medic, who likely received limited medical training in the army. He learned acupuncture himself from books and started practicing on patients, claiming outstanding results. It demonstrates the liberty and encouragement, at least in the early Communist years, for Western medicine trained low level personnel to self-learn acupuncture and provide healthcare to the impoverished masses. That this person publishes his experience with great pride testifies to the atmosphere of popularizing acupuncture at any cost as quickly as possible. In our articles we often see "Chinese medicine advanced studies", a misleading title that refers to the study of scientific medicine and Communist ideology. Today, when people go to TCM School they often call it "Acupuncture School", the origins of which begin here with mass popularization of acupuncture.

Page 26-27

I am a doctor working in a small clinic in a village. Previously, I didn't understand Chinese medicine. Even though I have witnessed a few aspects of Chinese medicine in practice on occasion, this was all confused in my mind. I heard some people say that Chinese medicine is not scientific and so I was under the impression that Chinese medicine is backward. Nonetheless, I have read reports that sometimes Chinese medicine heals diseases effectively and even better than Western medicine (like some acupuncture and moxibustion therapy clinical reports describe), and therefore I didn't dare conclude Chinese medicine to be good or bad.

In 1952, via the army, I was dispatched to work at the county commune hospital, which helped me get even closer to the people (Chinese medicine doctors). At this time I had already read a book titled *The New Acupuncture and Moxibustion Study Xin*

Zhen Jiu Xue 新針灸學 by comrade Zhu Lian 朱璉. I truly read it from beginning to end once; however, her emphasis (clinical efficacy) was hard for me to believe. Can there be so many diseases cured with one needle puncturing the skin and muscle? This was a problem constantly lingering in my mind but I didn't find the courage to start experimenting with it (as I was lacking a theoretical foundation). And so I didn't research it further, nor did I continue to study it. Even more so, during that time, new treatment methods (like tissue therapy) attracted me more, and so I neglected acupuncture study.

Not until I encountered, at the end of 1953, Pavlov's studies did I became clear about the nervous system (cerebral cortex) and the close relationship between the insides of the body and the outside layers. In addition, only when I grew aware of the Soviet "live points on the skin" research and foreign interest in our motherland's medicine, acupuncture and moxibustion, did I became enthusiastic about studying acupuncture.

At this point I already had Pavlov's theory foundations, as I was working at a local clinic and so, within a short period of time of self-studying the theory from books, I started using this treatment method. The results were fantastic.

For example, the first patient case was the director of the village farmers association comrade Liu 劉, who suffered trigeminal nerve pain. He could not feel half of his face, but with needling the point He Gu 合谷 he had an immediate and complete recovery. Until today he didn't suffer a relapse. Another case was a female patient name Yang 楊, who suffered numbness of the thigh nerve. She couldn't stand up and walk. Through diagnosis I decided to use acupuncture (points used were Huan Tiao 環跳, Ming Men 命門, San Jiao Shu 三焦俞, Small and Large Intestine Shu 大小腸俞, Xue Hai 血海, Xi Guan 膝關 etc points) altogether twice. People are telling me that she can walk now. (There was no long term observation done as of yet). Another case is of Mr. Li 李, a 48 year old military man, who contracted a severe infectious and acute conjunctivitis. He received acupuncture once and was cured (he fainted during the acupuncture treatment).

The masses welcome acupuncture because it is very cheap and the efficacy speedy. These cases got me excited. It got me wanting to pursue these studies with full trust. Until today, within one to two months I have already seen and treated 120 acupuncture cases (not included in this number quite a few other cases). Now, because I am a relative beginner, lacking experience and other conditions, I still didn't use moxibustion. I can say, however, that acupuncture and moxibustion have a definite clinical value. It is the crystallization of our forefathers' clinical experience over centuries. At present as our nation transitions its route to the beacon of light and expanding the health services and improving the people's health, promoting acupuncture and moxibustion therapy is a must and entails a special meaning. The accumulated experience I have from giving acupuncture to the 120 cases mentioned above I want to introduce here to my colleagues, hoping to consider together and receive corrections:

My little personal experience:

1) Before treatment, make it a habit to explain to the patient what acupuncture effects are, the mechanism by which it works and how it feels during the treatment. This allows the patient a situation overview and, with that, a secondary signal to the brain to establish preponderance and excitement. Using acupuncture and moxibustion therapy in such a way increases efficacy. It also helps improve patient compliance and may prevent fainting during treatment.

2) Before needling one should prepare well the acupoints. One cannot needle in a leisurely way because accurately preparing the acupoints can benefit the relationship and harmony between acupoints, which leads to higher efficacy. When selecting points it should be in order from top to bottom, distal to proximal, front to rear, internal to external, some acupoints are needled first, some after—this is also something requiring attention. According to my personal experience, one should first needle distal points at the nerve's periphery and only thereafter needle proximal points or local points. In this fashion, the ones being needled later can supplement strength to the earlier ones. Like a stomach patient case receiving acupuncture. When I needled Zu San Li 足三里 and Zhong Wan 中脘 I didn't see any effect—at best I could see slight decrease in stomach pains—but when I further needled stomach Shu point 胃俞 (on the back) the pains completely disappeared.

3) One should not choose too many points because this can cause the patient to be unsatisfied. This may also increase the difficulty next time to select points (one should avoid selecting same points). According to my experience, the least is 1–3 acupoints, the most is 10–12 acupoints.

4) One should pay attention to the patient's body condition and execute the needling accordingly. One cannot force it. Like a case of a patient name Li

李, to whom I gave acupuncture to for conjunctivitis. Because his age was advanced (48) and his body weak, and because he came from afar (five kilometers away), when I needled the point Jing Ming 睛明 he fainted and I had to deliver resuscitation methods and he recovered. But despite this, one should guard against such accidents.

5) Patient needling reactions include soreness, numbness, swelling, pain etc. Because each person is different, the nerves' sensitivity is different and one may not conclude that one feeling is better than another. Some people don't have reaction right away, so after each needling you should pause in that spot for a little while and twist the needle, after some time sensation arrives. Do not act recklessly trying to find it.

6) In most cases, one acupuncture session cannot lead to complete cure. On forms filled out as having effect or seeing cure, the patient came multiple times. In my work I am of the opinion that five sessions are one treatment course. Every 3–4 days when effect wears off they should come again for acupuncture. Because of this after 3–4 sessions patients are completely cured or see considerable improvement. Is it really accurate? I ask my colleagues to comment.

7) I have also used a method I read about in *Beijing Chinese Medicine* publication by comrade Liu Ronggui 劉榮貴, what he calls "burning the mountain method" and "penetrating heaven cooling method". Initially I felt that this application reached good results; however, I don't have many patient cases to prove it. Nonetheless, I feel that further investigation of it is a must.

Article end

Chinese medicine symposium convened in Xuan Hua City[392] People's Government (September 1954): Determining the plan for Chinese medicine work going forward

Yaron: The enthusiasm in the government takeover of Chinese medicine. "Increase their socialist education and allow them to understand better the future development of our society and the function that Chinese medicine needs to take within." How each individual doctor was impacted by this top-to-bottom pressure is incalculable, but it is certain that doctors inclined less to follow their own wish and instead followed what was expected of them.

Page 40

(*Xuan Hua* 宣化 *City News*) In order to carry out the party line and the four great principles of health work it was decided that, going forward, the plan for Chinese medicine is the following: Xuan Hua City People's Government convened a symposium from June 25th to 27th. Participating in the symposium were the city's government health branch, section chief, people's hospital director, city council and city government representatives, as well as Chinese medicine doctors from the entire city, a total of 35 participants.

When the conference started, first Xuan Hua City government health branch, section Chief Chen Bingzhang 陳秉章 delivered a report titled *The condition of Chinese medicine in the past four years and my opinion about its prospects into the future*. In addition, he educated the participants' thoughts about the Party's main policy line and the policy of merging Chinese and Western medicines. Through this conference, and especially the informal discussions, each Chinese medicine worker got to know deeply that the government's loving care is even in the smallest affairs and that current work is very important. There were many people eagerly wanting to participate in Chinese medicine advanced studies and professional studies, so they asked the government to swiftly establish Wei Xie Hui 衛協會[393] Association of Health Professionals and a Chinese medicine research association. There were also comrades making sugges-

[392] Xuan Hua city 宣化市 in 1955 became part of Zhang Jia Kou city 张家口市 in Hebei.
[393] Wei Xie Hui 衛協會 stands for Wei Sheng Gong Zuo Zhe Xie Hui 衛生工作者協會 Association of Health Professionals.

tions how to improve Chinese medicine work going forward and how to merge Chinese and Western medicines with vigor.

In order to curb Chinese medicine deficiencies and advance Chinese medicine work, as well as to supplement the Chinese medicine practical application, the conference decided the following: going forward, merging of Chinese and Western medicines must increase. Especially the different factions within Chinese medicine must merge (be eliminated). In addition, the Chinese medicine leadership has a plan to implement the four great principles of sanitation work. In addition, according to the number of fellows (in each locality) and expertise level, they will arrange small groups to research difficulties and patient records in order to advance Chinese medicine within the profession. They will establish group consultation controls. There is also a plan to have Chinese medicine doctors participate in the labor force, increase their socialist education and allow them to understand better the future development of our society and the function that Chinese medicine needs to take within.

Xuan Hua city, the people's government, health department, news report group

---

Article end

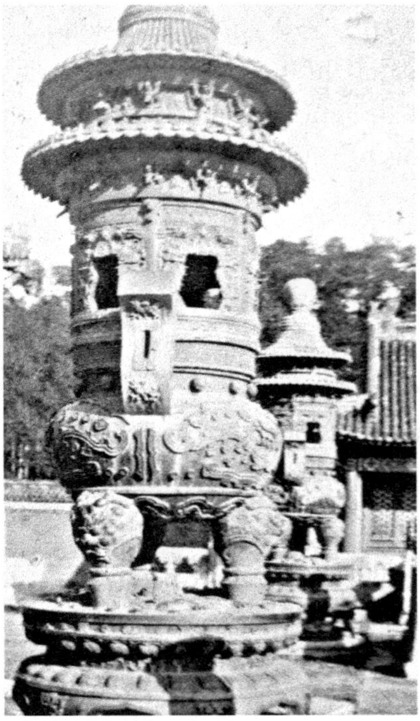

Photo by Mr P. Goux in early 1900s. "Incense burner (at the sacrificial room of the tomb of Emperor Quan Su He, 2nd emperor of the current dynasty)".

The benefit of Cheng Cheng 澄城 county convening Chinese Medicine Representative Congress[394]

1954 by Liu Zirun 劉自潤 and Ze Lie 昃烈

Page 40

In order to unfold the constitution draft study and propagation and to advance a step further in the merging of Chinese and Western medicine to create health work for the masses, the People's Government of Cheng Cheng county convened a grand conference of Chinese medicine representatives from the entire county. Altogether attending the conference were 95 delegates. The conference convened under the leadership of the county's assistant director Yang Jingshan 楊靜山. In the conference they listened to assistant director Yang's mobilizing report, the report by the Chinese Communist Party Cheng Cheng County Party Committee Ministry of Propaganda assistant director Gao 高, and Cheng Cheng County Commune Hospital director Liu Zirun 劉自潤 report on communicating his attendance in the third national health administration conference, the spirit of the event and going forward the tasks at hand.

These reports gave the delegates great inspiration. All delegates expressed a desire to increase efforts, raising the bar in regards to political affairs and skill level (of medicine) and to invest effort and labor increasing the people's health and serving the nation's socialism and industrialization. At the end, the Chinese Communist Party Cheng Cheng County party secretary Dang Qinshu 黨勤書 concluded with a summary, arriving at the following few benefits:

1) Every delegate on an entry level understood the constitution draft main points, furthermore they realized the importance and honor of the health labor force.
2) Everyone carried out even more the four main principles of the health care labor force.
3) They invigorated the merging of Western and Chinese medicines and made proper the attitude of medical treatment. They recognized that as our nation develops the health care labor force, importance will gradually grow.
4) In order to overcome the secrecy thinking process, they exchanged in public their secret recipes and experience.

Article end

[394] Cheng Cheng county 澄城縣 is a county of Weinan municipality, Shaanxi province 陝西省渭南市.

In order to meet our nation's socialist cultural construction we must increase the Chinese medicine allotted work

Source: *Beijing Chinese Medicine* (periodical), 1954 August (3rd volume 8th publication)
Published by Beijing Chinese Medicine Association Publication Committee
北京中醫
一九五四年八月號(第三卷第八期)
北京中醫學會出版委員會出版

[Printed as the article's subtitle] *(Editor's note) This article comes from opinions on how to undertake the Chinese medicine work by many of Shanghai's Chinese medicine comrades such as Shi Yiren* 時逸人, *Hong Guanzhi* 洪貫之 *etc. Even though in a few locations some of the concrete time-related statements are not valid anymore, but from within this article one can clearly see the aspirations for the Chinese medicine work. We therefore especially included it here in this publication.*

Yaron: Persons such as Shi Yiren,[395] the founder of Shanxi Research Society of Medicine during the Republic, were active during the scientification attempts of the 1920s and '30s. Here, their arguments and strategy for modern reform have, on the one hand, intensified and on the other, changed tone and even direction to reflect the Communist Party political line. I can only speculate that at least some practitioners were thrilled at the opportunities offered by the Communist regime, such as establishing Chinese medicine hospitals or departments within modern hospitals, mass scale advanced studies classes, standardized text books and schools.

There were many factors contributing to reshaping TCM, and point number 4 of this article is one of them. Many TCM practitioners today use patent herbal pills, also called Cheng Yao 成药. Why and from where these pills came about is here clearly explained.

---

395 For a short and interesting report about Shi Yiren, see *Neither Donkey Nor Horse* by Sean Lei, pages 178–180.

Point number 5 not only explains the rigorous standardization of textbooks and TCM knowledge, but it also highlights that all comrade practitioners had to follow the new standard in order to "elevate" their level. In Communist terminology, "not elevating the level" meant total and utter personal destruction. It was certainly not seen as "optional." Pressure was exercised upon individuals selecting and rejecting elements of Chinese medicine in order to fulfil the current needs: political, economic and logistic. It was not a group of scholars' "free meeting of the minds" discussing the medicine's best virtues according to scholarly or practical research.

Now, more than six decades have elapsed and many, if not all of us, have become used to the reality of TCM; it is already a 2-3 generations-old tradition. Today, people around the world wish Chinese medicine to be more than a second-class Western medicine alternative. Helping the masses today means finding a unique Chinese medicine perspective on health and life; it means that a potential for rediscovering Chinese medicine exists within the ancient philosophical theories that were dropped out of TCM. Having said that, I add a word of caution here: early 21st century China actively promotes Confucianism as a national heritage, which encourages the "reviving of anything classic" trend in recent years. Today, many things of old age become precious—including superstitions. This is another trap for us not to fall into.

Page 1–2

Since the Central Government put forth the general policy line and transitioned people successfully, in each professional circle, through learning and connecting to current political reality, one after the other they agreed and harmonized together with the general line plan. Each region launched ideological education of "strengthening the cultural education work" and "the health work is to serve the socialist construction". Under the spirit and guidance of the Fourth Plenary Session of the 7th National Congress of the Chinese Communist Party and the Third National Health Administration Conference, our medical work has made a clear advancement towards the construction of China's new medicine.

In order to support the general line needs, with everything we do and with every different kind of medical worker, we must break the boundary between Chinese and Western, old and new. On the foundation already established, we should emphasize more unification and even closer mutual help and hand-in-hand cooperation. First, we must prepare well for the exchange between Chinese and Western medicines.

This will allow the upcoming new medicine to open up brilliant and glorious flowers and form full-grown fruits. The motherland medicine is one of our cultural inheritances—it is an accumulated experience of our motherland workers struggling against disease.

Therefore, we must now use scientific methods and point of view to arrange it and accept part of its content that conforms to real principle. This will allow it to become a part of the new world medicine. At present, our new medicine already shook off mechanical materialism and the shackles of cell pathology theory. From now on, via strengthening the foundation of the "merging together", we should research constantly, criticize, expand and elevate the rich and accumulated experience of our motherland's medicine. In this way, we will gradually transition until reaching the goal of socialism, at which time there will be no difference between Chinese and Western, old and new.

In order for us to reach the above listed objectives, we propose a few recommendations below to serve as an energetic guiding principle for all of us. It is, as well, our task in this transitioning period!

1) Develop Chinese medicine advanced studies work, popularize and establish an advanced studies school in each province

Chinese medicine advanced studies is implemented according to the correct Chinese medicine scientification directive. In the past, because of objective conditions not being the same, organization of advanced classes took on different shapes in different regions. Now, through the selfless help of Western medicine comrades, and since they revealed Western medical treatment and preventive measures to everyone, it allowed Chinese medicine comrades to voluntarily repudiate the old secretive way of doing things. This not only increased everyone's level, but also impacted their "loving the motherland health and sanitation movement". From this we can see the progressiveness and correctness of the advanced studies system.

At present, advanced studies education is just slightly developed; it is not propagated everywhere and hardly fulfills the large-scale need of Chinese medicine. Advanced studies overall have only reached about ten percent of all Chinese medicine doctors in the country because there are still some low level cadres in local health ministries who don't see the importance of Chinese medicine, which leads to many areas still not offering advanced studies, or only offering few short classes and then stopping it. Even more so, there are Chinese medicine doctors in some regions who have graduated already from advanced studies but were not yet assigned appropriate jobs. This leads to "study having no application", which is a waste of human talent.

In addition, some Chinese medicine doctors are of lesser cultural capacity and as a result lack the ability to accept new things. Their political consciousness is inadequate. This, in turn, gave rise to cadres in some departments to excessively emphasize the deficiencies of Chinese medicine. They overlook the merging together of Chinese medicine and its improved work which, in itself, is leading Chinese medicine to "a divide between old and new". This truly is a mutual cause-and-effect relationship and the responsibility here is not limited to only one aspect. We must reflect upon and correct these deficiencies in order to accelerate the completion of advanced study in Chinese medicine. This, on its own, will implement the principle of promoting advanced education all around.

Therefore, our goal is that, in every region having adequate conditions, at least on the provincial level, there should form one Chinese Medicine Advanced Studies School. In cities of smaller population and on the county level, they should offer other advanced study classes, or resume operations of classes which were discontinued or, instead of resuming operation, offer other advanced classes of a higher standard. They should establish these classes with a view for constant improvement and allowing Chinese medicine doctors to have more work outlets.

2) Emphasis should be given to establishing Chinese medicine experimental hospitals

Establishing Chinese medicine experimental hospitals taps into the potential of the new perfect foundation of "our motherland medicine" and "the exchange of Chinese and Western medicines". For growing the force of Chinese medicine and better serving the Party line, there is a real meaning for diagnosing a disease in a scientific way and then having experienced Chinese medicine comrades delivering their specific specialized treatment. Not only that, while exploring the rich traditional medical experience, if one puts it through an "experiment phase" then he may extract the useful material out of it and be able to organize it. This may help spread the useful aspect of modern medical treatment and, even a step further; it may enrich the content of modern medicine. It will allow the new medicine of new China to become even more comprehensive. Our current need is to implement local bureaus of public health regional pilot schemes and within them, according to objective needs, step by step advance their[396] establishment in every province, or create a Chinese medicine department within comprehensive hospitals. This is, as

[396] Referring to Chinese medicine experimental hospitals.

well, one of the health plans of the transition period.[397] In this fashion, "merging together" and "exchange" can be implemented with great vigor.

3) Regulate Chinese medicine associations and organize them systematically

Since the Chinese People Political Consultative Conference Culture and Education Group and the Chinese Medicine Association unleashed the movement of "Chinese and Western medicines exchange", the task of each regional Chinese medicine association has increased in its importance. This also made the Chinese Medicine Association leadership unified in its pressing need to strengthen the organization. At present, different regional Chinese medicine associations have different names and their subordination is not standardized. In some areas they are called "Chinese medicine and pharmacology association". In some areas they are independent organizations, while in other areas they belong to the local association of public health works. Not only are the names not unified but also their status is different and their official power differs. We are of the opinion that, under the general need for strengthening the Chinese medicine work, the systematic organization of Chinese medicine associations must be appropriately adjusted.

When we compare the Public Health Works Association with Chinese Medicine Association, there are certain aspects which are different. The Public Health Association is composed of members who deal with public health and, while they do have a connection to each other, their subordination must not be connected. Now, in order to undertake the task of exchange between Chinese and Western medicines even better, Chinese medicine associations in every region of the country need to become independent organizations. From now on and without exception, all of them will accept the double tutelage of China's Medical Association headquarters 中華醫學會總會 and Beijing Chinese Medicine Association 北京中醫學會. In addition, specialized associations should partake in activities of China's Medical Association local branches in order to integrate. This will provide great help toward the exchange development between Chinese and Western medicines.

4) Change the form of Chinese herbals[398] and advance Chinese pharmacology scientification

China's national production of herbal products has been derived and developed by small agricultural economy and handcraft industry. Its professional direction lags relatively behind. Since the herbs' preparation and combination methods were often

[397] Into socialism.
[398] Instead of using raw herbs, make pills, powders and ointments that are easy to administer.

done the old way, many efficacious herbs have lost much of their efficacy and, to an extreme, even lost efficacy entirely. From another perspective, because herbs were originally used in the raw form, dosage used was huge. Adjusting the formula wasted time and administering it was inconvenient. For our working comrades participating in the collectivization work, in order for them to take it with ease at any given time, and since they know the efficacy of Chinese herbals and they also like to use Western drugs, this is then the natural development from here for Chinese herbal medicine. Therefore, changing the form of Chinese herbs not only answers the need to advance Chinese medicine but it also answers to the urgent need of the masses. After herbs have changed form and their usage is not limited to Chinese medicine alone, then it can be promoted to be used with modern medical treatment in the different departments. This conforms to the needs of our construction of a socialist society. In addition, this will have a distinct value in building our economy and so we must encourage it.

At present, even though some local small-scale privately-owned businesses are already doing this work, it is still, nonetheless, in the experimental phase and therefore their impact is minimal. We need governmental leadership and control and each of the administrative districts'[399] departments of health to plan the building of a modern Chinese herbal factory in each district. They should use a combination of public- and privately-owned enterprises to promote this objective. They should select efficacious formulas and commonly-used single herbs and, according to demand, emphasize the production and then, step-by-step, make it popular. In the future, the experimental Chinese medicine hospitals and the United Clinics will use this kind of "new Chinese pharmacology". This will be done in order to reduce waste and increase efficacy. It is also in accord with "increasing production while saving".[400]

5) Compile standardized and unified Chinese medicine text books

China's medicine has an entire system of its own. The medicine and its clinical application cannot be divided. However, because Chinese medicine comrades have different levels, it is not uniform. Their ability to master the accumulated experience of our motherland's medicine is incomplete.

It is also an obstacle that, in the past, Chinese medicine was influenced by the feudal society and transmitted within sects from teacher to disciple. Therefore, the first task at hand is to improve upon the accumulated experience of the past. There are some Chinese medicine comrades whose previous experience was insufficient and, therefore,

[399] This refers to the six administrative areas of the People Republic of China that were from 1951–1954 following the country's division from the late Qing dynasty. They were dissolved between June and November 1954.
[400] One of the government directives at the time.

after participating in advanced studies, felt that scientific theory and clinical practice could not link up[401] and, contrary to expectations, became improper abusers of Western drugs. Unavoidably, this caused a decline with the advanced studies anticipated result. We cannot ignore this. In order to remedy this shortcoming, we put forward the need to reorganize and unify the Chinese medicine text books. Even though this kind of work cannot escape difficulties, our request is not far beyond reach. For the time being, we don't have to "link" or "thread" all of it together. We simply need to take all the motherland medicine and pick and choose, discard what does not conform to logic and, instead, take the accumulated experience fruits and, with a critical approach, introduce it. Like this we will supply it to Chinese medicine comrades for review, which in turn will allow them to elevate their level. This task is not impossible.

In the past, there were also Chinese medicine scholars who had published works about Chinese medicine scientification. They already had rich clinical experience and familiarity with education and literary compositions. Even though their past accomplishments are not all of the same success, from now on, if we use a collective style of literary composition, then each single person's deficiencies can be overcome. This kind of unifying and standardizing the composition of text books will not only help in elevating the level of Chinese medicine practitioners, but it will also introduce our motherland medicine's concrete contents in a brief and to-the-point fashion, with modern and simple-to-understand language. This will furnish Western medicine comrades with written materials to consider. It will be done in order to help them make initial steps in understanding our motherland medicine and it is especially useful for the process of linking up Chinese and Western medicines at its initial stages.

6) The focal point of running a pilot scheme of Chinese medicine schools

In one country there is only one kind of medicine. Chinese medicine education does not require a separate course of development. However, because at present stage of medical education there is no existing curriculum for the original medicine[402] and, in addition, Western medicine comrades are still lacking the practical experience of the original medicine's "rational core", there is no contradiction between our socialist development and establishing Chinese medicine schools teaching mainly Chinese medicine. Our motherland originally had its own medicine and even though it lacked scientific explanations, yet some parts of it do contain scientific elements. More than simply Chinese pharmacology and acupuncture are worth serious consideration. Now that we study Pavlov's theories, we immediately recognize that

[401] Scientific theory could not link up with a Chinese medicine application.
[402] The medicine that was originally in China namely Chinese medicine.

Chinese medicine diagnostic and treatment system springs out of the view of wholeness. Indeed, it has a logical core to be explored. This was already proven by the success that the "new acupuncture" had with experiments and the subsequent popularity in Chinese medicine hospitals and clinics.

We are of the opinion that, after establishing Chinese medicine schools, the education therein will qualify Chinese medicine practitioners for registration. It will train many relatively high-level Chinese medicine doctors. For the vast group of Chinese medicine practitioners, this will afford another way to improve upon their prior experience and become better. These schools will be entirely different from Chinese medicine schools in the old society. If Chinese medicine comrades will rely upon their prior experience without having a high enough level, then exchange between Chinese and Western medicines will remain at the hands of a minority. This certainly is not ideal. At present, in Chinese medicine advanced studies classes, there are many people asking for expansion of instruction on "Chinese medicine research". Nonetheless, the prevalent problem is lack of qualified teachers.

Therefore, we are of the opinion that the ones who had previous experience in improving "Chinese medicine education" might as well share the workload in the Chinese Medicine Advanced Studies School. Following directly the Central Ministry of Health leadership, they will first conduct a pilot project in Beijing and recruit talent from the entire country to join efforts in planning, participating and teaching in the Chinese Medicine School. If it is successful, then a second and a third school can form in other major cities, all remaining under a unified leadership of the central government. In this fashion, education will improve and further incorporate clinical statistics from the experimental hospitals. This will certainly take the motherland medicine and systematically rearrange it. It will allow a foundation for inserting some motherland medicine courses into the new medical education curriculum, which will reach the end objective of converging Chinese and Western medicines.

Article end

My experience with Pavlov's theories and Chinese medicine scientification

1954 by Jing Xiaochou 荊小儔

Source: *Beijing Chinese Medicine* (periodical), 1954 August (3rd volume 8th publication)
北京中醫
一九五四年八月號(第三卷第八期)

Yaron: Scientification, Pavlov and other issues such as using small herb dosages—demonstrating the practitioners' overall attitude at that time.

Pages 3-8

1) Introduction

Before I start my discussion on the issue at hand, I want to introduce first my background of studying Pavlov's theories, the purpose of which is to allow readers a better understanding of my point of view towards Chinese medicine throughout the past and the transformation I went through after studying Pavlov's *Commentary on the Cerebrum's Two Hemispheres Functions* (translated by Ge Shaolong 戈紹龍) and why I put forth these few problems.

20 years ago, when I just started learning Chinese medicine, it was a moment in time when Chinese medical texts were being translated and introduced from Japanese into Chinese. There was one book, *The Big Iron Spear of Medicine and Pharmacology* 醫藥界的大鐵椎,[403] which criticized Western medicine deficiencies and caused the skin many bruises. At the same time, there was another book published by the commercial printing house, for which a foreword was written by the famous Western medicine doctor Yu Yan 余巖 (Yunxiu 雲岫). In this book they used Chinese medicine ancient texts to criticize Chinese medicine. They painfully extracted unscientific aspects of Chinese medicine and delighted in them in a sarcastic and uninhibited way. I was a youngster, possessing only slight knowledge of science and having

[403] Published in 1910 by Wada Keijuro 和田启十郎 (1872–1916). Translations into Chinese were published by Ding Fubao in 1911 and 1920. The "iron spear" is an allusion to a classical story in which a lord of Han, Zhang Liang, raised an army to fight the first emperor of China, Qin Shihuang, in order to reclaim his confiscated lands. He succeeded in getting close enough to throw his spear but missed Qin Shihuang's chariot, hitting a neighboring one instead. The message is that attacks on Kampo "Japanese style Chinese medicine" were aimed at the wrong target. Footnote credit: Bridie Andrews *The Making of Modern Chinese Medicine 1850–1960*.

interest in Chinese medicine, holding in my hands these two books, reciting and reading them with speed and I was undecided.

While undecided I connected with few friends, some studying Chinese medicine and some Western medicine. I was hoping to reach a final conclusion on whether studying Chinese medicine has value or not. Unfortunately, reaching this final conclusion was very difficult. Between these friends there was only ridicule and self-importance. Sometime thereafter, by chance, [visiting] a Western medicine doctor that I knew well, I saw his wife taking Chinese herbs. It seemed as though I had finally struck gold. I resolutely decided to investigate Chinese medicine further.

At that time I was of the opinion, "Chinese medicine has scientific value, yet the old theories were not scientific. One must rearrange it all from scratch with scientific methods, and only like this can it carry forward." I then used scientific methods to rearrange Zhang Zhongjing's 張仲景 *Shang Han Lun* 傷寒論. I used Yin Yang 陰陽 and the autonomic nervous system to explain it. I believed that "Yin holds the function of parasympathetic nerve[404] while Yang the sympathetic nerve. They coordinate with each other equally and this allows the smooth operation of all bodily systems. When we get to a state of disease, this mutual influence is being impacted. It loses its normal state of equilibrium and it becomes an abnormal situation that reflects outward, it becomes the myriad symptoms. The treatment principle of Chinese medicine, therefore, is to cause all these myriad symptoms to go back to the normal state. It targets these two types of nerves via the use of herbs. Other herbs that kill bacteria, lower fever, expel toxins, relieve inflammation etc. were not the main objective of Chinese medicine."

According to this point of view, I took the six conformations and viewed them as six levels of neurological pathologies. In my opinion, the old theory of "six meridians of hand and foot connect to the inner organs" is an addition by later generations and a strained interpretation of a mystical theory. It is not the original intention of Zhang Zhongjing. So how to divide these six levels then? I explained it as follows:

When there is a toxin, bacteria or abnormal weather that influences, attacks and injures the external part of the body and skin, this impacts the nerve periphery, which

[404] Vagus nerve also responsible for calming and slowing down action. Sympathetic nerves are mainly responsible for excitement and speeding up action.

induces a reaction in the nerve center.[405] When sympathetic nerve reaction reaches the ganglion, it brings into play a natural harmonizing and good effect. The sympathetic nerves of the entire body become excited and do not allow the nerve in the injured area to recede its action. Vitality of the entire body induces spring force in the sympathetic nerves' ganglions. The result is that the sympathetic nerve at the injured site becomes hyper-stimulated which causes symptoms such as bleeding, sweating, nasal discharge, salivation, or even fever, headaches, blocked nose, dry belching etc.

However, during this time, because the parasympathetic nerve is directly connected to the central nervous system and because the brain and central nervous system are accustomed to the patient's past experiences and ways of response, its reaction to the same stimuli appears different for different people. Sometimes it is strong while at other times weak and the level of strength is relative. When the reaction is strong it appears with no sweat and then it is Ma Huang Tang 麻黃湯 syndrome, when tendons spasm then it is Ge Gen Tang 葛根湯 syndrome and when the reaction is weak it appears to have sweat and it is a Gui Zhi Tang 桂枝湯 syndrome etc. This is the stage of Tai Yang 太陽.

If the virus attacks the respiratory system (includes the chest, ribs, diaphragm, and under the diaphragm lymph nodes, liver etc) it stimulates the sympathetic nerves in this region to react. Likewise the parasympathetic (Vagus) nerve is affected and, depending on its strength, one can see a variety of different symptoms. This is the Shao Yang 少陽 disease stage. If the virus advances to the digestive system and induces a reaction from the sympathetic nerves in this region, likewise the parasympathetic nerve reacts and, according to it being strong or weak, there are different symptoms visible. This is the Yang Ming 陽明 stage. These three Yang stages are all natural innate ability and spring-force reactions of the sympathetic nerve ganglia. They create resistance and excitement inflammatory syndromes. Chinese medicine calls these Yang syndromes. It is an acute and active pathological state.

If patient constitution is weak or disease lasts many days, the spring-force reaction of sympathetic nerve ganglia are surely defeated. They are not able to induce the natural innate ability of harmonizing and recovering. Or, even if there is reaction, it is not significant. These are called Yin syndromes. Yin syndromes are a deterioration of the inner organs' control and metabolic power. It is a passive pathological state. Tai Yin

[405] Central nervous system or brain.

太陰 disease is a decline of the digestive system metabolic function. Its controls become abnormal and it looks like the opposite of Yang Ming. Shao Yin 少陰 disease is a urinary system metabolic action decline. Its compensation and the body's toxic outcome of such a decline can be seen as an exterior/interior relationship with Tai Yang. Jue Yin 厥陰 disease is decline in the central nervous system itself and its signals. This creates chaos in signals coming from the central nervous system with symptoms such as "Yin Yang seen together, hot and cold are both present."

Whether or not my explanation was accurate is beyond the scope of this article. Nonetheless, at that time, I felt as if my own opinion was of a very capable person; it was conforming to science. 20 years later, I have used this point of view to explain and arrange Chinese medicine research. I felt, myself, that this can thread together the theory with practice. However, in some instances, I still felt that I rely solely on "inference" and "connected in my own mind" and it is not sufficiently scientific. Therefore, I refrained from publishing my research materials. I was afraid that others would immediately refute it. I was very keen to study Western medicine's neurological pathology in order to supplement my own. Unexpectedly, I could not find any satisfactory books on the topic. Even though I had a friend offering me to look at books in their original language, unfortunately my language skills were insufficient and I could not understand. This situation became my own heart suffering. I also tried to use my work and engage a discussion with other Chinese medicine practitioners in order to verify it, but they all felt that I went astray because my scientific arrangement of Chinese medicine had several aspects that they could not tolerate:

1) Naturally, I have used the above division of the six conformations and not the six meridians of hand and foot and their relationship to inner organs.

2) I sternly rejected the theory of five phases controlling and generating. I considered it as having started during the era of Song dynasty Ren Zong emperor 宋仁宗[406], when they established the official bureaucracy of Pharmacology and doctors were out of jobs. They had no option but to recruit mysterious doctrines to their aid and, with that, started all the nonsense.

3) I have opposed the pulse theory that "Cun, Guan and Chi 寸關尺 pulse positions reflect the heart, liver, lungs, spleen and kidneys". In my eyes, the pulse only has floating, sunken, slow and rapid phenomena that can be inspected.

406 Reigned from 1022–1063 CE.

> Where can one differentiate within the radial pulse what belongs to heart and what belongs to lungs!

There were a few old Chinese medicine doctors who, after discussing the topic with me, had the appearance of not being able to tolerate it, showing an embarrassing attitude.

I have also talked it over with friends who are Western medicine doctors. They would always never let me finish and burst in great laughter. This is because I didn't accept the all-powerful bacteria and didn't approve of the special effect therapy. From their point of view, my kind of science was too shallow and too limited. They did not even have a desire to argue about it.

In this situation it was really like the Bat in Aesop's fables,[407] or in a more pleasant-to-the-ear way, "being besieged on all sides, the isolated military force is struggling for the gate".[408]

In 1952, comrade Zhu Lian 朱璉 published her book *The New Acupuncture and Moxibustion* 新針灸學. I was thinking: This comrade Zhu has used Western medicine to craft acupuncture and moxibustion. This must possess a different and fresh view and maybe it is similar to mine. I contemplated it for a long time and then gathered courage and wrote her a letter. Not long after, I received her reply and here I narrate the main point of that letter: "All the paragraphs in your letter testify to your enthusiasm toward the future development of our nation's medicine. In another aspect, I am full of admiration for your explanation of the sympathetic nervous system to explain the "Yin Yang theory" as well as your rejection of the "five phases generating and controlling" as a mystical theory. (Skipping a part) However, from what we know thus far, using the autonomous nervous system to explain disease pathology and the recovery principle is still incomplete…Our aspirations and thoughts, being a high level of neurological function, testifies to the transformation of human life and disease."

---

407 A singing bird was confined in a cage that hung outside a window and had a way of singing at night when all other birds were asleep. One night a Bat came, clung to the bars of the cage and asked the Bird why she was silent by day and sang only at night. "I have a very good reason for doing so," said the Bird. "It was once when I was singing in the daytime that a fowler was attracted by my voice, and set his nets for me and caught me. Since then I have never sung except by night." But the Bat replied, "It is no use your doing that now when you are a prisoner: if only you had done so before you were caught, you might still have been free." "Precautions are useless after the crisis."
Footnote source http://www.aesopfables.com

408 There is a possible typo in the text as the original idiom is "when besieged on all sides an isolated force fights bravely 四面楚歌孤軍奮戰". Here the last character is replaced by 鬥.

This reply letter gave me much inspiration. On the one hand, what I understood in the past as a treatment method and my use of scientific methods to arrange it had its value. On the other hand, I understood that it is not yet complete. She gave me guidance, encouraging me to research further Pavlov's theory of higher nervous activity. At the time, I was ignorant of the contents in Pavlov's theories, so I immediately looked for a book on the topic. Only the following year did my son, who serves in the army, send me a translation by comrade Ge Shaolong 戈紹龍.

In the summer of 1953, the prefectural commissioner's office of Yuan Ling[409] in Chenxi county 沅陵專署在辰谿縣 established Chinese Medicine Advanced Studies Class 中醫進修班. More than 20 colleagues from my county participated. After they came back, some told me secretly that those who normally talk about Cun, Guan, Chi pulse theories, as well as the generating and controlling actions of the five phases, were heavily attacked and sternly criticized. Their intention was to compliment me, saying that my past theory was actually ahead of its time. When I heard this news I was not happy—to the contrary, I felt sad. How so? Because now, after studying the theories of Pavlov, I felt that my past point of view of science had many errors. Trying to expound and prove according to Pavlov's theories, not only that the Cun, Guan and Chi positions of the pulse are relevant, but also that the giving birth and controlling actions of the five phases may have a scientific basis as well.

Some may think that this is capricious of me or that I did not master well the theory at hand and just brag with new things. They are all wrong. I think that science has no boundaries. Its purpose is only to pursue true principle. Facing true principle, one cannot avoid errors of the past. One should not guard his shortcomings. Pavlov, after many decades of research, when publishing his work, still said "I am not ashamed of having mistakes". With humility, he was attempting—this is truly an attitude to be admired. For us, under the brilliant leadership of Chairman Mao and the Communist Party, we form the work of Chinese medicine, seeking the path of Chinese medicine scientification, which is a glorious affair. It is also a mighty difficult affair. We must come forth very honestly and explore it. There is no place for shyness or being afraid of making mistakes. We should acknowledge our mistakes with courage. Only then can we find true principle and truly undertake the scientification of Chinese medicine.

---

[409] This was part of Lishu Xiangxi administrative region 隶属湘西行政区, part of today's Hunan province.

The achievements of the advanced classes are great. But also a part of it is insufficient. Some think that the advanced classes, being led by Western medicine doctors, make the Chinese medicine doctors feel "there was not really anything new to study, but all the old beliefs were shaken". This statement is not without reason. The higher authority already noticed this upset and made necessary corrections. It is too early to make a final determination about the generating and controlling actions of the five phases. I have opposed the generating and controlling actions of the five phases and the Cun, Guan, Chi positions of the pulse for over 20 years and, without using them, I have treated patients for many years. Coming to today, I realize that my point of view was a mistake. I feel that the five phases generating and controlling still must be discussed. It is not that I dropped out or drive the car backwards, I am rather lowering my head in front of science looking for a true principle. If my current point of view is a mistake or not, I hope that all medical fellows will offer guidance. And so, following the spirit of Pavlov's "not being ashamed to have mistakes", I wrote this article. Following, I put forth a string of problems connected to the scientification of Chinese medicine. I hope that every advanced reader, after reading it, will offer me direct criticism and guidance, without too much politeness.

Yaron: In the 1930s, Chinese medicine antagonists discarded five elements theory as superstitious. Now, the antagonist turns around and approves of it. This gave hope to many old medicine practitioners, previously facing a total disappearance of this theory, now seeing a new scientific model that includes it. It was a big shift into TCM with five elements theory and Zangfu organ theory merged together "scientifically".

2) The issue of five phases generating and controlling actions

From Chinese medicine theories, the most repulsive is the five phases controlling and generating theory. This is because, according to five phases control and generation, each disease is clearly defined in a sly way. It is nothing but allowing the doctor's prescription to become plausible. I am not the only one to hold this point of view. After liberation I was still criticizing my colleagues' prescriptions, saying that they should not use language such as "liver wood horizontally attacking spleen earth". I was of the opinion that this was an irresponsible attitude.

Now, when I started to study Pavlov's materials, I have made myself a principle to incorporate this into Chinese medicine's practical aspect. Every article I learned made me contemplate. I took Chinese medicine treatment principles and made a comparison. The first article I read surprised me. I discovered that the five phases controlling and generating theory has a great value.

When we think of a problem the most worrisome is to be prejudiced, which in turn obstructs objectivity. In the past, whenever I saw "metal, wood, water, fire and earth" I immediately recognized it as a mystical theory and would not give it a second thought. I would not ponder deep how old Chinese medicine would use five phases controlling and generating actions in clinic. Naturally, I only looked superficially at the words "five phases controlling and generating is too mysterious". But upon careful inspection, from treatment and practicality point of view, five phases controlling and generating, according to the principles of Pavlov's theories, is logical in the following three ways:

1) Chronic bronchitis, for example, acts up every time during cold weather, but when it is warm it subsides. According to the common treatment principle one should expel phlegm and scatter cold, but according to five phases generating and controlling treatment principle one should strengthen the stomach, which is called "cultivate earth to generate metal". Herbs used are Xiang Fu 香附, Bai Zhu 白朮, Dou Kou 豆蔻, Guang Xiang 廣香, Hou Po 厚朴, Xiao Hui 小茴 etc and when these are combined with conventional treatment then recovery is speedy.

2) Pulmonary tuberculosis, at initial stage of spitting blood and then having white foamy phlegm, is often accompanied by abnormal sexual urges. The common treatment is to resolve phlegm, stop cough and arrest panting. According to five phases treatment the method is to strengthen the kidneys, which is called "moisten kidney water in order to receive lung metal Qi". The herbs used are Liu Wei Wan decoction 六味丸湯, Sha Yuan Ji Li 沙苑蒺藜, Ba Ji Tian 巴戟天, Gou Qi 枸杞, Che Qian Zi 車前子, Po Gu Zhi 破故紙, Hu Tao 胡桃 etc. These are often more effective than using herbs to target symptoms. It is like in the example of cough related to female menstrual cramps, you use Wen Jing Tang 溫經湯 to treat the cough, it is the same principle.

3) Tooth decay leading to toothache and trigeminal nerve inflammation pain, the normal treatment principle is to relieve inflammation and stop pain but, according to five phases generating and controlling treatment, it is to strengthen kidneys and solidify stomach. It is called "lead fire to return to its origin". The herbs used are Rou Gui 肉桂, Fu Zi 附子, Huang Lian 黃連, Xi

Xin 細辛, Liu Wei Wan decoction 六味丸湯 etc. With this, one often can see that as soon as herbs are taken the disease is gone.

The above three examples, and all other treatment methods following five phases theory, are united under one principle. Regardless of how old Chinese medicine used to explain it back and forth, they all utilized the sex and food desire in order to advance treatment. In other words, they increased one's desire to eat and sex by using strong herbs, with which excitement is created and disease weakened and so the healing objective is reached. It is exactly like using unconditioned stimulus in order to create conditioned reflex. It creates inhibition within the cerebrum function. Likewise, I believe, acupuncture and moxibustion therapeutic principle happens by stimulating the defense instinct. In the Soviet Union, the newly discovered tissue therapy is very much like acupuncture and moxibustion. It uses light stimulation, which is beneficial to the cortex function recovery. When the cortex receives a certain amount of stimulus then it helps control or weaken the stimulus inducing the disease. This is according to Pavlov's principle and scientific method where "When the first reflex arrives, then the second reflex becomes weaker or vanishes".

Also, in Pavlov's theories "external restriction" and "negative induction" etc situations can explain the treatment principle of five phases controlling and generating. For example, the above mentioned "liver wood horizontally attacks spleen earth" can be explained as the liver organ receives excessive excitation which influences the digestive system and creates a restrictive condition. This invokes a condition where nutrient distribution is impaired, absorption is lacking and digestive secretions are abnormal. The result would be indigestion and stomach pains. Another example is the saying "startling harms the spleen". This can be explained when there is a random and extreme stimulation from the external world, which in turn may cause digestive system and external restriction phenomena. This may lead to loss of appetite, aversion to food and nausea. "Startling harms the spleen" can be explained even better according to the principle that "as soon as defense reaction happens it excites an unconditional reflex to the central nervous system".

As for this five phases controlling and generating treatment modality, other than tissue therapy, Western medicine did not take notice of it at all. Even though, by chance, they may also use purging drugs to help inflammation in the head area or regulating the blood, it is unlike the depth of five phases controlling and generating treatment method. Like the aforementioned use of Rou Gui, Fu Zi etc very hot herbs to treat inflammation pains. From a theoretical aspect it is hard to explain the clinical efficacy of these. Therefore, this kind of treatment method holds great research value. How to eradicate its idealistic aspect and instead seek its scientific evidence from a materialistic view is truly an important issue. This will have a tremendous contribution to Chinese medicine scientification.

Yaron: The following illustrates a few technical points practiced today in TCM, such as minute herbal doses, using Gan Cao as a harmonizing herb and other food grade herbs as restraining tools of other more potent herbs; these ideas were selected into the TCM model. They reflected current politics and economics, as already explained.

3) A light dose treats a heavy disease—a Qi transformation issue

In Guangdong province there is a famous Western medicine doctor, a Mr. Zhang Gongrang 張公讓, who is very versed with Chinese medicine. He diagnoses using Western medicine methods and then treats with Chinese herbal formulas, his reputation being very high. He published an extensive book ten years ago titled *A Comparative View of Chinese and Western Medicines and Pharmacology* 中西醫藥比觀. In this book, he severely scolds the late Chinese medicine doctor from Shanghai, Mr. Yun Tieqiao 惲鐵樵. Scolds him in a very mean way. This is because Mr. Yun was one of Shanghai's famous doctors and after diagnosis, when he treated a patient, he would use in his formulas a very light dose of herbs. For example, Chai Hu 柴胡 he would use 3 Fen,[410] Su Ye 蘇葉 5 Fen etc. Mr. Yun would consider Chai Hu to be fierce if the dose exceeded 7 Fen. Mr. Zhang was of the opinion that such a small dose could not possibly have cured any disease. Accordingly, Mr. Yun could have only swindled the wealthy ladies and gentlemen of Shanghai, he could have only healed their cold-related headaches and that was it.[411] In the past I praised highly this article, as I too disliked Mr. Yun's case studies.

In addition, from clinical experience point of view, with old Chinese medicine doctors, the richer their experience the more they tend to use light herb dosages. In the past, I erroneously thought that they simply skimped along and escaped responsibility. However, often times they were able to treat serious conditions successfully. Their explanation was that this is "Qi transformation" and that "as soon as the grand Qi starts spinning all diseases are cured". In the past, I was of the opinion that

---

[410] Depending if the measuring unit was of ancient or modern times, 1 Fen equals 1/3 to 1/2 of one gram. 3 Fen equals 1 to 1.5 grams.

[411] Meaning he could not have treated any serious ailments successfully.

what really cured people was their reputation and not the herbs' force. So to say, it was a psychological treatment, such as the proverb "Medicine's fortune[412] is with luck". However, what we call "psychological treatment" cannot be applied at any place in any given time—it is hard to believe that truly there is such a thing as "medicine fortune". I cannot believe this.

Because of this situation, I developed suspicion towards Chinese herbs' efficacy. I also saw, in the past, that patients consumed prescriptions with 4 Liang[413] of Aconite and had no adverse reaction to it. An example quite to the contrary, when I concocted Li Ji Diarrhea powder, every time when using a heavy dose of herbs I could reach a cure. These kinds of facts caused me to reach inaccurate ideas about the limitations of herbs' dosages and their efficacy principle, such as the following:

1) I was of the opinion that if cooking time and method is not the same then the active ingredients remaining in the decoction varies greatly. Light dose of herbs then naturally should be cooked shortly in order to have some active ingredients left.

2) I was of the opinion that Chinese herbs' solubility has a certain degree of saturation. For example, 2 Fen of Shi Gao 石膏 requires 100 cubic centimeters of water to dissolve. Therefore, in formulas using 5 Fen or 5 Liang, the solubility is the same and therefore the heavy or light dose of this mineral makes no difference.

3) I was of the opinion that some Chinese herbal formulas simply swindle the patients. The fact that light dose formulas cure diseases is because diseases naturally have a recovery curve. They would recover even if they were no herbs taken.

These few opinions of mine of course cannot resolve this issue properly, and therefore my maze of doubts I could not resolve for a long time.

Only when I started learning Pavlov's theory of "abnormal time phenomena" (the 16th lecture) did I suddenly grasp it. After an initial strain, if it meets with a lengthy complex stimulus and differentiation, then the cerebrum's stimulating action becomes tired and, following that, there is an abnormal time phenomenon. At this time, to the contrary, a light stimulus will induce a heavy response while a heavy stimulus

[412] Fortune here means destiny, like in good fortune and bad fortune.
[413] Depending if the measuring unit was ancient or modern, 1 Liang equals 38-50 grams.

will induce only a weak response. This conforms completely to severe diseases being chronic. It is the stage where a Yang syndrome has just transformed into a Yin syndrome and here a light dose has great efficacy.

Nonetheless, duration of this time phenomenon is limited. Artificially created, it can last for 14 days but with disease development it lasts only 2–3 days. Mastering the timeliness is a crucial prerequisite. According to Pavlov's theory, following the "abnormal time phenomenon" is a "balanced time phenomenon". The feature of this balanced time phenomenon's external expression is semi-sleep state. After the balanced time phenomenon, it returns back to a normal state. If we combine this with disease development, the balanced time phenomenon is a state of coma (half-sleep) where the body's strength and the disease are in a stage of fighting a duel. If there is defeat then death follows and if there is victory then the condition improves. It is best if one does not reach to this very dangerous phase but, instead, from the abnormal time phenomenon it directly reaches to recovery of the normal state. This is the objective of "Qi transformation" treatment method. And so the experienced old Chinese medicine doctors have mastered this secret of success. How to transform this experience into a fixed theory is indeed one of Chinese medicine scientification's top tasks.

According to Ge Shaolong's 戈紹龍 study notes, using Pavlov's words, "The effective injectable dose of Bromine solution is according to individual nerve characteristics. It can range from one thousandth to five thousandths". This means that efficacy limitation of herbs depends on the ability of each individual nerve to receive it. The discrepancy can be as much as five thousand fold. This awakens us to the significance of patient's neurological receptiveness ability. At the same time, it also explains the phenomenon of "light dose can treat a severe disease". The patients of the aforementioned Mr. Yun were mostly wealthy people from Shanghai. Their neurological function was naturally weak, and so it is only a natural logic.

4) Combining herbs

Combination of herbs in Chinese medicine formulas has a definition of emperor, minister, assistant and messenger. For example: in Gui Zhi Tang decoction 桂枝湯, Gui Zhi 桂枝 is the emperor, Shao Yao 芍藥 is the minister, but in Xiao Jian Zhong Tang 小建中湯 decoction Shao Yao is the emperor while Gui Zhi is the minister. The herbs in both formulas are the same but within them the emperor and minister roles are not the same and the treatment objective is also not the same. Like the old Chinese doctors' secret verse "if in a formula there is Di Huang 地黃 don't use as well He Shouwu 何首烏, because two emperors can't stand in the same place." Or it is also like Po Guzhi 破故紙 can't be separated from Hu Tao 胡桃, Zhi Mu 知母 can't be separated from Huang Bai 黃柏, they simply become fixed sets. Where is the logic of this particularity?

In addition, there are some food-grade herbs which can be consumed daily, such as jujube dates, ginger root, licorice root, lotus root, seed and joints, Yam root, peach seeds, apricot seeds, walnut etc. How come when they are incorporated into a formula they can induce medicinal efficacy? The careless person would say, "it is a fake ingredient, one does not have to use it." However, when we study how to treat, we should not overlook any small link as insignificant, easily allowing it to slip.

In the past, in order to study well the use of Gan Cao 甘草, I have spent 2–3 months of toil analyzing all the ancient prescriptions. For example, from all the Ling Gui formulas 苓桂湯, why is it that only Wu Ling San 五苓散 and Zu Ling Tang 豬苓湯 don't use Gan Cao, where all the other Ling Gui Zhu Gan Tang 苓桂朮甘湯, Fu Ling Ze Xie Tang 茯苓澤瀉湯 etc do use Gan Cao? I collected many formulas, compared them and then from the difference between their treatment effects extracted one or two herbs and found out their specific role. This was one scientific method for arranging the material. It was easy to come to a conclusion that "when a virus did not reach a certain body part but the nerve is already in distress, then it is appropriate to not use Gan Cao". This conclusion made me feel very pleased like having a great achievement. I felt, "within the entire Chinese medicine community there is not another who studied it with such effort. I even used so much effort to research Gan Cao 甘草. "

However, what about jujube dates? What about ginger root? It seems like, throughout the generations, every formula used ginger and dates to guide the other herbs. What is the bottom line purpose of it? 3 slices of ginger and 3 dates—can they really invoke medical efficacy? I feel that this kind of problem cannot be resolved with a strike of the hand. This is because there are many other herbs which are also used to guide the formula such as Deng Xin 燈心, Zhu Ye 竹葉, Can Shi Sang Ye 蠶食桑葉 kind of herbs, they look like they are bland with no special action, but when they are missing from the formula it does not work.

There was this one time when I prescribed Xiao Jian Zhong Tang 小建中湯. When the patient saw the prescription, he inquired if he could substitute Yi Tang 飴糖[414]

[414] Maltose

with sugar cubes. I said he could but, to my amazement, this time the formula didn't work. I looked for the reason why it did not work and I came to the conclusion that it was because of the sugar cubes. When I used Yi Tang there was not one time that the formula was not effective. I was thinking that in the production of Yi Tang and sugar cubes the difference is that with Yi Tang, during its processing, they use soda[415] water, and soda water neutralizes acidity. Now Xiao Jian Zhong Tang has a large dose of sour Bai Shao and so from this point it became clear to me that many assistant and messenger herbs have a neutralizing effect on acidity. Licorice root, ginger root, jujube dates for themselves don't have a great medicinal value, but they harmonize the other herbs in order to avoid side effects.

This discovery was very important. Thereafter I received further confirmation in the clinic. This is a fact requiring one's utmost attention. For example, when treating tonsillitis, if one only uses cool herbs such as Sheng Di 生地, Xuan Shen 玄參, Mai Dong 麥冬, Jie Geng 桔梗, She Gan 射干, Huang Qin 黃芩 etc it is not effective. One must also add Su Geng 蘇梗, Jing Jie 荊芥, Fang Feng 放風, Bo He 薄荷, Sang Ye 桑葉 kind of scattering herbs, otherwise the sore throat becomes worse. This example is often seen in clinic. This is why ancient doctors always cautioned students and emphasized "when using herbs one should not be lopsided". In truth, what it means is that acidity and alkalinity need to be balanced. From my experience, balancing acidity and alkalinity in herbal formulas has reached the following secret rhyme:

> Scattering (exterior resolving) herbs are mostly alkaline, while clearing inflammation (cool) herbs are mostly acidic. Tonifying Qi herbs are mostly alkaline while tonifying blood herbs are mostly acidic. Scattering herbs cannot be used lopsided; they need be combined with clearing inflammation or tonifying blood herbs. Clearing inflammation herbs cannot be used lopsided; they must be combined with scattering or tonifying Qi herbs.

When looking at all the ancient efficacious formulas, discussions and arguments could not fully explain why Bu Zhong Yi Qi Tang 補中益氣湯 uses Chai Hu and Sheng Ma 升麻, Ren Shen Yang Rong Tang 人參養榮湯 uses heavily Shao Yao and Wu Wei Zi 五味子. How could it not be this principle we just explained? From this, one sees that combining suitable herbs like Po Gu Zhi with Hu Tao, Zhi Mu with

[415] Alkaline in nature

Huang Bai, Ma Huang 麻黃 with Xing Ren 杏仁, Ban Xia 半夏 with Chen Pi 陳皮, follow this principle.

This kind of harmonizing between alkali and acid in a formula, from Western medicine pharmacology point of view, is not according to principle because "when acid and alkali combine they reduce drug efficacy". If so, then does Chinese medicine turn its back on science?

When we carefully consider this problem, we can see the dividing line between Chinese and Western medicines. Originally, Western drugs' characteristic was the special effect aspect or, in other words, the direct impact on bacteria and infection. Therefore, the most worrisome thing would be to lessen their drug efficacy. Chinese herbs specialty, as I explained in point number 1 of this article, is to affect the nerves. In other words, they need not have a direct impact on bacteria and infection and instead, through acting upon nerves, they have an indirect action reducing inflammation and killing bacteria. Therefore, for herbs the most worrisome is to have them stimulate excessively the central nervous system.

Pavlov's theory states, "The differences in blood chemistry can be measured by laboratory equipment determining the state of the brain terminus. It can determine if the brain terminus is increasing or decreasing its excitement" (page 132). With this, one notices that when acidic or alkaline herbs are used alone then the brain nerves become over excited and brain damage occurs. For example, Atabrine[416] to treat malaria often induces side effects such as dizziness, deafness or tinnitus. People often criticize the lacking of Western drugs saying "their reaction is too strong, they don't consider the individual constitution". In reality, it is a lacking that Western medicine cannot remedy. The more special effect a drug has, the more it cannot prevent injury to the nerves. Now, if a Western medicine doctor can be cautious with the dosage to such a degree that he induces no side effect, then he is a good doctor. Chinese herbs are exactly the opposite. They are more precious when they have multiple actions. For example, Huang Qi 黃耆 is named the greatest of the hundred herbs, because "if there is sweat it can arrest sweat and if there is no sweat it can induce sweat."

This issue is not only a Chinese medicine scientification issue, but also the great issue of making Western medicine pharmacology better. Only recently did I hear of the director of a certain medical university hospital in Nanjing, Mr. Jiang 蔣. Since

[416] Western drugs also known as meparcrine and quinacrine.

learning Pavlov's theories he started to doubt special effect therapy. How to improve the drugs according to Pavlov's theories without utilizing excessive chemical analysis equipment fearing the decrease of drug effect? How to categorize Chinese herbs according to their chemical compounds? How to advocate the use of Chinese herbs by Western medicine according to Pavlov's theories? These are all worthy topics of deep investigation commencing today.

When we look at Pavlov's 17th discussion at the last few pages, we can clearly recognize that the most precious drug is not a special effect drug, but rather a drug that regulates and calms the nerves. From the main principle point of view, Chinese medicine in the Yang syndrome phase uses herbs that regulate the nerves like Gui Zhi 桂枝, Chai Hu 柴胡, Ge Gen 葛根, Fang Feng 放風, Jing Jie 荊芥 etc. However in the Yin syndrome phase calming the nerves herbs often used are Huang Qi 黃耆, Fu Ling 茯苓, Fu Zi 附子, Bai Shao 白芍 etc. This is another point where Chinese medicine herbs and prescriptions are in accord with Pavlov's theories.

5) The issue of Climax

In what I described earlier as correspondence letter with comrade Zhu Lian, I mentioned the neurological action climax and asked her to take note of that. I have not yet found materials discussing this issue in Pavlov's articles, only a slight logic in that direction. I feel that this is a shortcoming. Maybe this article is the very first summary of this topic. I have not yet seen research about this point of climax!

In Chinese medicine, the ones practicing acupuncture and moxibustion and external injuries therapy, if they are in a teacher-disciple relationship, must possess a hand-copied manuscript on top of which there would be a drawing of a human body with acupoints and meridians. In the commentaries on the side of the page would be time segments, which are called "time limits 時限". These explain that in a certain time of the day these acupoints are most prone to injury. If there is injury at that time then it is very difficult to heal. This "time limit" is the time period when climax arrives.

Pavlov, with great effort, avoided subjectivity in his research of nerve action. He only relied upon objective findings, which is the absolutely reliable method of science. What is the real reason that, as I said before, Pavlov's articles do not directly explain climax?

If we look at his third article page 40, Pavlov mentions the condition of "cyclicity". Cyclicity means that time becomes a factor in conditioned reflex. When it reaches a certain time limit reaction naturally occurs. Of course, this does not mean that time, in itself, is the factor but rather that the brain's cerebrum activity under the constraint of time turns into cyclical activity. How can time constrain the brain's cerebrum activity and make it cyclical? Pavlov did not explain, however, we can understand it. It is created by the cerebral cortex metabolic action that, within this time limit, develops a habit of repetitive motion. This understanding is very important because, when we study the entire experiments' materials of Pavlov, we easily forget that metabolism exists and, instead, erroneously think that the cerebrum simply is there without change.

As for the cerebrum metabolic action, does it happen simultaneously or in stages? This is a problem requiring investigation. Judging by our human daily life activities, such as sleeping, working, eating, they all have their habitual time. And so the brain's cerebrum excitement and rest phases, without even noticing it, have divided and became cyclical. This is a matter of fact. The metabolic function, however, accompanies daily life needs and at any given time may increase in a particular part of the body. In other words, it is very possible that it progresses in stages. For example, when we get to meal-time, naturally we feel hungry. The eating desire in the brain's cerebrum becomes excited. When food is introduced into the body the same part of the cerebrum, after reaching its objective, becomes restful. It then stops its activity until the next wave of hunger. This kind of action, when hunger arrives, is the time when climax arrives. It is the time when the cerebrum part responsible for food desire reaches its highest metabolic action.

Again, let's look at Pavlov's lectures, the 16th lecture this time, explaining the four different types of time phenomena. In a pathological state, there could be a time phenomenon where the auditory sense is clear but the visual sense is not, or the opposite in another time phenomenon, where the visual sense is clear but the auditory sense is not clear. However, in an equal time phenomenon, the time of half-sleep (hypnagogic state), both auditory and visual senses are equally functioning. This testifies to having a climax in a disease state, sometimes at the auditory region and sometimes at the visual region. However, in an even time phenomenon, where the disease may have aggravated and caused the patient to lose consciousness, similar to the half-sleep state, climax does not happen. After an even time phenomenon, a normal time phenomenon follows. One can, therefore, see that an even time phenomenon is a step in disease development toward the recovery phase; the entire cerebrum is in a rest-and-repair mode and therefore has no climax. This also testifies, in a reverse way, that climax is the individual's force that must be there as long as there is no exhaustion. What is called "undulant movement" and "refocusing" truly explains the man-made climax.

What is the treatment significance of all the explanations above? I sense that, when Western medicine treats a disease, there is no differentiation between what came first and what came later, what is inside and what is outside. However, Chinese medicine pays careful attention to what came first and what came later, what is inside and what is outside. What we mean with "not differentiating before and after, inside and outside" is not paying close attention to the existence of climax.

Using an example, Intestinal cold injury where external heat is coming and going. Western medicine will do stool analysis and if they have found eggs of round worms, regardless of the external heat symptoms they will give a formula to expel round worms. This kind of solution is prohibited in Chinese medicine. The reality is that even in Chinese medicine this prohibition is sometimes ignored and therefore the condition further deteriorates.

When the *Shang Han Lun* talks about "transmitting to next conformation, on the first day at Tai Yang, on the second day at Yang Ming, on the third day at Shao Yang…" etc, it exactly talks about the climax in the disease course. When climax is at a certain conformation then one uses a certain herb. If one uses the wrong herb then trouble arises. This is a kind of theory that Western medicine cannot pay attention to. For example, Chai Hu is an essential herb for treating the respiratory system. However, if disease is at Tai Yang, even if there is a syndrome in the respiratory system, using Chai Hu is prohibited. This is because Chai Hu is a herb for Shao Yang conformation. The fear is that, if Chai Hu is used, the pathogen then is led inward into Shao Yang. Saying the same a bit clearer, "The cerebrum reaction to a disease, if the climax is at an area corresponding to Tai Yang then one should resolve it from Tai Yang. One should not allow the virus to scurry the nerve reaction from a weak spot." In reality, if Tai Yang disease is resolved at Tai Yang then it resolves in a relatively straightforward way. For example, Ma Huang formula will resolve Tai Yang cough much faster than a Chai Hu formula. It is this principle.

This kind of theory is the strong point of Chinese medicine and the short aspect of Western medicine. How can we research this further according to Pavlov's materials already available which, in turn, will allow us to master in clinic the forecasting ability of climax, shorten the disease course and alleviate people's sufferings? In other words, how can we make Chinese medicine theory in this area more scientific? It seems that this is also a very important topic.

Yaron: The extent of using modern scientific knowledge, in this case from the Soviet Union, in explaining and developing Chinese medicine. While during the Republic, scientification mostly meant researching herbs and their efficacy by scientific means, here, in the Communist era, modern science of physical reality is melted into Chinese medicine old theories—what Sean Lei calls "mongrel medicine".[417]

6) Three Yin/ three Yang divide

I have already explained my position in point number 1 on the divide of three Yin and three Yang. I object to the old notion that the hand and foot six meridians accompany Zang Fu organs. I am of the opinion that the *Shang Han Lun* original intent for the six meridians syndromes is six-stage disease pathology. It is also six stages of neurological strains. When it reaches to nerve ganglions and stirs an innate spring-force response to make adjustments, then it is at the level of Yang syndromes. Opposite this will be the Yin syndrome phase. Relying on this kind of explanation to research the *Shang Han Lun*, versus the old Chinese medicine explanations, is much more reasonable. Therefore, I feel that this kind of divide is much more scientific.

However, in this topic, there is one point that should make people suspicious and want to refute. According to which materials can one explain the notion that, when reaching to the ganglion, there would be an innate spring-force response to make adjustments? This is a problem one should pose.

Twenty years ago, just from connecting it in my mind I said, "When reaching to the ganglion there would be an innate spring-force response to make adjustments," and this was my starting point to perform research. At that time I did not know, at all, the conditions by which the cerebrum creates reflex. So I set forth from this presupposition. I merged it with Chinese medicine theory and treatment and, often times, the facts matched marvelously. When I set out to explain this via Western medicine anatomy, looking for this marvelous proof, I could never find it. This got me very confused. When one does not consider the nerve action then there is no way to understand this just with anatomy. And so I blamed, again and again, Western medicine "science is not good enough".

---

[417] Lei, S. H.-L. (2014). *Neither Donkey nor Horse: Medicine in the Struggle over China's Modernity*. Chicago: University of Chicago Press.

When we study Pavlov's lectures, even though our study is still superficial, we can already grasp many principles explaining the accuracy of this presupposition. Following are a few examples:

a) According to one of Pavlov's principles, "because of external incoming conditioned reflex there is a temporary neurological relationship. The lower level center gradually transfers to the brain center." This principle testifies that disease pathology reaction begins in a lower level neurological center and not in the brain central nervous system. It also shows the innate ability of the nerves themselves to react.

   From what I understand, in dissecting inner organs' nerves, they belong to the scope of nervous systems vegetal law. Under normal conditions, the cerebrum maintains the struggle with, and reaction to, external stimuli. The main movement is introduced via the five sense organs[418] and there is control towards the inner organs' equilibrium. The larger part of this delivery happens between the self-regulatory nerves and the endocrine system connecting to each other and merging together. The cerebrum only slightly cares for the subconscious and the cerebral cortex fluid and cells. When it comes to the inner organs becoming sick, the subconscious voice overshadows the external stimuli. The cerebrum attention then turns inwards, and gradually replaces the lower nerves function in controlling the disease. Therefore, when a disease is severe the patient's recognition of the external world becomes confused. It is because the cerebrum attention is turning inward. And so the transfer from lower nerves to the cerebrum can serve as the explanation of the three Yang syndromes turning into the three Yin syndromes (especially Jue Yin disease).

b) Pavlov's rules have the following 2 ideas: "Negative reaction easily wavers, while positive reaction is relatively stable"[419] and "the control function is the highest realm of neurological action". These two rules confirm that my view, that the sympathetic and parasympathetic nerves' actions should be viewed independently, is correct. Because control function is relatively in a high realm, therefore the cerebral cortex pays close attention to the parasympathetic nerves. If it were not like this, then there would be no way to respond

[418] Ears, eyes, lips, nose, tongue.

[419] The Chinese term for negative reaction is Yin style reaction, while positive reaction is Yang style reaction. From language point of view this can easily fit with three Yin and three Yang hypothesis.

to external stimuli. However, if the cerebral cortex pays close attention to negative reaction why then does it easily waver? This is because the nerve action is naturally wavering, and negative action is closely related to the cerebral cortex pathways. Therefore wavering is in a direct ratio to that. When it comes to positive action, because it has to go through the sympathetic nerves ganglions' indirect pathways, therefore, compared to negative action it is relatively stable. Or, in other words, it is slow.

c) According to Pavlov's 17th lecture page 281 and the 18th lecture page 298, describing the principle by which disease forms, it claims "negative and positive stimulation struggle simultaneously in the cerebral cortex". This kind of argument I cannot understand. I am of the opinion that negative and positive stimuli cannot coexist at the same space at the same time. So to say, causes of two opposite functions cannot find themselves at the same time, on the same path, reaching to the same point. Using yet again different words, when a certain point of the cerebral cortex is inducing a positive action, it cannot instigate at the same time negative action. However, if the positive action comes from another source, then it is possible. So what is this other motive power? From the foundation that we have already, the only possible explanation that conforms to reality is the spring-force of the sympathetic nerves' ganglions.

The above few points are already impressive. I feel that this not only is a matter of Chinese medicine scientification but also a matter of a great revolution in disease pathology. This is not just for me, a single person who did not even receive proper education in this field, to investigate this. However, it is my achievement of being able to point out these issues.

Here I need to supplement one point. Sympathetic nerve function, even though stimulating in nature, yet inside the body in each part there is also opposite inhibitory action. The parasympathetic nerves, even though in each region it is inhibiting yet they transform into stimulation. In addition, in each particular spot the two coexist. This situation is very complex. Is there a problem with the current state of anatomy and physiology? Are there any other principles? I am ashamed that my intelligence has no ability to find out.

7) The pulse

As for pulse, up until 2 years ago I was arguing with colleagues that it is not possible that one pulse will show multiple phenomena at the same time. In addition, the feeling at one's fingertips is unreliable and often influenced by psychological elements. Therefore I was always of the opinion that pulse is only supplementary evidence. From pulse differentiation it is possible that, for example, Ma Huang syndrome pulse will be floating and tight, otherwise it is not. Cheng Qi syndrome pulse should be sunken and full, otherwise it is not. It is also possible to determine the herbal treatment from the pulse, for example, with floating rapid pulse one can use resolving the exterior herbs or cool herbs, when the pulse is floating and slow one should use tonifying and hot herbs. However, one certainly cannot determine from the three positions of the pulse—Cun, Guan, Chi—the heart, liver, spleen, lungs and kidneys. I was of the opinion that whoever talks about Tai Su pulse 太素脈[420] is a charlatan. This is because for one disease there would be an auspicious and inauspicious pulse, making it not possible to discover disease pathology from the pulse.

This opinion of mine invoked much resistance by my colleagues. It also displeased many of the patients. This is because most patients believe that "Chinese medicine doctor must rely on the pulse, where could there be a Chinese medicine doctor that does not talk of the pulse?" To the contrary, this achieved much appreciation by my Western medicine comrades, who also believe that pulse can only be supportive diagnosis. For example, by feeling the pulse one can tell if appendicitis has already festered, but one can certainly not determine from the pulse if there is appendicitis.

However, through retraining humbly for a whole year, I absorbed the experience of the older generation and then started realizing that the pulse positions Cun, Guan, Chi have their own logic. Some pathology, for example cough, can be detected and forecasted 1–2 hours before the onset. Not only can it be forecasted, using herbs at that time can have an action ahead of time, which also prevents one from losing his mind when it happens. This, from clinical applicability has a great value.

From Pavlov's theory of positive and negative reactions, the so called "inductive" and "mutative", when the neurological command system breaks off communication, it is not entirely impossible that from the radial pulse position, divided into Cun, Guan and Chi, it represents the inner organs' different phenomena. I am ashamed to admit that, at present, I am unable to produce material explaining systematically if Cun, Guan, Chi have scientific value. However, from what I have grasped above, I feel that it is worth opening the debate again about the logic contained within. This

[420] This refers to the pulse methods taught by Zhang Taisu 張太素 of the Ming dynasty, where via pulse one could forecast the person's good and ill fortunes

is actually an important issue for Chinese medicine scientification. Therefore my opinion is that it is worth twice and thrice to pay attention to the research of this.

8) Conclusion

The above issues I put forth are my small contribution to the great task of Chinese medicine scientification. Following the call of Chairman Mao, we, Chinese medicine colleagues, became very enthusiastic. Through advanced studies and technical exchange and other items of learning we already reached an adequate result in Chinese medicine scientification. This is a definite fact. At the same time, there are still great deficiencies we can't avoid speaking of.

The greatest deficiency is that Chinese and Western medicines are seemingly united but actually alienated. "Appear united" is a mistake violating the policy of merging together. The spirit of "in reality alienated" prevents any sort of professional collaboration. This is because, in the past, the health administration leadership was composed of Western medicine doctors, and from Western medicine point of view looking at Chinese medicine there was not one thing that was correct. Last year in a medical magazine in Jiangxi province, the first edition, a professor of herbal formulas thoroughly analyzed the Western medicine attitude toward Chinese medicine. He explained it thoroughly. It is worth our careful reading.

I feel that there is a wide gap between Chinese and Western medicines. They developed in completely different directions. Western medicine talks about special effect and there is a need for certainty. It diagnoses a "disease". For example, Intestinal cold injury requires Chloromycetin, malaria requires Quinine, and syphilis requires compound 914 kind of remedy; when the medicine arrives, the disease is resolved. There is no other word that can be said here. Chinese medicine does not speak of special effect. There is a need for chance. It diagnoses the entire patient. One only sees disease development and the direction of neurological reactions in order to seek and adjust the medicine. Taking the two and linking them together, in the past, was entirely impossible. See Mr. Ding Fubao's 丁福保[421] lifetime endeavor, what kind of a result did he reach to? But today, using Pavlov's theories, we can already see the possibility for this unity. It is: Chinese medicine must become scientific, and Western medicine is not entirely scientific. This should create a developmental target for a

[421] Ding Fubao 丁福保 (1874–1952) practiced medicine and was a Buddhist believer. He compiled many works on Buddhism and medicine, including the first modern dictionary of Buddhist terminology. He Established Ding's hospital and publication house. Altogether he wrote, compiled and arranged 80 medical works, later collected together as *A Collection of Medical Works by Mr. Ding* 丁氏医学丛书

new science following Pavlov's nerve action theory in order to reach a level of perfection. If one wants to create a Mao Zedong era Chinese medicine, one should know that if Chinese medicine does not undergo scientification, it has no future. In contrast, vague concepts, idealistic pathologies, make oneself clever assumptions, etc. all kinds of unscientific trash, all should, with one swipe, be wiped clean. The so-called "medicine is the art of ideas" nonsense should be avoided. Everyone should establish in their minds a scientific attitude struggling for scientification.

I am a small student of Chinese medicine's middle level. My understanding of Western medicine is also just at the skin level. My courage of posing the above string of issues comes from my studies of Pavlov's spirit of "no shame in admitting my mistakes". It is my hope of "throwing away the rock to bring in the jade". I hope to invoke the interest of advanced fellows and promote further discussion about it.

Article end

1954 first six months work summary of Beijing Chinese Medicine Association outpatient clinic

By Bai Xiaoshan 白嘯山

Source: *Beijing Chinese Medicine* (periodical), 1954 August (3rd volume 8th publication)

北京中醫

一九五四年八月號(第三卷第八期)

Yaron: During the early Communist years, such articles set the tone for diagnosis and treatment style. Specifically here, Beijing Chinese Medicine Association outpatient clinic is a model for the entire nation. Their TCM style included diagnosing a disease as a Western medicine disease and then using predetermined TCM protocols with specific acupoints or herbs to treat it. They hoped to demonstrate that Chinese medicine doctors were well acquainted with the "facts" of modern medicine and what they selected out of Chinese medicine was only the "experience based" clinical application. As we can see here, they also hoped to confirm the "experience based" clinical application efficacy with laboratory blood analysis. In sum, they demonstrated that Chinese medicine was becoming an integrated department within the bigger "new medicine". One can say that it is the evolution of earlier Chinese medicine scientification reformers, especially the Tan Cizhong 譚次仲 group. Note point 2)B: the environment that doctors had to comply with.

1) General situation

Beijing Chinese Medicine Association outpatient clinic was established in February 1952. Following the central government spirit of the time "organize and consolidate, emphasize development, elevate quality and advance with stable steps" there were only departments in the planning. The name selected was "Beijing Chinese Medicine Association Acupuncture Outpatient Clinic". In October 1953 we added an internal medicine department and the name changed to "Beijing Chinese Medicine Association Acupuncture Outpatient Clinic".[422] In June 1954 we have added a bone-setting department. In the near future we plan to add a surgical department.

[422] The name in the article should have dropped the word "Acupuncture" to match the title but is exactly the same as the original name. A probable misprint but we kept the mistake.

At the time of foundation in 1953 in the acupuncture and moxibustion[423] department there were seven Chinese medicine doctors, three acupuncture technicians, one nurse, 15 acupuncture beds and every day the clinic will see about 80 patients. At present there is one Chinese medicine doctor for diagnosis, in the acupuncture department there are seven Chinese medicine doctors, in the internal medicine department there are three Chinese medicine doctors, in the bone-setting department there is one Chinese medicine doctor, there are four acupuncture technicians, one nurse, one apprentice, three administrators and three personnel doing regular odd jobs. There are 37 acupuncture beds. Every day the acupuncture department sees about 200 patients, while the internal medicine department sees about 100 patients.

The clinic has assigned a director doing different tasks directly under the leadership of the Chinese Medicine Association chair. The entire personnel are divided into four groups:

a) Doctor group
b) Nurse group
c) Technician group
d) Administration group

Separately, one person is assigned to deal with human affairs, one person for literature, one person for cultural entertainment and one person for meals. Each group leader, under the leadership of the clinic director, leads his group's work and dictates the group's lifestyle discussions.

Because of the accurate leadership of Beijing's public health office and their great help, the clinic has developed day by day.

2) The different tasks performed

A. The treatment task

From the beginning of January to the end of June, between the different departments, only for initial visit there were 2655 patients, for repeat visits there were 26601 patients, the total patients seen was 29256. The majority of patients were cadres, workers and students. The majority of illnesses were chronic diseases. The treatment had definite efficacy. Following are a few examples out of the entire patients' base:

[423] Henceforth "acupuncture and moxibustion" 針灸 will be shortened to "acupuncture".

Yaron: There are 39 examples brought in the article; we translate here three of them. They all follow the same format, with a conclusion of full recovery. We made the following summary:

The table format for all 39 cases is as follows: Clinic case number, name, age, gender, diagnosis, main symptoms, acupuncture points (no mention of techniques or depth) or formula (only herb names are mentioned, no dosage or cooking instructions), number of acupuncture sessions or number of herb bags, result: all cases state 'complete recovery'. Total 10 patients used herbs, 28 patients used acupuncture, and 1 patient used both herbs and acupuncture. For 32 patients Western medicine terminology is used in diagnosis such as neurological weakness or inflammation. For 7 patients a combination of Chinese and Western terms is used, mostly wind damp plus inflammation. Chinese style diagnosis is mentioned for 3 patients. The diagnosis for 39 patients, multiple patients having same diagnosis, is as follows: Great Spleen disease (Banti's disease), for laboratory examinations see the attached summary. Neurological atrophy, heart organ atrophy, indigestion, facial nerve numbness, acute damp wind joint inflammation, joint inflammation of damp wind type, chronic joint inflammation, high blood pressure, shoulder and elbow damp wind syndrome, gastritis, chronic ulceritis, schizophrenia, neurological indigestion, colitis, chronic tracheitis, bronchitis, trigeminal nerve pains, bloody stool, varicosity, wind damp style sciatica, neurological stomach pains, neurosis, goiter, allergic dermatitis.

Case # 6135, name: Ma Binguan 馬賓光, age 38, female, diagnosis: facial nerve palsy. Symptoms: upper right toothache, right eye can't close, mouth slanting to the left. Points used: Zan Zhu 攢竹, Jing Ming 睛明, Ren Zhong 人中, He Liao 禾髎, He Gu 合谷, Di Cang 地倉, Xia Che 頰車, Yi Feng 翳風, Bai Hui 百會, Tong Zi Liao 童子髎, Cheng Jiang 承漿. Number of sessions 15, result: complete recovery.

Case # 6630, name: Gao Guangyuan 高光遠, age 26, male, diagnosis: esophagitis. Symptoms: Every time with food ingestion the esophagus experiences pain and the four limbs weak, the entire body is achy and lazy, after eating something patient throws up and experiences nausea, mouth ulcers. Herbs used: Cun Dong 寸冬, Pu Gong Ying 蒲公英, Yin Hua 銀花, Zhu Ru 竹茹, Dan Pi 丹皮, Xian Shi Hu 鮮石斛, Sheng Di 生地, Lian Zi Xin 蓮子心, Hang Shao 杭芍, Ze Xie 澤洩, Jian Qu 建曲, Wu Yu 吳萸, Huang Lian 黃連, Xi Huang Wan 犀黃丸. Number of bags 5, result: complete recovery.

Case # 6207, name: Xu Guirong 徐桂榮, age 40, female, diagnosis: chronic gastritis. Symptoms: sharp pains in the stomach and on occasion in the chest as well. Points used: Zhong Wan 中脘, Zu San Li 足三里. Number of sessions 2, result: complete recovery.

Endnote: A summary report of 3894 medical records laboratory test results:

A. November 27th, 1953: White blood cells 2300, red blood cells 4,260,000, blood platelets 95,000.

B. January 12th, 1954: White blood cells 2350, red blood cells 4,690,000, blood platelets 14.5g.[424]

C. January 20th, 1954: White blood cells 24350, red blood cells 3,570,000, blood platelets 14.5g.

D. February 8th, 1954: White blood cells 4400, red blood cells 4,230,000, blood platelets 105,000.

E. February 19th, 1954: White blood cells 3800, red blood cells 4,410,000, hemochrome 14.58, blood platelets 100,000.

F. March 19th, 1954: White blood cells 3300, red blood cells 4,440,000, hemochrome 14.5g, blood platelets 95,000.

B. The task of checking on work diligence and achievement

The political thinking leadership in our clinic was grasped very well. Every week a small group holds a meeting reflecting on past performance, and the entire clinic holds a summary meeting every month. In the meeting everyone can exercise criticism of others and self-criticism. The old Chinese medicine doctors who receive the admiration of the masses, with humility, are able to receive criticism and do the "change for the better" work. Building on this foundation, in January of this year, we checked upon diligence and achievement of the prior year 1953. We have spent more than a month and attained the anticipated result. Through this work of checking on diligence and achievement, the entire personnel advanced a step in mastering the criticism weapon and self-criticism. Self-reflection and criticism was done from top to bottom. Whatever seemed successful was still found lacking and plans to improve it were put forth. At the same time, exemplary persons and exemplary

[424] This unit 14.5g probably meant hemochrome as in point E, we have translated with the errors intentionally.

deeds were hailed. Nurses would wash uniforms, sheets and pillow cases after work hours. Technicians would take the used cotton balls, wash them and then steam sterilize them for reuse. This would save expenses for the clinic. Harmony between comrades has had marked improvement; the comrades have become a harmonious group, not talking badly to each other or misbehaving behind each other's backs. Through this mobilization they developed their self-criticism. The coming together was based on the official policy and so there was a notable improvement.

C. The task of electing model workers

In order to set up the banner and encourage the morale of everyone's work, on the basis of evaluating the work diligence and achievement, we have elected model workers. The standard for model workers included the following criteria:

A. Serving the people wholeheartedly

B. Working energetically and accepting assignments with courage

C. Be willing to study hard the professional work

D. Having serious and proper attitude towards patients

E. Coming together and helping each other

F. Being able to master the self-criticism tool

The way of selecting a model worker was done by self-assessment and public discussion of one's record. First the person put it forth himself, then it was discussed in the small group. Thereafter the entire personnel discussed it and then the leadership reviewed it and gave its final decision. For the first-rate model workers three were elected (Diagnosis Chinese medicine doctor Guo Xianya,[425] nurse group leader Ding Fengying, the general service group leader Zhang Jinsheng). For the second rate model workers four were elected (Apprentice Cai Zhenhua, administrator Wang Shiying, service person Jue Fengwu, internal medicine Chinese medicine doctor Liu Ruitang). For the third rate model workers three were elected (acupuncture technicians Meng Shaomin, Yuan Liping, acupuncture Chinese medicine doctor Xie Shaohou). In June 6th, 1954 we have held a model worker grand meeting where we gave material award, and at the same time we have disciplined and reduced salary

[425] Chinese characters omitted for personal names in this paragraph.

for comrades who were slacking and who did not correct themselves for the better. Through this work, the ones who received prizes expressed their willingness to succeed, to restrain their deficiencies, to avoid arrogance and recklessness, to work hard for the industrialization of the socialist society. The ones who were disciplined also recognized their own mistakes and the generosity of the leadership. They expressed that from that day on they will resolutely change themselves for the better. All in all, all the comrades were educated by this.

D. Political studies and professional studies

The styles of political studies, derived from the regional health branch leadership, are self-study, listening to reports and discussions. In normal times, workers rely on provided teaching materials to cultivate themselves. At fixed dates they go to the regional government to listen to reports. Once per week we lead discussions in the clinic. In addition, we also conduct studies of current affairs in order to elevate the knowledge of our nation's construction and the international situation.

Professional studies are divided into three areas: foundation studies, acupuncture research and treatment research. Foundation studies are based on the secondary medical school physiology curriculum; each chapter of their text is being explained one by one. The study objective is that the clinic's nurses and technicians will have basic foundation. At the end of each class there is a review examination. "Education and meetings" must take place.

The standard for acupuncture research follows the new acupuncture of Zhu Lian 朱琏. The target audience for these lectures are the acupuncture doctors and acupuncture technicians. The method of teaching is to follow each chapter one by one and research it, as well as use the practical experience of each doctor and add it to the class in order to research it.

The method of treatment research is to gather the clinic's every day case studies (including all departments) and research them thoroughly. This will increase in the future the level of Chinese medicine.

E. Establish medical relationships with industry and mining, state enterprises and schools

In 1953 there were six locations, factories, mining and schools that have established medical relationships with our clinic. In 1954 eleven more locations were added, in total 17 locations including the following: Western Beijing

Mining Bureau, Shi Jingshan 石景山 steel factory, Huabei 華北 agricultural equipment factory, Beijing building materials company and sandstone factory, Beijing automobile transportation company and repair factory, Beijing city public transportation company, Construction and engineering office, Xinhua 新華 printing factory, Beijing industrial school, Beijing university, Beijing wholesale company headquarters, Beijing wholesale company, Xidan 西单 business office, China machinery import company, China hardware electrical engineering import company, China technology import company, China import export company, The people's art publication house. Facing the factories and mines and the classification of medical services, we had a distinct impact.

3) The achievements of this work

With the great help of the leadership and the enthusiasm of the comrade workers, this piece of work had great achievement. From professional standpoint, we have added the bone-setting department and every day the patient number has risen by 300. We have added great help to the treatment of the masses and shouldered the heavy burden of hospitals. Through political studies, checking on work diligence and accomplishments and assigning model workers, the comrades advanced a step in self-criticism, emphasizing their good qualities and inspecting their deficiencies. Through every aspect of professional learning the comrades' professional skills have increased.

4) Problems that still exist

a) Political and professional studies are still insufficient: Since our clinic is a self-sufficient unit, therefore from Monday to Saturday we completely engage in treatment work. We use one hour before work to study political and professional studies. So time-wise it is not enough.

b) The problem of laboratory tests: In order to ascertain the diagnosis we plan to establish a laboratory. Even though we have already purchased laboratory equipment, the laboratory room is not yet suitable for use and so the laboratory was not established as of yet. At present we still rely on Beijing Chinese Medicine Advanced Studies School for our testing.

c) The problem of Chinese herbs: There are many workers and cadres who come to our clinic for internal medicine treatment. However, because we don't have our own pharmacy, the patients need to go to appointed herbal store in order to get their herbs, they waste time and it inconveniences the masses.

5) The plan going forward

With this kind of work we had a definite achievement but there were also not few deficiencies. In order to ascertain achievement and restrain deficiency we need to add more political and professional studies. In the second half of this year we plan to add surgical department and open a pharmacy. As conditions permit, we will gradually add laboratory and X-ray equipment.

In summary, Beijing Chinese Medicine Association Outpatient Clinic, from nothing became something, from small became big. Chinese medicine comrades from private clinics walked toward collective labor; within a very short period of time, be it political or professional, everybody improved. This certainly illustrates how it cannot be separated from the Chinese Communist party and the brilliant government leadership. Following the party line beacon of light we should develop the motherland's treasures and cultural inheritance. We should work enthusiastically toward the industrialization of our socialist society.

Article end

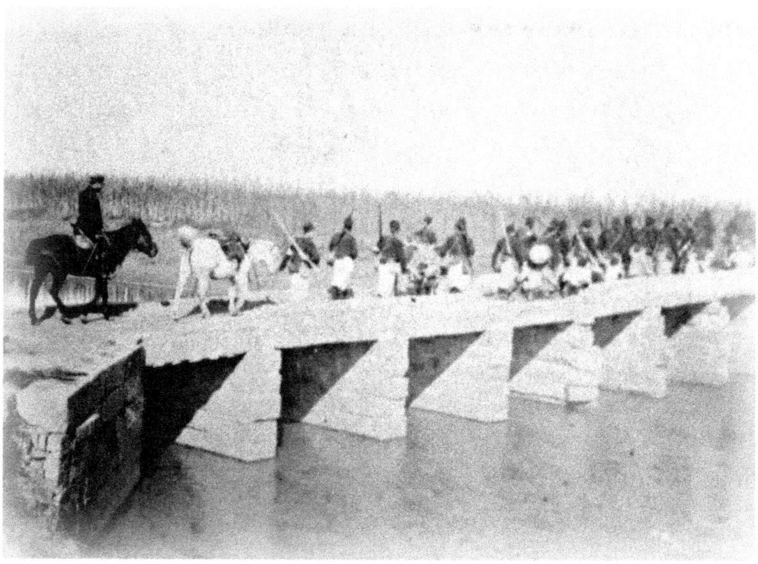

Photo by Mr P. Goux in early 1900s. "Bridge near Yang Tsen".

Tianjin Municipal General Hospital: Chinese medicine doctors are invited to participate in treatment work and exchange Chinese and Western medicines' experience

Source: *Beijing Chinese Medicine* (periodical), 1954 August (3rd volume 8th publication)
北京中醫　一九五四年八月號(第三卷第八期)

Yaron: How much did this kind of propaganda in media impact the minds of ordinary Chinese medicine practitioners, making them believe in something that is not?

Pages 34–35

In section: "Trends in the Chinese Medicine World"

In June this year, Tianjin 天津 municipal general hospital established an acupuncture and moxibustion treatment room. The hospital invited Chinese medicine doctors to participate in the treatment work and exchange experience between Chinese and Western medicines. By the middle of July, the Chinese medicine doctors in the acupuncture treatment room have already treated 120 patients using acupuncture and moxibustion treatment modality. The majority of patients reported excellent results. For example, a ten year old child, Li Guofan, was suffering from bed-wetting. He was bed-wetting every night. In the past he visited hospitals many times but was never cured. Recently he underwent 11 acupuncture sessions and recovered fully. In another example, one patient who has had neurological numbness in his face could not move any of his facial muscles. For eating he needed a doctor to administer nasal feeding. He needed to get milk through his nose, which was a great hardship. After the first acupuncture treatment in the acupuncture room he was able to move the corner of his mouth, and after the second acupuncture session he was able to move the upper part of his face. Currently he is still under treatment.

The Chinese medicine doctors participating in the hospital work have greater opportunity to exchange with Western medicine's experience. They began understanding the relationship between nerve distribution and acupoints as well as the connection between Pavlov's theories and acupuncture therapy.

Tianjin city municipal general hospital, in order to systematically research the acupuncture treatment modality, not only asked the Western medicine doctors to help with the acupuncture room work, but also dispatched a physiotherapist to survey each and every patient receiving acupuncture, recording carefully the disease changes. The accumulated material was then analyzed by both Chinese and Western doctors. Many Western medicine doctors, after seeing the effective results of acupuncture, gradually corrected their inaccurate opinions towards acupuncture. The contact between Western and Chinese medicine doctors becomes closer and closer every day.

Article end

Scientifically rearranging Chinese medicine learning and literature

1954 by Xue Ningsong 薛凝嵩

Source: *Beijing Chinese Medicine* (periodical), 1954 October (3rd volume 10th publication)
Published by Beijing Chinese Medicine Association Publication Committee
北京中醫　北京中醫學會出版委員會出版　一九五四年十月號(第三卷第十期)

Yaron: The reformers were separating "Chinese medicine art" from its literature. This article, of course, is not a government directive, but having been published by the Beijing Chinese Medicine Association it represented a banner to follow for the entire nation. Throughout history information regarding herbs' characteristics was not always uniform and, at times, even contradictory. These contradictions needed to disappear in order to make a single Chinese medicine standard. A large scale lengthy investigation of herbs and formulas, determining the nature of herbs and correcting all prior materia medica conflicts into a standardized herbs' textbook, never took place. I believe that many decisions to eliminate contradictions in ancient literature were done arbitrarily or, if opportunity presented itself, for ideological reasons. Coming down to the Communist era the theory of TCM became loosely attached to the application. The diagnosis was done with modern medicine while the application with predetermined protocols.

As we saw in a prior article *First Six Months Work Summary of Beijing Chinese Medicine Association Outpatient Clinic*, clinical studies had been done and published during this time, but such studies were closely knitted with the Party line and similar propaganda. The standard underlying such experimental studies was the absence of Chinese medicine theory. Even though it was done, it is actually illogical to extract theoretical conclusions from these studies. Of course, in these experimental studies there was a theory: a Leninist-Marxist dialectical materialism theory. People have judged the results by following this ideology and not ancient theories.

Pages 3–7

Scientific rearrangement of our motherland medical cultural heritage, extracting the essence and getting rid of the refuse, is indeed a significant Chinese medicine scientification step. Especially now during the transition phase, under the brilliant beaming of the Party line beacon of light, the state acts accordingly and cultivates talent in order to construct the new economy and build the new society.

Arriving at this climax is a work of great importance. In order to be a health worker and a Chinese medicine doctor struggling against disease for the health of the people, one should energetically study and enthusiastically labor, take the socialist mindset and change his own brain, take scientific technologies and elevate his own professional level. This may develop in all directions creating an outstanding work for socialism. It will become a brick in this beautiful building of socialism.

Chinese medicine scientification guarantees Chinese medicine development. Now, rearranging Chinese medicine and its literature will remove obstacles from Chinese medicine scientification and will allow a gradual buildup of optimal conditions for its development. Chinese medicine conceals within many things of great value. It is the accumulated experience of countless people even though, on the surface of it, it seems uncultivated and disorderly. It is exactly because it seems uncultivated and disorderly that it requires rearrangement.

Comrade Guan Xiangying 關向應[426] said the following statement in 1945: "Chinese medicine, acupuncture and moxibustion have good things in them. Arranging and researching them is a must. However, the objective is to go forward. If you only

[426] Guan Xiangying (1902–1946) a high ranking general in the Communist party army.

follow blindly trying to drive a car, believing that there could be miraculous prescriptions for all diseases in it, then this is wrong." These few very simple lines pointed to the direction Chinese medicine must go. If the rearrangement of Chinese medicine's art and literature is done well, the concealed things can express new applications and this is an immense contribution to the health of our motherland's people. It is also an immense contribution to the construction of our motherland's socialism. Therefore, the issue of rearranging Chinese medicine and its literature in a scientific way is an issue not easily ignored during this transitional phase.

Chinese medicine art and Chinese medicine literature, from conceptual point of view, belong to two separate realms. Chinese medicine art is the entire knowledge of accumulated experience by our ancestors struggling with disease. It includes not only texts but also oral transmission of prescriptions and their efficacy. Now, Chinese medicine literature refers to all materials connected to that knowledge. It refers to not only earlier medical works, but also to scattered pieces of information and short articles included in other texts like history books, novels and miscellaneous local gazetteers. Bronze and stoneware, pictures and rubbings from tablets can all be counted as material to assess the healthcare of the ancients. They are all part of the old medical literature. Rearranging the Chinese medicine art without rearranging the Chinese medicine literature is not possible. At the same time, only rearranging Chinese medicine literature without rearranging the Chinese medicine art has no purpose to it. Therefore the two cannot be separated.

Chinese medicine can become scientific; this is certain. Chinese medicine must become scientific in order to develop; this is also certain. The problem is, how to transform it? That Chinese medicine doctors will learn science, there is no doubt about that. That Chinese medicine doctors who have studied science will be the ones to make Chinese medicine scientific, there is no doubt about that either. The problem is, after Chinese medicine doctors have studied science well, how can they merge together with the Chinese medicine art? How can they expel the old and bring forth the new, making the old develop new applications?

If, for example, Chinese medicine doctors will hold the old in one hand and the new in the other but can't merge them together and use them as one, then they will come and go in the crossroads. Their suspicion toward China's medicine will deepen. How can this bring about new application? On the other hand, if they would be slacking in their criticism of the old, and then take the new and the old and combine them in an awkward way, blindly praising the ancients, believing that the ancients' words were always scientific, even if invisibly so, will this be able to create new applications? So how should we receive properly the motherland's medical inheritance?

This is, first and foremost, a mindset problem, a recognition problem; it is not entirely a technical problem. If we want to solve this problem, then we must strengthen the socialism leadership in Chinese medicine circles, we must strengthen their task of learning Marxism, Leninism and the transitional phase main Party line. In addition, we should develop Pavlov's and Lepeshinskaya's[427] theories and study them. The method for thinking Marxism and Leninism is to have a key first and then, with this key, one can easily open the vast door of this storage house. This key is the newest and most standard scale; after you have it, you can measure the goods inside the storage house, deciding which ones fit with this scale and which ones don't.

Therefore, for rearranging Chinese medicine art and Chinese medicine literature, one must use the Marxism-Leninism weapon. If we do well Chinese medicine scientification then China's medicine will expel the old and bring forth the new and so, to develop new applications, we must use even more this Marxism-Leninism weapon. Here, I want to clarify that I do not criticize the natural sciences, even not a little bit. What I am saying is that, in order to rearrange, we need to use dialectical materialism and historical materialism and we still need to use the natural sciences logic to explain it. If we cannot use the natural sciences logic to explain it, then it is useless.

The realm of Chinese medicine art and Chinese medicine literature is vast and the materials are abundant. Attempting to rearrange it is not an easy task. Not only does it require leadership, a plan and steps of progression, it also needs merging with reality and with the masses. It cannot be done with crudity and haste and with subjective, arbitrary decisions. I, the author, am ill-informed at present of my limitations; I took my thought of the rearranging methods and wrote them down. I was hoping to give some food for thought for all people concerned—Chinese medicine enthusiasts and comrades interested in rearranging Chinese medicine.

[427] Olga Borisovna Lepeshinskaya (1871–1963). A Soviet biologist who was a protégée of Lenin and Stalin. She rejected genetics and claimed to have made inorganic matter come alive, like crystals that can be converted into cells if one adds to them nucleic acids. She supported these claims by fabricating proofs which, in turn, were confirmed by other scientists eager to advance their own careers. One of her fake proofs was to film the dying cells and their decomposition and then project the film in reverse. In 1952 she received the Stalin prize and her ideas became mandatory instruction in Biology. In that year, in a special conference, the bourgeois Virchowian concept of cell development (only a living cell can produce another living cell) was replaced by a new dialectic-materialistic theory on the origin of all living cells from non-living matter. While her impact and dogmatic dominance have parallels to those of Lysenko, her claims were never officially renounced but just faded away. (Info for this footnote comes from Wikipedia)

1) Compiling a catalog of Chinese medicine literature

Our motherland's old medicine literature is like the distant ocean. If one wants to rearrange it, he must first have a guiding principle. I, the author, am of the opinion that we should first compile a catalog of all existing literature and prepare good summaries. Next, we should collect all sorts of medical fragments and records on bronze and stoneware, fractions of silks and pieces of bamboo slips, paintings, charts and rubbings from tablets, compile and revise a catalog for them with explanations. After we accomplish these two tasks then we can follow clues to locate things. At that time, engaging rearrangement becomes convenient.

2) Rearranging herbs and experience-based prescriptions

China's medicine and pharmacology has been constantly developing for several thousand years. The scope of herbs is vast and the number of experience-based prescriptions has increased. This is in direct proportion to production increase and working class struggle against disease and the accumulating experience resulting therefrom.

The earliest herbal work, *Shen Nong Ben Cao* 神農本草, was compiled around the Warring States period to the Western Han. It narrates 365 different herbs. Tao Hongjing 陶宏景 of the Liang dynasty compiled *Ming Yi Bie Lu* 名醫別錄, supplementing the Han and Wei dynasties famous doctors' use of an additional 365 herbs. Su Gong 蘇恭 of the Tang dynasty added 114 more. Liu Han 劉翰 of the Song dynasty added again 120 herbs. Coming to the Ming dynasty, Li Shizhen 李時珍 compiled the *Ben Cao Gang Mu* 本草綱目 (16th century) when the herb count had reached 1892. Within 2000 years, the herb count has increased more than fivefold. Medical prescriptions at the end of Eastern Han at the time of Zhang Zhongjing 張仲景 (3rd century), who compiled the *Shang Han Lun* 傷寒論 and *Jin Gui Yao Lüe* 金匱要略, uses only 225 prescriptions. However, Sun Simiao 孫思邈 of the Tang dynasty (7th century) who compiled *Qian Jin Fang* 千金方 and *Qian Jin Yi Fang* 千金翼方 already had more than 5000 prescriptions. After him came Wang Tao 王燾 (7th century), who compiled *Wai Tai Mi Yao* 外台秘要 and added additional 1000 prescriptions; all in all 6900 prescriptions. Within 500 years the prescriptions' number has increased thirty fold. After Li Shizhen, the herb number was still increasing and the herbal prescriptions have, as well, increased by a considerable number.

From the point of view of medical technique development, there was first pricking with stone needles and thereafter the burning of moxa. Only after that was there use of grass, roots and tree barks being cooked into a soup and consumed. These are called decoctions. At this time, the society had already developed into an agrarian society. After the invention of decoction treatment, as mankind struggled with disease, they attained a sharp weapon. China's medicine and herbals entered a new era. After that the medicine, in its pursuit of advancement, progressed and created different types of formulas: pills, powders, ointments and elixirs. They were produced according to needs of that time.

The methods to differentiate diseases and symptoms gradually improved. Seeing, hearing, asking and palpating became the foundations of clinical diagnosis.

From all these different aspects onwards, Chinese medicine has constantly developed. As for the rearranging of these materials, aside from compiling the historical development, we still need to accomplish the following two tasks: rearrange herbs and rearrange prescriptions. The experience of earlier people is reliable to a large degree. The records of herbs' efficaciousness and prescriptions' treatment experience are relatively objective, full and accurate. They have consultative value. However, this needs to be received in an accurate fashion.

In the past few years, the work of analyzing Chinese herbs in laboratory has been done by many and has yielded a distinct accomplishment. However, it seems that these have become somewhat disjointed from clinical research and their coming together with the predecessors' experience was even lesser than that. This way of doing things is very much departing from reality, it departs from the disposition of the masses. Analyzing the chemical structure of a certain raw herb must come only after a clear distinction of said herb; in such a way there will be no waste of effort and time.

In order to differentiate clearly the species, one must use the predecessors' records. This is because the predecessors already did this job well. They have already recorded in detail and handed down to us the variety, local growing area, shape, characteristics, the different names and methods of differentiating them. Adding to that the experience of farmers growing these herbs then the identification of species, to a large degree, cannot go wrong. If we do away with this knowledge, turn upside down everything and start anew, we will waste much time experimenting on so many herbs and still will not figure out which is correct which is not. In this fashion, will it still be possible to determine the herbs' effects? "Shen Nong 神農 tasted the hundred herbs" style of doing things does not merge with dialectic logic. The reason it was done like this in the past was the superficial view of reality. If we want to rearrange the herbs, we must first rearrange the materia medica. We should take all knowledge of herbs differentiated by different persons from different materia medica, repair and adjust and look for actual proof of efficacy. Then select the realistic part and discard all the mysterious theories. At present, this indeed is a task that must be done.

When it comes to experience-based prescriptions, what was left to us by our predecessors is truly rich. Even more, efficacious secret recipes transmitted by small groups of people are many. If we want to summarize this experience, it is not something that can be accomplished by a small group of people, nor can it be done well in a discussion during a meeting. This work must be merged with the masses. I believe that, at present, we can do it the following way: through the entire country's unified leadership of Chinese medicine research organizations, mobilize all local Chinese medicine groups (for example Chinese medicine associations), or Chinese medicine doctors with relatively long clinical experience. So to say, they should bring out the real and practical experience they attained with the experience-based prescriptions (secret recipes even better), write down patient cases, comment on and source the famous doctors' prescriptions.

The attitude must be honest and sincere, not exaggerated and not reduced. The entire country's unified leadership of Chinese medicine research organizations will collect these reports, select through them, research the reason why the selected ones are effective and decide which diseases they should apply to. Thereafter, compile them in batches and deliver it to each local Chinese medicine group to reprint and popularize and then experiment further with it. In this way, it comes from the masses and it goes back to the masses, experimented upon over and over. On the one hand it increases the exchange of things attained, on the other hand it popularizes the art. This must be effective and will gradually summarize the experience of the predecessors.

Yaron: The following point shows how the Communist ideology crafted the TCM theory; what was and wasn't allowed, what could and couldn't merge with Marxism.

3) Rearranging the progressively-changing theory of Chinese medicine

As for the development of Chinese medicine pharmacology, Chinese medicine theory had a distinct effect but it also had a distinct adverse effect. The effect was that it took herbs out of folk experience and gradually established a systematic theory, which made it a scientific art. The adverse effect was that these kinds of idealistic theories gradually took China's pharmacology from experienced-based to mystery-based. Like this, the more the theories matured, the more China's pharmacology was influenced.

During the earlier times of feudal society, the theory of Chinese pharmacology was not systematically mature and so its development was relatively fast. However, during the feudal society intermediate and late stages (from the Song and Yuan dynasties onward) Chinese medicine theories gradually matured and, with that, the development of pharmacology gradually slowed down and, to an extreme, even stopped completely.

This explains why, originally, Chinese medicine factual reality and theory were conflicting. On the one hand was the accumulation of practical experience, while on the other hand was the whitewashing of an imaginary theory. This conflict was always there and gradually even developed. The development and nurturing of imaginary Chinese medicine theories is inseparable from long-standing feudal rule. Before the feudal society, Chinese medicine had no theory.

During the Warring States period is when the *Ling Shu* 靈樞 and *Su Wen* 素問 (collectively named *Nei Jing* 內經) appeared and then came the *Nan Jing* 難經. The *Nei Jing* and *Nan Jing* are the earliest theoretical documents of China's medicine. All other later theories stem out of these two books. *Ling Shu* is an acupuncture treatment book written by occult practitioners. The *Su Wen* is the work of Daoist practitioners. *Su Wen* mainly speaks of nurturing life cultivation, it promotes "indifference to fame and dwell in emptiness" as well as "guard the spirit" in order to "avoid disease". There are also many places talking about disease, but these are just for the purpose of recognizing disease. The objective of recognizing disease was to guard against it and not to treat it. Guarding against a disease is one of the cultivation methods. Therefore *Su Wen* advocates the preventive viewpoint "don't treat the disease but rather treat it before the disease has formed" and so it does not discuss much treatment. Later people have merged the *Su Wen* and *Ling Shu* into one *Nei Jing*, and with that it became one complete medical work, it had prevention and it had treatment. Chinese medicine experience merging with theory had its beginning.

The basis of *Su Wen* theory was Yin Yang conflict of opposing each other and unifying with each other. From Yin Yang it developed to six conformations: Tai Yang; Yang Ming; Shao Yang; Tai Yin; Shao Yin; and Jue Yin. "Three Yin and Three Yang separating and merging" is the confliction and unification mentioned. It is the first and simple stage of dialectical thinking. Using this kind of logic to explain the relationship between human health and disease is plausible. Disease is an expression of conflict. When one takes a disease and heals it then the conflict reaches unification.

The human body's inner organs are all inter-reliant and mutually restraining. When they depend on each other it is called "merge" and when they control each other it is called "separate". If there is "merge" and "separate" then the person can exist, otherwise he will die. Using dialectics to explain this phenomenon is also possible. At the initial phases of Chinese medicine theory, Yin Yang changes have developed into five phases controlling and restraining, all these theories being product of imagination and still they don't depart from the spirit of dialectics. Ever since Daoist religion, Confucian thought and alchemists converged together, the study of "above the form", or formless, entered the realm of medicine and, ever since, there are many obscure influences.

Coming to the Jin Yuan dynasties, Chinese medicine entered the dark ages. Not only did the theory become more and more mysterious that one could not investigate it anymore, also the doctors' sectarian bias became very deep. The so-called four great physicians (Liu Shouzhen 劉守真, Zhang Zihe 張子和, Zhu Zhenheng 朱震亨, Li Gao 李杲) all simply clung to bias, attacked and resisted each other and became famous. They did not have any real understanding or new development. This was mainly because they received the absurd views and influence of the Song dynasty Confucians and the so-called Study of Principle.[428]

In the last 500 years, the only one that can be designated as an outstanding scholar was Li Shizhen 李時珍. His works, *Ben Cao Gang Mu* 本草綱目 and *Bin Hu Mo Xue* 瀕湖脈學,[429] do not have the polluted expression of forced and stray talk. They truly surpassed the other works of that time. The influence he gave to future generations was to focus on reality and use facts to correct the theory. Later works, such as Xu Dachun's 徐大椿 *She Tai Tu Shuo* 舌胎圖說, Ye Tianshi's 葉天士 *Wen Re Lun* 溫熱論 and Wang Qingren's 王清任 *Yi Lin Gai Cuo* 醫林改錯, in reality, are all works that had true attainment. After Li Shizhen, China's medicine again walked the path of practical experience.

As for China's medicine, its history is long, its content rich and its efficacy is considerable. It is only because of the long period of feudal rule that it had no way of

[428] The Idealist philosophy of the Confucian school 理學.
[429] *Compendium of Materia Medica* and the *Lakeside Master's Pulse Study*.

progressing, the main expression of which was the obstruction of clinical development by the imaginary feudal theories. This is because imaginary theories can only reflect inaccurately the accumulated experience in the clinic. They cannot serve as an accurate guide. They can only explain disease pathology and drug effects by imagination and they cannot research deeply, in a scientific way, from the expression to the intrinsic nature of things.

Therefore, Chinese medicine theories and facts are two separate things. There are Chinese medicine doctors with deep scholarship, but when they face a disease they can't use any of it. There are other Chinese medicine doctors with rich clinical experience, who can heal well many diseases but they can't explain the principle why. Because of this, there is the saying "after reading books for three years there is no disease that one can heal, and after treating disease for three years there are no books that one can read". Of course, the first belongs to dogmatism, while the latter to empiricism. One cannot avoid saying that Chinese medicine reality and theory are two different wooden stakes; however, is it possible to get rid of Chinese medicine theory with one kick? The answer is no. If one gets rid of the old Chinese medicine theory with one kick then the scientification of Chinese medicine becomes impossible! How so? It is because the old Chinese medicine theory, even though it has an awkward reflection of the pragmatic side of things, yet this kind of awkward reflection has its own type of pragmatic basis, which is one-sided subjectivity.

Lenin has said:

> Linearity and one-sidedness, inflexibility and rigidity, subjectivism and subjective blindness—these are the roots for knowledge of idealistic theories. And so the doctrines of monks and priests (philosophical spiritualism) of course have roots in theoretical knowledge as well. It is not that they don't have any basis. They, with no doubt, are a flower that does not bear fruits. Yet they grow and live, and their outcome is real. It is absolutely the human knowledge of this living tree that has flowers but doesn't bear fruits.

Chinese medicine's spiritual theories truly grow on this living tree that has flowers but doesn't bear fruits. However it has already, for so many years, become the reality of the "proper" path that must be taken. For so many years, the people who have studied medicine have walked this road toward receiving the predecessors' practical experience. And so Chinese medicine doctors' task took shape under the guidance of these awkward theories. Therefore, there are some Chinese medicine doctors with scientific inclination, who know that these theories cannot be explained. In clinic, when they write a prescription they have no choice but to battle against it. This is one great conflict.

If one wants to solve this conflict, one must bring an external influence into its core and make it change. Chinese medicine's awkward theories and the actual facts are, indeed, in conflict. Science is the influence coming from the outside. If one wants to do well with Chinese medicine scientification, he must first become familiar with this situation. In other words, one cannot take suddenly an explosive amount of scientific theory and replace the old Chinese medicine theory, and think that it will do the job. One must do well the merging of Chinese and Western medicines, cultivate well the scientific knowledge of Chinese medicine doctors, and with this kind of knowledge they should go ahead and resolve said conflict. One should take the old Chinese medicine theories, the ones that conform to science and the ones that don't conform to science, and separate and rearrange them, select the essence and get rid of the refuse. Like this, we can get Chinese medicine doctors to gradually use scientific theories and technologies to replace those inaccurate theories and supplement the diagnostic methods. Doing it like this will cause the Chinese medicine art to gradually walk toward scientification, on a path of development.

Konstantinov[430] said:

> No matter if it is natural sciences or social sciences, they all have not only their history, but also their pre-history. The pre-history of the relatively modern science of astronomy by Copernicus, where-the-sun-is-the-center theory, was Ptolemy's theory that the earth is in the center. The earlier body of modern chemistry was alchemy and its probing into "igniting metals and stones". Before there was historical materialism, the life expressions of society and the explanation of society's past records, was a special kind of history and alchemy—it was entirely controlled by opposing-science historical idealism and a social life view.

[430] Aleko Konstantinov (1863–1897) a Bulgarian writer. Known for creating the fictional character Bay Ganyo, one of the most famous fictional characters of Bulgarian literature (Wikipedia).

The old Chinese medicine theory of "above material knowledge" is the pre-historic body of modern scientific Chinese medicine theory. Seeking a scientific fetus in the unscientific earlier body of Chinese medicine, in order to cultivate anew Chinese medicine fresh foundations, has its own distinct impact. This grand historical task has befallen us, a generation of assiduous "Chinese medicine transforming into science" workers.

4) Rearranging the medicine's historical persons and their literature

Throughout our nation's history there are many medical persons and their written works are abundant. There are also those who did not leave behind written works but their achievement of treating disease was clearly shown. These people have had a definite impact on the development of Chinese medicine and pharmacology. However, the official histories of the different dynasties did not view them with great importance. In the past several thousand years, there were very few medical persons seen in the historical annals. Therefore, I suggest that we take the motherland's historical medical figures and their literature and rearrange it. We will line them up in chronological order and compose a book titled *The Annals of Medicine's Historical Persons* 醫史人物志 or *Review of Medicine's Historical Persons* 醫史人物述評. In addition to introducing their life and achievement, the historical backdrop of their time and their clinical experience, the most important would be to analyze their thinking and criticize their works. We should point out their good aspects as much as it was possible according to conditions prevalent in that time and, at the same time, use modern scientific standards to measure their lacking.

It may include mythical persons like Shen Nong 神農, Huang Di 黃帝 or Qi Bo 岐伯, whose transmission came down from antiquity or real people whose identity can be ascertained but their contribution to medicine is not certain, but it is possible that they had close relationship with medicine and pharmacology. We might as well compile a section according to mythological materials with added explanations. Our motherland's history is very long and its medicine developed very early on. There are many mythological stories and it is hard to avoid strained interpretations. In these mythologies, when trying to verify if persons and their works are true or fabricated, the attitude must be a cautious one. One must avoid relying on one person's subjective and arbitrary objection, but one must also avoid blindly believing the old arbitrary exaggeration. We should use historical materialism and dialectical materialism point of view to analyze and criticize the thoughts and writings of these historical medical figures.

When it comes to certain particular details of certain themes, they can be omitted and given to a few specialists to do research on. For example, the issue of Zhang Zhongjing being the prefecture chief of Changsha 長沙. This item is irrelevant for Zhang Zhongjing's contribution to medicine and pharmacology. However, for ones who specifically research the historical aspect, or for some other scholars, this maybe an issue of personal interest. After a systematic review of several thousand years of medical figures, the objective of publishing *The Annals of Medicine's Historical Persons* 醫史人物志 or *Review of Medicine's Historical Persons* 醫史人物述評 is to make a general introduction and analysis.

Even more so, we need to analyze and criticize the thoughts and writings of those persons who were standing out in their generation and who were impacting the medicine. Some people will surely be suspicious: "doctors are not philosophers, nor are they politicians or writers, why do we need to analyze their thoughts?" It is because the ancient doctors often were not only doctors. For them, the medical art was to serve the parents and help friends. In medicine, people who have written books certainly had literature accomplishments or political standings. Their thinking was appropriately complex and their knowledge was varied. These kinds of thoughts expressed in daily life as conduct and virtues and were reflected in their medical works. It is like the laughter of people, each person has a distinct sound.

Other than that, there are many other people who, because of personal beliefs and interest, understood medicine differently; the Buddhist understood it as Zen, the Daoist as Mysterious, the Confucian according to the Confucian principle, it is truly "ten thousand miles of the Yellow river, where clay and sand mingle together"[431]. One must analyze and repudiate the idealistic thinking. Only then can he base himself on materialism and objective facts, deeply researching the intrinsic value of things. Only like this can one bring forth the achievement of scientific medical persons like Zhang Zhongjing 張仲景, Chao Yuanfang 巢元方, Sun Simiao 孫思邈, Wang Tao 王燾, Li Shizhen 李時珍 etc. Only like this can one stimulate and smelt the past and present.

Therefore, *The Annals of Medicine's Historical Persons* 醫史人物志 or *Review of Medicine's Historical Persons* 醫史人物述評, this kind of book not only must give an objective introduction to medical persons but also a thorough analysis of right and wrong, highlighting the strong points and deficiencies. In addition, in China's medicine

[431] The meaning is that for thousands of years the good and the bad are always mingled together.

there was something called the "art of benevolence". A doctor must have a benevolent heart and only then can he practice this art of benevolence. This is to say that a doctor must possess a humanitarian spirit. Therefore the personal character of historical Chinese medicine persons was often excellent. There were also doctors who were not happy with current society and government and so they practiced in reclusion, while others always looked to increase the moral standing of society. These all have their strong aspects. They often showed loving care to their patients, which is admirable. Therefore their positive disposition must be promoted, which can help cultivate a good moral character of doctors. It can serve as a model for guarding the medical treatment rules.

5) Rearranging literature of historical medical cases

Patient case studies (the ancients called it medical cases) is the most precious part amongst Chinese medicine's literature. It is a record of clinical application. Even though there are some exaggerated ones, however, most are according to reality and are scientific in nature. There are many patient cases that not only record the symptoms, pulse and herbs, but also meticulously record the physical shape, emotions, work, lifestyle, environment, disease cause, past medical history and forecasted outcome. In these cases, there are very few empty-talk theories and mechanical copying of doctrines. They, rather, lend great help to future clinical medicine. It is a pity that these kinds of documents are rare.

In the book *Zuo Zhuan* 左傳 there is a record of Yi Huan 醫緩[432] who healed Duke Jing of the State of Jin 晉景公. In the *Records of Grand Historian*[433] there are records of Bian Que 扁鵲 and Cang Gong 倉公; these are the earliest medical cases. There are also quite a few others scattered throughout different historical books, however, these are medical records written by historians and amateurs, they are not systematic nor are they detailed; they can only be used as a reference material. Relatively complete patient records coming out of the hands of professional doctors, and often studied by medical professionals, include: *Ming Yi Lei An* 名醫類案 by Jiang Guan Fu Zi 江瓘夫子, *Yu Yi Cao* 寓意草 by Yu Jiayan 喻嘉言, *Hui Xi Yi An* 洄溪醫案 by Xu Dachun 徐大椿, *Xu Ming Yi Lei An* 續名醫類案 by Wei Yuheng 魏玉衡, *Gu Jin Ming Yi Lei An An* 古今名醫類案按 by Yu Zhen 俞震, *Ren Shu Zhi* 仁術志 and *Hui Chun Lu* 回春錄 by Wang Mengying 王孟英, and Hua Xiuyun 華岫雲 compilation of Ye Tianshi 葉天

[432] This is narrated in two places in *Zuo Zhuan*: 左傳·成公十年 and 通志.
[433] *Shiji* 史記 by Si Maqian 司馬遷.

士 cases named *Lin Zheng Zhi Nan Yi An* 臨症指南醫案, and Qian Shanshi 錢珊石 compilation of Chen Xiuyuan's 陳修園 cases titled *Nan Ya Tang Yi An* 南雅堂醫案 etc. Yu Yi Cao 寓意草 writes in a high-flown talk and does not reflect reality. The two books *Lin Zheng Zhi Nan Yi An* 臨症指南醫案 and *Nan Ya Tang Yi An* 南雅堂醫案 are mixed up in disorder, there is no proper methodology for the compilation. They also seem to plagiarize each other.

In the heap of paper, one can extract out here and there some things. From the mid-period of the Qing dynasty, in the area of Jiang Su and Zhe Jiang 江浙一帶, compilation of patient cases became increasingly important. Disciples of a certain teacher hand-copying his experience viewed it as precious. Many of them were not revealed to others or published. If we can extensively collect these kinds of scientific literature and rearrange it, then it will have a great application.

The rearrangement method should have the following three steps: First, collect patient cases from ancient and more modern literature, compile them tightly together and remove the refuse, select the essence of it. Second, standardize disease names and add to the compilation. Third, add scientific theory kind of commentary. Patient case literature contains mostly internal medicine cases, next to that gynecology and obstetrics, next to that pediatrics. External injuries, throat and eyes, acupuncture and moxibustion, bone setting etc cases are rare like phoenix feathers and beasts' horns. Yet, internal, gynecology and pediatric cases are complex and need to be simplified. Cases that involve complete treatment recovery, use new effective formulas or differentiate successfully difficult to treat disease, or cases that cannot be diagnosed and turn into hypochondria, have research value. We should select them all. The other refuse cases that require getting rid of include: cases recorded not clearly, exaggerated beyond belief or those in which the use of herbs don't follow the rules and this does not become a prescription, or that it does not help in the study process—these all need to be removed.

6) Compiling foundational reading material for youngsters starting their medical study

After we have finished compiling and rearranging the old medicine's literature, we need to compile a set of foundational reading material to give to beginner youngsters. Ignoring the next generation's cultivation is wrong. Youngsters are not entirely without interest towards Chinese medicine, however, they completely lack reading material on the topic. Flipping through the old medical books is difficult.

First is the ancient language. The ancients are very far from our generation, their language was very different. The ancient doctors were often very scholarly and loved playing with their brushes and ink.[434] Youngsters come only seldom in contact with such obscure language, therefore telling them to use this kind of literature to go and understand the ancients' ideas is a fruitless endeavor. In addition, they certainly will not have interest in that.

Second, much of the technical language belongs to times past. The ancient doctors had ancient technical terminology, modern doctors have modern scientific technical terminology. This is only natural. This is because the lifestyle of modern and ancient people is entirely different. There is really no reason for us to force youngsters to love technical terminology that has expired already. Should we ask youngsters to translate these terms themselves? This is another impossible thing. And so, for youngsters who love our motherland medical inheritance and yet can only feel inadequate and frustrated, there is no way to set about! Therefore, the responsibility to serve as the link between the past and the future falls on the back of our generation. The purpose of Chinese medicine scientification is to develop Chinese medicine. It is not to eliminate Chinese medicine. No one should be suspicious of that!

Chinese medicine inheritably has a beautiful aspect to it, however, it requires us to go find it, to go arrange it and push the masses of youngsters to study it. Youngsters that set their minds on Chinese medicine are a newly-created mighty force. If we ignore this one point we will be ignoring the developmental future of Chinese medicine and its grand contribution. In our nation, as Chinese medicine educational institutions have not formed yet, compiling foundational reading materials for youngsters, helping youngsters study Chinese medicine, is a task of utmost importance.

[Conclusion]

Rearranging Chinese medicine art and Chinese medicine literature is an arduous task. The above few points I wrote down as they came into my mind but they are certainly not exhaustive. However, this is unlike the design drawing of an engineer where, ahead of time, all the windows, doors, floors and walls need to be laid out to within-an-inch accuracy. There may be some problems that will only be discovered after the job has begun.

[434] Used extravagant, hard-to-understand language.

Our objective need is to have Chinese medicine become a medicine of "our nation, the masses, with scientific contents". When everybody takes action it should be long-lasting and with hard work it must conform to the bright light emanating from the Party general line. Enthusiasm and creativity should be put into play in order to bring forth Chinese medicine scientification. Only like this we will not let down our forefathers, not let down our leader comrade Mao Zedong and the Chinese Communist Party. I think that, for the construction of socialism and for giving better fortune to the people, diligently developing this health profession has a special meaning.

Article end

All major hospitals in Beijing recruit Chinese medicine doctors to participate in medical treatment work

1954 by Li Mohe 李墨鶴

Source: *Beijing Chinese Medicine* (periodical), 1954 October (3rd volume 10th publication)
Published by Beijing Chinese Medicine Association Publication Committee

北京中醫

北京中醫學會出版委員會出版

一九五四年十月號(第三卷第十期)

Yaron: Imagine! The US government issues a directive to Harvard medical school, forcing them to accept acupuncturists into their departments and teach the medical doctors about acupuncture, even forcing them to acknowledge that they like it. This to us may sound funny, but in China of the 1950s this was not funny at all. A crooked reality is the best term I can think of describing this situation. There is no way today to force Chinese medicine into hospitals, nor is there a need. There is, however, an urgent need to add to modern medicine elements they don't have, which in turn may benefit the people and our society. If this will happen to Chinese medicine then it will naturally exist alongside Western medicine like two halves of a scepter. The one half does not need to go into the other half or mix with it together—it simply needs to add the other missing half.

The following text is an announcement, framed on the page like an advertisement

In accordance with the resolution reached by the Third National Sanitation and Health Administration Congress—to strengthen the merging of Chinese and Western medicines, to copiously bring into play the force of Chinese medicine and to expand the scope of Chinese medicine professional work—starting at the beginning of September, Beijing Zhong Guo Xie He Hospital, Beijing Hospital, Central People's Hospital, The Dermatology Research Institute, Beijing City Number 3 Hospital, and the city's Number 2 Pediatric Hospital etc units have all recruited Chinese medicine doctors. They have established Chinese medicine offices. Likewise, directly connected to the Central Government Number 3 and Number 4 Hospitals' outpatient clinics have added Chinese medicine department. Directly connected to Central Government Number 5 and Number 6 Hospitals have added a Chinese medicine hemorrhoids department. Beijing Medical School is currently recruiting Chinese medicine doctors to help in the medical work of their hospital. Beijing famous old Chinese medicine doctors that have already been recruited include: Xiao Longyou 蕭龍友, Shi Jinmo 施今墨, Yuan Hechai 袁鶴儕, Zhao Bingnan 趙炳南, Tong Kuoquan 佟闊泉, Xu Hengzhi 徐衡之, Li Jingquan 李景泉, Sun Xushi 孫徐寔, Lu Shiru 陸石如, Jiang Qianan 姜潛庵, Shang Guyu 尚古愚, Shi Zhimo 施稚墨, Wang Pengfei 王鵬飛, etc.

Chinese medicine doctors were received warmly by doctors, nurses and personnel. This made all Chinese medicine doctors feel honored; they understood that only today, under the leadership of Chairman Mao, can they truly be respected. They all resolutely expressed their wish to do all in their power to serve the health of the people and repay for the loving care of the Communist Party and the Government. The Chinese external medicine doctor Zhao Bingnan 趙炳南 has revealed his external injuries secret formula in order to allow the department to research it. Because health department leaders viewed this with great importance, each hospital director personally arranged this task. Ahead of time they convened the physicians in charge and high level comrades, they arranged grand meetings with all hospital workers, they reported to them what is going to happen and they developed discussions about correcting the attitude because, in the past, there were some with wrong attitude. Through Chinese doctors' explanations and seeing them personally delivering effective results in clinic, Chinese medicine started to be looked at as valuable. Beijing Hospital made plans to have their specialists in each department learn Chinese medicine formulas that have proven themselves efficacious. First they would learn the efficacious formulas and herbs of Chinese medicine, then arrange discussions about them and thereafter gradually start learning also Chinese medicine theory.

In order to increase and deepen the interest of doctors, nurses and other medical workers in all the hospitals, Xie He, Beijing etc hospitals have asked Dr. Zhu Yan 朱顏 to come and report on the general rules of diagnosis and treatment in China's classical medicine. China's Medical Association and Ministry of Health directly-related units have asked the Chinese medicine doctor Zhao Shubing 趙樹屏 to come and report how Western doctors should learn Chinese medicine, as well as introduce the current condition of Chinese medicine development and clinical experience. He was received warmly and caused the doctors and nurses to understand better the general picture of what Chinese medicine is.

Even though Chinese medicine doctors have already started participating in the medical work of Beijing hospitals, yet the key progress is insufficient because the overall organization is still lacking. Each medical institute requires Chinese medicine doctors to treat too many patients, and so Ministry of Health leaders are currently investigating how to gradually expand this service.

Article end

Why our Western-trained doctors should learn Traditional Chinese Medicine

1955 by Fu Lien-Chang[435] 傅連璋

Source: *Chinese Medical Journal Foreign Language Publication*, September–October 1955
中華醫學雜誌外文版

Yaron: The following article was published in China in English targeting foreign readership. The term Traditional Chinese Medicine appears nine times coining the acronym now known as TCM. In contrast, modern medicine doctors appear here with a derogatory description as western-trained doctors ten times. Keep in mind that having the term "Western" attached to one's title, during that time, often meant social and personal disaster. Part of the psychological coercion exercised upon modern medicine doctors is to suggest that they belong to the foreign oppressors of China, and here explaining to them that if they come closer or "study" China's own medicine they will become less foreign.

Pages 363-367

Chairman Mao Tse-Tung more than ten years ago had called for close co-operation between Western-trained doctors and practitioners of Traditional Chinese Medicine in the service of the people. In his article on "United Front in Cultural Work" he said, "Modern medicine is of course better than old medicine; but if western-trained doctors pay no attention to the sufferings of the people, train no doctors to serve the people, and do not unite and work with the one thousand and more old-style doctors and veterinarians in the border regions, then, in fact, they are encouraging superstition and witchcraft among the people and are indifferent to the loss of large numbers of lives, both human and animal." These words show the importance and significance of solidarity among doctors of Native and Western medicine upon the health of the masses of the people. After the establishment of the People's Government, the principle of co-operation among old-time and modern-trained doctors was adopted, in line with Chairman Mao's directive, as one of the four basic principles of New China's health program. For many years the Central Committee of the Party and

[435] Fu Liangzhang 傅連璋 (1894–1968), a native of Fujian, was a medical scientist and a high ranking military officer in the People's Liberation Army. An outstanding party member of the Chinese Communist party and one of the founders of the health undertaking within the Chinese Liberation Army and the New China. At the founding of the New China he was named the army General of medical treatment.

Chairman Mao have repeatedly given specific instructions on the problem of helping and co-operating with the old-time doctors and developing and systematizing Traditional Chinese Medicine. If we had earnestly followed these instructions and put them into practice, we could certainly have had fruitful results in the direction of rational utilization of the service of our old-time doctors, of developing our ancient heritage, and enriching New China's medical science. But these results have not been obtained and up to now several hundreds of thousands of our old-time doctors are still being treated with indifference. What is the reason for this? The reason is that, although the leaders in our health administration have themselves adopted the policy of close unity between doctors of traditional and Western medicine, the fact remains that they have not implemented this policy.

In the past few years, our health departments, it is true, have done some work in advancing Traditional Chinese Medicine. There have been, for instance, the establishment of training schools, joint clinics for Western and Native medicine and clinics for doctors of traditional medicine, and the promotion of moxibustion and acupuncture, etc, and it cannot be denied that these steps have been attended with some degree of success. But, on the other hand, what we have done has not solved the fundamental problem of utilizing the service of old-time doctors to the fullest extent.

The work of the Chinese Medical Association in this respect has likewise been inadequate. The Association has held meetings with doctors of traditional medicine when papers on special subjects have been read and discussed, and it has organized a committee for exchange of medical knowledge between the two schools of medicine. But even this work has been superficial and much that should have been done has been left undone. Exchange of knowledge and experience has been limited to discussion meetings, and a great deal still remains to be done in promoting co-operation in medical practice and research. Even now, seldom do hospitals invite old-time doctors to participate in clinical work and consultations and even more seldom do Western-trained doctors earnestly seek advice from their Native confreres. It may be asked: How many Western-trained doctors since Liberation have studied Chinese medicine and have obtained successful results? Very few indeed! The great majority of Western-trained doctors have never considered the learning of traditional medicine as a task that should be undertaken seriously. The responsibility for this state of affairs lies with the health administration and the Chinese Medical Association for not having carried out their task of leadership.

Take myself for example. Although I have attended patients with practitioners of our Native medicine, I have never considered Chinese medicine as a subject I should learn. I have never seriously studied any books on traditional medicine. Hence, even today, I remain a complete ignoramus as far as our Native medicine is concerned. As a leader in our country's health work and as head of the Chinese Medical Association, I am ashamed to confess this. I must seriously take up the study of Chinese medicine.

Traditional Chinese medicine has a history of several thousand years and it has played a positive role in the preservation and development of our race. Even today, almost all the people in the countryside and one half or more of the urban population still depend on old-time doctors for medical care. That Chinese medicine has rendered and is rendering a very great service to the people in the prevention and treatment of diseases is absolutely irrefutable. Nothing could be more unscientific than to close our eyes to this fact. If, in ignoring this important fact, we neglect our old medicine and fail to unite and work with old-time practitioners, help them, and humbly learn from them, then we are neglecting the people's welfare and cannot claim to have any concern for the health of the people.

Traditional Chinese medicine with its long history is a part of China's ancient culture. Our culture has made rich contributions to the world, and, among these, the contributions of Chinese medicine have been outstanding. Not only in the past have other countries learned from Chinese medicine, but even today it is a subject of research in many countries. These are undeniable facts, and they testify to the rich treasure we have inherited, well worthy of preservation and further development. To disregard them is to be unscientific. If we do not start out from the realization of these facts and seriously learn, experiment, and help to systematize the traditional theory and practice of our native medicine, then actually we are casting aside our rich heritage, and are rendering an ill service to our people, our ancestors and the generations to come. The immense and difficult task of developing our traditional medicine in order to enrich New China's modern medical science must fall, and rightly falls, on the shoulders of medical workers of the present generation.

Therefore, whether or not we conscientiously carry into practice the basic principle of co-operation between doctors of traditional and Western medicine has an important bearing on the health of the people, the development of our medicine, and our country's contribution to world science. Our medical workers should with all seriousness face this problem.

In the past we have organized training courses for old-time physicians to learn Western medicine. This, although necessary, is not of the greatest importance. The Central Committee of the Party and Chairman Mao have enjoined us that the key to the problem is that our Western-trained doctors should study Traditional Chinese Medicine. If emphasis is placed solely on the learning of modern medicine by our traditional doctors, then the result will be that they all become doctors of Western medicine. This is tantamount to retaining only Western medicine and discarding our native medicine. It must be emphatically stated that not only should doctors of traditional medicine learn Western medicine but, particularly, Western-trained doctors should study Chinese medicine. Only thus can there be a merging of the old and new, native and foreign, and only thus can this union of empirical knowledge with modern science blossom forth into New China's medicine that will be an integral and vital part of modern medical science based on the natural sciences. In the past, this policy was not understood and most of our comrades in the health administration were content with the establishment of more training schools for old-time doctors. I am also not free from blame. As for the Chinese Medical Association, it did no more than urge modern-trained and traditional doctors to learn from each other, and beyond this it made no plan to enable the former to learn Chinese medicine. I am strongly of the opinion that hereafter our Association should actively help the Ministry of Health in the work of promoting the study of traditional medicine by Western-trained doctors.

The main obstacle in the way of modern doctors learning traditional medicine is that they look down upon old-style doctors. This attitude must be done away with. There are two possible reasons for this erroneous thinking. Firstly, there are those who believe that everything foreign is good and nothing old in China is worth retaining, which is a reflection of the semi-colonial comprador mentality. It is certainly true that industry and the natural sciences in China are backward because of past oppression under feudalism and imperialist exploitation, and that therefore we must make a special effort in learning from the scientific achievements of other countries. And here it must be pointed out that to develop science in New China we should first of all learn from the scientific achievements of the Soviet Union, as otherwise we shall still remain backward. But merely to learn from other countries is not enough. Besides this, we must also fully realize that our ancient cultural heritage is the fruit of the genius and creative labor of the Chinese people, and that many of our contributions to culture are worth preserving and developing. To refuse to accept what is good from abroad is wrong; to ignore good things of our own is equally wrong. Secondly, there are those who take the view that only modern developments of this age are worth learning and all things of the past are not. They believe that our native medicine is a thing of the past, is backward, and need not be bothered with. As a matter of fact, to consider that the past is something dead is entirely unscientific and violates the very concept of history. Which branch of science has no history of development? Is there a modern science that does not have its roots in past experience and experiments? How can history be separated into airtight compartments? The study of contemporary culture is to guide its future development and the study of culture in history is also bound up with its future advance. Further, to say that present knowledge includes all past knowledge is also wrong. This is especially true where Traditional Chinese Medicine is concerned. It extends over such a wide field that it is difficult to say how much of it has been scientifically investigated. Probably very little. Facts show that the little research we have undertaken has already produced good results (for example, studies on *ch'ang shan* 常山 *Dichroa febrifuga Lour; ping lang* 槟榔 *Areca catechu; ya tan tze* 鸦胆子 *Brucea javanica* (L.) Merr.; *tang kuei* 当归 *Angelica sinensis; yi mu ts'ao* 益母草 *Leonurus sibiricus* L.; acupuncture and moxibustion). If only we would enlarge the scope of our studies in Chinese medicine, rediscover the hidden treasures in our ancient science and art of healing, and make them available to the people, great achievements could result. But it must be remembered that this immense task can only be carried out by the joint efforts of traditional and Western-trained doctors through learning from each other and conducting a common program of research, and, further, that the study of Chinese medicine by Western-trained doctors must now be emphasized.

There are some who think that, while much may be gained from the study of native drugs, there is little to learn from old-time doctors. This way of thinking is also erroneous, for how could the empirical value of the drugs be separated from the doctors who prescribe them? Are not our effective remedies the result of the experience of Chinese doctors throughout the centuries? Furthermore, Chinese medicine does not mean only drugs. There are, besides, many Chinese methods of clinical observation and treatment of disease, including the proper attitude towards patients, that are well worth our learning.

Of course, we do not imply that all things in Traditional Chinese Medicine are good. A critical attitude is necessary. We should reject what is useless and unceasingly search for scientific explanations for methods that show good empirical results. But, first, we must study Chinese medicine. Unless we do so, we are not qualified to criticize it.

Some hospitals in Peking already have traditional doctors participating in their clinics and giving lectures. I firmly believe that, in response to the call of the Central Committee of the Party and Chairman Mao, there will soon be a nation-wide movement in the study of Traditional Chinese Medicine and that the spirit of co-operation between our doctors of Western and native medicine will be further enhanced. The labors of our medical workers will surely provide the groundwork for the opening up of new vistas in China's medical science.

Article end

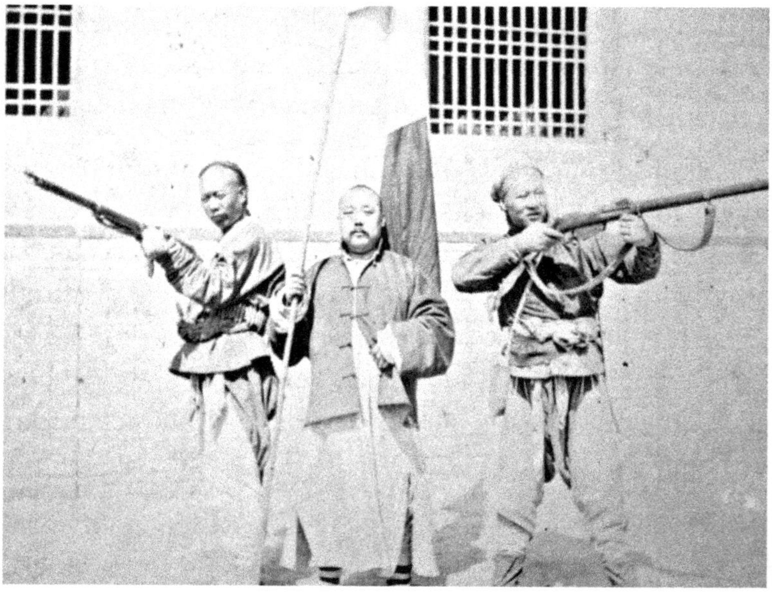

Photo by Mr P. Goux in early 1900s. "Father Paul Ouang and two Catholics".

We must swipe away ideological obstructions in order to promote Chinese medicine therapeutic experience

1955 by Qi Luyu 漆魯魚 and He Yuruo 何雨若

Source: *Chinese Medicine Magazine*, Published 1955, the 12th issue
The People's Public Health Publishing House
中醫雜誌
1955 第十二号
人民衛生出版社

Yaron: This article places Chinese medicine, or at least the idea of a Chinese kind of medicine, on the side of the Communist party. With no doubt there is, here, an attack against the Ministry of Health leadership and Chinese medicine is being used as the weapon of choice. Being used as a weapon of "the people" to target "Rightists" is something Chinese medicine enjoyed during those years. "Western-trained doctors must study Chinese medicine" was often a kind of political attack rather than a scientific endeavor. This certainly impacted the nature of the new medicine. In my opinion, in a war everybody loses, even if there is an apparent winner. This too I find as a problem that TCM needs to confront; in the 1950s Chinese and Western medicines were forced together not only to help the masses and provide cheap healthcare but also for political agendas. So while today we try to dress it beautifully, this does not change the fact that under the dress there is a problem.

Pages 5-7

Ministry of Health decided to promote the accumulated experience of Chinese medical treatment for epidemic Japanese encephalitis in Shijiazhuang 石家莊. We are of the opinion that this is one of the Communist Party and the government's important measures in implementing Chinese medicine. Due to erroneous opinions about Chinese medicine, it will be hard for us to promote Chinese medicine experience until we clear up all these obstacles.

For example, some cadres and technicians in Ministry of Health still look down on Chinese medicine. People like Wang Bin 王斌 regard Chinese medicine as a placebo instead of therapeutic medicine and they object to it blindly without reading any Chinese medical books or realizing true facts. Therefore, there are all kinds of ideological obstructions preventing us from promoting Chinese medicine's accumulated experience. The Party's Chinese medicine policy can't be implemented until these obstructions are gone. There are two measures for us to start changing the current situation. The first measure is that people of capitalist class who disrespect and discriminate against Chinese medicine should be criticized severely. In addition, we should point out the importance of newly reorganizing and researching our motherland's medical legacy. The second measure, we should show those cadres many practical examples of diseases that have been cured with Chinese medicine, and educate those people that their past opinions were wrong. The two measures I mentioned above relate to each other and they both help clear the ideological obstructions, which then will help achieve the goal of unity between Chinese and Western medicines and further develop our traditional medicine. At present, the Ministry of Health is working on these two measures.

From the past until the present, some administrators in the Ministry of Health and other medical workers still think it's incorrect to unite Chinese and Western medicine and to inherit our motherland's medical legacy. In their opinion, Chinese medical therapy is outdated or ineffective. Some believe that Chinese medicine can only treat general diseases instead of acute contagious diseases, therefore the organization of Chinese medical treatment for Japanese encephalitis in Shijiazhuang 石家莊 is the best example to prove them wrong. The efficacy of Chinese medicine has been proven by Chinese people for thousands of years. As long as one is willing to open their eyes and see, diseases cured by Chinese medicine are seen everywhere, including acute epidemic diseases. Some of these diseases seemed difficult to treat by Western medicine doctors in big hospitals, and at the end were cured by experienced Chinese medicine doctors. The example above shows that our motherland's medical legacy is vast and has large variety. All along, the Communist Party policy to unify Chinese and Western medicine 团结中西医 in order to develop our motherland's medical legacy was proven correct.

However, there is one critical point if we want to develop further our motherland's medical legacy. It is that Western medicine doctors need to learn Chinese medicine. This is needed because Western medicine doctors can't organize and develop Chinese medicine, not even mentioning the unity job, if they don't know Chinese medicine. However, when speaking of Western medicine doctors learning Chinese medicine, some people object immediately and question us, "Should we learn advanced or outdated things?" They think that Chinese medicine is out of date and that it only existed in feudal times. They liken Chinese medicine to an oxcart and Western medicine to a car or even a plane, making such a point that since we have cars and planes, why bother with oxcarts? They regard the idea of learning Chinese medicine as going backwards. Other people ask "which should our current medical scientific research emphasize: antibiotics or tree bark and grass?" Obviously, they are against researching tree bark and grass. This kind of opinion is totally wrong.

We should put it in the following way: antibiotics are an advanced product so naturally it requires research. Nonetheless, our motherland's medical legacy has abundant and varied content, which is a fact as well. The development of medicine should base itself on its inherited scientific legacy so it can move forward. Otherwise, we cut out the medical history and deny the necessity of research of "tree barks and grass", meaning we deny the efficacy of Chinese medicine. The epidemic Japanese encephalitis in Shijiazhuang 石家莊 was cured by "barks and grass" kind of herbal medicine. How can these be defined as outdated and backward when they can actually cure diseases? Therefore, the first priority for the Ministry of Health and medical workers is to inherit and develop our motherland's medical legacy and combine it with Western medicine in order to enrich the current medical science, instead of blaming Chinese medicine theory for being too old. Some say that the fundamentals of Chinese and Western medicine are different—that Chinese medicine was produced in a feudal society while Western medicine was produced in a capitalist society—and they ask, how can they unite together? Answering this question, we should know that there is no difference in society for diseases. Not one disease happens in either feudal or capitalist society. No matter which disease in which society, the treatment should always be the same. A doctor who can cure diseases is a good doctor, no matter if he uses Chinese or Western medicine. This is the truth and it is a scientific attitude.

The experience demonstrated with Chinese medicine formulas including Qing Wen Bai Du Yin 清瘟敗毒飲, Bai Hu Tang 白虎湯, An Gong Niu Huang San 安宮牛黃散, Ju Fang Zhi Bao Dan 局方至寶單 curing epidemic Japanese encephalitis is a very obvious fact. However, due to capitalistic thought, some people fail seeing this fact. They already had a bias and blocked themselves from accepting new things. Even when the new thing is an obvious fact, they still don't admit it. They turned their back on an important principle of Marxism and Leninism, which is "The objective fact comes first in priority, while our own knowledge is second in priority". Aren't they turning to total idealists?

Science constantly develops and so does people's knowledge. This is the rule for everything in a society. The mission of scientists is to find out new perspectives and conclusions and to replace old ones in order to enhance scientific development. If we stick to old rules, science can't propel forwards. Take gypsum Shi Gao 石膏 as an example: in Western medicine people use it for bone fracture, while in Chinese medicine we use it to treat epidemic Japanese encephalitis. There is here an ideological conflict and people believe that Western medical knowledge is more reliable than the Chinese kind. However, Chinese medicine cured epidemic Japanese encephalitis, which shows an objective opposite result to what people have believed in. As a matter of fact, in science, an old perspective or old principle can be replaced by a new one.

There are other similar examples. In the past, Novocain was only used as a normal anesthesia drug. After Pavlov discovered classical conditioning, people realized that Novocain not only has a local anesthetic function but it can also mildly stimulate a nerve to cause a beneficial cycle. Thus, Novocain became popular in internal medicine and surgery for its blocking therapy Feng Bi Liao Fa 封閉療法.

In the past, tuberculosis could only be treated with symptomatic treatment, surgical treatment and adequate rest plus nutrition. Now we can use streptomycin, para-aminosalicylic acid and other medication to treat tuberculosis—isn't it more advanced than before? Inflammation is very commonly seen clinically, at first it could only be treated with methylene blue, phenyl salicylate, mandolin acid and Urotropine; now we have sulfonamide, Prontosil, salazosulfapyridine to treat it, which is more advanced than before. But now we are broadly using sulfadiazine, penicillin, albomycin, chloromycetin, aureomycin and other kinds of medicine to treat inflammation—isn't it great progress?

During the development of science, new perspectives keep replacing old ones and new conclusions replace old ones all the time. Besides, any kind of science needs to battle with its own old content in order to create progress. Otherwise, scientific development will be stuck in the middle. About this theory, the discourse of *The*

History of the Communist Party of the Soviet Union has better explanation: "Be proficient in Marxism and Leninism. This means you should enrich the content of theory with revolutionary experience and new principles and conclusions, and you should also develop the theory. Don't be afraid to shift to a new principle or a new conclusion." Stalin also said, "Since it's a kind of science, it will keep growing and refreshing itself. Therefore it needs new experience and knowledge to fulfill itself during this development. The individual principle and conclusion will definitely differ from time to time, therefore a new conclusion and principle come up to help it adjust into a new environment." These instructions work not only for socialistic science but also for natural science. It proves that a scientist should have an objective attitude and shouldn't be afraid to get rid of old stuff, all along learning from practical experience. Only when we are able to acknowledge the facts and the truth can we treat science with a correct attitude. Being prejudiced is always the number one enemy of scientists.

Some people question: "do you want to return to the old ways or do you have a nationalistic point of view?" Our answer is no. We are neither reviving antiquity nor are we nationalists; we don't develop Chinese medicine because it was produced in China in the past. There are many useful parts in Chinese medicine that we want to use in order to serve the people. As long as we newly reorganize and research it, it can enrich the modern medical development. This is exactly why we want to inherit and promote it.

Why don't we advocate witchcraft and why do we only advocate the new unity Chinese medicine 團結中醫? There is a clear distinction between witchcraft and Chinese medicine. Therefore, people who regard Chinese medicine supporters as ancient revivalists or nationalists actually mistake the policy of the Communist Party. Some even think that unity Chinese medicine is derived from political and personal points of view, but when it comes to scientific technical angle they think that it's incorrect. People who have this kind of thinking don't understand the essence of the Party's policy, so in their minds political unity differs from scientific unity, which is the wrong thing to think.

Chinese medicine has contributed a lot to our nation's existence and development. Even now, it is still the main means for medical treatment for the population majority in China, especially in rural areas. It's correct to unify Chinese and Western medicine politically but less correct if we only focus on political and personnel unity but not on how to reorganize and research Chinese medicine in order to devote it to the masses. Mr. Song Daren 宋大仁, in an emotional article, said:

> Under any condition, add a measure of "cooperation between Western and Chinese medicine in order to build a united front". Now, Chinese medicine people are enthusiastically encouraging unity between Western and Chinese medicine based on this principle, however, this principle is referring to personal unity instead of academic unity. The current cooperation is due to the lack of Western medicine doctors. If we really combine the Chinese medical theory with modern medical knowledge, then it equals combining idealism with materialism, which is very funny and impractical.

His thought is absurd and people who have this kind of viewpoint regard Chinese medicine as nonscientific empirical medicine. They deny the academic status and treatment value of Chinese medicine saying that it lacks epidemiology knowledge. Furthermore, they deny the Party's policy for Chinese medicine, hoping to limit and exclude Chinese medicine.

From accumulated current experience, it is necessary to reorganize and develop our motherland medical legacy in order to have long term cooperation between Chinese and Western medicine. There is an abundant clinical experience in Chinese medicine lacking clear explanations due to deficiency in modern scientific foundations. Western medicine has very strong natural scientific background and in this respect it is better than Chinese medicine. Therefore, if we want to develop Chinese medicine and promote it further, we have to depend on and use Western medicine and make a big effort to research it.

For example, during the process of the Chinese medical treatment of epidemic Japanese encephalitis, when a patient was unconscious, nasal feeding from Western medicine worked much better than oral intake. Also in Chongqing 重慶, Chinese medical treatment Ku Zhi San 枯痔散 for hemorrhoids and anal fistula had a new development thanks to the tight cooperation between Chinese and Western medicines. The white arsenic in Ku Zhi San 枯痣散 is a very strong poison and it gives pain and burning sensation and even intoxication when it's applied to the skin. After the cooperation of Chinese and Western medicine, they injected Novocain intravenous while applying Ku Zhi San. On the one hand it decreased patient's pain, while on the other it prevented intoxication and made the entire procedure safer. They even improved the ingredients and process of making Ku Zhi San so now it is easier to apply. These examples show the importance of tight cooperation between Chinese and Western medicine.

However currently, the one critical point is still Western medicine doctors learning Chinese medicine. Only when Western medicine doctors understand Chinese medicine theory, and seriously research it, will they be able to develop this treasure. Being a lazy person who doesn't want to invest any effort in order to take over this precious legacy and instead just wants to blame the ancient people when they realize they can't get it themselves, is incorrect. On the other hand, some say that Chinese medical books are too difficult to understand and this holds them back; this is incorrect as well. As scientists, we should have the right attitude to face and overcome difficulties and obstructions. Due to having a marked difference between Chinese and Western medical theories, terminology, medication and instructions, if we want to seriously study Chinese medicine, we need to follow its own narrative and eventually will get used to it.

Generally speaking, only if we keep sweeping away all ideological obstructions toward Chinese medicine can we promote Chinese medicine accumulated experience and implement the Chinese medicine policy. It is not the right attitude to beat down Chinese medicine doctors by asking controversial questions. All we need to do is totally focus on studying Chinese medicine in order to develop the precious motherland's medical legacy. It is proven that we cannot promote Chinese medicine accumulated experience without swiping away ideological obstructions. Ideological work is a powerful weapon to promote every kind of duty. We should tightly grasp onto this Marxism ideological weapon in order to get rid of all obstructions and in order to win the final victory.

Article end

Chinese medicine scientification commentary

1955 by Zhu Hegao 朱鶴皋 and Lu Kuisheng 陸奎生

Published in June 1955 in Hong Kong by China's Medical Press

中醫科學化講義

朱鶴皋 陸奎生 著

中國醫學出版社

Yaron: The following excerpt is from a book by noted Chinese medicine practitioners in Hong Kong, who, while not directly impacted by Communist political pressure, were still influenced by the mass-scale scientification unfolding in the mainland. We, Chinese medicine practitioners, often look to China to see what they are doing. This was the case then and is still the case today. However, as Chinese medicine becomes a global phenomenon this should change too.

Foreword by Liu Dazhi 劉達志

In the modern era, scholarly research advocates experiments. The art of Chinese medicine is the accumulation of experience. Within it, there is no shortage of scientific principle. Certain herbals that cure ailments and time-tested prescriptions are truly Chinese medical science's true essence. Appropriately, I arranged it in order to expound and propagate it and, with it, fix resolutely the position of our Chinese medicine.

April 1955

Foreword by Zhu Hegao 朱鶴皋[436]

Medicine is a benevolent art. Naturally, one should spare no effort in this duty and attend to it with his whole strength.

Sincerity is the foundation for scholarly research. Hegao (myself) fully made up my mind to make this art public. When getting hold of complete sincerity, one cannot take what he does not know and pretend he knows it and absolutely can't assume extravagant appearance. Take, for example, ancient things where one, without examining it himself and while it has no efficacy like Bai He Hu Huo 百合狐惑 disease[437] still, with effort, inserts it into his book in order to look profound.

[436] Zhu Hegao 朱鶴皋 (1903–1995), born in Jiangsu 江蘇, emigrated to Hong Kong during the Communist takeover, served as Hong Kong's Chinese Medicine Society president, Hong Kong Chinese Medicine Hospital president and other positions.
[437] From Jin Gui Yao Lüe

In this book, each prescription comes from the late master Nanshan,[438] and passed through my clinical experience. Prescriptions that were tested much were used tens of thousands of times, while prescriptions that were used less were tested only several thousand times. Even though I don't dare to say that they all will work every time, these can be named time-tested prescriptions. The Dao of medicine is the art of saving people. Accomplishments need to be preserved and not lost. Horizontally it needs to be spread in the four directions, while vertically it needs to be transmitted to future generations. I follow my heart's desire to create an art of saving people and this is my only wish. Last fall in September, China's Medical Academy established the research institute in Hong Kong. I then collaborated on this book with Mr Lu Kuisheng 陸奎生 taking prescriptions from our clinical experience as the core and adding modern scientific commentary as supplement, naming this book *Chinese Medicine Scientification Commentary*.

Foreword by Lu Kuisheng 陸奎生

Science's focal point is experiments. It is exactly the process by which Chinese medicine has developed where accumulated experience explains its clinical efficacy and time-tested prescriptions are its focal point. This is the hidden treasure of its scientific value. Chinese medicine experiments were directly and extensively developed with the human body over a long period of time and only then did it become trustworthy and established its curative efficacy. In this commentary book, one immediately sees that treatment methods look like case studies and prescriptions come out of experience. The art of Chinese medicine has several thousand years of accumulated rich experience; this is a fact. However, theories differ, treatment methods differ and the use of herbs differs. This gave rise to considerable confusion and errors and this is also a fact. In modern day medical circles, scholars set their hearts on new discoveries in order to advance by exchanging old with new. Yet whatever new and old theories you want to link and flow together, it is appropriate first to take one's own experience and reveal it in public and then smelt them in the oven of this era. Therefore, the working of this commentary book has two aspects to it; benefiting future students and serving the entire medical world.

Here, linking and flowing together the new and old medicines has its merit and benefit. Printing new terminology may help understand the situation better, but as we arranged it we use our nation's own theories first and, thereafter, bring the new

[438] Zhu Nanshan 朱南山 is Zhu Hegao's father, who was known as one of the ten famous doctors of Shanghai Chinese Medicine College 上海中醫學院 十大近代名醫.

theory supplementing it. This will help doctors unfamiliar with the new theories and make it easy for them to memorize it which will, later on, benefit them as they diagnose patients. Chinese medicine's strong point is to match herbs to symptoms, so as we compile this prescription collection we use symptomology first.

The book contains 28 chapters as follows: headaches, cold hot, summer heat disease, dampness diseases, wind strike, cough, vomiting blood, hiccup, diarrhea, constipation, incontinence and retention of urine, stranguria complicated with hematuria and painful urination, emissions and impotence, abdominal and chest pains, lower back and feet pains, menses ailments, leucorrhea, during gestation, after labor, measles and rubella, small pox and chicken pox, sudden wind, worms and parasites, ear, nose bleeds, throat, red eyes and toothache.

All chapters contain the following subheadings: modern theory, pathology, differentiation of symptoms, effective prescription, expanding (the prescription), simultaneous treatment (of other symptoms).

Excerpt end

A study into Traditional Chinese Medicine

1955 by Zhu Yan 朱顏[439]

Published by The People's Health Press, Beijing third print January 1955 (First print March 1954)

中醫學術研究

朱顏著

人民衛生出版社

Yaron: An influential book during the early years of the People's Republic. The first edition circulated 14,000 copies and by 1955 third print, a year later, a total of 50,000 copies were sold. In class 1 we can see the detailed logic behind creating TCM. We have already mentioned these points, but bring them here again since Zhu Yan was a prominent figure at that time, so let's see how he describes the task at hand.

---

[439] Zhu Yan 朱顏 (1918-1972), a person from Jinhua, Zhejiang 浙江金华, studied Chinese medicine early on in his life and practiced in Jinhua. In 1950 he graduated from the 4th Military Medical University 第四军医大学. He then served successively in Beijing as the Chair of the Chinese Medicine Advance Studies School, and Deputy Director in the Ministry of Health—Chinese Medicine Research Institute, Chinese Pharmaceutical Research Department and Pharmacodynamics Laboratory, then in Xi Yuan Hospital Internal Medicine Department Chair of Hematology Department, was a member of the Ministry of Health Pharmacopoeia Committee, a member of the Medical Sciences Committee. His influence on Chinese medicine development in the early days of the republic is noteworthy.

Pages 1-7

Class 1: Chinese medicine research direction and phases

1) In order to advance Chinese medicine research we must master dialectic materialism thinking weapon

Chinese medicine development is closely tied to China's social development. Chinese society's development was stuck in the feudal era for a long period of time. Metaphysical thought, prevalent in feudal societies, ruled the land. Chinese medicine began its development in a feudal society and so could not avoid accumulating, on top of its basic foundation, the pollution of metaphysical theories. These kinds of theories belonging to spiritualism cannot reflect objective reality. From a practical point of view, it cannot master the intrinsic qualities of the action of things. For a long time it obstructed the advancement of Chinese medicine and, when comparing it to the technological advancement of modern medicine, on grounds of spirituality it forever runs in circles without finding an exit point. We must discard this spirituality aspect.

At the same time, we must avoid the influence of the bourgeois mechanical materialism. We should not, on mechanical basis, find in Chinese medicine some erroneous theories and, as a result, not expound on its core ability to deliver reasonable efficacy via its experience. We should also not ignore present conditions of objective reality, and we should pursue future possibilities for putting it into practice in today's world reality.

If we want to advance Chinese medicine research then we must oppose the thinking of "pulling the wagon backward", we must also avoid departing from the high and noble way of reaching far within reality. In other words, we must begin our way from reality. We must, within the foundations of present reality, using large scale workforce, advance more practice and, step by step, elevate the level. We must rearrange practice and theory to merge into one cohesive system in order to advance. Only if we do it like this, only if we study it well and effectively master it, that a scientific society will have the practical characteristics of Marxism and Leninism—it will be the military thinking weapon of dialectic materialism.

2) One should recognize clearly the characteristics of Chinese medicine

If one wants to research Chinese medicine, the first step is that one must know clearly its characteristics:

A. Chinese medicine is a kind of medicine coming from practical experience. It developed over a long period of time through accumulated experience. This is to say that it went through countless experiments and its curative techniques were practically applied to humans and its experience accumulated over thousands of years. This, what we call experience-based medicine, did not pass through initial animal experiments but, rather, it is a medicine that was directly applied to humans. From its developmental process we can also say that it is a kind of medicine that used human testing instead of animal testing. Therefore, its treatment methods are extremely rich and the scope of its safety is quite large. However, for the medicine's techniques as a whole, evidence for the efficacy rate is still lacking.

B. Chinese medicine theory is an accessory to the curative techniques. In some instances, theory does not match reality. The principle by which it developed was first a collection of therapeutic techniques coming from experience, and only thereafter a theory developed. Since some theories cannot accurately reflect actual reality, sometimes the practical aspect is one matter while the theory is another separate matter. Even when one reaches curative effect in practice, the theory is not necessarily correct. In other words, the theory may not be scientific, but there is still curative effect. This phenomenon of disjointed practice and recognition is often seen in Chinese medicine.

C. When comparing some aspects of Chinese medicine to modern scientific medical techniques, from practice point of view, it has the high level of viewing the body as an organic whole. Its target is the patient's entire body and not only the physical disease elements. It is a functional treatment modality (what we describe as following syndrome treatment modality) and special effect treatment modality.[440] However, explaining the efficacy of these treatment modalities has limitations. It can only be explained by practical experience and only with great difficulty solely by the scheme of their theories. This is because experience-based medicine has dregs mixed in together, all these things that are not accurate and are not based in objective real facts, which have been recorded and transmitted together.

[440] Also described in a different chapter as using specific herbs to reach a specific effect.

3) Chinese medicine's position and its prospects within the present health system

The use of Chinese medicine in our nation has a long history and its spread is deep-reaching; with traces in every corner, it is closely tied with the people. If we want to develop it in a truly valuable way then it is from this basis of the masses.

Our nation discarded already the half-feudal half-colonialized position and now became a new democracy. In addition, our society has already advanced beyond into socialism. At present, within the national production quantity, agriculture occupies a central role. Chinese medicine's equipment and materials, such as herbs, are, to large degree, agricultural products. The quantity produced is vast and so, from local trade point of view, it has a definite economic position. It also carries the benefit of medical equipment industrialization.

However if we don't improve the Chinese herb production style, then it will gradually fall out of sync with the collectivism requirement. Our society advances by leaps and bounds without interruption going forward towards socialism and production style is moving gradually from a scattered individual production to a collective production. Therefore, the shape of medicine must transform into easy and convenient and medical treatment facilities must undergo modernization. If the old-style Chinese medicine does not transform and advance, then it cannot produce a marked effect on the advancement of the new collective production and collective lifestyle of our society.

Describing Chinese medicine as a medical science on its own is incomplete. It is only an accumulated experience of folk treatment modalities. We must adopt and implement scientific theories in addition to its proven clinical efficacy. We must also expound and realize its medical spirit and aspiration for prevention as in "the sages treated the disease before it formed not after it formed". If we supplement and expand the techniques and applications of preventive medicine, only then will it become the people's scientific medicine of our new democracy.

4) The concrete research work of Chinese medicine is part of the entire medical work and part of the entire natural sciences work

Some people think that Chinese medicine research belongs entirely to Chinese medicine circles, and that other people should not research it. This kind of indifferent attitude is wrong. Chinese medicine is one of our nation's cultural inheritances. This inheritance belongs to the masses and everyone should be concerned about it. Especially is the case for the medical community in its entirety; it should not be divided into Chinese medicine and Western medicine. Even more than that, all other natural sciences should partake in this work, because this work requires assigning away parts of the work to others and collaborations as follows:

A. Chinese medicine doctors that have real clinical experience, especially those who received modern scientific education and participated in the advanced classes of Chinese medicine, should engage energetically in dissemination of their accumulated practical experience. They should continually furnish their research materials. Simultaneously, hand-in-hand with the help of proper scientific diagnostic techniques and completely absent of pre conceived ideas, they should perform clinical efficacy studies in order to confirm the true nature of Chinese medicine's experience-based clinical efficacy. At the same time, they should also dispose of these parts of fuzzy influences Chinese medicine had in the past.

B. Western medicine clinicians as well as all other medical workers, teachers and researchers, on the one hand should engage energetically in the advanced classes of Chinese medicine in order to assist in the studying of Chinese medicine. This, in turn, will help them analyze and utilize their own experience via the "military" tools of modern science they previously acquired and mastered. On the other hand, they should deeply enter into the contents of Chinese medicine, select one topic of research and make it their own. They should bear together the research analysis responsibility.

C. Chinese medicine herbal production workers should study even more government policy and their professional responsibility in order to improve themselves. They should prepare to invest their entire effort in the advancement of Chinese medicine's herbal production.

5) Concrete phases of Chinese medicine research

Chinese medicine concrete research phases should follow its main characteristic, which is being experience-based treatment modality. Using reality as our starting point, one should merge clinical efficacy observation with laboratory experiments. One should take result of numerous practical experiments with many participants, simplify it, integrate it and standardize it. As for using herbs for treatment, we can go through discussions and selections by the masses,[441] and then fix the commonly used herbs, their median nature of efficacy as well as the criteria for processing them. At

[441] Meaning by many professionals related to the research.

the same time, we will simplify the prescription selection process and select only clinically efficacious prescriptions. These will include folk remedies and single-herb prescriptions. We will determine the disease a prescription is appropriate for and its efficacious dosage. Thereafter, according to needs on the ground, we will advance clinical applications and decide the appropriate form of administering a prescription.[442] In other words, we need to use modern-day scientific drug preparation techniques to advance and replace Chinese medicine's ancient preparations techniques. This will gradually elevate the level of Chinese medicine drugs formulation.

As for other treatment modalities not involving herbs—such as acupuncture, massage and other external techniques—we can first fix a few distinctive diseases that it is appropriate for and others that it is prohibited for. The federal organization, through Chinese medicine advanced classes, rallied together the professional work and collaboration with Western medicine. Through their initial steps of treatment and prescriptions' standardization, and with the help of modern scientific diagnostic techniques, they have created a new medical treatment style, one that advances clinical usefulness. At the same time, they also encouraged precise observations and analysis and initially calculated the curative effect. The prescriptions and medical techniques that initially displayed curative success should be used and promoted.

Integrating laboratory research, we should take clinical evidence or a value found in curative efficacy of a certain prescription and other treatment modalities then, with an objective in mind and a plan, perform animal testing and bacteriology experiments. We should utilize physiology, pathology and even knowledge of physics and chemistry and its technology to discover the curative cause and the medicinal pure active ingredients and compounds. As for the herbs themselves, through steps identifying toxicity and fixing dosage we can keep on using them in clinic until eventually we can use chemistry techniques to analyze and replicate them.

In this process of clinical observations and discovering prescriptions' efficacy we need reference materials. First and foremost, this reference material needs to incorporate, to a large degree, modern experience of Chinese medicine treatment. Next to that, it needs to incorporate modern scientific research reports on Chinese herbs and medicine and, lastly, a few excerpts of old Chinese texts. When selecting and arranging the old Chinese texts, one must first comprehend well dialectic materialism point of view then, merged together with clinical experience, analyze and scrutinize its possible value.

[442] Liquid, pill, injection etc

6) How to avert a few possible erroneous tendencies

In the process of researching Chinese medicine, one must first guard against strained interpretations. This erroneous tendency happens easily at the initial stage of incorporating scientific medicine. It is because a strained interpretation, linking Chinese and Western medicine, cannot extract the valuable component of Chinese medicine and elevate it to the level of science.

In addition, we must guard against ever-expanding tendencies of secrecy and returning-to-antiquity points of view. This is because science is ever propelling forward. We must build upon the experience of the ancients, scrutinize and step-by-step improve it and not be complacent and conservative, forever treading in the old level.

We must also avert research in the lines of doctrinarism. Sitting in the office and only drawing a circle on a piece of paper, write a few books or make a few plans. Only hear the thunder but can't see that it is raining. Attempting this kind of idle research to achieve practical results is not needed.

Lastly, we must avert a lofty and arrogant style of research. Take the upcoming research steps, not follow current needs and instead just desire to create something new and be different, or follow one's own interests and research them, this also cannot attain a satisfactory result.

7) Conclusion

Chinese medicine research must fall under the guide of dialectic materialism. Only after mastering the thinking process behind this weapon can one avert erroneous tendencies. We must recognize clearly Chinese medicine's special qualities and its position in present times. What is effective must be promoted, what is refuse must be discarded. Its progressive steps must use practical efficacy as its guide advancing and reforming treatment and herbs' formulation styles, combining clinical applications and their observations with experimentation and, with that, determining efficacy rates. We must change it in a way to fit with collectivism and, at the same time, avert empty talk and lofty and arrogant behavior. We must be earnest and down to earth, the starting point should be reality and, like this, we will take Chinese medicine and advance it one step forward.

Discussion outline

Publish everyone's opinion towards the research of Chinese medicine. The focal point should be: where is the value of Chinese medicine? And how to arrange it in order to improve it?

Table (folded) between pages 6 and 7 with title at the bottom of page: The steps for Chinese medicine research

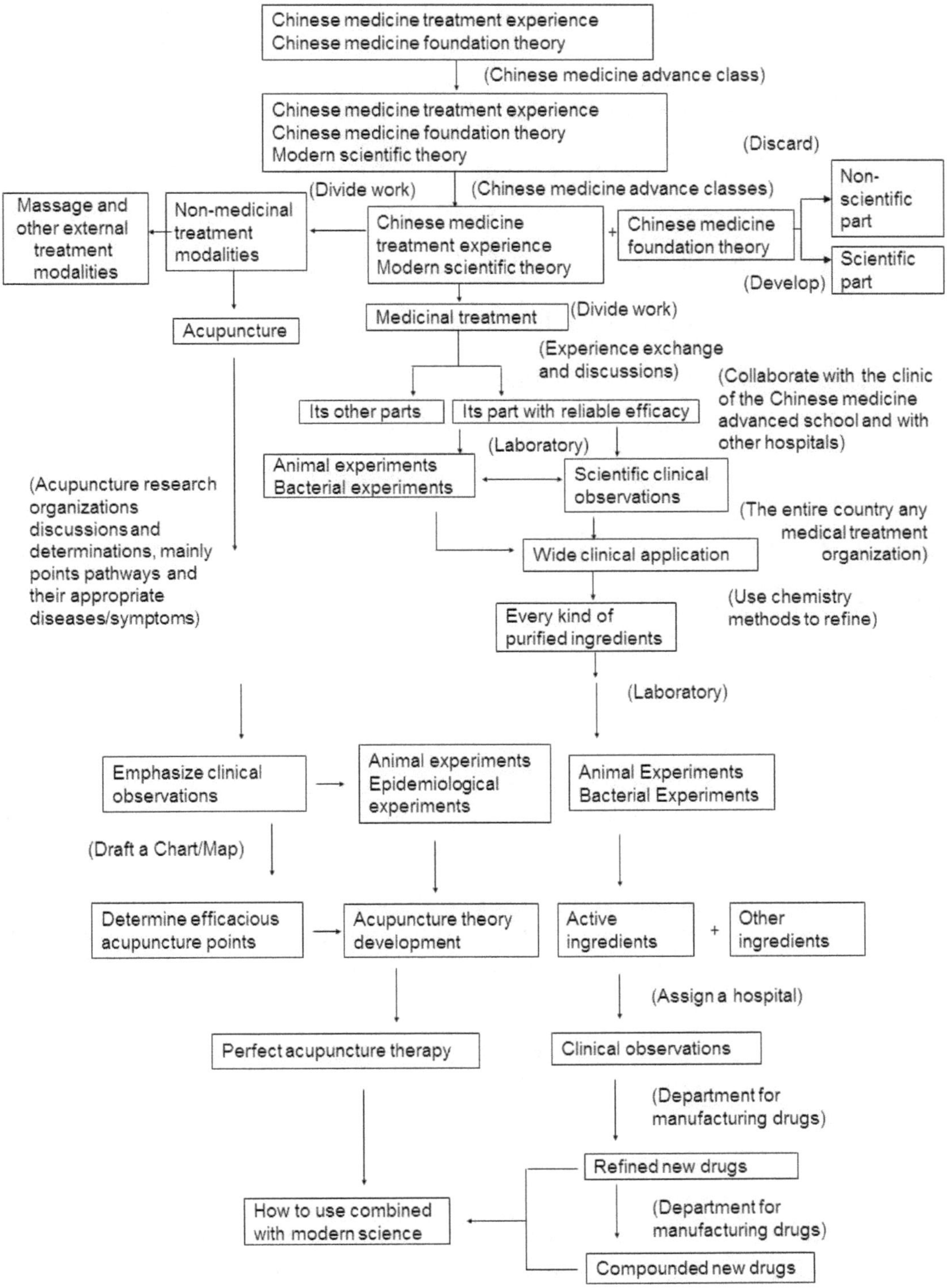

Yaron: Following are the subsequent Class titles discussed in the book, then an excerpt from Class 8

Class 2: General Understanding of Chinese Medicines

Class 3: Disease Treatment According to Patterns in Chinese Medicine

Class 4: Chinese Medicine Special Efficacy Treatment

Class 5: Chinese Medicine Development Path

Class 6: Anesthetic and Analgesia Pharmacodynamics Experiments

Class 7: Medicines Exciting Respiration and Animal Experiments

Class 8: A deliberation on calming cough and resolving phlegm medicines

Subchapter 4: Clinical value of Chinese herbs calming cough and resolving phlegm

Yaron: Using herbs and old information in a new way—the following excerpt shows an example, out of many similar suggestions, of how to become "scientific".

The boldest statement in this example is that Chinese medicine needs to remove from its principle the idea of "individualism", concluding that all humans are built the same and therefore treating cough should be the same for everyone.

It is following strictly the Western medicine model, which requires reproducible results in order for a treatment to be considered "scientific".

Page 37

Chinese medicine prescriptions treating cough, phlegm and asthma kind of diseases are many. Judging by their experience they have certain efficacy. We should take these kinds of prescriptions and, following the aforementioned principle of treating cough and resolving phlegm, sum them up and simplify it, allowing us to use it universally for all diseases that display the same symptom. In addition, we should take the administration method, changing and improving upon it in order to allow for the patient's ease of administration.

Among western drugs, Zong Se He Ji 棕色合劑 Brown Compound (mainly distilled Gan Cao particles) and Tuo Fo Shi San 陀佛氏散 (Compound Ipecacuanba Powder) are clinically often-used drugs for calming cough and resolving phlegm. Chinese medicine prescriptions with similar effect can be compounded according to the methods described in Pharmaceutics. This will allow easier clinical use and efficacy observations.

Class 9: Summary of digestive system treatments with medicines

Yaron: How TCM diagnostics transformed into "thinking of symptoms" style, which when grouped together were called patterns. This style encourages single herbs fitting specific symptoms, and adding herbs according to symptoms logic.

Pages 39-41

The main function of the digestive system is to digest food, absorb nutrients and expel feces. At the same time, the digestive system is the gate and pathway to receive toxins, which include medicines entering into the body. Therefore the digestive system is extremely important, regardless if it is from physiology, pathology or treatment point of view. Because of this, digestive herbs in clinical practice contain a distinct value. It can be divided in the following way:

1) Expelling harmful or undesired things from the digestive system, one uses induce-vomiting and diarrhea-causing herbs.

2) Correcting digestive system pathological changes like calming-vomiting herbs, stopping-diarrhea herbs, resolving-wind herbs, arresting-acidity herbs etc.

3) Helping digestive system inadequacy like helping-digestion herbs, strengthening-stomach herbs. However, the human body is a highly organized organism, each

bodily system is closely related to another system, and so all the digestive system abilities are closely related and influenced by the central nervous system. When we discuss and apply digestive herbs we should absolutely not forget this point.

Herbs to induce vomiting:[443]

Plant material: Gua Ti, Li Lu, Xiang Sizi

Minerals: Dan Fan, Tong Qing

Herbs to induce diarrhea:

Plant material: Da Huang, Fan Xie Ye, Lu Hui, Gan Sui, Qian Niu Zi, Qian Jin Zi, Ba Dou etc

Salt kind: Pu Xiao (Mang Xiao and Xuan Ming Fen)

Herbs to strengthen stomach

Arrest vomiting: Er Chen Tang, Huo Xiang Zheng Qi San, Ju Pi Zhu Ru Tang etc

Stop diarrhea: Huo Xiang Zheng Qi San, Ping Wei San, Ge Gen Qin Lian Tang, Li Zhong Wan etc

Help digestion: Shen Qu, Mai Ya, Gu Ya, Shan Zha, Ji Nei Jin etc

Expel wind Qi from digestive tract: Dou Kou, Sha Ren, Chen Pi, Pei Lan, Sheng Jiang etc

Cure stomach ulcer

Chinese medicine treating stomach ulcer normally doesn't use machine-made antacid drugs, instead it uses "calming the liver and harmonizing stomach" method. Following are a few prescriptions to treat stomach ulcer:

1) Xia Bangke Fen (baked clam-shell powder): This is a folk remedy. Baked clam-shell powder contains large amounts of calcium and can harmonize excessive stomach acid; however, it often creates constipation and is not an ideal solution.

[443] We have intentionally excluded all Chinese characters from the remaining article to allow a better flow of text.

2) Zuo Jin Wan: Huang Lian is the main ingredient, Wu Zhu Yu is assisting it and it has the effect of controlling acid and calming pains.

3) Gan Cao Jin Gao (Gan Cao extract): Originally from a Dutch doctor Rever (1946) who developed a special remedy to treat stomach ulcer. How valid it is, still remains to be seen in clinic.

Class 10: Observation of Chinese herbs promoting urination in a dog

---

Yaron: Experimenting on animals in the name of medicine and progress is still done today in TCM in China. This is simply not appropriate for life-medicine. Zhu Yan on the one hand says that Chinese medicine has been tested for thousands of years on humans and on the other hand advocates animal testing in the name of progress. It is inconsistent.

1) Treat edema

    a) Fang Ji Fu Ling Tang treats four limbs edema, water Qi is at the skin. One uses Fang Ji, Huang Qin, Gui Zhi each 3 Liang, Gan Cao 2 Liang, Fu Ling 6 Liang, water 6 sheng, cook until reduced to 2 sheng, divide to three portions and administer.

    b) Wu Pi Yin treats puffy face and eyes, four limbs full, heart and abdomen feel bloated, Qi agitated, use: Wu Jia Pi, Di Gu Pi, Sheng Jiang Pi, Da Fu Pi, Fu Ling Pi in equal quantities. Each time use 3 qian, boil and drink hot.

2) Treat gonorrhea: use formulas like Pi Xie Fen Qing Yin, Wu Lin San, Ba Zheng San etc. It is possible that a single benefiting-urination herb has the effect of killing the gonococci bacteria.

3) Benefit urination

    a) Wu Ling San: Ze Xie, Zhu Ling, Bai Zhu, Fu Ling, Gui Zhi grind to paste, with boiling water swallow one square inch spoon full, three times per day, drink plenty of warm water.

    b) Zhu Ling Tang: Zhu Ling, Fu Ling, E Jiao, Hua Shi, Ze Xie, each 1 Liang, use 4 sheng water to cook.

c) Fu Ling Xu Yan Tang: Fu Ling half Jin, Bai Zhu 2 Liang, Xu Yan 1 piece pellet size. Water 5 sheng, cook and reduce to 3 sheng, drink warm three portions.

4) Using anti-urination herbs

Suo Quan Wan (Shrinking the Spring Pills), treats frequent urination: Wu Yao, Yi Zhi Ren, each equal quantity and ground to flour, cook with wine and Shan Yao paste to make pills the size of dryandra seeds. Each time 50 pills, drink on empty stomach with salt water.

5) Experiments on benefiting-urination herbs' pharmacodynamics

Single herbs like Fu Ling, Ze Xie, Che Qian Zi, Zhu Ling, Mu Tong, Ju Mai.

Patent formulas like Wu Ling San etc were all pre cooked into a decoction, every 100ml of liquid included 100 grams of herbs, a dog was used in the experiment. To the dog ureter was attached a drip calculator device. Into his veins were injected the abovementioned decoctions, the impact on its urination was observed.

Class 11: Circulation formulas and their impact on a frog's heart

Yaron: Is it really Chinese medicine anymore? Researching and contemplating life was always difficult. Here, there is simply no life left.

A. Chinese medicine understanding and handling of circulation-decline

Circulation-decline, even though a new name, had its symptoms already recognized in the day of Zhang Zhongjing. For example, in the Shang Han Lun, Shao Yin symptoms and Jue Yin symptoms look very much like circulation-decline symptoms. There are many reasons for circulation-decline, for example heart disease, circulation blood quantity decrease and nervous system pathology etc. Because of this, Chinese medicine handling of circulation-decline has different methods, for example:

1) Si Ni Tang: treats sunken pulse and body aches, quietly wants to vomit, diarrhea with undigested food, cold hands and feet, inside cold outside heat, pulse small wants to vanish etc symptoms. Use Gan Cao 2 Liang, Gan Jiang

1.5 Liang, Fresh Fu Zi one bulb, water 3 sheng, cook and reduce to 1 sheng 2 Ge, remove residue, drink warm in 2 portions. If, after diarrhea, blood perishes add Ren Shen, it is called Si Ni Jia Ren Shen Tang.

2) Ma Huang Fu Zi Xi Xin Tang: treats Shao Yin disease that just started, to the contrary there is fever and pulse is sunken, Ma Huang remove the joints, Xi Xin each 2 Liang, baked Fu Zi 1 bulb, boil in water and drink.

3) Tong Mai Si Ni Tang: treats diarrhea with undigested food, pulse vanishing, sweating and faint, it is Si Ni Tang with double dose Gan Jiang plus scallions.

4) Bai Tong Tang treats Shao Yin disease diarrhea with small pulse. Scallions 4 stems, Gan Jiang 1 Liang, fresh Fu Zi 1 bulb, water 3 sheng, cook and reduce to 1 sheng, remove residue, drink warm in 2 doses.

5) Bai Tong plus urine and pig bile: treats symptoms after giving Bai Tong Tang whereby diarrhea doesn't stop, sweating and the person is faint with no pulse, dry belching and agitation, after drinking the decoction if pulse abruptly comes out there is death, if it is small then there is life. It is the previous prescription plus human urine 5 Ge, pig bile 1 Ge, drink warm in 2 doses.

The abovementioned 5 prescriptions' treatment scope all have sunken pulse, small pulse about to extinguish or no pulse, four extremities are cold etc symptoms. It is like when heart function deteriorates, and the five prescriptions all use Fu Zi (aconite), therefore it is possible that Fu Zi is a drug benefiting the heart.

1) Dang Gui Si Ni Tang: treats cold hands and feet, pulse is thin and about to perish. Use Dang Gui, Gui Zhi, Shao Yao, Xi Xin each 3 Liang, Gan Cao, Tong Cao each 2 Liang, Da Zao 25 pieces, water 8 sheng cook reduce to 3 sheng, remove residue, drink warm 3 sheng, three times per day.

2) Zhi Gan Cao Tang (also called Fu Mai Tang "Recovering Pulse Decoction"): treats exhaustion and deficiency, sweat and oppression feeling, pulse irregular with heart palpitations. Use Zhi Gan Cao 3 Liang, Sheng Jiang, Gui Zhi each 3 Liang, Mai Dong half Jin, Sheng Di Huang 1 Jin, Huo Ma Ren half Jin, E Jiao Ren Shen each 2 Liang, Da Zao 30 pieces, wine 7 sheng, water 8 sheng, cook down to 3 sheng. Remove residue then add Jiao and dissolve completely, drink warm 1 sheng three times per day.

3) Shen Fu Tang: treats Yin Yang blood and Qi abrupt separation symptoms. Use Ren Shen 1 Liang, prepared Fu Zi 5 qian, Sheng Jiang 3 slices, Hong Zao 3 pieces. Above three prescriptions probably treat circulation-decline due to decrease in blood volume.

B. The search for heart-strengthening medicines

1) Seeking out from ancients' prescriptions, we have mainly Si Ni Tang, Shen Fu Tang, Zhi Gan Cao Tang.

2) From single-herb prescriptions we have Wan Nian Qing and Lai Zhu Tao etc.

3) In order to prove medicinal efficacy, we advanced an experiment with a frog's heart, using the suspension method from L. D. Heiner. Or we used abdominal vein irrigation method. The method of irrigation into the frog's abdominal vein was as follows:

a) We impaired the frog's brain and laid it on a frog board and fixed its four limbs.

b) We excised open its thoracic cavity and pulled out the heart, we cut open the pericardium, we used a hook to fix the apex cordis.

c) We cut open the abdominal cavity skin to expose the abdominal vein, we sliced open the abdominal muscle, we used Ringer's solution and with a needle injected it into the abdominal vein and then we fixed the artery with a needle to the abdominal wall.

d) We used a thread to connect the heart hook to an all-purpose lever, first injected a little bit Ringer's solution, then recorded the heartbeat rate.

e) Through the abdominal vein we gradually injected the different herbs decoctions we wanted to test, like Si Ni Tang etc, the injected liquid didn't surpass 1ml per minute.

f) We observed how the frog's heart behaved upon receiving the herbal decoction.

Class 12: Medicines adjusting the menses and decreasing blood pressure

---

Yaron: The ancients were confused.

Page 47

From accumulated traditional experience, one can see that herbals regulating the menses are many. However, as we investigate carefully the so called "regulating menses herbs", and try to find what the pharmacodynamics are, we see that there is a great confusion.

Subchapter 2: Herbals reducing high blood pressure

Yaron: How to follow the Soviets and make a correlation between Chinese medicine terminology and Western medicine diagnosis.

Page 48

Chinese medicine often uses herbs with effect for "calming liver"; within these, many are similar to lowering blood pressure herbs like Xia Ku Cao, Huang Qin, Du Zhong etc which have been used in the Soviet Union to treat patients with high blood pressure. Currently there is no absolutely successful treatment for high blood pressure. In the past, high blood pressure was seen as caused by blood vessel and kidney pathology. Since the Soviets advanced a sleeping therapy for high blood pressure, inspired by it, we should also pay attention and address the central nervous system role too.

The experience accumulated in Chinese medicine treatment of "resolving stagnation" may also play a role in reducing high blood pressure, for example:

Xiao Yao San treats the liver function group suffering from blood deficiency and fire rising, headaches and blurry vision, red cheeks and bitter mouth, curled tired and agitated, thirst, oppression and depression, ribcage pains on both sides, cold and heat alternating, lower abdominal pulling, irregular menses, pulse wiry, large and empty. Formula contains: Dang Gui, Shao Yao, Bai Zhu, Fu Ling, Chai Hu, Sheng Gan Cao, each 2 qian, Gan Jiang 3 slices, Bo He 1 qian, cook and drink. When analyzing this formula's symptoms and pulse, it looks like high blood pressure. Out of this formula we can make a modern form of drug and begin clinical observations. At the same time, we can perform animal experiments.

Class 13: A sketch of endocrine and nutritional herbs

Class 14: Animal experiments with Chinese medicine's effective resolving heat formulas

Subchapter 2: Common formulas in Chinese medicine to resolve heat

Pages 51-52

a) Chai Hu Tang treats alternating heat and cold, bitter fullness in chest, agitation and nausea, abdominal pains and heart palpitations. Formula contains: Chai Hu half Jin, Huang Qin, Ren Shen, Gan Cao each 3 Liang, Ban Xia half sheng, Sheng Jiang 3 Liang, Da Zao 12 pieces, cook in water.

   According to the Japanese Mr. Jin Teng, Chai Hu decoction (ratio 20:1000) introduced into a rabbit stomach 25ml has a resolving fever effect. According to Zhou Muchao and Huang Dengyun reports, Chai Hu can stop reproduction of malaria parasitic protozoan and eradicate it.

   Huang Qin, in a test tube, can inhibit growth of many kinds of bacteria. Therefore Chai Hu decoction targets both the disease's symptoms and cause.

b) Bai Hu decoction is used to quell thirst, knotted heat in the interior, when interior and exterior both hot, tongue is dry, pulse is surging big. The herbs are: Zhi Mu 6 Liang, Sheng Shi Gao 1 Jin, Gan Cao 2 Liang, rice 6 Ge, cook in water. Shi Gao is a crystalized calcium sulfate and is difficult to dissolve in water. Does it really have a resolving heat effect? It is worth investigation. Zhi Mu has an inhibiting effect on bacteria growth.

c) Research methods

   1. Induce fever in a rabbit, first establish rabbit normal temperature in rectum, then use Si Lian vaccine 0.5-1.0ml intravenous and cause it to have fever.

2. Use Chai Hu decoction, Bai Hu decoction or other decoctions, and inject it through to the stomach, every kilogram [body weight] use 15ml.
3. Every 15 minutes read rectum temperatures, produce a curved line (of results on a chart).

Class 16: Treatment of infectious parasitic protozoan

Class 17: Treating variety of parasites

Class 18: Various external treatments in Chinese medicine

Yaron: In TCM, learning acupuncture's physiological effects defined the meaning of the therapy. This, as we can see next, matched and followed Zhu Lian's *New Acupuncture* and the Soviets' Pavlovian theories of neurological stimulation. So to say, the technique is ancient but now we can explain it with modern science. After the original theory was discarded, acupuncture simply became an act of inserting fine needles into the skin. This is how, following the Party line, they savored acupuncture as an ancient treasure and yet modernized it with a new theory. Even if they kept on using the idea of meridians, these had now the meaning of nerve-like channels that connect to the inner organs, just like nerves connect all parts of the body. It remains for us, modern practitioners, to rediscover and reevaluate all the information lost during the early years of Communist China.

Pages 61–64

Subchapter 1: Basic theory and meaning of external therapies

The efficacy of external therapies relies on external stimulation. Its effect is delivered via the nervous system and the circulation system. Therefore, what it can be used for in treatment is limited. It cannot be outside the scope of physiological stress to the nervous and circulatory systems.

Subchapter 2: Acupuncture

Acupuncture is a kind of economical, simple and easy-to-use physical therapy. It can treat many types of diseases (for detailed explanation, see special acupuncture books). The therapeutic functions of acupuncture are as follows:

1) Calming effect: It has a calming effect towards nervous ability and excitation, hormonal hyperfunction, hyperemia, muscle spasms etc.
2) Exciting effect: It has an exciting effect towards feeling of numbness, slacking muscles etc.
3) Inducing effect: this means its tenet can reach far places. While using stimulation and via the reflex system it can heal a disease in a remote place in the body. The main therapeutic effect of moxibustion is to increase the exchange of old with new and improve circulation.
4) A suggestion for research methods:
    a) According to old experience, determine the few most appropriate diseases to treat and the appropriate acupoints for them. Complement it with scientific diagnostic methods and observations, and then calculate the efficacy.
    b) We can use electrocardiogram, brain wave diagrams and oscilloscope etc instruments of physiological electricity in order to observe the impact acupuncture exerts over the body.
    c) Use physiological chemistry, bacteriology and immunology as well as diagnostic methods to determine acupuncture effect on the blood and the immune system.

Classes 19–20: Chinese medicine diagnostics I and II

Page 70

Subchapter 3: Observation

The face area conforms to five Zang organs. *Neijing* 內經, in chapter *Ci Re Lun* 刺熱論 states: "in liver heat disease the left cheek is red first, in heart heat disease between the eyebrows is red first, in spleen heat disease the nose is red first, in lung heat disease the right cheek is red first, in kidney heat disease the chin is red first." This kind of pairing facial areas is very similar to the astrologers pairing five phases kind of spirituality. It has nothing to do with science and its diagnostics have no value.

Class 21: Chinese medicine foundation studies

Yaron: Emphasizing the uselessness of CM theory, as a whole and on a national scale, started in the Republic and continued full force during the creation of TCM with Communism. What originally were faint voices became stronger and coming to this point in time forced everyone else silent. Zhu Yan, as we see next, was pitching the same ideology as everyone else. It was a time where different voices and debates ended. This is why bringing the 1930s debates back to life in this book is so critical for us. We should not view it as water under the bridge but rather re-live it. We don't have a gigantic government behind us that can manipulate or control us as one group, but instead, and far better, we have our Chinese medicine hearts and we are all connected together in this one place. This is why, when we become aware of these events unfolding in the 20th century, that we, Chinese medicine practitioners all over the world, can forget our small differences and work together on making Chinese medicine more alive in the 21st century. In my opinion, what happened in the 1920s and 1950s was necessary for Chinese medicine to survive and to a degree even beneficial. However, keeping it today as if we are still in 1950s is a terrible mistake. This medicine can contribute so much to the world if it could only allow and free itself to discover new things, developing its life-style medicine.

Page 78

Subchapter 1: A general survey of Chinese medicine foundation studies

1) "Heaven and man unite into one" kind of spiritual theory gradually replaced the original standard method of dialectical materialism. Chinese medicine foundation studies based on spiritual theory established a "plausibility" stand-alone system. It departed from the original scope of "experience-based". It became a "mature" trend, where all phenomena in the medical field could be explained in a very subtle, mysterious way. In reality, not even one problem could attain one true solution. Because of this trend, scientification of medicine was obstructed.

2) A feature of Chinese medicine foundation studies is that, through superficial observations of changes, unrefined recordings and lack of experiments, rarely could its theory accurately reflect the objective reality. With strained interpretation of spirituality and a strained interpretation that nature's phenomena reflect

physiological and pathological transformation of the human body, it is often the case that, even while observing the phenomena, it cannot reach to the intrinsic value of things.

3) Chinese medicine foundations and its use in clinical applications: Chinese medicine is a kind of experience-based medicine. Its treatment principle, application and mastery lies entirely within its practical experience. To a large degree, it knows that something acts like this but does not know why it acts like this. For example, when a disease is cured with Chinese medicine, other than using Chinese medicine's own invented theories to explain why, it is very difficult to come by a true explanation of why the cure took place. Taken from another angle, Chinese medicine cannot make a correct scientific diagnosis of a disease, yet, by its appearance, it can treat it and often times reach a cure. This explains plenty that Chinese medicine's clinical practice has no true bond to its foundational theoretical studies. Chinese medicine's foundational theory contains plenty of wrong hypotheses that somehow paired with clinical experience. However, only after the treatment was implemented were some criteria for that experience created. For us, its theory cannot serve any purpose from an objective reality of physical evidence.

4) Summary: Since Chinese medicine foundation theory contains many unscientific elements and unfounded assumptions, in clinical application it cannot dominate nor have a pushing forward ability.

Class 22–23: Chinese Medicine clinical study part I & II

Page 84

1) Chinese medicine's deficiency is that it doesn't have scientific diagnostics; no matter whether it reaches a cure or not, it cannot thoroughly explain what the disease is. However, even before the diagnosis was established, it can still implement a treatment and often reach a cure. This is the main characteristic of experience-based medicine.

2) Treatment of the spirit in Chinese medicine is also one characteristic. What we call "spirit treatment" means that by using words, attitude and other methods one can cause the patient's thoughts and emotions to change in order to benefit the patient and reach a cure for an ailment. It can lead the patient out of mental

situations like oppression, stress, depression, confusion etc and into a state of mind of happiness, positive outlook and wellbeing. In the past these kinds of treatments were considered tricks of the quacks. However, according to Pavlov's theories we recognize that the person's mood does impact his body greatly. Therefore, altering the patient's mental attitude in order to reach a cure for his disease has a scientific basis. This is especially the case for mental patients, chronic patients and pulmonary tuberculosis patients.

Page 89

Conclusion [of this class]

Chinese medicine clinical studies, strictly speaking, are fragments of medical experience. Chinese medicine theory is indeed a complete theoretical system. However, judging it with modern medicine scales it is indeed a deficient and incomplete one. We must follow the rules of a scientific medical development, take Chinese medicine's clinical and scientific parts and add to it the strong points of medicine coming from foreign lands. Only then can we improve upon Chinese medicine, reaching to modern medicine's current level.

Class 24: Analysis of Chinese medicine thought and criticism

Page 93

In Western medicine developmental phase we can find stepping-stones similar to Chinese medicine development. For example, there were theories comparable to the Chinese five phases such as four fluids and four elements etc. European countries and their societal institutions followed the feudal system's development until reaching capitalism; production methods changed with industrialism and, naturally, science made rapid progress. It gave intellectual developments optimum conditions. Because of this, Western medicine was able to rid itself of the four fluids and four elements kind of spiritual theories. It entered the scientific realm. Even though it acquired capitalist thought in many places, it also received significant mechanical materialism ideas. All in all, this established the foundation of modern science and, in comparison to Chinese medicine, its evolution had advanced a step further. From developmental principle point of view, Chinese and Western medicines should not have carried two forms. It is only that Chinese medicine had paused at an earlier developmental stage than Western medicine. Chinese medicine should not pause any more at this inferior step but, rather, it should absorb the medical scientific accomplishments coming from abroad. We must march on a path towards the Soviet medical advancement. We should take the plain accumulated experience and, from the realm of the old-style thinking, elevate it to the new scientific level.

Yaron: For Communism, getting rid of the most dominant and significant "old" Chinese medicine principle was top priority. Following, Zhu Yan explicitly explains that TCM has to get rid of the old principle in order to become Soviet scientific. Today, this "old" principle is the first thing that we must bring back into the medicine. In other words, when Zhu Yan says get rid of the "circular principle" it actually translates to "stop talking about life principle". If we want to make Chinese medicine talk about life again then the circular principle is the first thing that needs to come back into the medicine. I call this the Hunyuan principle of medicine.

Page 94

The development of the circular principle. Chinese medicine logic is often stuck with "when a thing reaches extreme it must return" and "when cold is extreme it turns to heat, when heat is extreme it turns to cold" kind of ideas. It thinks that the development of things is "like a ring with no end". From this circular idea, which was exercised in the old ways, getting self-entangled was often the result (literally going in circles). Other than "returning to antiquity" and "going back to the origin" kind of rhetoric, there were no new solutions to be found. This kind of logic only knows to 'respect the classics" and "revere the ancient" but cannot criticize and scrutinize the ancient culture and, because of that, it obstructed any kind of new developments.

Appendix: Chinese medicine research—Summary discussion excerpt (arranged by Luan Zhiren 欒志仁)

Yaron: Among many problems inflicting TCM transformation, the following was probably the worst: "So to say, if we take one herb or one herbal prescription and try to determine chemically its active ingredients plus seek the proof via animal testing, we need three to six months, or even one to two years or even longer. The people's needs cannot wait such long months and years." Not only did Chinese medicine discard its generations-long theories, it

> needed a new theory and needed it quickly; the people have no time to wait. So if they teach in TCM schools that Chinese medicine was created over thousands of years and is time-tested, in reality, the opposite is true. Modern TCM was created in a short period of time, untested, or at least very poorly tested. Today, in TCM hospitals doctors dispense herbs with steroids, acupuncture with electricity. There are no thousands of years of testing. We should all know that!
>
> Pages 97-98

Chinese medicine research 24 lectures were taught at Beijing Chinese Medicine Advanced Studies School to the second and third classes. On October 5th 1952, thirty seven graduating fellows—including Luan Zhiren 欒志仁, Duan Yongquan 段永泉 and others and led by Dr. Zhu Yan 朱顏—convened a summary discussion conference. In attendance was the education director Yu Daoji 于道濟.

First, Dr. Zhu Yan gave a simplified summary of the Chinese medicine research course. In addition, he gave a detailed description of the research work done on stomach ulcer treatment, stopping cough and resolving-phlegm medicines and a brief and to-the-point description of the state of affairs with animal testing. Thereafter, towards his fellow students, he put forth his opinion on the content of the curriculum, teaching methodologies and the necessary steps for advancement, in order to conveniently change and improve the required work going forward.

Fellow students expressed their enthusiasm and put forward their feedback via abundant discussions, a summary of which follows:

They expressed complete satisfaction toward the contents and teaching methodology of this course.

This kind of arrangement and tackling problems can truly reach the objective of Chinese medicine scientification. Chinese medicine's strong points are not few; however, investigating exactly "where they are?" is very difficult to answer. Dr. Zhu pointed out these problems and the study material associated with it plus the methods to deal with it. We believe that these are the basic steps for making Chinese medicine scientific.

Raising problems and seeking scientific answers is, with no doubt, a difficult affair. In many places in these 24 lectures there are limitations of the subject matter. As we consider the entire Chinese medicine material, one cannot avoid deficiencies. After every lecture we proposed that there would be a discussion segment, in which every fellow student should question extensively and put forth his opinion and outlook on things. We should do this in order to collectively consider and supplement this research work.

Chinese herbalism is effective towards some diseases. Therefore, in this phase, rearranging Chinese herbs and investigating them has a pressing need. Here, we delivered the research material and methods. Fellow students agreed that it was ideal. At present, Chinese herbs first need to be simplified and easy to use. Using the herbs' effective parts, emphasis should be put on advancing a change in the drug form in which it is used.

Next to that, chemical analysis and reconstruction of drugs should take place. However, in such a short period of time, attempting to chemically analyze so many Chinese herbals, pills, powders, ointments and elixirs and find out their active ingredients, we are afraid is not such a simple task. So to say, if we take one herb or one herbal prescription and try to determine chemically its active ingredients plus seek the proof via animal testing, we need three to six months, or even one to two years or even longer. The people's needs cannot wait such long months and years. At the same time, the advancement of science is at a pace of a thousand miles per day. Following the leaps and bounds of reconstructing our new nation, the need for our Chinese medicine and herbalism must take on new development.

Therefore the majority of our fellow students advocated: "emphasis should be on taking the most effective known formulas and herbs, change and advance them into drug form in order to be administered easily. At the same time, put into place animal testing and determine its toxic dose limit, its fatal dose and its efficacy level and then publish this as reference material. First use it in clinic for emergency cases then, through clinical practice, determine if it is useful or not."

Other discussions and their results were omitted here.

Book excerpt end

Experimental research on Qigong therapy

1956 by Liu Guizhen 劉貴珍

Source: *Xin Zhong Yi Yao*, January 25th 1956

新中醫藥

一九五六年一月

第七卷第一期

Yaron: While Qigong exercises have their root in ancient times, here, government encouragement of cheaper health care options is certainly at play. Qigong, or Neigong as it was previously called, involved a high degree of spiritual practice. During Communism, spiritual practices had no standing and dialectic materialism was the dominant accepted doctrine. Here, I simply bring the example of Qigong to demonstrate that any and all aspects of Chinese medicine underwent the TCM transformation.

Page 42

Our nation's medicine has thousands of years of history. It contains tremendous content and valuable clinical experience. It had great impact throughout the dynasties on people fighting against disease. Chairman Mao has instructed us the main direction of sanitary works, "combine Western and Chinese medicines and gear it toward workers, farmers and soldiers". Under the guidance of the Communist Party there is a big improvement in Chinese medical work. For example, since acupuncture has been very effective in treating Japanese encephalitis and anal fistulas, Chinese medicine treatment for these problems recently has been promoted all over the country. (The above example is just a part of Chinese medicine academic advancement, and there will be more discovery in the future.) Hence, developing Chinese medicine, our national legacy, to enrich the medicine of the world is very meaningful.

Qigong is one of our national cultural legacies being used for strengthening the body since long ago. Many Chinese medical books, talking about health care and life extension, have incorporated research with experiments to discover its therapeutic effects. Qigong therapy, under a doctor's supervision, aims to control posture and breath. In a peaceful environment only by practicing Qigong one's physiological mechanism may recover back to normal without any medication, injection or surgery. It has been proven with clinical experiments that this kind of therapy is based on Ivan Pavlov's theory main idea. It also matches the guiding principle of "One ounce of prevention is worth a pound of cure". Not to mention that practicing Qigong doesn't need any equipment, so it's a simple and cheap therapy.

I used to have stomach ulcer, and I had been through long-term medication and nothing worked for me. At the end I was cured by Qigong therapy. The Communist Party and people's government value the cultural legacy so they sent me to learn about this therapy and, in addition, enthusiastically supported my experimental research work. There have been some hundreds of people cured in south Hebei 河北 area since 1949 while the second cadre nursing home 第二幹部療養院 in Hebei province started a Qigong department in 1953. In 1954 the Qigong sanatorium 氣功療養所 was established in Tangshan 唐山 with support from Tangshan City municipal committee, Board of Health and the general labour union. This is from where Qigong therapy started being promoted. In Tangshan, Qigong was not only used to treat patients, but there were also two Qigong training classes. Since September 1954 until now, after the first group of Western medicine doctors graduated from the first Qigong training class, they cured more than three hundred patients with chronic and debilitating disease. In June 1955, Western medicine doctors from hospitals in Shanxi 山西, Wuhan 武漢 and other places came to attend the Qigong research and training. After they went back to their home town, some started to practice Qigong therapy in their hospitals, while others are still at the preparation phase before practicing it.

During the one year it has been doing Qigong experimental research in Tangshan, the Qigong sanatorium had received more than a thousand letters from other medical institutes, cadres and the masses asking to learn Qigong or get treated. Many of the letters were from border areas and different working positions, which shows how much people believe and feel comfortable with our national legacy. Since the president of Chinese Medicine Research Academy 中医研究院院長, comrade Lu Zhijun 魯之俊, published an article, *Seriously Studying and Researching our National Medicine* 認真学習和研究 祖國的医學,[444] it has aroused people's attention to Qigong therapy and we have received much encouragement and support. Today we follow the suggestion of the *New Chinese Medicine* editors and introduce Qigong therapy methods and some case studies.

Article excerpt end

[444] Recorded in *Xin Zhong Yi Yao*, 5th volume, issue 9 新中医药五卷九期.

Qi Gong and Preserving Health Gong

1959 by Hu Yaozhen 胡耀贞[445]

Source: Published by People's Sanitation Publishing House 1959, Edited by Beijing City Acupuncture Department

气功及保健功　人民卫生出版社　北京市针灸门诊部整理

Yaron: Another Qigong book excerpt, three years later, brought here together for reference. All practitioners of Chinese medicine and Qigong had to conform to the party line.

Preface

Qigong healing is one of China's inherited medical treasures. It has a very long history. This treatment modality can cure disease, prevent disease, keep the body healthy and prolong life. In the past, Buddhists and Daoists named it stillness cultivation Jing Gong 静功 while martial artists named it inner cultivation Nei Gong 内功. It is said that Lao Zi transmitted this kind of cultivation. Lao Zi transmitted it to Guang Cheng Zi 广成子 and Guang Cheng Zi transmitted it to the Yellow Emperor. As a result, in the *Yellow Emperor Inner Canon* there is An Mo massage 按摩, Dao Yin 导引 exercises and other nurturing life and benefiting longevity exercises.

From age sixteen I began my study of medicine, martial arts and Daoism (Daoist cultivation methods). My style of acupuncture is also derived from the Daoist "Wu Ji Acupuncture 无极针". The art of Wu Ji Acupuncture is the art of using one's own essence, Qi and spirit and applying it while pricking with needles. When pricking and using tonification and sedation methods the patient feels inside his body numbing heat, or cool distension spreading all over the body. This kind of acupuncture is carried out by using Qigong. In order to study Qigong, during the prolonged times of the old society, I have asked to study with many teachers and visited many friends.

My teacher Peng Tingjun 彭庭隽 (a disciple of the old Daoist recluse Huo Chengguang 霍成光) transmitted to me Dao cultivation, inner cultivation, heart mind boxing and Hua Tuo's five frolics exercises. Later on I became a disciple of the monk Li Hong 立宏 from Shan Xi's Chong Shan monastery 山西崇善寺. He transmitted to me the Buddhist cultivation methods. In addition I also learned "Zhuang Zi exhaling old and inhaling new" method.

[445] For more Hu Yaozhen translations and his life story refer to the Hunyuan Research Institute www.ChineseClassics.org.

For 40 years now I have carried the practice of medicine without interruption. In my spare time I practiced martial arts. The practice of inner cultivation was as well never interrupted. The testimony of time shows that my practice of martial arts and inner cultivation helped my practice of medicine greatly, especially so was my practice of Hua Tuo's five frolics exercises. Regardless if it was my stillness cultivation, martial cultivation or medicine skills it helped in all directions. My teacher gave me the classic of the five frolics exercises and it was never published. As time becomes available I'll arrange and publish it in a separate booklet (others like Xin Yi classic, Tai Ji classic, Mai Zhuang Tu Xin Yi Quan classic, preserving health and prolonging life methods etc, one after the other I will arrange and publish).

China has a very long history. Throughout the ages people struggled with disease and the experience accumulated is great. Chinese medicine doctors, martial artists as well as Confucians, Buddhists and Daoists all have their methods of nurturing life.

In 40 years of practicing martial arts and inner cultivation I certainly walked a round-about way and also experienced great hardship. The above mentioned arts I have practiced throughout (even though never practiced well). Through the grinding work and the long process of cognition I began seeking out the rules of practicing cultivation, especially the rules for "stillness" and "movement". Based on these rules plus integrating it with the inner cultivation of martial art I synthesized a kind of "Stillness and Movement Qigong" practicing method. This kind of practicing method is what we currently use in clinic to treat patients.

After liberation, through the correct instruction of the Communist Party and chairman Mao, the application of Qigong healing in clinic got popularized and reached great results. Our clinic since 1956, utilizing Qigong therapy, attained good success with treating difficult to treat chronic diseases such as duodenal ulcers, stomach prolapse, chronic hepatitis, liver cirrhosis, neurasthenia and heart disease. It has a definite action in improving the curative effect.

I recognize that under the leadership and education of the Party, through the different arrangement steps, progressively there is an improvement. Under the Party's utmost effort and striving for progress, to achieve greater, faster, better and more economical results for constructing socialism, the glory of this general Party line shines down, for me and for the entire people likewise all elated by this work, gradually to take these practicing cultivation methods and transmit to patients in order to increase the curative effect. Especially after attending Bei Dai He's Qigong Experience and Exchange

Conference 北戴河气功交流经验大会 in October this year, in which I received direct and meticulous loving care from the organizing committee, and much respect from the other comrades, I feel extremely grateful and inspired. Therefore, after coming back to Beijing I decided not to keep any secrets of whatever I know about Qigong healing, and whatever cultivation methods previously I did not teach. I record and narrate them here in order to allow everyone to consider and use them.

Believing in the leadership of the Party, Qigong healing going through research and arrangement of everyone, certainly can be more beneficial for constructing a service for socialism. As there is a time constraint, we still didn't bring out other exercise methods and content, and from the theory aspect also didn't explore further. I'll await the second print of the book to supplement it.

For the tenth year anniversary of our country I wrote this small booklet, the hand moved hastily and especially because my level is limited, that in it the deficiencies and errors are certainly many, I respectfully invite doctors of Chinese and Western medicines and the general public to kindly correct me.

November 1959 in Beijing.
Hu Yaozhen

Book excerpt end

Miscellaneous words about acupuncture therapy

1956 by Li Youshen 李幼申

Source: *Xin Zhong Yi Yao*, January 25th 1956

新中醫藥　一九五六年一月　第七卷第一期

Yaron: A clear and easy way to understand acupuncture. Practical and concise approach, using sterilization techniques and a realistic view of therapy are indeed beneficial and fit the modern day. However, what is lost here are things which are not physical. In reality, the treatment modality described here is entirely Western medicine physical modality, and still of an inferior type; a second class Western medicine modality. It is not pure physical science because it is ideologically influenced and it is not Life-medicine kind of Chinese medicine for the same reason. It is not here and not there, hanging in mid-air.

1) The close relationship between acupuncture and the workers

Acupuncture is one of the earliest inventions among physical therapies in our medical history. Because this therapy is easy to apply and has instant effects, it has been popular and influential among the workers, and therefore closely related to the workers in China for thousands of years.

2) The origin of acupuncture

Although there is no clear description of the origin of acupuncture in history, according to ancient medical literature, it can be traced back to around the New Stone Age, when people were leading a primitive life. In order to adapt into a tough environment, they struggled to survive and resisted natural disasters. When falling ill, witchcraft was the only way to get rid of diseases. If this didn't help, they took a needle made of stone (actually the sharp edge of a stone, which was called Bianshi 砭石) and cut their skin as to let it bleed a bit, which magically helped the patient feel better. Afterwards, the form of needles improved to bamboo needles, copper needles, tinplate needles, gold needles and silver needles. This is the origin of acupuncture.

3) The discovery of moxibustion

Moxibustion was accidentally invented from an unexpected burn after people knew how to utilize fire. As the burn happened, people realized that it reduced some body pains, so they expanded on the use of heat from fire to treat disease. Then the method was improved to burn moxa. This is the beginning of moxibustion.

4) What is an acupoint?

Acupoint (stimulating point) is the basic unit of acupuncture therapy. Regardless if acupuncture or moxibustion is used, acupoints on the body need to allow through sensation with different strengths in order to cure disease. (Stronger stimulation causes inhibition while weaker stimulation arouses excitatory effects.)

5) The effect of the nervous system inside a human body

After Ivan Pavlov 伊瓦巴甫洛夫 discovered classical conditioning, people realized that a human being is a complete organism, which has a single part leading the other parts to work together. Cerebral cortex, which is at the highest level in the central nervous system, is in charge of every movement of every single part of the body. Once the body encounters external stimuli it reacts properly and in a timely fashion. For example, when it's hot the skin pores and blood vessels dilate and then the body perspires in order to lower its temperature. This prevents body temperature from rising up too high. On the contrary, when it's cold skin pores and blood vessels contract to reduce spreading out heat. This prevents the body temperature from dropping too fast.

The reason a human body adjusts to different external conditions is that the central nervous system orchestrates the entire body to regulate itself. This also explains how our nervous system, while functioning normally, can ensure normal physiological function.

6) Viewing disease pathology from the point of dialectic materialism

In the past, many people were influenced by the old medical theory, or cell pathology,[446] and therefore they believed that every disease is caused by stimulation, such as bacteria or toxins, directly damaging tissues and cells. Their research focused on changes resulting directly from reaction of cells and tissues to bacteria and toxins. However, if we criticize this concept based on the great Soviet Pavlov's accurate theories of conditioning, we will find that their theory is only one-sided and not complete. From a dialectic materialism point of view, a disease course should be regarded as a battle between an external invasion and the body tissues under the tutelage of its central nervous system. Any concept without seeing the entire picture is improper.

7) What is the logic behind acupuncture treatment of disease?

Acupuncture can cure disease not because the needle is able to extinguish the invading toxins or bacteria, but rather because acupuncture stimulates (stimulation actually means conforming to what the body needs) and regulates the nervous system function and indirectly facilitates metabolism and invigorates the body to kill bacteria by itself and therefore heal. For example, most of malaria patients can heal after four or five acupuncture treatments applied two or three hours before relapsing fever and shivering. This is because at this time malaria parasites become active and interfere with the nervous system. If we strengthen the nervous system exactly at that time to resist the invasion of malaria parasites then the patient won't need to suffer from recurrent fever and shivering. The parasites will lose a suitable environment to function and therefore will be extinguished inside the body and the patient will recover.

8) Is acupuncture really a "cure all"?

Some people think that acupuncture can cure all diseases. As a matter of fact, the therapeutic effect of acupuncture in some way is better than that of herbs in clinical

[446] USA-Europe modern medical theories on cell pathology.

practice, such as rheumatism of muscles and joints, neuralgia, malaria etc.; acupuncture has surprisingly good results for these diseases. But some other diseases might need herbs or Western medication.

For example, for bone fracture, acute appendicitis and cross-birth, best is to use a surgery; for meningitis and pneumonia sulfamido or penicillin works faster and better. We should apply the proper measure to each disease and not hold the mistake that acupuncture is good for all diseases. Furthermore, we should research the therapeutic effect of acupuncture and combine it with scientific techniques, focus on diagnosis, pay attention to anatomic structures and administer strict disinfection. We should apply other treatment modalities to diseases, which are not suitable for acupuncture. The concept "acupuncture cures everything" doesn't fit the mindset of dialectic materialism.

Article end

Encouragement of apprentice system: Health daily editorial

Source: *Xin Zhong Yi Yao*, March 25th 1956 新中醫藥 一九五六年三月 第七卷第三期

Yaron: During the early years of Communism, an apprenticeship system was promoted. One may erroneously conclude that a more traditional Chinese medicine was sought after but, in reality, mass education of affordable healthcare personnel was the reason. An apprenticeship system explicated that every practitioner and every United Clinic could train new Chinese medicine medical workers without relying on schools. It was about urgent breeding of a large number of practitioners.

It actually stood in contrast to a traditional apprenticeship method where a disciple will serve many years by the master's side before being qualified. In a way, it was mocking the old discipleship system. The author emphasizes "The main thing to be done is the 'reinforcing of political leadership'. Before those Chinese medicine doctors start training apprentices, we should separately and in advance instruct both sides. Let apprentices know the correct way of Chinese medicine and point out to them the future direction of their career, which will raise up their confidence. For those doctors who will be training the apprentices, educate them

> to know better the mission and change the invalid thoughts of 'teach the son and not the son-in-law, teach the daughter-in-law and not the daughter'." Like many things at that time, it meant to look traditional but was not traditional at all.
>
> Pages 97–98

In recent years, the Department of Health corrected the wrong thoughts of comrade He Cheng 賀誠. The Communist Party, while implementing the sanitary work medical policy, advanced for the better merging of Western and Chinese medicines and, with that, raised rapidly the work quality of Chinese medicine. Chinese medicine practitioners are thankful for the care and attention from the Party and the government. They treasure Chinese medicine even more, do more research about it, and also teach it with passion. Furthermore, more Chinese medicine doctors reveal not only many secret and experience-based formulas, but they also take on more disciples. Even secret disciples they now make public.

With encouragement from the prefecture Party committee, Chinese medicine doctors in Tianjin Cang County 天津滄縣 have almost two hundred apprentices; the ones in Shanxi Taigu County 山西太谷縣 are also training up apprentices. The famous Suzhou 蘇州 acupuncturist You Bomin 尤舽民 has recruited ten apprentices recently. The famous Chinese medicine ophthalmologist Fei Haoran 費浩然, who previously had stopped his children from studying Chinese medicine, now encourages them to pick it up again. All these kind of situations should be encouraged and supported.

It is Party and government policy to develop Chinese medicine. The Ministry of Health needs to implement every aspect of this policy. We should explain to Chinese medicine doctors that training apprentices, in order to pass down the Chinese medical knowledge, is an honorable responsibility and, if needed, we should provide aid. Only like this could we preserve our precious Chinese medicine and amplify the people's health industry.

In order to develop our medical legacy, we encourage Western medicine doctors to learn Chinese medicine. However, there are not that many Western medicine doctors, plus they can't systematically learn Chinese medicine. Although the Chinese Medicine Research Center has been established and it includes experience of numerous famous Chinese medicine doctors, it cannot bring together one hundred thousand Chinese medicine doctors.

Medical experience recorded in books is only one part of the ancient wisdom, while the other, modern Chinese medical knowledge, is only in the modern Chinese medicine doctors' brains. If we want to pass down the entire Chinese medical knowledge then every single Chinese medicine doctor needs to share his or her knowledge and experience, otherwise we will lose this chance. There were many brilliant doctors in the past that didn't have the chance to pass down their precious experience, which is an enormous and preventable loss for us. This is how to prevent losing Chinese medical knowledge.

Furthermore, as for sanitary work, our country is moving forward with socialist construction and so people's demand for health care increases. We cannot meet the demand until we have enough support for our sanitary work. The most significant strength in our current health care system is having numerous Chinese medicine doctors who are, in fact, able to take charge of most people's health care needs.

For now, most of our Chinese medicine doctors are elders. According to an investigation, more than 75% of them in Shanxi Changzhi City 山西長治市 are above age 50, and about 90% are above age 40. Therefore we should pass down our Chinese medical knowledge as soon as possible. It is not enough if we solely rely on schools to train up Western or Chinese medicine doctors. We should encourage Chinese medicine doctors to train up apprentices, in which case we could develop five hundred thousand Chinese medicine doctors in a short period of time. It is absolutely important and necessary mission.

However, thus far, local departments of health did not recognize the importance of it; some of them even instituted improper regulations prohibiting personal apprenticeships. This should be corrected immediately. The main obstacle for this job is, at the moment, the Ministry of Health's contempt for Chinese medicine. They seem to have "infinite concerns" about educating more Chinese medicine doctors. Their attitude blocks the development of this work. They don't understand well enough the influence, which might come about by every industry (including Chinese medical work) on social reformation. They also under estimate the political progressiveness of Chinese medicine. Some of them even set the unreasonable restriction on the apprentice system.

One should know that a "master training apprentice" is not the objective itself but rather it is one part of the entire Chinese medical work. If we do well the entire Chinese medical work then we basically can solve most problems related to the apprentice system. The main thing to be done is the "reinforcing of political leadership".

Before those Chinese medicine doctors start training apprentices, we should, separately and in advance, instruct both sides. Let apprentices know the correct way of Chinese medicine and point out to them the future direction of their career, which will raise up their confidence. For those doctors who will be training the apprentices, educate them to know better the mission and change the invalid thoughts of "teach the son and not the son-in-law, teach the daughter-in-law and not the daughter". The prefectural Party committee in Cang County 滄縣 has relieved many of the Chinese medicine doctors' concerns and now they are more willing to train apprentices and pass down their experience and knowledge. The apprenticeship system will definitely not facilitate feudalism or anarchy. These are just unnecessary concerns.

Some people can't understand the apprenticeship system. They think that if we continue developing Chinese medicine in this way then it is incompatible with the merging (He Liu 合流) of Western and Chinese medicine. In their minds, extinguishing Chinese medicine is the only viable way to "merge" Western and Chinese medicine. In other words, as long as we extinguish Chinese medicine, we achieve a "merged medicine"—which is totally incorrect. They don't understand that merging the two is a high-level development of our national medical science, which includes both Chinese and Western medicine; it contains the essence of both Western and Chinese medicine. It is proper today, for the "merging" to enthusiastically encourage Western medicine doctors to learn Chinese medicine and to encourage Chinese medicine doctors to train apprentices. If no one researches it or inherits it then it will be the failure of Chinese medical knowledge, not to mention a failed "merging".

Conforming to the development of a new cultural education and the agricultural cooperative transformation, there are many young intelligent people with good cultural backgrounds that can become the troops for supervising the cooperatives and lead sanitary works. Many people are still willing to learn Chinese medicine as long as the rules are explained properly and there is support of the political leadership. Today, Chinese medicine United Clinics in the countryside and cities, medical centers and health centers develop quickly. They are good locations for the apprentice system.

According to current information, training of apprentices varies in different locations. For example, doctors in Shanxi Taigu County 山西太谷縣 train up apprentices mostly in United Clinics. Apprentices do part of the work in the clinic and then listen to doctors' lectures in the morning and at night. The United Clinics provide meals and some pocket money so that the apprentices can learn Chinese medicine wholeheartedly. Some learn and teach only after hours, while the priority remains their own work in clinic, and the apprentices can have other production jobs. Some recruit apprentices privately; the doctors work in the clinic during the daytime and teach the apprentices at nighttime, while the apprentices do their obligatory work which is decided by both sides. Some are fathers teaching their sons.

As for the teaching methods, some doctors use ancient classical books, while some give oral instruction, some even work on annotating the ancient books to make them like an easier textbook for the apprentices' convenience. This is even a more appropriate method; however, all the above methods can be used. It is even better if local Health Departments and government offices on all levels provide political leadership and guidance; it then can provide an optimal condition for this system.

As to how many years of learning and at what level can an apprentice start seeing patients independently, the teaching doctors should be deciding it. Also, past experience in apprenticeship can be used as a reference. Nowadays, though, conditions for teaching and learning have changed a bit; teaching today is more advanced than in the past, so the learning curve should be faster. These problems can be solved with that.

Generally speaking, it is necessary to build up Chinese medicine schools and develop more Chinese medicine doctors; however, we can't rely solely on schools while ignoring the better and broader way to train up doctors. Setting up Chinese medical research, encouraging Western medicine doctors to learn Chinese medicine, founding Chinese medical schools, encouraging the apprentice system etc. are a series of necessary works to develop our motherland medicine. We should "plan comprehensively and strengthen political leadership", do thoroughly and systematically the Chinese medicine work to assure no loss to our motherland medicine and to improve the sanitary works in order to meet demand in our reconstruction of socialism.

Article end

My opinions about how deeply to needle Fengfu 風府 [Gv16] and Yamen 啞門 [Gv15]

1956 by Chen Dazhong 陳大中

Source: *Xin Zhong Yi Yao*, March 25th 1956

新中醫藥　一九五六年三月　第七卷第三期

Yaron: 'Acupuncture must be proven to work via nerves' was the instruction; the following article is the result.

Page 128

Preface

Fengfu (Gv16) and Yamen (Gv15) are two acupoints commonly used for central nervous system disease. Ancient literature explains that neither can be deeply punctured, and so some doctors are too scared to use these two points or, if they do, only with shallow insertion, which reduces the therapeutic effects.

The location and anatomic structure of Yamen and Fengfu

Yamen (Gv15): on the nape mid-line, 5 Fen 分 upward above the hair line. It's between the first and second cervical vertebrae, deep inside the vertebral canal and is close to the lower edge of medulla oblongata and upper part of spinal cord.

Fengfu (Gv16): 5 Fen upward from Yamen (Gv15), in the sunken part of a big muscle. It's between the occipital bone and the first cervical vertebrae, deep inside the vertebral canal by the spinal cord and medulla oblongata.

The local anatomical structure around these two points relates to trapezius, splenius capitis, semispinalis capitis, rectus capitis posterior major muscle, rectus capitis posterior minor muscle, and innervation of greater occipital nerve, third occipital nerve, and the branch of occipital artery and occipital vein.

Medulla oblongata, the vital center, hides deeply inside

Medulla oblongata is an inviolable brain tissue, which is also the part sending out the sixth, tenth, eleventh and twelfth cranial nerves. Inside lies the most important brain center of the entire body responsible for things such as respiratory, cardiac and vasomotor centre.

The functions of medulla oblongata come from the brain motor nerve fiber which consists of important brain center sending branches to the spinal cord and distributing farther all over the body. If medulla oblongata suffers injury, this can be immediately fatal, which might be the reason for ancient literature always recommending not to deeply puncture these two points. They tried to avoid damaging the medulla oblongata.

How deep to generate therapeutic effect

The goal of acupuncture therapy is to stimulate the nerve inside the points. During acupuncture, there is no efficacy until patients start feeling achy, heavy or distension. According to ancient literature, these points can't be needled deeper than 4 Fen, which anatomically is at depth of the first tissue layer; the trapezius. If we want to touch the main nerve stem of these two points and have a therapeutic effect, we certainly need to puncture them deep enough, which is about 1 Cun in proportional body units. What is the distance between skin surface to medulla oblongata? For a normal medium shape, it's about a bit less than 3 Cun proportional body units, which is around 5 centimeters.

Discussion

Why was it prohibited to needle deeply these two points in most ancient acupuncture literature? Ancient intelligentsia got their knowledge from clinical experience instead of making it up. As we can see in exhibitions of ancient items, probably because their tools for acupuncture were thick and rough, the old needles being six to ten times thicker than the ones we currently use, that the stimulating effects generated by the old needles must have been very strong. Once the experience resulted in danger, unfortunately, it became prohibited to needle these two points deeply. People recorded it in books to remind others not to make the same mistake again. This is just my assumption and experts can find out if that's true.

Now we already know the local anatomical structure of the two points, and we mostly use no.28 to no.30, which is 0.30 to 0.35mm thick needles and they are clean and smooth. With these conditions in mind, in order to generate sensation while needling these two points, as long as we sterilize the skin and the needle and the needle is in a good condition, the needle should be inserted 1 Cun proportional body unit deep. This will induce the correct therapeutic effect if the acupuncturist is skillful.

Now we're going to introduce the proper depth of these two points shown as below for others' reference. Yamen (Gv15): 5 to 8 Fen. Fengfu (Gv16): 8 Fen to 1 Cun, both following proportional body units. Using this standard will induce most patients to feel the achy, heavy and distended sensation. Above is simply my opinions and I'm happy to have some advice and comments from other experts.

Article end

People's Daily Editorial

Source: *The New Chinese Medicine Magazine*, June 1956

新中醫藥

第七卷第六期

Yaron: The apprenticeship system should not be in the old unregulated way but instead have new rules. Let's remind ourselves of the "big plan" starting in the Republic and continuing here without interruption with the words of Song Daren[447] in 1937:

"Now that Chinese medicine doctors enjoy equal legal status with Western medicine doctors, they are certainly obliged to promote public health. Instead of obstinately placing themselves at the opposite side impeding the progress of society, they should bear our responsibilities and fight with us together. Although there is still no clear regulation as to whether the system of apprenticeship should be abolished, such a system should be repealed sooner or later as apprentices cannot gain comprehensive knowledge and it would be difficult to obtain a practicing license that way. From now on, the only way for those who would like to learn Chinese medicine is to receive education from Chinese medicine schools that are established and approved by the government and taught according to the standard curriculum, in order to learn about Western medical knowledge as well as traditional Chinese medical skills. In the future, people will not distinguish between a Western doctor and a Chinese one. If there were any differences between the two, it will only be in the application of drugs. One uses herbs while the other uses synthetic drugs. As time goes by, Western and Chinese medicine doctors will converge and people will not be able to distinguish the two. These new Chinese medicine doctors will no

---

447 From: *Review of "How to learn Chinese Medicine Well" and "Chinese Medicine Doctors Thereafter"* by Song Daren 宋大仁.

> longer be picked on, as what they do has become more reasonable and detached from superstitious beliefs. As for those Chinese medicine doctors who are already practicing, they should at least know the basics of the new scientific medical theories. Otherwise, they would not be able to compete against the new Chinese medicine doctors and would inevitably be eliminated."
>
> Page 241

Develop Chinese medicine ambitiously, reinforce hygiene work team

At present, our hygiene work team consists of Western medicine modern knowledge and the profound knowledge of Chinese medicine and our country's healthcare industry depends on them. With development of the people's healthcare industry, we should train up more Western medicine doctors as well as Chinese medicine practitioners, so that we can meet demand of the masses and carry our ancient traditional medicine forward. This is a critical mission for developing our hygiene industry, as well as being an historical act. Nowadays, the Ministry of Health has already decided to develop new Chinese medicine practitioners to reinforce the hygiene work team. According to the Ministry of Health plans, some Chinese medicine practitioners will train in Chinese medicine schools, while the rest through apprenticeship programs. Therefore, organizing an apprenticeship system is now the most important item for the Ministry of Health.

Why did apprenticeship system become the new main method to train up Chinese medicine practitioners? Because Chinese medicine knowledge has been passed down for thousands of years without being organized systematically. Precious clinical experience was recorded in ancient literature and spread to millions of practitioners' hands. It will be hard to pass down Chinese medicine and inherit this tremendous knowledge only by school education. There have been many ways to hand down Chinese medicine knowledge for thousands of years, the main method being the apprenticeship system. It has a very important effect, so for now we still use it to train up new Chinese medicine practitioners. Under the leadership of every department of health in the entire country, we should ambitiously encourage and organize the apprenticeship system and develop it.

In the old society, there was a lot of flexibility in the apprenticeship system. They didn't consider how to teach, how to learn and how to practice what you've learnt. Now, although we still adopt the apprenticeship system, we can't follow it in the old way. Instead, we need to train up apprentices strategically and help them practice Chinese medicine. We need to consider the masses' needs and the medical progress in our country, as well as the career plan and future of the Chinese medicine practitioner. We need to think about the quality and quantity of Chinese medicine practitioners that we train. For those newly trained, we should not only sensibly arrange their work place, but also ensure their improvement into the future.

In order to conserve what was mentioned above, first of all, there should be a minimum number of apprentices able to inherit Chinese medicine knowledge from experience of current Chinese medicine practitioners. After working for a fair amount of time, they should receive further education to absorb a certain degree of modern medical knowledge to enhance their skill. In an apprenticeship program, we should emphasize both quality and quantity evenly; it is incorrect to do it in a shoddy way. Any Chinese medicine practitioner who is willing to lead an apprentice, whether in a health center or a United Clinic, should be applauded. Yet, their apprentices should inherit completely their experience and become proficient in a certain subject or skill, and be able to treat patients independently. After the apprenticeship is completed, the local department of health will issue a degree certificate and be in charge of arranging their duty.

All departments of health have started already the arrangement of apprenticeship programs; the problem in the future will be to empower those who are leading the program. We should follow the Party line in deciding the many problems that may arise; for example, who teaches apprentices, who leads them, how do they learn, how do we lead them? Furthermore, regarding different methods for different subjects, if we try to set up one solution for all problems, it would never work and it's not appropriate. As for the health department main function, it should provide specific help, for example, register the number of apprentices, determine supplementary teaching materials and help teachers solve problems encountered during the teaching process. Furthermore, all departments of health in our country should plan meticulously according to local needs, and put it at the top of their working schedule. In order to complete the mission, we should know the current situation well, plan the work ahead on a reliable foundation, according to local demands and possibilities, and process a series of thinking and organizing to facilitate the main work.

It's our generation's mission to train up new Chinese medicine practitioners. It's also the honorable job of health departments in every level, Chinese medicine practitioners and the masses. We should try our best to accomplish it.

Article end

Under the policy of debates among different schools of thoughts, we should debate on what most people agree with and what should be developed

1956 by Song Airen 宋愛人

Source: *The New Chinese Medicine Magazine*, September 25, 1956
新中醫藥第七卷第九期

Yaron: We get now to a brief moment in Chinese Communist history when freedom of debates was afforded and encouraged. It was shortly thereafter that tides turned and whoever dared speaking his/her mind against the Party's policy became a target: an anti-Party Rightist. From that point on, there were no more debates in Chinese medicine, just a delicate maneuvering of "what is allowed and what is not allowed".

Pages 389–391

One night we had a meeting on "encouraging the development of all academic schools".

Yesterday I read an article from May by Lu Dingyi 陸定一 about the May 26th speech, "Debates among different schools of thoughts, and let a hundred flowers bloom", acknowledging that the Chinese Communist Party supports development of different forms and styles of art and welcomes all debates among different schools of thought about scientific work. Let me discuss the policy of "letting a hundred flowers bloom". Mr. Lu said in his article, "Take a most recent example; drama. Several years ago, there were still some people against Peking Opera. During that time, our Party decided to support the development of different forms and styles of opera. Now, as everybody can see, this policy was correct. Because of all kinds of competitions, assessment and learning from each other, the progress of drama is huge."

From this angle regarding scientific work, the government suggests that we should open the "debates among different schools of thought". We believe this is as important as the policy of "letting a hundred flowers bloom" for art work, which inspires popularity and much progress, bringing it closer to our needs in the area of arts. After we start this policy, we can expect not only the improvement of our scientific technique but also the production of excellent scientific work. Besides, through all sorts of communication and interaction in these debates, we can inspect and learn from each other, help each other, work as a team in the scientific field and improve ourselves so our scientific development can continuously propel forward.

Following, I present two suggestions for "debates among different schools of thoughts":

1) Emphasize what most people agree with
2) Emphasize what should be developed

1) Emphasize what most people agree with

Mr. Lu said, "Two thousand years ago in our country was the Spring and Autumn and Warring States Periods. There were debates among different schools in academia, which made this period a golden period for academia. But, during that time, society was in turmoil and debates were spontaneous instead of being led."

As we know, debates among different schools during Spring and Autumn and Warring States Periods did exist, and it was a golden peak era. Yet, why couldn't it stop the jostling between supreme powers? To the contrary, statements by School of Diplomacy figures, such as Suqin 苏秦 and Zhangyi 張儀, facilitated the separatist regime and instigated a situation where the weaker was the prey of the strong. This made civilians destitute and homeless.

It is because during this era, debates were spontaneous without a uniting leader. Although some schools of thought grew larger, other grew smaller or lasted only a short while and, while receiving no support, receded. Quyuan 屈原 from Chu State 楚國 had sighed, "The golden bell was abandoned and replaced with earthenware pots", which meant the government was not using talented people and instead was letting mediocre people into the higher ranks. We can imagine the situation during that time.

We can conclude that some of those debates aimed to weed out malpractices and improve techniques of different industries and all people's health, so they represented most of the masses. There may have been some small debates not representing the masses' demands, so these didn't get much support and disappeared soon thereafter. Therefore, today, we should emphasize what most people need and agree with, and then we will be able to achieve progress in all kinds of industries.

Mr. Lu said, "In order to strengthen our country, we should not only consolidate people's political rights, develop the economy and education and facilitate national defense, but also improve the cultural art and scientific industry, otherwise there is no way for a prosperous development." This is the necessary trend for our social development. So, while encouraging debates among different schools of thought in the field of science, we should start with people's real needs. Like this, we can gain many advocates and much support, even if we just begin with a simple sentence on a piece of paper.

2) Emphasize what should be developed

Mr. Lu said, "We have a great national legacy, such as native medicine, agriculture, philosophy, history, literature, drama, painting, music etc. We should learn them intensely and accept others' criticism, as we didn't do much of it yet." Our original science is varied and colorful. We should have specialists remove the rubbish and retain the precious in order to meet the masses' demands. Then we could apply it to real practice. In the debates among different schools of thought, we should emphasize what should be developed.

Mr. Lu instructed us, saying: "While facing our national cultural legacy, we should carefully choose the items we wish to protect and develop and honestly criticize its mistakes and shortcomings."

Let's talk about our traditional medicine.

Traditional Chinese medicine was recorded in debates during Spring and Autumn and Warring States Periods, *Neijing* 內經 being one of the examples.

The *Book of Han Han Shu – Yiwenzhi* 漢書藝文志 states that there were four kinds of books of medicine Fangji 方技: medical books Yijing 醫經; prescriptions Jingfang 經方; bed chamber Fangzhong 房中; and Gods and deities Shenxian 神仙. We know that the reason Han Dynasty medicine could achieve huge progress is because there were debates among different schools. One school even contained seven groups, as recorded in *Book of Han*, and included two hundred and sixteen articles, although the names of these seven groups have already disappeared. The *Suwen* 素問 and *Lingshu* 靈樞 that we read today don't have two hundred and sixteen articles and so we know that many ancient schools of medicine did not survive; this is an incalculable loss of our cultural legacy. Although the current *Neijing* is incomplete, we can still confirm that it had a status in our medical legacy, shown by a statement of the seven groups prevalent in ancient medical books of those debates.

Wang Yan 王炎, in *Xin An Wen Xian* 新安文献, said, "*Suwen* is ancient words of Qin Dynasty, and although it might not be all Huangdi 黄帝 or Qibo's 岐伯 words; during Spring and Autumn and Warring States Periods, there were people who were good at medicine such as Hesui 和綏 or Qinyueren 秦越人, however, their description of the function of Yin-Yang and five elements was not as incisive as *Neijing*."

Song Lian 宋廉, in *Wen Ji* 文集, said, "Although *Huangdi Neijing* 黃帝內經 was suspected to have been falsified by Qin Dynasty scholars, its words are profound and its idea is overwhelming and worth promoting. According to textual research it is reliable and borne out of evidence. It should be the main classic among different schools of medicine."

Lü Fu 呂復 said, "*Neijing Suwen* was called Huangdi Qibo's 黃帝岐伯書 book, however, its ideas do not seem from one time and one place and how it was recorded not from one person. Liu Xiang 刘向 said it was made by aristocracy in Han 漢 State, and Chengzi 程子 said it was accomplished around the end of Warring States Period."

Gu Congde 顧从德, in the preface of Song version *Su Wen*, said, "*Neijing Suwen* is actually Huangdi's book of pulse, which got broadly spread by Qinyueren 秦越人, Yangqing 陽慶, Chun Yuyi 淳于意 and other respectable people."

Huang Xingzeng 黃省曾, in *Neijing Zhu Bian Xu* 內經注辨序, said, "Since Shennong and Huangdi it's been practiced for long and we found that many people from many dynasties had assumed Huangdi's book as the ancestor."

From this literature we can see that traditional Chinese medicine, no matter in which aspect—lifestyle, herb decoction, massage or acupuncture—came from the accumulated experience of the great working people. Also experienced doctors such as Yihe 醫和, Bianque 扁鵲, Yangqing 陽慶, Canggong 倉公 etc., passed down their knowledge and experience orally and in writing to later generations in order to put their theories into practice. Only then did Chinese medicine become prosperous and competent during debates of that time. These debates represented medicine, what people needed the most, and therefore it became very popular and passed down for more than two thousand years.

Our chairman Mao has instructed us, "If Chinese culture is to contribute to this world, then Chinese medicine must be included within." Since we inherited traditional Chinese medicine, we should aim to pass down this knowledge as did Bianque and Yihe and other respectable people, emphasizing what should be developed.

I'm going to provide my undeveloped opinions based on comrade Lu's 陸 words. Comrade Lu said, "It has been shown in our history that if there's no encouragement of independent thinking and free discussion, academic development will stop. On the other hand, if we encourage independent thinking and free discussion, our academic development is able to achieve great progress." Today, our debates, independent thinking and free discussion already received the people's encouragement. We should be passionate, learn from and criticize each other, speak for the masses and emphasize what should be developed and what are people's needs. Conservative thoughts and exaggerating styles are not allowed. Then, no matter whether our statement of medicine is big or small, it can fit in the debates we have.

People want rapid development of science, a conscious plan for the entire science work and they want us to take the policy of debates and, with it, facilitate academic development. This is also the conclusion of every scientific worker after going through these debates. Scientific workers want to cooperate and work more like a team in order to fortify the foundation of our academic development.

Article end

Unify Chinese medicine and Western medicine to head in the direction of scientific technique

1956, by Chen Susheng 陈苏生

Source: *The New Chinese Medicine Magazine*, September 25, 1956
新中醫藥第七卷第九期

Yaron: No freedom of opinions. The independent Chinese medicine practitioner is categorized as one of the "conservatives who think themselves heirs." It became clear that having an individual opinion about Chinese medicine is not going to end up well for one's person. All practitioners unanimously must think "through combining Chinese and Western medicines, soon there will be a medical scientific 'New Chinese medicine'". They must understand that following orders is a higher cause: "We can raise up the level of our sciences only when we have political agreement, and then Chinese and Western medicines can work together to expound and develop our science for the people's benefit and like this earn honor in the world for our country." It is the time when an intensified selection process begins for TCM schools and curriculum. It is now becoming a new medicine.

Pages 392-393

"Unify Chinese medicine and Western medicine to serve all people" has been a principle of hygiene work by our Chairman Mao for more than ten years. However, during these last few years—and due to lack of traditional medicine culture knowledge—the supervising department of hygiene administration didn't follow or carry out the policy of unifying Chinese and Western medicine. Instead, it rejected and discriminated against Chinese medicine and limited its practice. Like this, it defeated the passion of Chinese medicine doctors and also affected the development of our hygiene industry.

The Chinese Communist Party and People's Government often pay attention to the Chinese cultural legacy, and their Chinese medicine policy is very clear. Whether we can unify Chinese and Western medicines well influences all people's health, the development of medicine in our country and the development of science for benefiting people of the entire world.

In order to carry out the correct Chinese medicine policy, our Party and government have done much research on the topic; they also criticized Wang Bin 王斌 and He Cheng's 賀誠 thoughts. Now, it's fashionable for Western medicine to learn from Chinese medicine. This shows that our Party's policy is correct and matches Truth.

We know that our traditional medicine has been passed down for thousands of years and it includes abundant content and precious experience. How to inherit this cultural legacy and make it help the people more efficiently should be executed by all medical personnel. It is a difficult but also glorious mission.

Medicine is a science that people use to fight diseases. Hygiene work masters this science to get rid of upcoming disease threats and so it wins people's love, esteem and respect. Medical science belongs to the people. All people working to strengthen people's health should not have divergence among them.

As people know, the objective of both Chinese and Western medicines are the masses. The goal is to extinguish diseases and maintain people's health. Although there are some differences in terms of tools and forms of execution, they both help people fight diseases. They have the same goal and same mission; obviously they are "battle companions" on the same front.

Since Chinese and Western medicine are "battle companions", they should have worked together and been friendly to each other. However, feudal thoughts and capitalism left from the old society, which is expressed as conservatism and sectarianism, separated these two battle companions and made divergence between them. This divergence blocks medical culture development and affects the hygiene industry achievement. It's no doubt a huge loss for the people.

Chairman Mao, in *On Coalition Government*, has said, "any scientist, engineer, technician, Chinese and Western medicine doctor, and other intelligentsia, as long as they serve the people, they deserve respect from the government and society and to be regarded as precious treasure of our country." We can see that the government regards both Chinese and Western medicines as very important. So if you ask someone a question about Chinese and Western medicines, the masses will reply that we need both Chinese and Western medicines as long as they serve the people wholeheartedly and solve people's problems and reduce people's pains from diseases. On the other hand, if either Chinese or Western medicine treats us poorly, we will be upset. This means that Chinese and Western medicines are regarded as equal by most people.

A small number of conservatives regard themselves as heirs of our traditional medicine, which otherwise has been solving diseases for thousands of years. These people don't care if Chinese medicine makes sense or not in a scientific way as long as it cures diseases.

A small number of sectarians hold the opinions that Chinese medicine has no scientific value at all and it will be rather an obstacle for the development of science. Therefore, in order to have a better scientific growth, we should extinguish Chinese medicine.

Because of these two kinds of incorrect thoughts, there have been many unnecessary conflicts for decades. This has increased the difficulties in implementing medical practice and has confused people about it.

We know that both Chinese and Western medicine each have their own advantages and shortcomings, and difference in quality certainly exists. But, in short, either one has value to be preserved and disadvantages to improve. They both serve the people and take care of people's health by using different ways to fight with a mutual enemy: diseases. Meanwhile, they can complement each other's shortcomings, learn from and support each other. Only like this can they both improve their ability to serve the people.

One should acknowledge that if we use Western medicine diagnostic methods in Chinese medicine practice, then we can obviously treat diseases in a more accurate way. Likewise, if we adopt Chinese medicine experience in Western medical practice, then we can expand the treatment scope (ie, acupuncture therapy).

It doesn't make sense that Chinese medicine cannot apply scientific diagnosis and that Western medicine cannot improve by using Chinese medicine.

Comrade Liu Shaoqi 刘少奇 has said that the conflict between Chinese and Western medicines is like the Peking opera play *San Cha Kou* 三叉口, having people trying to hit each other in the dark, which is totally useless.

The plot of *San Cha Kou* tells of two groups of people both trying to protect Jiao Zan 焦贊 but they fight each other due to misunderstandings. Similar is the conflict between Chinese and Western medicines. In principle they have the same objective, which is to take care of people's health. Now, because of conservatism and sectarianism, they become each other's enemy. This misunderstanding should be solved; Chinese and Western medicines should learn from each other and remove all shortcomings. This is the scientific attitude and spirit of seeking truth from facts.

There is an old Chinese saying, "It's a good cat no matter whether it's black or white, as long as it kills rats." This can be the metaphor for Chinese and Western medicines. They have the same goal, which is disease; as long as it can cure disease, it works. So they should work together to cure diseases.

Comrade Xie Juezai 謝覺哉, in the health report, said, "Mysterious phenomena should be in the past. Now, as a modern doctor, it's unacceptable to have no scientific knowledge. As a Chinese doctor, it's unacceptable as well to have no traditional medicine knowledge." He also said, "About medical knowledge, some came from abroad and some came from our own culture, doctors shouldn't have different titles such as Chinese or Western medicine doctors. Instead, Chinese and Western medicine should work with and learn from each other." He pointed out that through combining Chinese and Western medicines, soon there will be a medical scientific "new Chinese medicine".

Dear Chinese and Western medical comrades, the era is calling the intelligentsia; we have twelve years to work on unifying Chinese and Western medicines to welcome the peak of socialist construction. We can raise up the level of our sciences only when we have political agreement, and then Chinese and Western medicines can work together to expound and develop our science for the people's benefit and, like this, earn honor in the world for our country.

Article end

Presidential Address

1956 by Fu Lien-Chang 傅連璋

Source: *Chinese Medical Journal Foreign Publication*, September–October, 1956
中華醫學雜誌外文版

Yaron: This is a foreign language publication so we keep the language without corrections other than obvious typos. It is a translation by a native translator of that time. This may help us see how China wished to present itself to the West. Chinese medicine played a role in presenting the new China to the West: "The subscription of the *Chinese Medical Journal* in English has also increased, and it has exchange relations with 270 journals abroad, an important factor in our country's international interchange of information and research in medicine."

As for the forced cooperation between Western and Chinese medicine doctors, this article explains it clearly. Not only were opinions within Chinese medicine silenced, but also Western medicine was no exception; everyone needed to accept what they were told: "A change finally came about upon repeated instructions from the Central Committee of the Party, and in 1953, a Committee for Exchange of Experience between traditional-style and Western-trained doctors was established at the head office. Forums were held on traditional Chinese medicine, and traditional-style doctors were invited to attend academic meetings. In 1954, our Association began to accept traditional-style doctors as members. Meanwhile, enthusiasm rose throughout the country for studying traditional medicine."

Chinese medicine practitioners may have wanted this recognition but Western trained doctors certainly did not. In the end and despite the oppressive state of Western doctors, most influencing for TCM was the forcing of Western doctors to learn Chinese medicine who then needed to produce scientific discoveries: "We call upon those western-style doctors who have been successful in learning from Chinese medicine to tell us of their experience and ideas, for this will be a powerful means of promoting further study of Chinese medicine."

The activities of the Chinese Medical Association and its future tasks[448]

Four years have passed since the Ninth General Conference of the Chinese Medical Association. During these years, under the leadership of the Communist Party and the government, the people of our country have made great strides along the path of socialist construction. Now, with the First Five-Year Plan approaching fulfillment, great changes have taken place in our society and work of all kinds is developing with great rapidity. Economic construction, national defense and cultural development are making new demands on the scientific workers of the whole country and are opening up to them ever wider fields of activity. We, the medical workers, are facing much heavier tasks than ever before.

Before discussing the further development of our academic activities, let us first summarize and take stock of the work of our Association since the last general conference.

Our work during past four years

During the past four years, the patriotic feeling of the medical workers of our country has risen higher than ever under the stimulus of socialist construction. As a result of their deepened political and philosophical understanding, the quality of their professional work has greatly improved. Unity among medical workers has been strengthened, especially between western-trained and traditional-style doctors. A tendency to disparage our medical heritage has been severely criticized, and study and research in traditional Chinese medicine have been fostered throughout the country with some fruitful results. Planned research in medical science is spreading on a wider scale in response to the needs of national construction and the health of the people. Exchange visits with medical circles abroad are becoming more frequent. These, together with the fostering care given by the Party and the government, are responsible for the steady progress of medical science in China in the period under review.

In the past few years there have been several new developments in the Chinese Medical Association. First of all, there has been a great increase in membership. At the time of the Ninth General Conference there were 6,819 members, but now the

[448] [Original footnote] Summing-up report presented at the Tenth General Conference of the Chinese Medical Association held in Peking from July 23 to 29, 1956.

number is 15,059. The rate of increase has been especially marked since 1954, when our Association opened its doors to traditional-style doctors, whose membership now numbers 1,037. This has not only increased the cooperation between doctors of traditional and Western medicine but is a promising sign that, in the future, there will be a great upsurge in the development of medicine in our country.

In order to promote the further development of academic activities, it was decided at the Ninth General Conference to establish special scientific societies. Fourteen such societies in the fields of internal medicine, surgery, pediatrics, obstetrics and gynecology, public health, ophthalmology, otorhinolaryngology, tuberculosis, radiology, dermatology and syphilology, neurology and psychiatry, stomatology, pathology and medical history have already been established. In addition to the above there is also a Committee for the Study of Hospital Administration. The 43 local branches of the Chinese Medical Association have established branch scientific societies according to the specialties of the local members. The organization of the headquarters of the Association has been strengthened, and there has been an improvement in maintaining connections with the local branches.

An overwhelming majority of the members of the Chinese Medical Association has actively participated in the various patriotic movements and in social activities. Regarding other important problems of both internal and external significance—such as the cease-fire negotiations in Korea, opposing the use of the atomic weapon, the New Constitution, the policy towards intellectuals and analysis of the ideological errors of Ho Ch-eng 賀誠 and Wang Pin 王斌—the headquarters of our Association has organized forum discussion for medical specialists and members of our executive committee. The various local branches have also engaged in activities in this direction.

Academic activities

Regarding the extension of academic activities, we have, during the past two years, laid emphasis on raising the equality of our work. The branch scientific societies have intensified methodical planning of their work both on a long-term and a short-term basis. For instance, the Societies of Internal Medicine, Surgery, Public health, Dermatology and Syphilogy, Obstetrics and Gynecology and Pediatrics have started on a large number of specialized subjects for study and have made concrete plans for division of work toward this end. Many of the subjects proposed are related to public health, occupational diseases and the common epidemic diseases. Recently, a considerable amount of work has been done in different localities in the eradication of schistosomiasis. The various local branches of the Society of Ophthalmology have engaged in wide discussion on the classification of trachoma. The Society of Tuberculosis has adopted the Soviet classification of tuberculosis. The Society of Radiology has proposed research into problems of early diagnosis and treatment. The Society of Otorhinolaryngology has examined and analyzed the possibilities of using acupuncture in the treatment of ear, nose and throat diseases. The Society of Obstetrics and Gynecology conducted, in 1954, an analysis of 33,000 cases of ovarian and uterine tumors collected from thirteen hospitals in nine cities dotted throughout the country. A number of societies have proposed setting up standard procedures for diagnosis and treatment of certain important diseases and compiling statistical data for physiological norms in Chinese. The Societies of Stomatology, Pathology, Medical History and Neurology and Psychiatry have all been active, although the membership of some is comparatively small and some have been established only recently.

Since 1953, the headquarters has organized forum discussions on selected topics with the participation of specialists from all interested departments. The proceedings have been published in the journals and have been of great help in our practical work. The branch scientific societies have organized many meetings on medical subjects, which may be divided into two categories according to their character and content:

1. Discussions on specialized medical subjects in different forms—reports on special subjects, forum discussions, analysis of case histories, clinical and pathological conferences, review of literature, while some of the branch societies have even organized ward rounds and inter-professional consultations in special cases; and

2. Meetings for the spreading of medical knowledge and for assistance in the professional studies of the general run of medical workers. These meetings mainly took the form of discussions on selected subjects, study meetings or training classes held in conjunction with the local public health authorities. The Shanghai branch of our Association also organized a lecture group in cooperation with the Shanghai branch of the Chinese Society of Physiological Sciences which gave lectures at Ch'angchow, Wuhsi and other places, receiving a warm welcome wherever it went.

The editing of medical journals is an important aspect of the work of the Chinese Medical Association. At the time of the Ninth General Conference, the Association published eight different journals; the number is now sixteen. In addition, quarterlies have been transformed into bi-monthlies, bi-monthlies into monthly publications. At the moment, the total yearly issue of the sixteen journals numbers ninety-five issues, with a total subscription of 210,000. These journals provide useful information and study material for our medical workers. The subscription of the Chinese Medical Journal in English has also increased, and it has exchange relations with 270 journals abroad, an important factor in our country's international interchange of information and research in medicine. Improvements also have been made in editing our journals. Articles are now coming in from a much wider field and there is more planning in the editing and selecting of material. What is specially worth mentioning is that the contents of most of the journals have been strengthened as regards our traditional Chinese medicine.

There have also been striking developments during the past few years in learning from the advanced medical science of the Soviet Union. Enthusiasm for the study of Pavlov's theories has increased greatly since the Ninth General Conference and in both medical research and clinical work, Pavlov's views are becoming the basis of medical thought. The problem before us is to apply these theories in a real, and not in a superficial, manner in our practical work.

Cooperation among medical workers

Here we must emphasize the work we have done in bringing about cooperation between Western-trained and traditional doctors and in studying the traditional medicine of our country. Firstly, in spite of an appeal from the Central Committee of the Party to study the ancient medical heritage of our country and put it at the service of the people, it must be admitted that the Association paid insufficient attention to the matter. At the time of the Ninth General Conference, all that we did was to help health organizations to promote further study and training for traditional doctors; little was done to utilize fully the service of traditional doctors or in research in traditional medicine. A change finally came about upon repeated instructions from the Central Committee of the Party and, in 1953, a Committee for Exchange of Experience between Traditional-style and Western-trained Doctors was established at the head office. Forums were held on traditional Chinese medicine, and traditional-style doctors were invited to attend academic meetings. In 1954, our Association began to accept traditional-style doctors as members.

Meanwhile, enthusiasm rose throughout the country for studying traditional medicine. Many of our branch associations followed the example of the head office in organizing Committees for Exchange of Experience between Traditional-style and Western-trained Doctors, and scientific societies of the branches of our Association in various places began to learn from, and adopt the experiences of, traditional doctors and to study the history and special achievements of Chinese medicine in their particular fields. More recently, some branches have organized groups for the study of special subjects in which old Chinese methods of healing are particularly efficacious. The Peking branch, under the leadership of Professor Li T'ao, has compiled a catalogue of books on Chinese medicine in the five big libraries of Peking; our regional association in Shanghai and the Society of Medical History and the Pharmaceutical Association in that city have held an exhibition of Li Shih-Chen's books; these activities being coordinated with the movement to learn from Chinese medicine. Now that a large number of hospitals throughout the country are inviting traditional-style doctors to participate in their work, cooperation between traditional-style and western-trained doctors has become closer as regards both the study and practice of medicine.

Criticism directed at disparagement or underestimation of the role of traditional medicine has had considerable effect in promoting the coming together of traditional-style doctors, in bringing about a fuller use of both Chinese and Western medicine, and in the joint study of Chinese medicine by both traditional-style and Western-style doctors. It may be claimed that the hiatus between old-time and Western-trained doctors has now been bridged as regards medical studies, medical practice and medical organization; thus a foundation has been laid for further and ever closer cooperation in developing the medicine of our country. However, we are not completely satisfied with what we have done in this work. Henceforth, we must still consider it to be one of the most important tasks of the Association.

Internal cooperation

Lastly, we have done a certain amount of work in promoting international contacts. During the past few years, owing to objective factors, and the great development of the World Peace Movement, there has been an increase in our contacts with medical organizations in other countries. In 1953 a group of representatives of Chinese medical workers, headed by Dr. Fang Shih-Shan, vice-chairman of the executive committee, was sent out by our Association to take part in Vienna in the World Congress of Doctors for the Study of Present-Day Living Conditions. On their way back, in response to invitations from the Soviet Union and Czechoslovakia, they visited Moscow, Leningrad, Prague, and Brno. Dr. Pai Hsi-Ch'ing, member of our executive committee, who was elected secretary of the World Congress of Doctors, has taken part regularly in the work of the secretariat of the organization.

Living Conditions and Health, the medical journal published by the World Congress of Doctors, will be distributed by six countries, in six different languages, and the Chinese Medical Association will be responsible for the Chinese edition which will be distributed from Peking. During these past years, we have frequently acted as host to medical friends from abroad. We have organized discussions and exchanged information with them, invited them to give lectures on medicine and given them opportunities to see all aspects of our society. We have also sent delegates abroad to attend medical conferences in many different countries. In 1955 alone we had contacts with medical workers of twenty different countries; a French, a Franco-Belgian, and a Japanese delegation to exchange specialists to give lectures. In April and May this year, a medical delegation from Argentina was received by us. We have sent medical groups to the Soviet Union, Yugoslavia, Poland, Switzerland, Japan, Sweden, England and Pakistan to attend international medical conferences. Among our medical specialists, Dr. Wu Ying-K'ai has been elected an honorary member of the U.S.S.R. Scientific Society of Surgeons. Drs. Chung Huei-Lan, Wu Juei-P'ing, and Ch'I Chuang-Huan were made honorary members of three Soviet Scientific Societies at the Thirteenth All-Union Congress of Hygienists, Epidemiologists, Microbiologists and Infectionists. Drs. Shen K'o-Fei, Huang Chia-SSu, Wu Ying-K'ai, Lan Hsi-Ch'un, Wu Chieh-P'ing and 24 others have become members of the International Society of Surgery. All this shows closer cooperation between medical circles of our country and our medical friends abroad.

Shortcomings

The above are our achievements but, of course, there are still defects in our work.

As has been indicated, what we have done in cooperating with the traditional-style doctors and in studying our medical heritage is only a beginning and has not yet, by a long way, attained what is required of us in this respect. The attitude of indifference, or even disparagement, towards our traditional-style doctors and medical heritage has been criticized, but evidently not severely enough. This can be seen from the fact that very few articles of a profoundly critical and analytical nature have appeared. The movement calling upon Western-trained doctors to learn from traditional-style doctors was launched two years ago, but no periodical summing-up of experience has been made in order to further the movement. No clear decisions have yet been made as to the most effective method of learning from traditional doctors or the best order in which Chinese medical books should be studied. Up til now, there has been no consistent plan in arranging our ancient medical books and their explanatory notes and introductions. Although traditional-style doctors have been admitted as members of our Association, the number is still too small and should be increased.

There have been deficiencies also in our academic activities. This is shown by the inadequate discussion of conflicting or different views; scholarly discussion or argument has not been sufficiently widespread. There is too wide a gap between our academic activities and the actual needs confronting us. For instance, not much guidance has been given in industrial hygiene and the prevention and treatment of endemic diseases. Too little has been done in introducing to our members the current accomplishments of medicine throughout the world.

The contacts between headquarters and the branches of our Association are not sufficiently close and for this the former must be held responsible. Headquarters has insufficient understanding of the work of the branches and has not given them practical guidance in solving some of their difficulties. In the case of those branch associations which have done good work, we in the head office have not sufficiently examined the reasons for their success so that their experience can be widely adopted. In regard to increasing the membership of our Association, the work has been dilatory. A great many people qualified to become members have not yet joined our Association. The reason for those deficiencies is to be found partly in insufficient personnel at the head office, and partly in defective working methods. Also, the work of our regional associations is not all on a high level; some of them are very active and others just the reverse.

The tasks before us

Alongside the socialist construction of our country, and the raising of the cultural and living standards of the people, there has been unprecedented development in science, including medicine. The tasks before us are to utilize to the fullest extent the medical personnel, both traditional-style and Western-trained, in the forward movement in medical science and promote cooperation among our health workers in service of the people.

To raise the level of medical science

To actively and energetically improve the level of our scientific work, to institute and develop scientific study and research, is the common direction in which all scientific workers are moving. The Association must organize all our medical workers to concentrate their efforts in this direction.

The health administration, together with scientific organizations, are now formulating a twelve-year plan of scientific research. As regards research in medical science, we need to direct our attention primarily to the following: prevention and cure of the most prevalent diseases; arranging and systematizing the theories of Chinese medicine and studying its practical experience; inquiry into the uses of new drugs and new medical equipment; further research into labor hygiene; and improvement of environmental hygiene and the nutrition of the people. The headquarters and local branches of the Chinese Medical Association and all the scientific societies should place their whole energy at the disposal of the health authorities in this research program.

We must clearly realize that research in medical science is not the function of medical institutes and societies alone, but is also the concern of the mass of medical workers. In the field of scientific research, in addition to relying on scientific research institutes, the great bulk of medical workers must also participate. All our members should play an active part. Only by a thorough implementation of the policy, "let all schools of thought contend", by encouraging original thought in scholarship and learning, by advocating free discussion and argument, can the progress of science be promoted. The aim of controversy is to stimulate study and research, to explore deeper into science and to raise continuously our scientific level. There should be this kind of controversy not only between traditional-style and Western-trained doctors, but also between members within these schools. The bringing forward of different theories and views by different schools of thought in free and open discussion can only help the development of medical science.

Before liberation, there were in our country the "English", "American", "German", and "Japanese" cliques in medicine which existed to "contend" for their own fame, benefit and position. We oppose such "schools", for they are deleterious to the welfare of the people and obstruct the progress of science. But we are by no means against schools of thought arising from differences of opinion in study and research. The "contention" of such schools can only be of benefit to the people and promote the progress of science; Pavlov's ideas are undoubtedly the most advanced in medical theories but we should not promote them to the exclusion of other theories and ideas. From now on, while still concentrating on learning from Soviet medicine, we must at the same time study and learn from the medical achievements and contributions of all other countries. We should learn not only from the People's Democracies but also from the capitalist countries. The "contention of all schools of thought" is not restricted to fully developed theories but also includes the expression of partial or incomplete views and fragmentary ideas, as long as they are apposite. Henceforth the task of our various medical journals will be heavier; their editorial boards must become the hub around which scientific "contention" will revolve.

To study and utilize Traditional Chinese Medicine

To learn from the medical heritage of our country is an important part of our struggle on the scientific front. The movement for Western-trained doctors to learn from traditional-style doctors has only just begun and we must continue to promote it with all our strength. We must continue to criticize disparagement of our traditional medicine and contempt for traditional-style doctors for such behavior obstructs cooperation between the two schools. We must attempt to persuade those Western-trained doctors who do not yet recognize fully the importance of learning from our traditional medicine. We call upon those Western-style doctors who have been successful in learning from Chinese medicine to tell us of their experience and ideas, for this will be a powerful means of promoting further study of Chinese medicine. There are many methods of study but the most important is humbly to seek out traditional-style doctors as teachers and to learn from their practice.

Under the unified leadership of the Ministry of Health, research institutes and schools in Chinese medicine are being established. The Chinese Medical Association should have close contacts with them, coordinate its work with theirs, hold frequent meetings for interchange of experience and publish regular reports of study and research in traditional Chinese medicine in our journals and papers. As for specially effective cures practiced by Chinese medicine, we should help the health authorities to spread them widely. The Ministry of Health is preparing to establish, in various places, committees to promote study of traditional Chinese medicine by Western-trained doctors. The local branches of the Chinese Medical Association should have close relations with these committees and help them in their tasks. Research into the history of medicine is also important. We must make the history of the development of Chinese medicine available to all medical workers.

The Association should take the initiative in enrolling all the traditional doctors of wide experience and knowledge as members.

And how should traditional-style and Western-trained doctors "contend"? "Contention" between them certainly does not mean that each school should obstinately harp upon its own merits and criticize the point of view of the other. It means that each school should not only develop its own particular merits but also study the merits of the other, thus helping to raise the level of both. The task before us is that the two schools should learn from each other and more especially Western-style doctors should learn from traditional doctors.

To strengthen international exchange of medical knowledge

The development of the World Peace Movement and our notable contributions to that cause, together with our socialist economic and cultural construction, have succeeded in drawing increasing numbers of foreign friends to visit our country. It is necessary for us to establish friendly relations with all scientific circles abroad who wish to have contacts with us. Visits between the Chinese Medical Association and medical organizations abroad will undoubtedly increase. This is an important aspect of our work. These visits will not only promote the development of medicine through interchange of medical knowledge, but also serve to strengthen world peace.

As has been mentioned above, foreign medical delegations and individuals who have visited us have carried back with them very good impressions. But in our work as host there is room for improvement.

The *Chinese Medical Journal* in English, edited by our Association, is the only foreign language publication we have for exchange with foreign countries. Henceforth it should be fuller in content and obtain a wider circulation.

Much of the material on medical subjects that we have sent abroad in the past has not been carefully enough prepared and has not fully reflected the conditions of health work and the development of our medical science; neither has it been scientific enough in character. This has been due to insufficient preparation in the collection of statistics and other materials. From now on, we should seek to strengthen our relations with the health authorities in order to improve this aspect of our work. Attention to this should also be given by our regional associations throughout the country.

Unity and cooperation

To carry out properly the tasks enumerated above, closer unity is of paramount importance. The "contention of all schools of thought" can only be achieved on the basis of solidarity and cooperation. Although in the past few years there has been a marked improvement in cooperation between traditional and Western-trained doctors, as evidenced by the rapid development of the work of the Association, yet we cannot say that cooperation is close enough in every institution or administration, or in every aspect of work. It is necessary for us to oppose anything inimical to unity and solidarity, and we should concentrate more on our political studies so that our ideological level will be further raised.

Unity covers a wide field. It includes all who are ready to contribute their efforts for our country and people. Our socialist construction is in urgent need of scientific personnel. The chief difficulty before us in health work is insufficient personnel. We cordially invite those medical workers and specialists who are studying abroad to return and work with us in the common cause of promoting the health of the people. Unemployment of trained personnel is a thing of the past and will never come back again. Independent, democratic, free and exuberant New China is opening up, with inexhaustible power, a road for culture and science with ever widening horizons.

We fully understand the feelings of envy and admiration with which our health workers now stranded in Taiwan regard the tremendous progress on the mainland in the reconstruction of our country. Taiwan will certainly be liberated. We are doing our best to achieve this peacefully and we would like to bring about its realization through the joint efforts of our colleagues now in Taiwan. We welcome them, whenever they are ready to come to the mainland, and will put their abilities to mainland but who would like to see with their own eyes the developments in health work during these past years and other aspects of our construction are welcome to visit us. We also wish to establish connections with them for exchange of medical knowledge and experience.

Article end

[Book] Chinese medicine knowledge

1956 by Li Tao 李濤 and others

Distributed by: Hong Kong Scholarship Bookstore, Printed: December 1956
中醫的知識李濤等著香港學問書店印行 12 月 1956 年

Yaron: Being traditional was China's main problem; Li says it's time to change this attitude.

Page 13

China's medical science development and accomplishment

By Li Tao 李濤

In the middle of the 17th century, the Qing government adopted a stern policy of closing up. There was no exchange with foreigners. The result was that Europe developed as a capitalist society from the 17th to the 18th centuries, while Chinese people continued a small scale agricultural and household industry. The feudal economy stagnated and the culture adopted an air of secrecy. These were entirely the workings of the government at the time. The Qing government's cultural policy adopted the Ming's eight-part essay 八股文取士 of selecting talented persons to official positions, which tied down the scholars' ways of thinking. In a different aspect, it encouraged textual criticism. It meant taking the literary person's spirit and wearing it down in a hip of musty old books, causing his thoughts to depart reality. This general atmosphere was adapted by doctors as well, making them believe that "revering the ancients" is the skill needed. Many doctors polish their style via the *Neijing* 內經, *Shang Han Lun* 傷寒論, *Ben Cao Jing* 本草經 and these kind of works, holding them as genuine. One can say that their work and the true purpose of medicine have nothing in common.

However, the people of China all possess the sense of acquainting true principle. No matter how sternly the Qing government enforced closing-down policy, prohibiting the import of Western knowledge, educated persons still had the courage to absorb true principle like Zhao Xuemin 趙學敏 and Wang Qingren 王清任 (1767–1827) etc. When Western people introduced Chinese medicine to Europe, to the contrary, reception was ever-continuous. It had the ability to help Western medicine develop.

Chinese Medicine Style and Content

By Chen Susheng 陳蘇生

Yaron: Chen lays out exactly what the scientists of TCM need to discover.

Page 21–27

Look at acupuncture and moxibustion—in the past there were people who thought that this therapy model was discovered fully by the ancients, and yet modern people still acknowledge its efficacy in the face of this fact. However, it is still not easy to explain the mechanism by which acupuncture works, how it can heal infectious diseases and diseases that modern medicine still stands helpless against. If we follow modern scientific theory of neurological diseases in order to research acupuncture's clinical efficacy this may lend a hand in explaining this one point. For example, when advancing acupuncture's clinical efficacy research, it is possible that modern medicine's theory will write a new page. To an extreme, there might be a whole new understanding for human health and the adjustment of patient's organic activity and its nerves. This will mean that, for this external acupuncture therapy, not only will it have actual content but rather this will be very deep content!

There is no need for many examples. To summarize: The content of Chinese medical and cultural heritage is rich without equals. Each expression of the different medical styles contains different kinds of accumulated experience. From all different kinds of medicine styles and medicines by different people of different nationalities, extracting their true contents, analyzing their expressions, exposing their roots is in order to know nature and, with that, benefit from nature. Still a step further, it is in order to change nature. This is the task and purpose of arranging medicine and culture.

Informal discussion about Chinese herbal medicine

By Tu Dengbang 涂登榜

Yaron: Tu lays down the TCM principle that treatment is done by symptoms, which later were called "pattern differentiation". No matter if one was a Confucian doctor or a quack, if he followed the symptoms he was successful.

Page 23-25

As for all the different kinds of formulations, even though there are places that cannot be explained scientifically yet, amongst them, some more some less, directly or indirectly, come from the masses' practical experience. No matter if it is from a long line of doctors, Confucian doctors or even the quacks, they all master, some more some less, the medical prescriptions. As long as they treat the disease in accordance with the symptoms, they will have the efficacy of "miraculous medical skills". Practice and experience is the foundation for all types of science and therefore Chinese medicine is very scientific. It conforms to its most basic requirement. However, Chinese medicine was born and developed amongst the people and, therefore, one cannot avoid the people's customs being attached to it, for example, the Daoist and Buddhist influences. Its theory also acquired, at times, an outer garment of mysteriousness, which hindered its progress. Yet its essence is still scientific. Until today, many health-preservation folk customs, according to modern scientific medical theory and practice, all testify to abundant scientific value.

From our nation's medical quintessence to examples from the peoples' customs, I narrate the following: From the peasant and cities in the Yangzi river basin, every time when they get to the Dragon Boat Festival[449] each household has the good custom of sweeping their house clean. After sweeping they use realgar 雄黃 to fumigate inside the house in order to eradicate the Five Toxins. Each household during this festival soaks garlic heads and realgar in liquor, to be used during the upcoming summer months to rub toxic insect's bites with. Every child in the household hangs on his chest one or more fragrant bags in order to expel and pestilent Qi (infectious diseases). Or they hang on the door Mugwort leaves Ai Ye 艾葉 to show that they swept the interior of the Five Toxins. The medicines used in the above example, when scientifically analyzed, are found to contain antibacterial effects.

Tea, tobacco and wine were first discovered in China. Small dose of tea, smoke and liquor has an exciting effect on the body. Tea also has a diuretic effect. Liquor has anti-bacterial and anesthetic effect. The regular folk of China use water pipes to smoke, which is very scientific. When tobacco smoke goes through water some of the nicotine is being absorbed by the water. This helps preventing smoke intoxication.

[449] On the fifth day of the fifth lunar month.

No matter if in the cities or countryside, folks in the heat of summer like to sip tea in order to prevent passersby from drinking unboiled water and contracting a disease.[450] Also in the countryside some farmers know that when they labor in the heat of summer, to drink salty tea, in order to supplement the body's salt the deficiency caused by sweat.

During meals adding vinegar has anti-bacterial effects, which prevents infectious diseases.

In the recent 100 years our country received considerable negative influence from foreign countries, and so the people are not likely to view our nation's own folk medicine as so important. In the recent few years, our country appealed for uniting Chinese and Western medicine and for Western medicine to learn from Chinese medicine 團結中西醫, 向中醫學習. And so, in many parts of the country, there established Chinese medicine research organizations. Even though their research period is yet very short, however, their achievements already startle people. Like in Heibei's Shi Jiazhuang 石家庄 city hospital in their Chinese-Western collaboration group. They reported several dozen cases of curing type B encephalitis. This disease is as of today considered hard to treat anywhere around the world; every year the mortality rate is very high. Experiencing our country's medicine with these kinds of examples, if one would add more research experience to it, it will be then possible to reach an international scientific level of our medicine.

Other examples for application of Chinese medicines there are: Bai Tou Weng decoction 白头翁汤 can treat amoeba dysentery, Huang Lian 黄连 can cure bacterial dysentery, Chang Shan 常山 and Ya Danzi 牙胆子 can cure cholera, Du Zhong 杜仲 tincture and Xue Mo decoction can treat high blood pressure.

In recent years, we found out that Yin Qiao San tablets 银翘散片 can cure the common cold. When washing the skin with this formula it can also relieve toxins and itchiness.

These few examples of accomplishment above are all not so simple to attain. Many ailments still don't have cure in modern medicine and yet Chinese medicine can cure them. We cannot be but very thankful to our ancestors for handing down to us the most precious family treasure. What is sad is that we, sons and grandsons, because of receiving such a negative educational impact from foreign lands, turned

[450] From contaminated water.

our own education to a family whose fortunes were dissipated, sons and grandsons. As if the accumulated family treasures we gathered over the history are now all of a sudden looked upon as useless antiques.

All the slanderous attacks in the past against Chinese medicine and herbs now have facts to prove them otherwise. If only we could study and research it with humble hearts, we will discover our nation's most precious, richest and most scientific treasure. Now we can only wait for the entire country's Western and Chinese medicine to collaborate, and together formulate scientific research path. Expose the richness of our treasure from every angle. Not only will it be able to solve swiftly most of the health hazard people are suffering from, it will also enrich the international scientific medical knowledge.

Talking about moxibustion therapy

By Li Youshen 李幼申

Yaron: Just like scientific medicine, Li finds a physical reason for moxibustion and acupuncture efficacy. The new "scientific" discovery supersedes the older primitive explanations showing that there is no real difference between acupuncture and moxibustion; they both simply stimulate nerves.

Page 122–123

The curing principle of moxibustion

From our rudimentary understanding of the neurological action theory by the great scientist Pavlov, we can understand that the nervous system is the organizational unifier of the human body and that the cerebrum's two hemispheres of the central nervous system (the cerebral cortex) is the supreme command. At the same time, explaining further inside the cerebral cortex, the nervous system's normal action is either a process of "excitement" or "restraint". Under normal conditions, these two processes stimulate and lead each other and therefore at all times can adjust the body's internal transformations.

As for the development of disease according to the Pavlov principle, it is like this as well; pathological developments are all the same. It is always a conflict between the excitement process and the restraint process. In other words, it is because the normal balance of the two becomes upset. Because of this, it is easy for us to explain the principle behind moxibustion's curative effect. It is mainly via the use of heat to stimulate the skin surface in specific locations (acupoints, also called stimulating points) in order to arouse and adjust the body's higher nervous system mediating function and controlling function.

The difference between moxa treatment and acupuncture treatment

The difference between moxa treatment and acupuncture treatment is the methodology. In moxibustion we use heat to stimulate the skin receptors, whereas acupuncture is a mechanical stimulation. Aside from the application to the skin receptors, acupuncture can also directly impact deeper-lying nerves. However, the two—acupuncture and moxibustion—from stimulating the central nervous system point of view, are identical.

Yaron: Other articles in this book compare Chinese and Western medicine or explain merging them together:

Seeing the scientific nature (of medicine) from the records of vessels in the Neijing 內經, by Geng Jianting 耿鑑庭

Informal discussion about high blood pressure by Sheng Zhonggui 沈仲圭

Chinese medicine view and treatment of rheumatism by Sun Shuqi 孫書棋

Chinese medicine understanding and treatment of kidney inflammation by Yue Meizhong 岳美中

How does Chinese medicine treat Type B epidemic encephalitis? by Liu Zhiming 劉志明

Some experience in Chinese medicine treatment of neurasthenia by Zhao Timeng 趙惕蒙, Li Zhensan 李振三 and Wang Zhanxi 王占璽

Achievements of Chinese medicine with external injuries by Li Yisan 李益三

The superiority of Chinese medicine treatment of hemorrhoids and fistulas by Zhou Jimin 周濟民 and Chen Zhihan 陳之寒

Chinese medicine knowledge of painful periods and its treatment by Yu Ruifeng 于銳鋒

Chinese medicine contribution to obstetrics by Zhu Shimo 朱師墨

Discussion about nausea and vomiting during pregnancy by Yu Daoji 于道濟

Chinese medicine prevention of trachoma by Wei Wengui 韋文貴

Chinese medicine massage by Lu Yinghua 盧英華

How to learn well the *Nei Jing Zhi Yao* 怎样学習內經知要

1956 by Qin Bowei 秦伯未

Source: *The New Chinese Medicine and Pharmacology Magazine Xin Zhong Yi Yao* 新中醫藥, December 1956, 7th volume 6th issue, Published by the New Chinese Medicine and Pharmacology Society

一九五六年十二月號第七卷第六期新中醫藥雜誌社出版

Yaron: The following two article excerpts are from Qin Bowei in Communist 1956 and from Qin's student Ma Shizhi in the Republic 1929. Both excerpts talk about Yin Yang and here are brought together for comparison purpose. During the 1950s, medicine was navigated toward the prevailing ideology of "dialectical materialism", whereas during the 1930s the struggle with Western medicine and modern science triumphed and so, as we see, Chinese medicine steered in the overall direction of the time. I have marked several lines in bold for easy assessment.

Chinese medicine was always subjected to a "some" process of selection: some people selected some of its content for some reason.

Excerpt page 249, point (2)

About Yin Yang

The ancients experienced and observed the objective contradiction-unity phenomena of nature. They had **a sort of perceptual knowledge and from this they arrived at a rational knowledge**. These became the rules for the sense of principle that came to explain the myriad problems. This is the origin of the Yin Yang theory. The *Nei Jing* borrows this Yin Yang theory to understand and address the myriad problems within the medical field, mainly using the **mutual connectedness and mutual restriction** of it. Since the *Nei Jing* uses Yin Yang to represent **varying degrees of opposites in phenomena**, it is not like a fixed entity. Therefore, in addition to descriptions such as "when Yang accumulates it's heaven, when Yin accumulates it's earth", "the outside is Yang, the inside is Yin", "the back is Yang, the abdomen is Yin" and "Yin is quiet, Yang agitated" etc explaining the meaning and location of Yin Yang, other descriptions go on to describe the functions of it like "when Yang is born Yin grows, when Yang dies Yin conceals", "Yang transforms Qi, Yin makes form", "when Yang wins there is heat, when Yin wins there is cold", "clear Yang exits the upper orifices while turbid Yin exit the lower orifices", "when Yin wins then Yang is diseased, when Yang wins then Yin is diseased" etc. Therefore one can see that **Yin Yang is a name describing mobility**. In any kind of situation one can describe Yin and Yang, however in medicine it is not so simple and stiff.

It is exactly for that reason that if one merely puts forth the term Yin and Yang, it is not possible for him to resolve carefully a more complicated problem. And so, with this, Yin and Yang were divided further into another Yin Yang. It became "in the midst of Yin there is Yin, in the midst of Yin there is Yang, in the midst of Yang there is Yang and in the midst of Yang there is Yin". One must be clear-cut, however, that **no matter how Yin Yang change, forever they are relative opposites and not absolutes. They are mutually dependent, unable to be separated or stand alone. Specifically, they require the equilibrium between the two**. The *Nei Jing* puts forth:

> The essence of Yin Yang, that Yang condenses then it becomes resolute, if the two don't harmonize, it is like the spring without the autumn, like winter without summer. Because of this, when one harmonizes them it is called the extent of the sage. Therefore if Yang is stiff and can't condense, Yin Qi then perishes, when Yin is even then Yang condenses, the spirit essence is then in order.

This explains the balance inside the body and that only then one can respond to the external surrounding stimuli. The opposite of it, is that if one's body loses the internal balance then it creates physiological chaos. It is the main reason why one will become sick. This is the *Nei Jing* extremely important holistic point of view of Yin Yang. Chinese medicine, while using a definite objective view of phenomena and things, applies these abstract nouns: Yin Yang. **It establishes a simple and unadorned dialectical materialism point of view**, creating the basic system for China's medical theory.

End of *Chinese medicine knowledge* book excerpt

About Qin Bowei 秦伯未

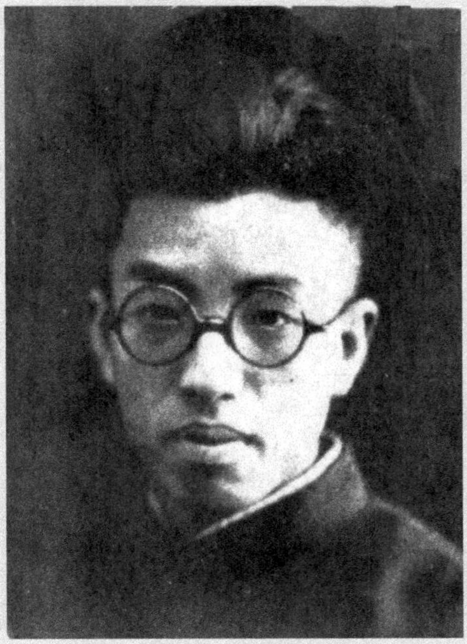

Qin Bowei 秦伯未 (1901–1970): In 1919, enrolled in Shanghai Chinese Medicine Specialized School 上海中醫專門學校 and studied from Ding Ganren 丁甘仁, graduated in 1923 and remained in same school as teacher. In 1927, with several other practitioners (Wang Yiren 王一仁, Zhang Cigong 章次公, Wang Shenxuan 王慎轩, Yan Cangshan 严苍山), founded Shanghai Chinese Medicine Academy 上海中国醫學院 and served as the academic dean.

In 1930, founded the Chinese Medicine Guiding Society 中醫指導社. He compiled *A Collection of Chinese Medicine Guiding Books* 中醫指導叢書 and published the *Chinese Medicine Guiding Records* 中醫指導錄 magazine. In 1938, founded Chinese Medicine Caring Hospital, which had 100 patient beds and served as base for many students' clinical training.

In 1955 he moved to Beijing and served successively as a Chinese medicine advisor to the Central Ministry of Health, a committee member of Beijing Chinese Medicine College, Zhong Hua Medical Sciences Association vice president, the chief of the National Science and Technology Committee and a committee member of the Chinese People's Political Consultative Conference.

About Ma Shizhi 馬師贄

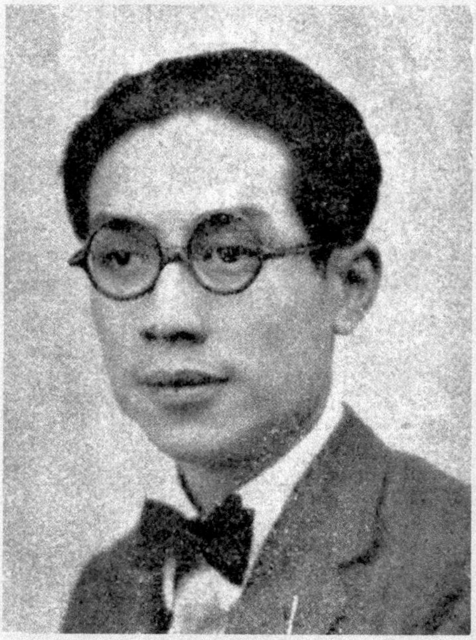

Ma Shizhi 馬師贄, a student of Qin Bowei who graduated from the first class, was also active at the May 4th movement in Guangdong.

Birth place (included in the graduation book): Guangdong Shunde, age 25, address: Guangzhou city, Nanguan Daxiangkou 9 Hao.

A general discussion about Chinese medicine theory

中醫學說概論

1929 by Ma Shizhi 馬師贄

Source: *Chinese Medicine Academy: The First Graduating Class Commemorating Publication,* Published in July 1929 by the Chinese Medicine Academy

中國醫學院第一屆畢業紀念刊

Comparison article from Qin's student Ma Shizhi written in 1929

The physiology of Yin Yang, water fire, blood and Qi

The pathology of wind, cold, summer heat, damp, dryness and fire

The basis for Chinese medicine theory is that man reacts to Heaven and comes in contact with the material Earth. Chinese medicine always paid attention to experience and yet neglected a principle for future generations to follow as a set routine. Even though **throughout the generations there were many commentators, what they recorded were strained interpretations.** As time went by, **the more they did it the more it became mysterious**. Now in all earnest, **how can this kind of mysteriousness treat people's diseases? Normally medical science is a very complicated kind of research. Medical science must get physiology in its grip and only thereafter can it understand pathology. Now since the medical science of the West uses dissection for experimental observations on pathology, they fly and advance compared to their knowledge prior to the 18th Century**.

Now **if we take the Western medicine** and summarize it and observe it a little, we see that they have two aspects. From physiology point of view they set up the nerves and cells as the two foundation blocks. From pathology point of view they have bacteria and physiological reaction that creates their pathology theory. This allows the student to feel that he knows what he has learned. With this, one can see their revolutionary spirit. **It is unlike my Chinese medicine theory which is different from clarity and logic**. In contrast, how astute is Western medicine. Absolutely, when they diagnose a patient, they cannot swallow a situation where "the manifestation to the contrary is claimed as cause". **Western medicine with its diagnostic methods** may sometimes find the cause itself as the disease, how come it is so? **I do not reject Western medicine theory** as being "untrustworthy," because it is not partial and not leaning to one side. Chinese medicine can have a principle though. Because of this, my suspicion of Chinese medicine is even greater than my suspicion toward Western medicine.

I use my suspicion attitude to contemplate the content of Chinese medicine theory. I want to see in it the true principle that Western medicine up to date did not discover yet. **I want to follow our own Chinese medicine treatment experience and compare it to Western medicine treatment**. I want to find the strong points of each one. Therefore, when I think of the earlier people introducing mysteriousness into Chinese medicine, they caused the people to know very little about Chinese medicine, which is a great deficiency. Any kind of theory cannot shape up just from looking at the surface of things. **The foundation must have concrete methods and only after that can it become a medical science and treat disease.**

The cause of disease of course finds itself in physiological changes. The physical body comes in contact with the external environment's stimulation and then it starts to change. These are called diseases. Of course, disease can start from physiological changes occurring within the body. However when it comes to external stimulus, both Chinese and Western medicine recognize the following causes: "seasons, local features of a place, daily life, food and drink" etc influences. These may promote physiological activities but can also harm the body.

Since both Chinese and Western medicines **observe the physiology** and have experience with pathology of the human body during its birth and growth, it is known that Yang alone cannot give birth and Yin alone cannot give growth. The myriad things in the universe rely on both heaven and earth. Heaven and earth have their root in Yin Yang, the place where the two Qi accumulate. The core of Chinese medicine theory is Yin Yang principle. It is used to assess every situation. In addition, the creation and formation of a human indeed starts with a merge of Yin Yang "father and mother exchange essence, attain spirit and then there is life". This is how *Nei Jing* explains the beginning of physiology. **What we call water, fire, blood, Qi are names that Chinese medicine derives out of experience with physiology**. As for analyzing pathology, it divides even further into wind, cold, summer-heat, damp, dryness and fire all sorts of physical phenomena that impact the body from outside and cause pathological changes in the body and so they have these disease names. **This is what we call experience-based development of Chinese medicine theory.**

Now, **earlier people often pretended themselves smart** and when explaining things didn't rely on physical evidence. They only followed the texts and teachings and turned it into what we see today as a mysterious kind of a thing, a lock that has lost its key. Therefore, **my feeling is that Chinese medicine is in the error of earlier people's explanations**, causing the society as a whole to have doubt in it. I cannot but speak to our society and people about Chinese medicine principle and not go through the Western scholar's knowledge. I explain for a moment and allow them to understand the foundation of Chinese medicine, allow students to have a standard for research and, even more, regroup Chinese medicine people and the people that believe in them, allowing all to get at a resolution. Now, my research of Chinese medicine is just of few years and so I write *A General Discussion About Chinese Medicine Theory* and take the following physiological items to discuss briefly: Yin, Yang, water, fire, blood, Qi, wind, cold, summer-heat, damp, dryness, fire etc.

1. Physiological assessment of Yin-Yang, water-fire and blood-Qi.

Yin-Yang physiology

What kind of a thing is Yin Yang exactly? "Looking at it, it has no form", "listening to it, it has no sound". **Chinese medicine using it in order to deduce human physiology, no wonder people describe it as unreal and absurd**. Unreal is not a mistake, sure enough its trace is close to unreal. Therefore, it is said that Yin Yang itself can have endless and inexhaustible transformations. One sentence absolutely cannot explain its entire function. And so, in our Chinese medicine, when Yin Yang are mentioned it always has founded and trustworthy truth that can be relied upon and substantiated.

Yang—it is not the Yang of "Tai Yang" kind of Yang, but rather it is the Yang Qi inside the body. **This kind of Yang Qi is what Western medicine calls "body temperature". It is an ability that the human body has**. This is the explanation of Yang.

Yin—it is not the Yin of "Tai Yin". Yin is the "counter representation" of Yang. It is the opposite side of Yang. **In the human body, it is a kind of ability to mediate the body temperature.** After it harmonizes with Yang Qi it becomes a kind of "life force". This is the explanation of Yin.

Water-Fire physiology

So what kind of thing is "fire and water"? Water and fire is much easier to understand than Yin Yang. In the body, blood, sweat, mucus and saliva are all fluids. **Inside the body, everything contains a water component that can be analyzed by a scientific method. It is something that can be seen, not something made up**. So what can we say about fire then? **The use of fire is a kind of electric and heat function**. Any movement in the body, be it blood circulation, limb movement, organ metabolism, all stem out of the electric and heat action of the body. In the West, they say that nerves are responsible for sensory and motor actions. **So may I ask, the nerve action—does it not rely on electric and heat action? However, the nerve distribution is only in threads, therefore water and fire merge together and only then it generates electric force and heat force.**

Water—water physiology is soft, harmonious and able to be tolerant with all organs. **In the human body it is like the steam of the locomotive** that because of it, it can come to life. This kind of application is the explanation of water.

Fire—**the physiology of fire is like the heat force and electric force that comes out of the engine**. This kind of application is the explanation of fire.

Article excerpt end

Destroy Rightists' conspiracy: Health Daily Editorial

Source: *Xin Zhong Yi Yao*, August 25th 1957

新中醫藥　一九五七年八月　第八卷第八期

Yaron: If there was ever any doubt in a doctor's mind that he should not innovate things other than exactly what he was instructed to, then this article sure explained it to him well. In a scientific experiment, one develops a theory and then puts it to the test—if the test fails the theory collapses. In a way, the newly-created hybrid scientific TCM was the opposite of science: the results were predetermined, regardless of the test. It was an ideological construct, in which anything and everything was permissible as long as the predetermined objective is reached. Today, we simply cannot keep doing this. If we want to develop our medicine we need to find a way to undo this awkward construction.

Pages 341–342

The public health anti-Rightists battle is already in full swing all over the country and it will become bigger and broader in the future. Anti-Rightist revolution movement is political and socialistic and can ensure the leadership of the Communist Party and also become the basis for victory of our medical work. Therefore, medical workers should wisely attend to this battle against Rightists' schemes in order to win a victory.

Rightists are aggressively attacking the Communist Party; their conspiracy is to steal the leadership of sanitary works and follow capitalism. First of all, they communicate with reactionary people and say that all the directorship positions are occupied by Communist Party members, so there is no use to it. Jin Baoshan 金寶善 is so arrogant that he even slanders the Communist Party by saying "from the Ministry of Health to the leaders of the Central Communist Party there are no thoughts about prevention", implying that all Health Departments and the Central Party are unprofessional and don't understand the industry so they should change to someone who is a professional to lead the team. (Yet the suggestion for prevention was actually brought up by the Party and the Party is also executing this suggestion). They not only ask the Health Department to invite more "scientific experts to attend the administrative leadership" and "add some scientists", but also "ask scientists to join automatically". They are so eager to steal the position of leadership. Now their conspiracy is revealed; the Rightist students in Beijing Medical School health department suggest Jin Baoshan 金寶善 to be the chief of the Ministry of Health. Xue Yu 薛愚 also said "Ministry of Health should get rid of some people who don't understand the profession and add some who do…", which actually implies that the chief of the Ministry of Health is very unprofessional and should be replaced by a professional Rightist. Li Zongen 李宗恩 took the Ministry of Health leadership seal from Zhang Bojun 章伯鈞.

In order to materialize their reactionary scheme, they even lied about the facts, made up rumors by saying "there's no execution of prevention policy", "hospitals and pharmacies got endless damage", "Union Hospital is a child bride", "Union Hospital is worse than before being taken over" etc. They distorted all facts and the Communist Party's policy about sanitary works; for example, they said "the Party's instruction to Chinese medicine in 1954 was overcorrection", "the regulation of hospitals is a mistake", "the teaching reformation is wrong", "Ministry of Health pays too much attention to doctors and too little to drugs, too much to treatment and too little to prevention" etc. They even objected the "resist America" aid[451] and our support to Egyptian war.

Other than distort facts and enchant crowds, Rightists have tried to associate with other anti-Communist and anti-socialist organizations through the Chinese Peasants' and Workers' Democratic Party to attack the Communist Party. It is proven by facts that Rightists are not pure scientists but rather aggressive politicians and are very passionate about anti-Communist reactionary political activities. Li Zongen 李宗恩 is not eager to attend political activities of the New China but he is helping with developing an organization by Zhang Bojun 章伯鈞 and trying to lure more people in.

---

[451] Aid to North Korea in the resistance war against the United States.

Rightists know that they need to develop organizations and recruit new people to achieve their ambition of at least sharing equal status with the Communist Party or even replacing it. Li Zongen 李宗恩 had said, "With organization and opinions the power will be strong"; apparently, what he truly meant was "with organization the power to attack the Communist Party will be strong". We should be aware that Rightists are against socialism and the Communist party when they plan an organization; we shouldn't regard their tricks as a personal scheme.

Another way Rightists attack the Communist Party is to drive a wedge between the Party and the masses and incite the masses' dissatisfaction toward the Party. They take advantage of reputation and positions, such as representatives of people and political consultative committee members, to spread rumors and make up things. For example, they say epidemic prevention workers don't receive much attention, pharmacists have no chance to escape from oppression and discrimination, they challenge the Ministry of Health leadership in public and set the worst example in the entire country. Not only in Beijing 北京 but also in Tianjin 天津 and Wuhan 武漢 they try to instigate medical schools' students to be against the Communist Party. These are all their conspiracies.

After medical and public health circles had attacked back, Jin Baoshan 金寶善, Li Zongen 李宗恩 and Xue Yu 薛愚 have revealed their true faces. Under the guise of experts or scientists, they are, in reality, evil aggressive politicians trying to steal the leadership of the medical industry and take it on the road to capitalism, which is similar to the time when Kunmintang and American imperialism ruled together. We certainly can't repeat the sorrowful history and let the medical industry go backwards. Therefore, the anti-Rightist battle is the battle for the fate and future of the people's medical industry; it also relates to who will lead this industry and what path it will follow. Do we want our medical industry to go back to a leadership of bureaucracy and capitalist class or do we want the Communist Party to lead us to socialism? We can only choose one of the two options. Indeed, this is a battle about choosing socialism versus half-feudalism half-colonialism.

Therefore, at the frontline of the anti-Rightist battle, it is a good opportunity to strengthen ourselves and it is also a good test to see if we can firmly follow socialism and make a clear distinction for every single medical worker being a Rightist or not. We should uncover fake masks of Rightists and attack them and break all their schemes with no mercy. We should strongly advocate the leadership of the Communist Party and know that it takes us toward developing socialism.

Article end

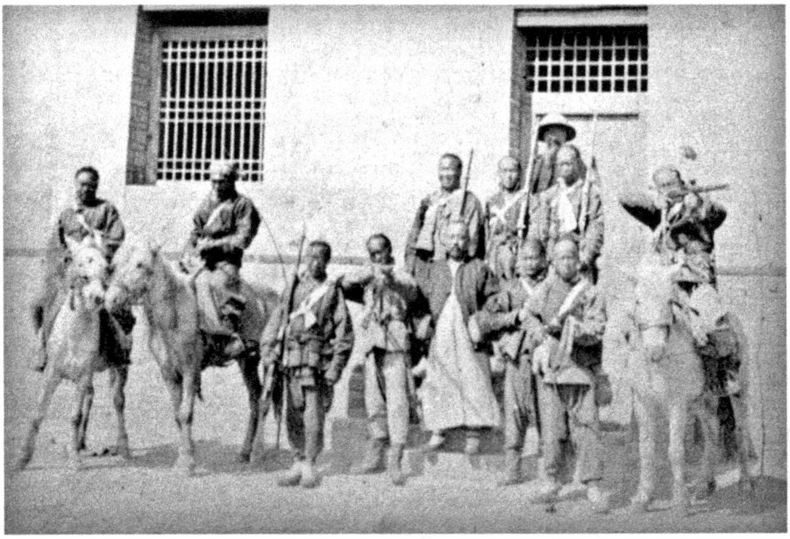

Photo by Mr P. Goux in early 1900s. "Armed Chinese Christians coming back from an expedition against the Boxers".

The Party's policy brings a new face to Chinese medical work

1957 by Lu Bingkui 吕炳奎

Source: *Xin Zhong Yi Yao*, August 25th 1957

新中醫藥

一九五七年八月

第八卷第八期

Yaron: The mass popularization on a national scale of this new and ideologically-influenced style of medicine. Because of this mass popularization, five decades later to newly-arriving students, this will seem as the Traditional Chinese Medicine; a medicine that was always like this since times immemorial.

Pages 342–343

Lu Bingkui 吕炳奎, Chief of Chinese Medicine Department of the Ministry of Health

In old China, Chinese medicine was objected to and attacked and although Kunmintang's plan of stopping Chinese medicine totally failed, Chinese medicine was in a worse position. After liberation and under the leadership of the Communist Party and People's Government, the political status of Chinese medicine has risen. Especially after the Party executed the *Chinese Medical Work* policy in 1954, that the old thoughts to extinguish Chinese medicine, prevalent during Kunmintang ruling period, disappeared. Chinese medicine turned positive and served socialistic construction more effectively.

Chinese medicine status has obviously risen

Due to correct execution of the Party's Chinese medicine policy, its political and social status improved and now there are Chinese medicine representatives among current people's representatives and political consultative members. In many health administration departments or medical centers there are a few Chinese medicine doctors in position of leadership. According to an uncompleted statistic, the heads of twelve provinces are Chinese medicine doctors and there are two thousand Chinese medicine doctors as members in the Chinese Medical Association. Chinese medical status is higher than at any time in the past and doctors are more willing to provide their books, experience and proven formulas. These years, more than 17,600 proven formulas were collected.

Obvious development in Chinese medical work

Chinese medicine has a new character following the Party working with the new Chinese medicine policy. As for Western medicine learning Chinese medicine, six classes of two years have been established in Beijing, Tianjin, Shanghai, Wuhan, Guangzhou and Chengdu. More than three hundred Western medicine doctors joined the classes and one year later they were already able to compose academic essays, see patients and prescribe formulas.

Meanwhile, in order to adjust to different situations in different places, there are also half-year classes and on-the-job training classes of which both can provide some Chinese medical knowledge to Western medicine doctors. As for the aspect of clinical practice, 144 Chinese medicine hospitals and more than 450 Chinese medicine departments have been established. Other public medical centers also recruited roughly 29,000 Chinese medicine doctors (about 21,000 in health administration departments and 8,000 in other departments).

In order to develop new personnel, other than the apprentice system which has brought us 44,000 new doctors, four Chinese medicine colleges (Zhong Yi Xue

Yuan 中医学院) were also established in Beijing, Shanghai, Guangzhou and Chengdu in order to train new Chinese medicine doctors. Chinese medicine schools (Zhong Yi Xue Xiao 中医学校) were established in many provinces such as Guangxi, Hebei, Tianjin, Shanxi, Jiangsu, Jilin to train professional Chinese medicine workers. In order to elevate the level of Chinese medicine, there are twenty-three Chinese medicine training schools (Zhong Yi Jin Xiu Xue Xiao 中医進修学校) in all provinces and cities, some starting Chinese medical correspondence classes and training classes.

To adjust to the need, Chinese medicine publications progressed as well. 209 kinds of Chinese medical books, 3.82 million books in total, have been published. Furthermore, Chinese medicine has a distinct impact on society as well. There are more than 80 United Chinese Medicine Hospitals 联合中医医院, more than 50,000 United Clinics 联合诊所, about 10,000 agricultural health centers and about 200,000 Chinese medicine doctors are working for them. The combination of the full-time and half-time people's health organization and other Chinese medicine services can facilitate the deficiency of public hospitals and also provide opportunities for Chinese medicine to practice.

Chinese medical prevention is very effective

Chinese medicine, through the experience of Chinese and Western medical collaboration, has been found effective in the treatment of not only chronic diseases but also some acute and chronic contagious diseases.

For example, Chinese medicine shows clear efficacy treating epidemic encephalitis B using the treatment principle of epidemic febrile diseases 温热病. This treatment principle has been applied in the entire country and saved many lives. In Hunan Province Yiyang City 湖南益陽市, Chinese medicine cured thirteen Japanese B encephalitis patients without recurring symptoms using lying-in-mud therapy which won praises from Russian experts. Four hundred leprosy patients of different types had obvious improvement from Chinese medical treatment in a leprosy hospital in Liaoning 遼寧 Province. The most dangerous and virulent is Schistosomiasis. Chinese medicine has devoted many proven formulas which are very effective for ascites. For example, in Hunan Province's Yuanjiang City 湖南沅江市, doctors treated 130 ascites patients with advanced Schistosomiasis using modified Wei Ling Tang 加減胃苓湯 and Jiang Pan Wan 絳磐丸 and the therapeutic effect was up to 80–90% without recurrence. In Zhejiang Province Hangzhou City 浙江杭州市, fifty Schistosomiasis patients were treated with compound prescriptions for seven months, 48% of them becoming negative afterwards. In Shanghai in the 11th People's hospital, bacillary dysentery patients are treated with Bai Tou Weng Tang 白頭翁湯 which is 100% effective and regarded even better than sulfanilamide and without side effects.

Furthermore, there is a large enough number of patients in the statistics of diseases treated by Chinese medicine to prove it has good therapeutic effect, such as influenza, cirrhosis, digestive ulcer, poliomyelitis, cataract, epidemic meningitis, pneumonia, brucellosis, malaria, scarlatina, diphtheria, filariasis, ancylostomiasis, syphilis, hepatitis, nephritis, diabetes, hypertension, measles, pertussis, menoxenia, pelvic infection, vomiting of pregnancy, bone tuberculosis, quinsy, neurodermatitis, keloid, arterial embolism etc. As for acupuncture, Qigong therapy, bone setting, and Tuina, they all have high medical value.

Chinese medicine is valued in many other countries

Due to its practical therapeutic value and plethora of scientific research, Chinese medicine has been taken seriously in other countries. People from Russia and other democratic nations often study Chinese medicine and travel to China to inspect Chinese medicine and herbs, which is a good starting point for international academic interaction. We should dedicate more effort towards it in the future.

Chinese medicine work has gotten already great accomplishment. However, there are some mistakes in the execution of Chinese medicine policy. Those mistakes were caused during the developmental process of Chinese medicine and are easy to revise. After we rectify incorrect styles of work and subjectivism, bureaucracy and sectarianism, then the Party's policy for Chinese medicine will be executed in a better and improved fashion.

Article end

Prove measurements and method of Quchi 曲池 point in anatomy

1957 by Chen Dazhong 陳大中

Source: *Xin Zhong Yi Yao*, September 25th 1957

新中醫藥

一九五七年九月

第八卷第九期

Yaron: The instruction given was that acupuncture must be proven to work via nerves; the following article is the result.

Page 436

Quchi [Li11] is a commonly used acupoint and also He 合 point of hand Yangming 陽明 Large Intestine Meridian, which is located around the center of upper limb outside of elbow. With the elbow bent, the point is at the concave of the origin of the line of the elbow cress. Locate the point with the hand touching against the chest.

The anatomy description of this point in *Chinese Acupuncture and Moxibustion Zhong Guo Zhen Jiu Xue* 中國針灸学 is "on radial muscle, on the branch of back arm cutaneous nerve and radial nerve, there's radial recurrent artery."

In *New Acupuncture and Moxibustion Xin Zhen Jiu Xue* 新针灸学 the anatomy description is "it's around the lateral epicondyle of humerus and radial side of the joint, the origin of extensor carpi radialis longus muscle, outside of brachioradialis, there's radial recurrent artery and innervation of radial nerve and posterior cutaneous nerve of forearm."

The two paragraphs largely describe the anatomical location of the point Quchi 曲池 and clinically when we needle the point Quchi 曲池, according to patients' statements, there is an achy distended feeling radiating down to fingertips of index finger, mid finger and thumb. Some patients feel the sensation only going to the fingertips of index finger and thumb. As for the sensation mostly going up around the shoulder, only a few patients can feel it up to the face. Hand Yangming Large Intestine Meridian 手陽明大腸經 starts at the point Shangyang 商陽 [Li1] on the radial side of the index finger and ends at the point Yingxiang 迎香 [Li20] next to the nose on the face.

Its large collateral connects to the point Pianli 偏歷 [Li6] communicating with the point Lieque 列缺 [Lu7] of hand Taiyin Lung Meridian's 手太陰肺經 large collateral, which demonstrates that lung and large intestine are interior-exterior related. Based on the description above, we may assume that the sensation should radiate to the fingertips of index finger and thumb. However, the result of clinical experience is mostly radiating to the fingertips of index finger, mid finger and thumb. Is that because the needle also punctures hand Jueyin Pericardium Meridian 手厥陰心包經 at the same time? In order to get the answer, we did an experiment on a cadaver, and we dissected it four times in total.

Instructions: Let the cadaver lie facing up, both elbows bent in front of the chest. Use an injector to withdraw colorful liquid so pretending to be a gold needle. Puncture the needle in the point Quchi 曲池 as when doing acupuncture, insert one drop of the colorful liquid every 0.3 unit until the insertion is one and a half unit deep.

We found out through dissection that when puncturing the point Quchi 曲池 with the elbow bent, before it went one unit deep, it hit the main stem of radial nerve. After it went to a depth over one unit, it hit the median nerve. The innervation of radial nerve is around hand Taiyin Lung Meridian 手太陰肺經 and hand Yangming Large Intestine Meridian 手陽明大腸經, and that of median nerve is around hand Jueyin Pericardium Meridian 手厥陰心包經. So through this experiment, it became clear that doing acupuncture on the point Quchi 曲池 is simultaneously stimulating the three meridians mentioned above: hand Taiyin 手太陰, hand Yangming 手陽明 and hand Jueyin 手厥陰 meridians, and different postures such as bent or extended elbow can cause different distribution of internal tissues inside the point.

The diseases' range that Quchi 曲池 can treat is very broad; it can treat things like "painful pharynx and not be able to talk, distention and agitation in the chest" according to description in ancient medical literature, which proved that hand Yangming Large Intestine Meridian 手陽明大腸經 has certain relation to hand Taiyin Lung Meridian 手太陰肺經 and hand Jueyin Pericardium Meridian 手厥陰心包經. Therefore, in the medical literature it says that doing acupuncture on the point Quchi 曲池 is definitely with elbow bent and depth of one and a half units and only then will therapeutic effect be achieved.

Every detail in the literature means a lot; every character is a valuable accumulation of experience. Since we're discovering and developing Chinese medicine legacy, we can't neglect any part therefrom. We need to think thoroughly and discuss every character in order to develop it in the best way. I would like to hear some advice from other experts as well.

Article end

Scientific development cannot be separated from political affairs: People's Daily Editorial

Source: *Xin Zhong Yi Yao*, October 25th 1957

新中醫藥

一九五七年十月

第八卷第十期

Yaron: A final warning to any and all medical workers to comply: "Generally speaking, they didn't realize the connection between the anti-Rightists battle and the future of our nation, the connection between this battle and their profession."

Excerpt from *Anti-Rightists Battle in Health Industry*

Pages 439–440

At present, the battle against the anti-Rightists in the health industry is in full swing. More and more medical workers are devoting themselves to this major debate concerning our nation about what is right and what is wrong.

Rightists hiding within the health industry were rampant during the beginning of rectification. They joined the Rightists in the political arena and intelligentsia and pretended to be concerned about the development of medical and sanitary works. Then they distorted the Communist Party's foundational policy of medical and sanitary works and they hid the achievements the Party has made. They first of all criticized the leadership of the Communist Party, saying that the Party doesn't know about scientific techniques and so is unable to lead medical sanitary works. They claimed that for the past few years, under the leadership of the Communist Party, our medical sanitary works have been going backwards. They intended to use a despicable way to pick fights between medical workers and the government and also to instigate them to overthrow the leadership of the Communist Party and change the socialistic direction of our medical sanitary works.

For people who take a firm stand and understand the situation very well it's easy to see through the Rightists' tricks and, indeed, they did see through the tricks. However, some medical workers and experts can't see the Rightists' true faces.

Why did it happen? The main reason is that they didn't solve the problem of finding the proper relationship between politics and scientific development. Not only do they think that there is no relationship between politics and science, but even more so they think that experts and scholars shouldn't ask about politics. They disapprove of all political movements, especially ones which are in scientific technical departments. They think that political movements can't fix scientific technical problems and only interfere with the scientific work process. Generally speaking, they didn't realize the connection between the anti-Rightists battle and the future of our nation, the connection between this battle and their profession.

This situation exists in the health industry and might also exist in other scientific industries.

The dispute between us and the Rightists should focus on whether we want proletariat dictatorship and the leadership of the Communist Party. Can we say that this issue only applies to regular people but does not apply to scientific workers? Of course we can't, because this is about nationalism. If we want proletariat dictatorship and the leadership of the Communist Party then socialism will rise—and so will our nation. Otherwise, we will face the oppression of imperialism once more. China has been controlled by imperialism in the past and I'm sure that many scientific workers had experienced this personally.

In the past, all patriotic intelligentsia wanted the country to become a prosperous and powerful one with independence and freedom. Now this great ideal has become a reality for our socialistic nation, which is currently powerful and in which people are having a peaceful, happy and constructive life. However, at this point in time, Rightists stand out to oppose the leadership of the Communist Party and proletariat dictatorship. They intend to bring back capitalism and imperialism. How can this be tolerated by patriotic scientific intelligentsia? How can battling with Rightists not be part of the scientific workers' battle?

As for whom to serve from science point of view, it is also part of the anti-Rightists battle and it is related to scientific workers. Everyone knows that there's no class division in the scientific technique itself but in a society with class division, people who control scientific techniques should have class consciousness. If scientific knowledge is controlled by the reactionary political class, then it couldn't freely serve all the people and instead it will be used for negative purposes. A good example is imperialists using the achievements of medicine and biology to create biological warfare. Another example is the medical scientific situation during the reactionary days when Kunmintang was in power. Every medical worker, working during that period, knows only too well how little the Kunmintang used medical knowledge to serve the people. So we can easily see that if Rightists were to control the power, then the entire scientific situation will become miserable as before.

Some might ask, during the Kunmintang period, didn't medical workers attend to labor patients? Yes indeed, but think about this, who can serve the people better, the old reactionary China or the New China? During that time in Kunmintang controlled areas, there was no medical care in the countryside. People had no money to see doctors—so when they fell ill, they were ruled by heaven's fate. The infant mortality rate was two hundred out of a thousand and that of the general population was twenty-five out of a thousand. Cholera, black plague, smallpox, kala-azar, schistosomiasis and other extremely dangerous diseases were rampant among regular people, but Kunmintang didn't ask about it or solve it. To the contrary, its reactionary reign created even more disease and death. This was seen by the people's miserable experience during that time. During that period, every time a natural disaster struck, epidemic diseases followed. However, Kunmintang provided no disaster relief, and made no efforts to treat sick people either. Therefore, many disaster victims died from not only the lack of food and clothing, but also from lack of medical care.

After the establishment of New China, under the leadership of the Communist Party, we eliminated many serious epidemic diseases and took many measures to reinforce the people's constitution in order to resist disease. After natural disasters happened, the people's government sent a lot of food and equipment to support the distressed and medical workers to treat the sick people immediately; therefore the death rate from diseases decreased a lot.

From medical research point of view, during the Kunmintang period, there was only one Central Health Experiment Institute 中央衛生實驗院 and not many people were doing research there. Likewise, medical publications were few. However, in New China, we have established Parasite Disease Research Center 寄生蟲病研究所, Epidemic Research Center 流行病學研究所, Labor Health Research Center 勞動衛生研究所, Tuberculosis Research Center 結核病研究所, Dermatology Research Center 皮膚性病研究所, Hainan Malaria Research Center 海南島瘧疾研究所, Chinese Medicine Research Institute 中醫研究院, Southwestern Chinese Herbal Research Center 西南中藥研究所 and other research centers. There are roughly 3,000 people who work in these research centers and medical schools. Also, the number of large medical publications is sixty times more than in the Kunmintang period. Would all of this development be possible if we had no socialism or the leadership of the Communist Party?

To a scientific worker, the relationship between scientific technique and politics is an old problem which has been resolved already by many people. Yet there are many others who haven't thoroughly understood and solved this problem. We hope that the majority of scientific workers can positively join the anti-Rightists battle. On one hand make a clear division between themselves and Rightists and reveal the Rightists' true faces. On the other hand, try their best to reform themselves and discard the capitalist class standpoint and stand on the workers' side in order to become socialistic intelligentsia that serve the people.

Article end

Learn from Soviet experience to contribute to our health industry: Celebrating the 40th anniversary of October Revolution.

1957 by Li Dequan 李德全, Ministry of Health Director

Source: *Xin Zhong Yi Yao*, November 25th 1957
新中醫藥　一九五七年十一月　第八卷第十一期

Yaron: Not only was TCM forced to develop according to the Party line but also Soviet advisors helped the Chinese determine how to do it. In a way, some parts of Traditional Chinese Medicine are not only *not traditional* but even *not Chinese*:

"Soviet medical science is the most advanced. It is based on dialectical materialism and the combination of theory and real practice. Our country is learning and practicing Soviet medical scientific theory and skills. Many Chinese medicine scientific workers studied Pavlovian conditioning theory 巴甫洛夫學說 and other Soviet medical achievements, which caused obvious changes in our medical academic thinking and based our medical science on the dialectical materialism foundation."

Pages 487–489

This November 7th is the 40th anniversary of the great October Revolution. All Chinese people are celebrating this day with great excitement, regarding all victories as our own victory. At this great moment, I congratulate the Soviet medical workers and all Soviet people.

The October Revolution started a new era in human history and created a brand-new social system with happy lives, liberating the proletariat and all laborers. For forty years, Soviet achievement has clearly shown people that socialism is much better than capitalism. There are so many socialistic countries from Europe to Asia at present and they constitute a strong worldwide socialist system. Everything that happened in the world in the last forty years has proven that Marxism and Leninism is a Truth which is applicable everywhere.

The Chinese revolution developed under the influence of the October Revolution. Chairman Mao 毛主席 said, "The October Revolution gave us Marxism and Leninism. It helped the entire world and also helped Chinese intelligentsia to see the destiny of our nation from the proletariat angle, then reconsider their own problem and then follow the Soviet way. This is the conclusion." The Communist Party is now leading the masses in the entire country to follow the path of the October Revolution in order to get the victory of our revolution, and also successfully build a great socialistic country.

The Soviet is the most loyal friend of China; it generously provided aid to the Chinese people's liberation efforts, which was an important reason for our success. During the domestic revolutionary wars, the Soviet Communist Party, government and people gave us sympathy, support and assistance. After the People's Republic of China was established, the Soviets helped us recover our economy and assisted with the great economical construction.

The Soviet Union helped with our sanitary works generously and comprehensively. Everyone knows that before liberation, the northeastern part of China was a plague- and epidemic-stricken area; it significantly destroyed people's health and lives during an outbreak every year. The Soviet Red Cross and Red Crescent sent people to help prevent plague every year from 1947 to 1949. Their aid was a complete set, including experts, epidemic prevention workers, disinfection workers and nurses, and they also brought a lot of medicine, plague preventing suits, and hospital equipment. All of them had professional scientific knowledge and skill and they worked with passion, not only helping us to extinguish the plague and, with that, decrease death rate and control the plague but, even more importantly, they helped us train many epidemic prevention workers to form a good foundation for future epidemic prevention work. Today, the plague has been almost extinguished and a big part of it is due to Soviet assistance.

After the People's Republic of China was established, Soviet Communist party members and the government sent people, including the vice president of Ministry of Health, chairman of academic committee and many other experts, to help with construction of our own medical industry. Soviet experts regarded our medical industry as their own and devoted their knowledge and experience with passion.

One of the experts, comrade F. S. Bikuof 佛斯比闊夫, comprehensively introduced Soviet healthcare achievements and experience and especially the socialistic medical education system. He consistently sacrificed rest days and holidays in order to work for the Chinese people's health industry. Even after suffering a serious heart disease, he cared so much about the situation of the Chinese health industry that he refused to go back to his country. Although he passed away, his spirit will always live in our minds.

The former director of the Ministry of Health, comrade Boldyrev 波爾德列夫, systematically introduced their advanced experience of healthcare organization, and he also did an inspection tour in China. He then combined the Chinese overall situation with his experience and provided us his suggestions for industry-wide sanitary works, sanitary supervision, development of urban medical prevention network and other aspects. As for schistosomiasis, comrade Boldyrev 波爾德列夫 provided his opinions for comprehensive measures, which were very important for extinguishing schistosomiasis.

Another example is the Soviet medical group of malaria headed by the professor comrade Ishayev 依沙耶夫. Through observation, analysis and research, they discovered and confirmed some problems we were unaware of and also gave us suggestions and measures to extinguish malaria. Many Soviet experts attended our meeting about a 'twelve-year scientific medical development plan" and provided many valuable opinions. The Soviet expert group headed by comrade Kochergin 柯切爾金 is now working on the Chinese medicine industry with experience and passion.

Five years ago, in order to strengthen the friendship between China and Soviet Union, the Soviet Red Cross and Red Crescent founded Beijing Soviet Red Cross Hospital in China based on proletarian internationalism and revolutionary humanitarianism. Rights were transferred to our government this March. There have been more than 120 Soviet medical workers coming to this hospital and working with Chinese medical workers to treat hundreds of thousands of patients, including many with difficult and complicated diseases. For the five years, many patients from all over the country came to see them and wrote them more then 64,000 inquiry and thank you letters. Those who had been cured by the Soviet experts happily got back to their work position. Furthermore, Soviet medical workers in that hospital took care of Chinese medical workers, helped them learn the advanced Soviet medical technology and trained more than two hundred specialist advanced medical personnel. In 1956, young doctors working at the hospital wrote 79 essays with assistance from Soviet experts. Soviet medical workers showed us the spirit of proletarian internationalism, good socialist ethics and medical treatment style and set a positive example for Chinese medical workers.

Soviet health industry is the most advanced in the world; they earned fabulous achievements for forty years. The principle of their healthcare industry is prevention policy with unity and planning, plus it should be based on scientific theory. Therefore, it's very meaningful to us to learn from their advanced experience.

For example, since 1953, we have learnt from Soviet experience and started a national supervision system of sanitary works. We have also established a series of specific centers for supervision of preventive medical work, plus drafted different kinds of laws to manage sanitary works. The national supervision system of sanitary works is an important measure to implement prevention works. Due to this measure, on the one hand it helps the construction of new industrial cities and new factories; these will be able to follow the socialistic principle and fit sanitary standards. On the other hand, it gradually changes the unreasonable and unsanitary conditions of factories built during old China, thus helping maintain workers' health.

As for prevention works in hospitals, we combine Soviet experience and on-the-ground situations to implement "medical service divided to areas". So far, there are more than twenty cities applying this measure and thus preventive medical centers are able to arrange the work and serve the people more effectively. The protective medical system based on advanced Soviet medical experience has been well carried out by preventive medical centers. It improved medical workers' attitude and the relationship between medical workers and patients. It also helped the management of hospitals to increase efficiency of medical service.

As for industrial sanitary works, many factories have learnt the factory-doctors system from Soviet experience, which helped raise medical quality and implement prevention policy. As for medical education, we implemented the policy of "enthusiastically learn the Soviet advanced experience, combine it with the actual situation in China and start the education reform". We gradually determined the national uniform professional setting and education system. We also drafted professional uniform teaching plans and outlines to systematically reform the higher education system and organization, teaching contents and methods. This measure changed our medical education from the ground up, which previously was half-feudalism half-colonialism in old China and now is turning into socialism in New China. For these couple of years, due to the combination of Soviet experience and our actual condition, the health industry in our country has been fast growing and had vast achievements.

Soviet medical science is the most advanced. It is based on dialectical materialism and the combination of theory and real practice. Our country is learning and practicing Soviet medical scientific theory and skills. Many Chinese medicine scientific workers studied Pavlovian conditioning theory 巴甫洛夫學說 and other Soviet medical achievements, which caused obvious changes in our medical academic thinking and based our medical science on the dialectical materialism foundation.

With the growing friendship between Soviet Union and China, there is more and more medical academic interaction and medical scientific cooperation between the two countries. During these several years, our country has sent ten delegations and thirty-seven medical experts to attend all kinds of Soviet medical academies at their invitation. In order to learn from them, we have sent six delegations and eighty-one people to visit Soviet Union. Meanwhile, we have invited nine delegations headed by the director of Ministry of Health, Kovrigina 科夫里金娜 and thirty-seven people to visit our country. During their visit, they delivered over a hundred academic reports and multiple special symposia. Through academic interaction between us and Soviet Union, we can learn more about their experience and facilitate the friendship between China and Soviet Union.

Soviet Union highly values our traditional medicine. Their Ministry of Health director, Kovrigina 科夫里金娜, during a visit to a Chinese medicine treatment and research center had said, "I have no doubt about Chinese medicine research. I know Chinese medicine is very important to our healthcare and I have already dispatched experts to learn more about it." Last year, three experts who came to inspect acupuncture returned to Soviet Union and started practicing acupuncture therapy. The two Soviet doctors Odessa 奥德薩 and Stalin 斯大林 visited China, brought back some Chinese medicine for hemorrhoids and used it on their patients. Soviet doctors also asked for Chinese medicine for pertussis, measles, and diphtheria for research purposes. Not long ago, the Soviet Union had invited our Chinese medicine experts to the Soviet Union to do a group consultation.

No matter if it is in the past, present or future, Soviet constructive socialistic experience and Soviet assistance is very meaningful to us. The patriotism of their people and scientific experts and the spirit of proletarian internationalism set a good example for us. In order to improve our socialistic construction, we should implement Chairman Mao's 毛主席 instruction to continually learn socialism construction from Soviet Union experience. Like them, we should advance our medical industry and skills, medical workers' patriotism, proletarian internationalism and virtue. We should learn from their people the passion for Communism and constructing socialism and work together for the great socialistic construction.

Article end

Learn from the advanced Soviet medical science with resolution and persistence

1957 by Fu Lien-Chang 傅連璋

Source: *Chinese Medical Journal Foreign Language Publication*
中華醫學雜誌外文版

Yaron: I dare you to not follow the Soviets in constructing this new medicine! "There are still a minority, especially the bourgeois Rightists, who doubt the advanced nature of Soviet medical science. They slander and distort facts and try to belittle the achievements of Soviet medicine, obstruct our learning from the Soviet Union, and undermine Chinese-Soviet friendship. They often claim, on grounds of isolated technical problems, that the Soviet Union cannot compare with the capitalist countries."

Fu Lien-Chang said, in the September 1956 *Presidential Address*, "From now on, while still concentrating on learning from Soviet medicine, we must at the same time study and learn from the medical achievements and contributions of all other countries. We should learn not only from the People's Democracies but also from the capitalist countries."

Here, in November 1957, this was no longer an option. In making Chinese medicine scientific, one could not even follow the world's science, but rather only ideological science of the Soviet Union.

The Great October Socialist Revolution of the Soviet Union celebrates this year its Fortieth Anniversary. During the forty years, the Soviet people, under the correct leadership of the Soviet Communist Party and lighted by the beacon of Marxism, have attained great and glorious achievements in every field of construction. Recently, in launching the first artificial satellite, the Soviet Union has once again proved to the world the high level of her science and technology and the peerless superiority of the socialist system. The working class and the oppressed peoples of the whole world all rejoice in the Soviet Union's achievements and consider the Anniversary of the October Revolution as their own celebration. The victory of the Soviet revolution gave a tremendous impetus to the Chinese revolution, and the generous and unselfish aid given us by the Soviet Union has greatly accelerated the pace of our construction. The friendship of the Chinese and Soviet people is everlasting and indestructible.

We, medical and health workers, will forever remember with gratitude all the aid that the Soviet Union has given us. As early as the War of Resistance against Japanese Aggression, the Soviet Union sent some of her best medical experts to help us in our health and training work, contributing much toward raising the efficiency of our medical service and the technical level of our medical personnel. Since liberation, the Soviet Union has given us still greater assistance. Each time we have asked for help, the Government and people of the Soviet Union have readily and generously supplied us with technical and material aid. Aside from this, the Soviet Government has also accepted a large number of our students for special training in the Soviet Union. The achievements we have made are inseparable from the Soviet Union's fraternal aid, and our zeal in learning from her.

We learn from the Soviet Union as from the closest of friends and the best of teachers. First of all, following her experiences in sanitation and prevention, we have established more than 600 specialized prevention centers and stations and more than 1,500 anti-epidemic stations, teams and groups. These have greatly contributed toward the prevention of communicable diseases.

Supervision and control over sanitation and hygiene have also developed under the expert guidance of Soviet specialists. This has made town planning and industrial installations conform to health standards beneficial to the health of the people.

In treatment and prevention, we have learned from the advanced Soviet system of district health service, initiated the system of medical stations in industries and laid special emphasis on prevention.

In the field of medical training, we have carried out reforms in our educational system, revolutionized our ideology in medical theory and practice, enriched our curriculum and improved our educational methods. In maternal and child health we are also profiting from Soviet experience.

Our great army of medical workers is enthusiastic in learning from Soviet medical science. Since liberation, a great many lectures and study meetings have been held on Soviet medical science. In 1953, Pavlov's teachings were studied all over the country. A considerable amount of Soviet medical literature has been translated and published. In order to gain access to Soviet medicine directly, a large number of medical workers have taken up study of the Russian language.

In short, the organizational systems, methods of work, scientific theories and technology in Soviet medicine are what we learn from the Soviet Union. Learning from the Soviet Union has been of great help to us in improving our style of work and ways of thinking. In respect to ideology in medical theory and practice, we have come to realize the close relationship between medical science and the development of society and the social system and the guiding role of dialectic materialism. All these are very important gains.

But in the course of learning, we have made mistakes and have taken unnecessary detours. Sometimes we did not fully consider the actual conditions in our country in relation to certain problems, but mechanically applied Soviet methods to them; sometimes we promoted incomplete and immature experiences; sometimes our understanding and applications of advanced Soviet medical theories were too superficial; and sometimes we overemphasized emulation of the material conditions in Soviet medical work, neglecting the austere and steady methods of Soviet medical workers. But most of these faults, though arising at different times, have been quickly rectified; the main thing is the knowledge we acquired in the process of learning.

Of course, not all medical workers fully appreciate the importance of learning from the Soviet Union. There is still a minority, especially the bourgeois Rightists, that doubts the advanced nature of Soviet medical science. They slander and distort facts and try to belittle the achievements of Soviet medicine, obstruct our learning from the Soviet Union and undermine Chinese Soviet friendship. They often claim, on the grounds of isolated technical problems, that the Soviet Union cannot compare with the capitalist countries. This is substituting a part for the whole. If we take isolated technical problems and compare them, then all countries are advanced in some respects and retarded in others.

All industrially-developed countries have their own system of medical practice and research and, therefore, in such a wide and varied field as medicine, all countries stand a good chance of making discoveries or improving techniques. We consider that the proper evaluation of a country's scientific level and progress should be made from an over-all and developmental approach. Seen from this point, Soviet medical science is certainly superior. The advanced nature of Soviet medical science manifests itself in the fact that it is really serving the welfare of the people. Soviet medical workers, inspired by a noble goal, are able to exert their utmost in creative achievement and, applying dialectic materialism to their scientific world outlook, delve into the mysteries of medical science and attain distinctive results.

It is an established fact that Soviet medicine not only is foremost in guiding principles and organizational systems but also is unsurpassed by capitalist countries in many academic and technological aspects, such as health protection, physiopathology of the nervous system and the application of atomic energy in medicine.

With regard to the pace of development, pre-revolutionary Russia was a comparatively backward country. During the forty years since the founding of the Soviet Union, for a long time she was within capitalist encirclement and during World War II she suffered the heaviest loss in manpower and materials. Yet, in spite of all these handicaps, Soviet medical science still forged ahead and, in some respects, surpassed the United States—an earlier industrialized country which not only escaped the ravages of the World War but made fabulous wartime profits. Thus considered, the advanced level and superiority of Soviet medical science is even more irrefutable. There are some skeptics who see, in some of our mistakes in learning from the Soviet Union (such as mechanical application), evidences of inferiority or backwardness in Soviet medicine. Obviously this is even more erroneous.

Our resolute and persistent policy is to continue earnestly learning from the Soviet Union. Aside from learning the advanced Soviet organizational system, methods of work and academic theories, we must, in particular, emulate the wholehearted spirit of service to the people that is a fundamental characteristic of Soviet medical workers. It is precisely because of this selfless spirit of service that they can share the sufferings and joys of the people, dedicate themselves wholeheartedly, overcome difficulties, take pains to be precise, constantly improve and attain distinctive results in preventive, curative, educational and research work.

We must also emulate the international spirit of Soviet medical workers. The generous and unselfish aid given us by the Soviet Union and the attitude of Soviet experts working in our country in making our cause their own are all real manifestations of this noble spirit of internationalism. We must learn from the Soviet Union, consolidate Sino-Soviet friendship and strengthen the unity of the peoples of the socialist countries and the rest of the world.

We must also emulate the Soviet Union's practice of thrift. Her great achievements are all won by long and hard struggle on the part of the people. Although their material conditions have greatly improved, the Soviet people have still retained their thrifty habit of work, emphasizing substance rather than form, and making use of all serviceable equipment. To us, who are still in the first stages of construction and still faced with all kinds of difficulties, emulation of this thrifty habit and hard work is absolutely necessary.

In order to learn better from the Soviet Union, we must completely shatter the slanders and attacks of the Rightists, take a firm working class stand, master dialectic materialism and thoroughly reform our ideology.

Let us learn from the advanced Soviet medical science with resolution and persistence, develop the heritage of our traditional medicine and study on a critical basis the advanced medical sciences of all countries. Under the leadership of the Communist Party, the medical science of our country will certainly attain greater and more rapid development.

Article end

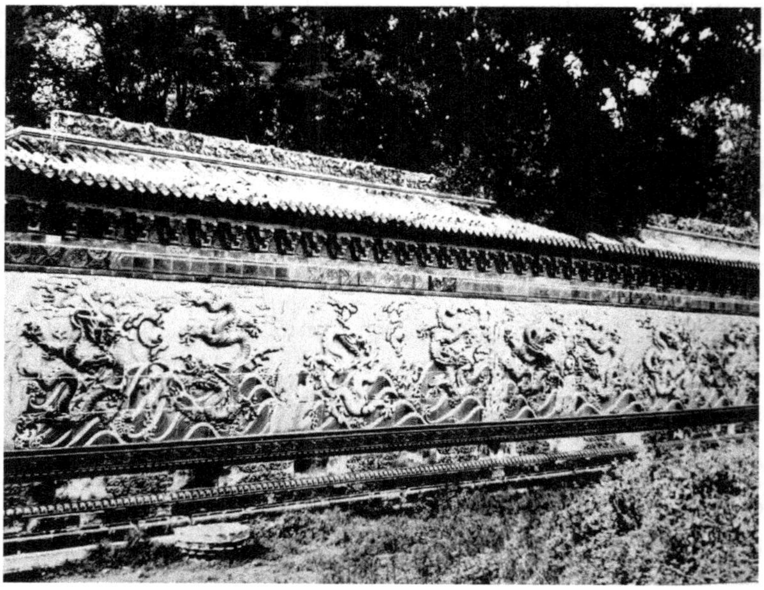

Photo by Mr P. Goux in early 1900s. "Imperial City – Ceramic Wall".

Reinforce the management of Chinese medicine

1957 by Lü Bingkui 吕炳奎, Director of the Chinese Medicine Department at the Ministry of Health

Source: *Xin Zhong Yi Yao*, December 25th 1957

新中醫藥

一九五七年十二月

第八卷第十二期

Yaron: By the end of 1957, and even though all opposing voices were silenced, there were still unhappy Chinese medicine practitioners to be found: "A few Chinese medicine practitioners do not understand the strategy and instructions regarding Chinese medicine and still think that the issue is just about their income. They don't understand that it is about the development of our traditional medicine, not to mention the historical chance that exists to merge with Western medicine and in the future create a new medicine" is a description of practitioners not wishing to follow the Party's plan.

In this article, there is a description of how the Party cracked down on those practitioners. Naturally, these non-conforming practitioners are described as criminals, but see for example, Tian Qiuping and his electric acupuncture reaching tens of thousands of people. Who decided that his electric acupuncture technique was a lie? Tian being innocent of criminal actions is certain, and we can see it by this statement: "Finally, he was arrested after refusing the advice from the government." It was only after Tian was given a warning to obey the Party's advice and he refused that he was arrested. Real criminals don't get advice first from the government, not to mention that electric acupuncture became very popular in TCM later on.

Pages 535-536

Since criticizing He Cheng 賀誠 and Wang Bin's 王斌 mistaken thoughts and revising the wrong measures they took in limiting Chinese medicine in the past, we correctly executed the strategy of the Communist Party, which made some changes in Chinese medicine at a fundamental level. Chinese medicine can occupy a better place politically and socially. However, quite a few Chinese medicine practitioners do not understand the strategy and instructions regarding Chinese medicine and still think that the issue is just about their income. They don't understand that it is about the development of our traditional medicine, not to mention the historical chance that exists to merge with Western medicine and in the future create a new medicine. In the Ministry of Health administration, there are some people with these types of confused thoughts. They regard the Communist Party policy for Chinese medicine as a united front. They view the current arrangement plan of Chinese medicine as the Party's entire Chinese medicine plan. These one-sided opinions cause poor management of Chinese medicine.

Due to this reason, some chaotic phenomena exist in the Chinese medicine field. Some people try to sneak in with a legal loophole in the execution strategy. For example, Niu Wuqing 牛梧青 and Wang Kunshan 王昆山, the Chinese medicine Rightists from Henan, were originally reactionary politicians. They took advantage of opportunities to sneak into the Chinese medicine field and tried to steal power in order to do something against the Communist Party and socialism.

Also there are some dicey people who claim themselves to be Chinese medicine practitioners and concoct various excuses to open Chinese medicine crash courses and recruit jobless vagrants and reactionary army and police people who start seeing patients after a couple of weeks' training.

There were dozens of cases in Beijing before it was banned, such as the law offender Tian Qiuping 田秋萍, who organized a "Chinese Medicine Scientification Research Society 中国医学科学化研究社" and distributed different handbooks to spread his "electric acupuncture therapy 电针疗法" and taught disciples by correspondence. More than forty-five thousand people were tricked and tens of thousands of Yuan were collected. Finally, he was arrested after refusing the advice from the government.

Another case was in Xüzhou City 徐州市. One guy failed his business and started studying acupuncture for a few days with a local Chinese medicine practitioner, then tried to apply to open his medical practice, but got rejected by the Board of Health. So he saw patients for free to attract people, all along even asking horizontal inscribed boards or flags from patients in order to create a buzz. These are examples of people pretending to be Chinese medicine practitioners. They're everywhere—in cities and in the countryside. This situation is serious and should be utterly banned. Otherwise, it will affect the people's view of medicine and even the development of our health care system.

I think that before the central government announces the uniform rules, local government could draft regulations for Chinese medicine management based on local situations and then report it to the People's committee of the city or province. For example, they have examined all Chinese medicine practitioners in order to arrest the ones a without license in Beijing 北京 City. In Shanghai 上海 City and Jiangxi 江西 Province they made Chinese medicine management interim regulations. In Gansu 甘肃 Province they made regulations to examine Chinese medicine. These are methods to reinforce the management of Chinese medicine and it's good and necessary that local governments can take measures in time.

It is the main goal of the Communist Party to develop the proper political view and a concept of Chinese medicine practitioners. The objective is to inherit and develop our domestic cultural legacy and make it useful to the socialist construction and for serving the people. However, behaviors which are against this purpose exist and we need to oppose them. We can't give those deceivers a chance to get away with it. Instead, we need to report these cases to the government when it's more serious or persuade the offenders not to do this when the circumstances are not so serious.

Some people who have a specific skill, good reputation and can serve as Chinese medicine practitioners, even without having much academic knowledge, we should protect and help them to serve patients in a better way. People who have studied from a master or family and were practitioners for a while in the past but stopped for some reason and now want to come back into this industry, we should allow them to practice. Currently, people who have been learning Chinese medicine officially either from a master or from family for four to six years can apply to be practitioners, however, the application should be presented by both master and apprentice and the apprentice needs to pass an exam.

The management of Chinese medicine is very complicated and new work, and it should be under the guidance and strategy of the Communist Party. With earnest research and investigation we can control the situation and do the best management job.

Article end

Defeat Rightist Long Bojian's 龍伯堅 attack on the Party

1957 by Zhang Cigong 章次公, Department of Health TCM consultant

Source: *Xin Zhong Yi Yao*, December 25th 1957

新中醫藥

一九五七年十二月

第八卷第十二期

Yaron: The Communist Party danced any way it wanted in order to reach the power grasp objective: "Long Bojian's 龍伯堅 arguments demonstrate not only his rejection of Chinese medicine's important status in research but also his disrespect to the value of Chinese medicine theory."

The Communist Party had very little respect for the theory of Chinese medicine and it only used and manipulated parts fitting into the dialectic materialism model. Here, "cherishing Chinese medicine theory" is used as a weapon against the Rightists, represented in this particular moment as Western medicine doctors who don't cherish the motherland. This political duress made possible a new Chinese medicine theory to not only flourish but also be supported by modern science as "scientific."

Clearly, Western science did not support Chinese medicine theory but was forced to. If we wanted to make an imaginary analogy to the Republic, this situation will equal a scenario in which Yu Yunxiu, the great opponent of Chinese medicine theory, will be forced to change his views and now claim to agree with its theory. A false and coerced act indeed. In fact, this actually did happen in the early 1950s in Shanghai before Yu Yunxiu's passing in 1954. Yu changed his opinion saying that Western medicine should become for the masses and Chinese medicine should not be looked down upon.

Pages 538–539

The Rightist Long Bojian 龍伯堅 published an article *A Few Questions about Chinese Medicine Research* 中医研究工作中的几个问题 in *Health Daily* on January 25th and 29th this year, in which there are many academic mistakes. These have been criticized harshly by other comrades. The article was aiming to attack the Communist Party Chinese medicine policy from the Rightists' point of view and Long Bojian 龍伯堅 is a Rightist pretending to do Chinese medicine research and development. Let's take a look at his proposition.

Attempting to deny Marxism leadership in an academic research field

When Long Bojian 龍伯堅 talked about the main problem of Chinese medicine research work, he refuted the Russian professor Vadim Gabrielevich Vogralik's[452] 華格拉立克 opinions and tried to avoid the four conditions for Chinese medicine research set by the professor, such as "the right thinking in the work" and "the positive and energetic cooperation between Chinese and Western medicine" etc. Professor Vogralik emphasizes that dialectic materialism philosophy is the most advanced and scientific and this was totally dodged by Long Bojian 龍伯堅. He one-sidedly emphasized that "the leader of scientific work should be skillful and experienced in scientific research" and gave further emphasis that "Only a first-class Western medicine doctor with a high-level scientific knowledge can be the leader." It is really clear that his objective is to steal the leadership rights of Chinese medicine research work.

Long Bojian 龍伯堅 also took Guo Moruo 郭沫若 as an example and said that the reason Guo could be an expert of Oracle bones and Chinese bronze inscriptions was because he used scientific methods while he was studying medicine. Everyone knows that medicine is a kind of science and although it can help us understand some parts of science, it is not at a leadership position. In the entire world only Marxism is the real truth. Long Bojian 龍伯堅 deliberately avoided Marxism and put Western medicine in a position to lead everything, in order to build a vague impression and to make people believe that knowing Western medicine is equal to knowing everything, which even though it may sound right, in reality, it is actually wrong.

[452] Vadim Gabrielevich Vogralik (1911–1997) was a professor of Nizhniy Novgorod Medical Institute. During the times of the Cultural Revolution, together with a group of Soviet specialists, he supervised the health of the Chinese Communist elite, who often refrained from treatment by Chinese doctors. After learning Chinese medicine at that time he returned to the Soviet Union and started teaching and further developing acupuncture in a scientific way.

Attempting to reject Chinese medicine within the Chinese medicine research work

Long Bojian 龍伯堅 was trying to make a monopoly of Chinese medicine to steal some parts of it to impress the Western world. However, he knows nothing about Chinese medicine. So he claimed "only Western medicine doctors with a high level of scientific knowledge are qualified to research Chinese medicine." He drafted a measure *The Task Assignment Between and Cooperation of Chinese and Western Medicines* 中西医分工合作, in which this is what he said: "...set up a group of doctors for monographic study—doing specific research work for things known to have certain effects in the hospital". Isn't this obvious? According to his statement, in his definition of research work, Chinese medicine doctors just go around doing some "certain effect work" in front of Long Bojian 龍伯堅. In this way, Chinese medicine doctors are the object being studied instead of actively joining the research work.

Real Chinese medicine research work may include the therapeutic effect conclusion, but it must be based on a sincere cooperation between Chinese and Western medicines, and the absolute respect for the motherland's medical theory. One must realize that Chinese medicine diagnosis and treatment rules stem out of its theory and only if we follow this we can get the correct scientific conclusion. Long Bojian's 龍伯堅 arguments demonstrate not only his rejection of Chinese medicine's important status in research but also his disrespect for the value of Chinese medicine theory.

Yaron: The following paragraph shows the massive Soviet influence on selecting TCM theory. Yin-Yang and five elements merged with Zang-fu matched well with dialectic materialism. The Communists simply valued a theory that fit their purpose. Here we can also see Yu Yunxiu turned into the villain character, Long Bojian being his inheritor. It is the time where everyone—traditional or scientific—was submitting to ideology.

Attempting to tear apart the integrality of the Chinese medicine system

Opposing research of Chinese medicine theory, Long Bojian 龍伯堅 said, "There are three parts for Chinese medicine research work: clinical research, herbal research and historical research." People know that Chinese medicine theory is based on long-term medical practice and that it can lead Chinese medicine clinical work. The Russian expert Vadim Gabrielevich Vogralik, who is qualified to be a Western medicine doctor with a high level of scientific knowledge, said "Through centuries of experience, Chinese medicine theory has been proven to be correct; 'Yin-Yang' and 'five elements' theories are the foundation for viscera theories and treatment. All of these theories are correct and advanced as testified by deep research, and they totally fit the principle of dialectical materialism." According to this statement, we can see the value of researching Chinese medicine theory.

However, Long Bojian 龍伯堅 has the opposite opinion, saying, "If we can't confirm the therapeutic effect, then everything about the theory is just moonshine." This is upside down and being unreasonable. If a theory can't be tested by experiments of course it's wrong, but Chinese medicine theory has been working for thousands of years and has achieved brilliant results, so how can it be regarded as wrong? This kind of arbitrary statement will definitely die down. Long Bojian 龍伯堅 intended to inherit the work of Yu Yunxiu 余云岫, who totally failed academically and politically, denying the value of Chinese medicine theory for clinical application, and also denying the fact that the motherland medicine is a unique system of science. His purpose is to build a nonscientific image for Chinese medicine and then use it as an excuse to destroy it. This intention to extinguish Chinese medicine is really going backwards politically.

Yaron: The following section shows the freedom of no-speech and freedom of no-thought.

In an evil way attacking the Communist Party Chinese medicine policy

Like other Rightists, Long Bojian 龍伯堅 doesn't admit that the Communist Party is able to lead scientific work, neither does he reveal his real objective. Therefore he quoted a decision from the political report of the Chinese Communist Party 8th National Congress to prove he's right, but omitted important content from the report such as "should inherit and absorb the ancient cultural legacy" and "the work of Chinese and Western medicines learning from each other". These were emphasized in the second five-year-plan proposal, in order to help our nation's economic development. He makes a garble, quoting, "it's necessary to organize our national cultural legacy in a modern scientific way" and "seriously organize Chinese medicine and herbal medicine" and making it his political basis, and then pretends to be a loyal scientific follower of the Communist Party while actually twisting the facts which in turn lead people to misbelieve Marxism and the Communist Party. He also refused Chinese medicine doctors in the research work and discouraged Western medicine doctors from learning Chinese medicine in order to destroy the Party's Chinese medicine policy.

The Communist Party policy of "letting a hundred flowers bloom, letting different schools of thoughts debate" clearly explains that we never object real academic debates, no matter what they are about. Whether about Chinese medicine theory, Chinese medicine research work or other things, the debates will always be approved. But we highly insist to object to what Long Bojian 龍伯堅 did—used the freedom of debates as an excuse to aggressively attack Chinese medicine and current policy. We should destroy the attack from Rightists such as Long Bojian 龍伯堅.

Article end

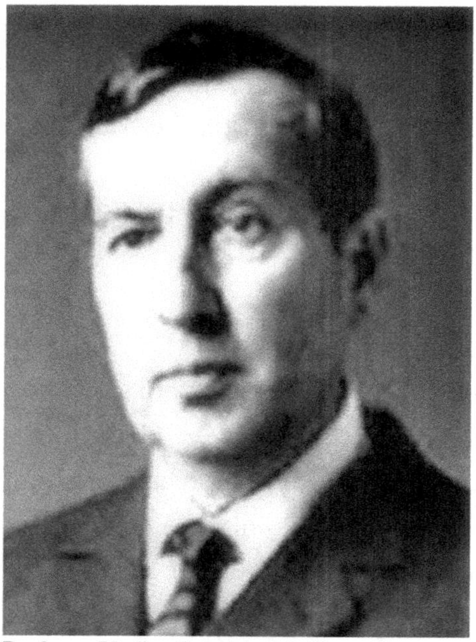

Professor Vadim Gabrielevich Vogralik

Do away with superstitions and liberate the mind
Health Daily Editorial

Source: *Xin Zhong Yi Yao*, July 25th 1958

新中醫藥 一九五八年七月 第九卷第七期

Yaron: Even though, coming to this point, the reader may feel that this awkward ideological situation cannot get any worse, it actually does as we can see below. It is shortly after the four big TCM colleges were established in Beijing, Shanghai, Guangzhou and Chengdu as well as many other smaller schools around the country. What was allowed in TCM for years to come, who decided the curriculum and why? We should contemplate these and other critical questions while reading the following article. At one point, which in my opinion is this point, we can no longer ignore the ideological forces behind the remaking of the new TCM. What does "develop real science for normal people" mean? According to this statement "The health industry is the masses' business, and so is the medical scientific technique; both should follow the masses line and be accomplished by the masses," who really created and promulgated TCM? During the Republic and while creating Chinese medicine specialized schools, Chinese medicine reformers were hoping to eradicate the uneducated from the medical circles. Was this element reintroduced here?

Pages 1–3

In the Chinese Communist Party second meeting of the 8th National Congress it was announced that the revolution of our country has gotten into a new historical period: a period of China's socialist construction centering on technical and cultural revolution. In this great era, "Our Party, our country currently needs a big group of people who dare to speak and act, dare to do away with superstitions, dare to create, dare to insist on the truth and fight for it. Only with these kinds of people can we lead the masses to make a great progress and accomplish the greatest socialist construction." (Extracted from Liu Shaoqi's 劉少奇 statements in the Chinese Communist Party second meeting of the 8th National Congress). If we use the same standard to check our sanitary works, we will discover that "superstition" has become an obstacle and so liberating our minds from it is a critical step for our sanitary works.[453]

[453] "Sanitary works" (Wei Sheng 衛生) means all activities related to public health.

What kind of superstitions do we have in sanitary works? First, we only believe the Western world and disbelieve ourselves. Whatever is foreign is good. We learn everything from the Western world, including systems, organizations, work methods and foreign equipment and we even follow the English names of medicine, diseases and machines, while all along disrespecting our own culture. In the work of disease control and scientific research, we always check if it's been published in foreign literature or experimented in Western countries instead of doing it in our own way. This is, as far as Chinese medicine is concerned, because we always dispose and deny our motherland medicine which has been passed down for thousands of years and we enslave our minds to Western medicine.

Second, we superstitiously believe in experts and authority and ignore the masses and the new generation. People are afraid to do things when they're in front of an expert. They even don't dare say anything even when they know that the expert is making a mistake. We emphasize too much academic degrees and reputation and so young people don't have an opportunity to show themselves.

Third, we superstitiously believe scientific techniques and ignore politics. We treat scientific knowledge as high-end goods and we assume that only high-end intellectuals can get it; common people have no access to it. Some people even claim that medical scientific techniques are too complicated to learn in a short period of time.

Fourth, we superstitiously believe in systems and regulations and ignore reality. All systems and regulations should be flexible and adjustable for people who follow them. However, currently it is the opposite situation in our country. Some people even believe that those systems and regulations can make everything work.

Fifth, we superstitiously believe in formal rules and pursue formality too much. Sixth, we superstitiously believe in official documents and files too much. Furthermore, some people only superstitiously believe in their own abilities and refuse to work with others, for example, in the scientific research and disease control work. They over estimate themselves and don't look for the benefit of the people. In any case, there are too many superstitions limiting our thoughts.

What will be the result of having these superstitions in our work? We think that the following will happen: First, good things will become bad things. We ought to learn advanced experience from foreign countries, which is a good thing, but if we only believe in other people and underestimate ourselves then it's a bad thing. All the scientific techniques and systems should be controlled by people but, instead, now we are controlled by the techniques and systems due to our superstitions.

Second, leaders of every position rely on experts, authority, science and techniques too much and then ignore the masses. The more we superstitiously believe those experts and authority, the more difficult it will be to develop real science for normal people, and the more constrained people's minds will become.

Third, the more superstitions we have, the more we incline to non-politics, which will facilitate the development of wrong points of view, such as "Technique is the first priority", "Technique is above everything" and "Politics can't lead techniques". Fourth, we work in a small world due to those superstitions and can't see the great creation of the masses, which therefore will result in lack of confidence and determination with other effective and efficient methods in our sanitary works. Generally speaking, the outcome of superstition is to become slower and more costly. So we definitely need to get rid of these superstitions.

Why do we have such superstitions? Why does our Ministry of Health have so many superstitions? Comrade Shaoqi 少奇 said, "Our country has been invaded and oppressed by foreign countries for more than a century, which is why we are currently lagging behind in so many aspects. Although we were liberated already and have made big progress and much development, we still feel deeply inferior and superstitiously believe in foreign stuff." This problem has existed in our Ministry of Health for a long time and as long as it's not resolved, it will facilitate the development of those superstitions.

If we want to crash superstitions thoroughly, we need to set up the mass viewpoint and trust the masses' infinite creativity. The health industry is the masses' business, and so is the medical scientific technique; both should follow the masses' line and be accomplished by the masses. Historical materialism shows us that the world was created by the masses—and so were scientific techniques, which are not reserved for intellectuals and experts.

Those great scientists in history, to a large degree, were not from the higher strata of society. For example, those great Chinese doctors Li Shizhen 李時珍, Bian Que 扁鵲, Hua Tuo 華佗, Sun Simiao 孫思邈 etc., were not from noble families and did not have special education; they were all common people. Leeuwenhoek 利文霍克, the first person who discovered bacteria, wasn't highly educated. Selman Waksman 瓦克

斯曼, who discovered streptomycin, was only educated in primary school; Charles Nicolle 尼古拉, who found that lice were the transmitters of epidemic typhus, even didn't get into primary school; Friedrich Sertürner 塞特歐納爾, who first isolated morphine from opium, was just a trainee in a pharmacy.

There are many similar instances in other professional areas and we witnessed many miracles created by the masses during our huge leap forward. For example, Li Shimei 李始美, who went to junior high school only for one year, solved the problem of termites, which had remained unsolved for long time; Wang Baojing 王保京, who went to primary school only for three years, created a miracle in agricultural production and got hired to be a researcher specialized in agricultural science. There are some similar cases in our sanitary works, such as the solution to the infection problem of penicillin, the automated drug-dispensing machine. These were created by common workers. In the Campaign against The Four Pests, the masses regularly researched the four pests and invented many methods for their elimination. Some of their discoveries and inventions impressed the experts.

These facts demonstrate that there is no mystery with scientific techniques. All scientific inventions are simply the product of laborers' production. Everyone can handle scientific skills, especially with our current social system. The key point is to liberate the people's mind and eliminate all superstitions, such as "Chinese is not as good as foreign", "common people are not as good as experts", "regular people are not as good as famous people", "not according to the rules is not as good as being according to the rules" etc. We should make our efforts aim directly at technical and cultural revolution. We have our own hands and feet and our own minds, so we are doing what foreigners are doing but we also can do what foreigners did not do before. Simultaneously, we can surely learn from other laboring people and from our own laborers. If we invest more effort than other people, then we can learn more. Everyone can be an expert or a scientist.

A real authority or expert should never consider themselves to be an authority or be superstitious about Western people. No scientific technique or knowledge belongs to any single individual. Although achievement is regarded as the result of one's work, it is still created by the masses, because once we leave the masses, we can't create anything. The masses are the ocean of knowledge and the resource of every invention. All experts and authority should acknowledge this fact and do away with superstition about the Western world and themselves and cooperate with the masses to create a bigger progress.

When we insist on eliminating all superstition, we don't deny anything. We may still learn from the Western world wisdom. We can learn all the advanced experience from every country and everyone as long as we have confidence in our own. We should believe ourselves to be able to create new things. Our ancestors passed down a lot of precious traditions and wisdom to us and we are diligent and brave people. So we should put faith in ourselves that we can definitely catch up to others and even surpass them. We should not think that others have good abilities but we don't. If we want to eliminate superstitions, we need to check if we have the great spirit of six hundred million people.

Not being superstitious about the experts doesn't mean that we belittle them. To the contrary, we're doing this in order to seek the truth from experts. The idiom "Modesty helps one advance, whereas conceit makes one fall behind" should be our motto forever. Not being superstitious about systems and regulations doesn't mean to destroy all systems. We still need them, need to follow them and need to put them to better use.

Every scientific technique is the outcome of labor and is created by laboring people. It's wrong to have superstitions about scientific techniques. But in order to use it in a better way, we need to research it hard and make labor efforts and spend energy. It's also wrong to underestimate scientific techniques.

The technical and cultural revolution has just begun; we should catch up in sanitary works. So we need to reinforce the Communist Party leadership, eliminate all superstitions and liberate our minds, combine wisdom of experts and creation of the masses and, like this, promote the style of the Communist Party, which is the new trend in sanitary works. As long as we eliminate superstition and liberate our minds, the intelligence of the masses will be like the nuclear fission process generating infinite power, leading our medical scientific sanitary works into the next phase.

Article end

Traditional Chinese Medicine in Treatment of Tabes Dorsalis

By the Institute of Dermatology and Venereology of the Chinese Academy of Medical Sciences and the Peking College of Traditional Chinese Medicine, Peking

Source: *Chinese Medical Journal Foreign Language Publication*, April 1960. 中華醫學雜誌外文版

Yaron: In this foreign language publication we see the term "Traditional Chinese Medicine". Here, Chinese medicine practitioners are referred to as traditional medicine specialists. These traditional specialists modify an ancient formula for a disease diagnosed in a modern way. In fact, there is no trace of Chinese medicine theory or why and how the formula was modified, nor is there a Chinese medicine diagnosis involved. This article wishes to demonstrate that Chinese medicine formulas can be integrated into Western medicine and help Western medicine yield better clinical results. It shows the perfect "new medicine".

Considering the political and social pressures surrounding these kinds of studies one doubts the patients' and doctors' objective reports. Even if true and Shengti formula had a certain efficacy for this particular disease, is it Chinese medicine at all? The second half of the 20th century was full of studies showing Chinese medicine formulas fitting into modern medicine, which, as we have seen before, was Tan Cizhong's vision some 30 years earlier. At that time they called it scientific investigation of Chinese medicine, but in my opinion there was no investigation of Chinese medicine at all.

Pages 347–350

The current treatment of tabes dorsalis cannot be considered satisfactory, inasmuch as some of the distressing and disabling neurologic symptoms cannot be alleviated by antibiotics or the standard arsenicals and heavy metals in the present antisyphilitic armamentarium. It is only natural that we should have turned our attention to traditional medicine, looking for additional effective therapeutic measures to improve upon the results.

Under close cooperation between doctors of Western and traditional medicine, researchers in the past year have brought forth some fruitful results. It is the purpose of this paper to make a preliminary report on our clinical observations on the treatment of tabes dorsalis by specialists in Traditional Chinese Medicine.

Choice of patients and treatment program

We purposely chose the more severe cases, including a good number in which the response to western antisyphilitic treatment had been unsatisfactory, in order to give the traditional drugs a more rigid test and make it easier to draw conclusions. The first series consisted of 11 cases. In each instance, prior to treatment, the diagnosis of tabes dorsalis was firmly established by history, clinical symptoms and signs, together with serologic, neurologic and spinal fluid examinations. Some of the patients were so incapacitated that they could not walk without support, and most of them had to use a cane. Other symptoms such as lightning pains, urinary incontinence, impotency, constipation or girdle sensation, etc., were both frequent and marked.

The duration of tabetic manifestations varied from three months to 17 years (Table 1). It was more than ten years in 5 cases; 6-8 years in 4, three years in 2, and less than one year in 2. 8 cases had received more than 6 million units of penicillin before the initiation of this treatment, 3 of them having had arsenicals and/or bismuth in addition. 2 patients received penicillin (6-12 million units) and *Ti huang* decoction concurrently. 1 patient received *Ti huang* decoction alone (Table 1).

This plan of treatment was designed by our specialists in traditional medicine. The patients were first classified according to the methodology of traditional Chinese medical practice. According to this methodology these selected patients were subjected to the treatment with a special prescription which for the sake of convenience will be called "*Ti huang* decoction" here.

Ti huang decoction is a formula of long antiquity. The original prescription comprised some 15 drugs. In the course of our investigation, we have simplified the prescription to six constituents as follows:

Rehmannia glutinosa (cured) 地黄	9.4 gm
Polygala reinii 远志	"
Cornus officinalis 山茱萸	"
Orobanche ammophyla 肉苁蓉	"
Aconitum fischeri 乌头	"
Cortex Cinnamomi cainensis 肉桂	2.5-3.1 gm

This was the daily amount given to each patient in the form of a decoction. To this prescription, other supportive Chinese herbs might be added as required, or the dosages varied, according to Chinese therapeutic regime.

The duration of treatment varied from two to six months. The period of post-treatment observation was from 14-103 days. Other details are given in table 1.

Table 1. Status of patients before treatment

Case no.	Age	Sex	Duration of syphilitic infection (yr)	Duration of tabetic symptoms (yr)	Previous antisyphilitic treatment	Prominent symptoms on admission	Blood serology*	CSF change	Plan of treatment
1	*43*	*M*	*19*	*15*	*20 injections of '914' in 1944, many penicillin injections in 1954*	*Ataxia, incontinence*	-	*Normal*	*Ti huang*
2	45	M	25	10	7 courses of penicillin with bismuth in 1956-58	Ataxia, incontinence, girdle sensation	+	"	"
3	57	M	15	6	Penicillin 21 mil. units in 1956-58, penicillin 24 mil. units in 1958, '914' 5.8 gm in 1957	Ataxia, incontinence	+	"	"
4	48	M	28	10	Penicillin 9 mil. units in 1958	Ataxia, incontinence, lightning pain	+	WaR**+	"
5	29	M	?	3 mos	None	Ataxia, girdle sensation	+	"	Penicillin 12 mil. units, *Ti huang*
6	*43*	*M*	*25*	*17*	*Penicillin 3 mil. units in 1950 penicillin 12 mil. units with bismuth in 1957*	*Ataxia, incontinence, lightning pain*	+	*Normal*	*Ti huang*

7	59	M	20+	6	4-5 injections of '606' 10 yrs before, penicillin amount unknown in 1958	Ataxia	-	"	"
8	57	M	19	1	Penicillin 6 mil. units in 1958	Ataxia, lightning pain	+	"	Penicillin 6 mil. units, *Ti huang*
9	*43*	*M*	*15*	*3*	*Penicillin 14 mil. units in 1959*	*Ataxia*	-	"	*Ti huang*
10	53	M	24	3	None	"	+	WaR†	"
11	45	F	18	8	"	Ataxia, incontinence	-	Normal	Penicillin 12 mil. units, *Ti huang*

* Wassermann and/or Kahn reactions.

** Also increase in cells and protein.

† Also increase of cell and protein in addition to a paretic curve.

Results of Treatment

The results of treatment are listed in Table 2. All cases receiving the *Ti huang* treatment showed varying degrees of improvement, the most marked being in ataxia and sphincter control. Evident improvement in symptoms and signs began to appear in the first or second week, and became most marked within the first two months. Further treatment after the second month brought very little additional improvement. In 4 cases cessation of treatment for longer than four weeks witnessed a recurrence of symptoms; usually those that first disappeared relapsed first. However, the relapse never regained the former severity during the period of our observation—the longest being 103 days after termination of treatment.

It should also be pointed out that the duration of the disease seemed to have no effect on the rate or degree of improvement. Among the 11 cases receiving the *Ti huang* treatment, 2 cases of one year's duration and 1 of eight years (receiving simultaneous penicillin treatment) showed no better improvement than the other 8 cases—in fact the improvement seemed to be slightly less than the others.

Retreatment with *Ti huang* decoction after a recurrence usually restored the original level of improvement. Continued treatment with this formula caused no untoward side-effects on the blood, urine or liver function. The longest period of treatment in this series was eight months.

According to our specialists in traditional medicine, *Ti huang* decoction is not an antisyphilitic remedy. In our small series of cases, we did not observe any influence on blood serology or the CSF during the period of observation.

Table 2. Symptomatic improvement after treatment

Symptoms	No. cases with symptoms	No. cases improved	Remarks
Lightning pain	10	9	Only decrease of frequency of attacks or in severity
Urinary incontinence or difficulty in urination	10	8	In 4 cases symptoms disappeared but recurred after cessation of treatment and disappeared again after retreatment; 4 cases with marked decrease of symptoms only
Impotency or inability of erection	9	7	4 cases became nearly normal, 5 cases regained power of erection
Constipation or loss of rectal control	5	4	3 cases became normal, 1 case improved
Girdle sensation	3	3	Disappeared in all 3
Tabetic gait	11	11	Marked improvement, 5 cases nearly normal
Heel-to-knee test	11	9	–
Finger-to-nose test	3	1	–
Romberg's sign	11	11	4 cases nearly normal, 5 showed very slight sign, 2 markedly improved
Passive movement sensation	8	4	Partial recovery
Vibratory sensation	8	5	Partial recovery
Achilles tendon reflex	11	0	–
Testicular reflex	5	3	Recovery
Argyll-Robertson pupils	9	2	From complete loss of reflex to sluggish reaction

Discussion

Although the number of cases is small, we were much impressed by the uniformity, rapidity and degree of improvement in symptoms and signs; for instance, marked improvement of ataxia appeared in all of the 11 cases. Owing to the difficulty in finding a larger number of cases for investigation in Peking, we made observations on another series of 8 cases of tabes dorsalis collected in Tientsin. There again, the improvements were both prompt and striking. Unfortunately detailed analysis of therapeutic results cannot be made now, a longer time observation being needed.

We failed to find more patients with previous antiluetic treatment. In the earlier part of our investigation, we had 2 patients who had not received antisyphilitic treatment, but to give them the benefit of combined antibiotic and traditional drugs treatment, penicillin was given just before starting *Ti huang* decoction treatment.

Since many of our patients had received penicillin and/or arsenicals prior to the use of *Ti huang* decoction, the question naturally arises whether the improvement is due to the traditional drugs in our *Ti huang* prescription or to the delayed effect of penicillin which most of the patients had received before our study—6 of them had had penicillin within two years. We are inclined to the former interpretation for the following reasons:

1) After using *Ti huang* decoction all of our patients showed prompt and striking improvement of symptoms and signs, which in our common experience was rather unusual for modern antisyphilitic agents.

2) In 1 case treated with *Ti huang* decoction alone the clinical improvement was as marked as in any other case.

3) Cessation of treatment caused a return of symptoms and retreatment achieved improvement again.

4) In 4 cases, though there was a history of some improvement of symptoms during or shortly after penicillin therapy, by the time of the traditional drug treatment their symptoms had become worse or had been stationary for some time. *Ti huang* decoction alone brought about definite improvement in these cases. On the other hand, 2 other cases of proven tabes dorsalis with lightning pains which failed to respond satisfactorily to penicillin therapy for a period of nearly two years, were treated with a traditional prescription other than *Ti huang* decoction (because our specialists in traditional medicine considered them as not belonging to the same category as the tabetics show-

ing marked ataxia); both failed to show good response, thus in a way serving as controls for the *Ti huang* decoction treated group. Unfortunately these cases could not be called back for a trial on *Ti huang* decoction therapy.

5) In the *Ti huang* treatment series, 3 cases received simultaneous penicillin treatment (because in the earlier part of the investigation, the efficacy of the traditional drug alone had not yet been established), but their improvement was not any more noticeable than in the other 8 cases in which penicillin treatment was given much earlier or not at all.

Is the *Ti huang* decoction antiluetic in nature? We do not believe it is spirocheticidal because:

1) It contains no spirocheticidal component as far as is known. According to traditional medical specialists, this prescription is not used as a remedy against syphilis.

2) Within the period of our observation, no changes were produced on the blood serology or on the spinal fluid picture, as would have been the case with western antiluetics. Clinical improvements appeared in some cases in which the blood serology or CSF picture no longer showed any sign of syphilitic reaction. Furthermore, the clinical effect came on after the standard western antisyphilitic regime had failed to bring about further clinical improvement.

However, the mechanism of the treatment is a subject for further study. At present, we can only venture to suggest that this regime probably has a stimulating effect on the remnant fibers in the dorsal column of the spinal cord which are usually not completely destroyed in tabes dorsalis. This seems to be indicated by the rather prompt appearance of positive effect and, in the cases showing relapse of symptoms, restoration of positive effect as a result of retreatment. However, a sustained effect lasting four weeks is rather unusual for ordinary stimulating drugs on the nervous system. In the *Ti huang* decoction treatment the effect can be partially retained even for 100 days or more. These seemingly contradictory phenomena need further studies.

Summary

1) This investigation points to the value of integration of modern and traditional medicine and to a new approach using a *Ti huang* decoction in the therapy of tabes dorsalis.

2) The drug brought about striking and rapid clinical improvements of varying degrees in all of the cases in this investigation.

3) It has no untoward side-effects even after prolonged use.

4) Its effect on the nervous system is more prolonged than the ordinary stimulating drugs.

5) Its exact mechanism and application to other nervous diseases of similar nature merit further study.

Article end

Book advertisement

1960

Source: *Chinese Medical Journal, Foreign Language Publication*, May 1960

中華醫學雜誌外文版

Yaron: The beginning of standardized textbooks. It is now twelve years into the Communist rule and ideological influences, social and political pressures that have dictated a selection process for the new Chinese medicine. What is here called a Synopsis of Traditional Chinese Medicine actually means "the result of our selection process"; the topics, theories, formulas and logic we have decided should become Chinese medicine going forward.

Book announcements

Synopsis of Traditional Chinese Medicine (in Chinese)

Compiled by the Nanking College of Traditional Chinese Medicine

The first part of this book presents the fundamental theories and the therapeutic principles of Traditional Chinese Medicine, including Yin and Yang, the five elements, Yun Ch'i and ching luo as well as herbs and their prescriptions. The second part deals briefly with internal medicine, acupuncture and moxibustion, gynecology, pediatrics, surgery, traumatic wounds, ch'i kung and massage.

The first edition of this synopsis, compiled by the Nanking College of Traditional Chinese Medicine, was published in October 1958. It was very well received by the medical profession. Since then, it has been extensively revised by the original compilers in collaboration with the Peking College of Traditional Chinese Medicine and the Academy of Traditional Chinese Medicine. The book is now being used tentatively as a textbook in medical colleges and schools.

Synopsis of Traditional Chinese Pharmacology (in Chinese)

Compiled by the Nanking College of Traditional Chinese Medicine

Since its first publication in October 1958, this book has been revised and enlarged. It is now being used as a textbook in medical colleges in China.

Besides the history of traditional Chinese pharmacology, the book gives a detailed account of 285 commonly used herbs, classified according to the principle of traditional Chinese therapeutics, with explanations on the nature, active principles and use of each herb. Also, after each group of herbs, a short summary is given with annotations of the terms and synonyms usually employed.

Published by: Peoples' Medical Publishers

Sold by: Guozi Shudian P.O Box 399, Peking, China

Article end

Advance the great work of protecting the people's health

1960 by Hsu Yun Pei 徐运北

Source: *Chinese Medical Journal, Foreign Language Publication*, Volume 80 No. 5, May 1960.
中華醫學雜誌外文版

Yaron: Since the Communist "liberation", Medicine in China developed rapidly toward science and modernity. Chinese medicine too moved rapidly in the same direction: "A good start has been made in the research in ching luo and acupuncture and moxibustion; indeed, we are beginning to find the way of utilizing modern scientific methods for their study and systemization."

TCM prides the fact that now Chinese medicine is scientific and not primitive. However, the following line reveals the problem with this "scientification": "The leadership we give is, first and foremost, political leadership; hence we must do our ideological and political work properly. Professional and technical activities must be subordinated to politics. Without political leadership, being correct and effective in science and technology is not possible."

The scientification of Chinese medicine and especially the selection process dictating it was not according to science alone. Therefore, today when we learn a kind of mix of Zang-fu, five elements and Yin Yang, it is not the selection of modern science, nor is it a selection of "traditional experts"—rather, it is an ideological selection. Today in medicine, we don't follow ideology and even if we firmly believe in science, the selection of Chinese medicine needs to start again. Ideological influences in Chinese medicine were of long duration: "Such struggles will disappear only when the bourgeois political and ideological influences are finally wiped out. Therefore, a long-term task of the medical, pharmaceutical and health fronts is to persevere in the struggle between the socialist and capitalist road and continue with the socialist revolution in politics and ideology." Ideology presided over Chinese medicine for too long.

Pages 405-414

Hsu Yun Pei 徐运北, Vice Minister of Public Health, People's Republic of China

Under the correct leadership of the Central Committee of the Chinese Communist Party and Comrade Mao Tse-tung and the inspiration of the Party's general line of socialist construction, the great work of protecting the people's health in close coordination with the great leap forward in industrial and agricultural production has made tremendous achievements.

During recent years, the mass health movement has been extensively developed; literally every member of the population—man, woman and child—has taken part in the fight against the four pests and disease. As a result, the pest nuisance has greatly diminished and diseases from which the people suffered most seriously, such as smallpox, bubonic plague and kalaazar have been eradicated. In the prevention and treatment of schistosomiasis, endemic in 12 provinces and municipalities in South China, a tremendous victory has been won; the number of patients treated to date has topped the 4.9 million mark. Malaria, ancylostomiasis, filariasis and other serious diseases are being rapidly controlled and stamped out. Areas formerly desolate and laid waste by disease are now prosperous and healthy. In diseases such as Kaschin-Beck disease, goiter, pulmonary tuberculosis and trachoma new effective methods of prevention and treatment have been found, thus providing favorable conditions for their ultimate eradication.

To meet the new demands arising from the establishment of people's communes, health work has been strengthened in collective production on farms or working sites and in collective welfare facilities such as public dining halls, kindergartens and nurseries, resulting in a decrease in infectious diseases. Remarkable development has been seen in the health organization in the communes. At present, United Clinics (or hospitals), maternity centers and clinics (or health stations) operated by the communes in the countryside number over 270,000. Besides, there have been trained a vast army of skeleton health workers and activists among the masses who take up this work in addition to their ordinary occupation to form the backbone of the movement. A beginning has been made in the formation of health protection networks centering around the communes; and a great many communes have instituted collective medical care, thus ensuring better health for the commune members.

Urban health has also taken on a radically different aspect. We have fundamentally transformed the appalling conditions of the working people inherited from the old society. In mines and mills, labor protection and prevention and treatment of occupational diseases have made marked progress; silicosis, heat exhaustion, benzolism, etc. have basically been brought under control.

There are at present upwards of 390,000 medical units of various forms, equipped with more than 570,000 regular beds and 760,000 "simple" ones. The area of cultivated land for medicinal plants exceeds 200,000 hectares. A great many sources of wild plants and animals of pharmaceutical value are also tapped. A number of western drugs which previously had to be imported such as cortisone and hypotensive drugs are now being produced in China. In the field of medical research, effective methods have been formulated for the prevention and treatment of the five major parasitic diseases (schistosomiasis, ancylostomiasis, filariasis, malaria and kala-azar). The application and study of radioactive isotopes are also being steadily developed. Our work in intra-cardiac surgery and vascular prosthesis has reached the current world level. As for the management of burns, our technology has surpassed it, the cure rate obtained in extensive burns being 70.2%. The integration of traditional and Western medicine and the enhancement of our traditional medical heritage are proceeding rapidly. Preliminary results have been obtained in the study of the rationale of treatment for hypertension, chronic nephritis, etc. A good start has been made in the research in ching luo and acupuncture and moxibustion; indeed, we are beginning to find the way of utilizing modern scientific methods for their study and systemization.

In the wake of the momentous development in the country, our army of medical, pharmaceutical and health workers is growing daily. At the end of 1959 there were 1.46 million specialized medical and health workers in the country, excluding the core of several million health workers and activists among the masses; the enrollment in the medical and pharmaceutical colleges reached 90,000 and in the corresponding intermediate schools 150,000. Under the Party's guidance and in the course of steeling themselves in practical work in the outlying regions and mines and factories, our medical and health workers have been totally transformed in political ideology. Not a few of them, after abandoning their bourgeois outlook, have started on the road being "ideologically red and professionally expert" step by step dedicating themselves whole-heartedly to the service of the people. The unity among the ranks of medical and health workers has been greatly strengthened; the nihilistic tendency to reject our ancient legacy has been effectively counteracted and the unity of traditional and Western medical workers has entered a new phase. A vast army of red and expert medical, pharmaceutical and health workers is mustering. It is composed of workers in both traditional and Western medicine, high, intermediate and low grade medical cadres and whole time and part time health personnel.

II

The tremendous achievements in our health work have been gained as a result of the Party and Mao Tse-tung's leadership and guidance, of perseverance in the socialist revolution on the political and ideological fronts, and of repeated hard-won struggles in the choice between the capitalist road and the socialist road in health work. Over the years the struggle between the two roads in health work has centered in the fundamental issues as to whether, in health work, the Party should lead, the mass lines should be followed, and our ancient medical legacy should be inherited and developed.

PARTY'S ABSOLUTE LEADERSHIP—THE BASIC GUARANTEE OF VICTORY IN HEALTH WORK. In health organizations there used to be the erroneous view that health work is a special field of science which laymen are not fit to lead. A great many medical and health workers who were seriously imbued with bourgeois ideology resisted the Party's leadership, thus causing the health work in their organizations to become divorced from politics and reality. Led by the Party, we resolutely carried out in the health organizations the socialist revolution on the ideological front. Consequently, following the successive political campaigns, especially the anti-Rightist struggle and the rectification campaign in 1957 and the rectification campaign within the Party in 1959, we obtained decisive victories. The Party's leadership has once and for all been established.

The successive struggles waged by us against the Rightists and all those having erroneous tendencies, while differing in character, invariably boiled down to the issue of whether or not the Party should lead. The calumnies directed against the Party's leadership of health work always monotonously followed the refrain that health work was a special field of science which laymen were not fit to lead. This of course is sheer nonsense. In divorcing politics from professional work they have adopted a point of view completely irreconcilable to the Party and Mao Tse-tung's constant teachings. Time and again the Party and Comrade Mao Tse-tung have taught us that we must put politics in the leading role and place the relationship between politics and the vocational activities on a correct basis. In its directive to Party committees at all levels on the subject of strengthening their political leadership in health work, the Central Committee of the Party pointed out that: "The leadership we give is, first and foremost, political leadership; hence we must do our ideological and political work properly. Professional and technical activities must be subordinated to politics. Without political leadership being correct, effectiveness in science and technology is not possible." Health work has always been considered by the Party and Comrade Mao Tse-tung to be a "major political problem" and has received their closest care and attention. Guiding principles were laid down and clear and definite directives were put forth for each historical period. In the early post-liberation years we drew up the four cardinal principles of health work, viz., service to the workers, peasants and soldiers, prevention of disease as the primary task, close cooperation among medical personnel trained in the traditional and western schools, and integration of public health work with mass movements. These principles of the Party and Comrade Mao Tse-tung have been the guiding principles in all our health work and also an effective weapon in our struggle against the capitalist road in health work. Over the past years, it is precisely because we persevered in the Party's leadership, faithfully carried out the Party and Comrade Mao Tse-tung's directives, implemented the Party's general line and each and every policy, and incessantly criticized bourgeois ideology that we managed to bring about a fundamental transformation in our health work and marched from victory to victory.

In hospital work, for instance, we criticized the bourgeois ideologies and practices of "dictatorship of experts", supremacy of technique, disregard for the patient's needs and interest and neglect of preventative work. In implementation of the spirit of the Third Plenary Session of the Party's Eighth Congress, we carried out radical reforms and established the Party's leadership in hospital work. In pursuance of the policy of running hospitals economically and expanding prevention work with hospitals as centers of technical guidance for the districts and local mines and factories, we instituted round the clock clinical service and simple sick beds and strengthened the preventive work. Also, our hospital workers have gradually dedicated themselves wholeheartedly to the service of the people. As a result of all these, the hospital work has considerably improved in quality and is advancing swiftly along the road of socialism.

In medical education, we have discarded the bourgeois policy of letting professors and experts run schools, disregarding the masses and training students to be proficient professionally but devoid of proletarian ideology, thus divorcing medical education from politics, the masses and reality. Instead, we have established the Party's leadership in this field and carried out the Party's policies in education. We follow the policy of simultaneously developing large, medium and small-scale schools. Consequently, large numbers of medical and pharmaceutical schools of every size and type have sprung up across the country. The staff and students go from the confines of their schools and work among the worker and peasant masses, participating in labor production and mass health campaigns. Also, extensive study and systemizing of traditional medicine is carried out. As a result, medical education is realizing the aim of accomplishing greater, faster, better and more economical results.

In the field of medical research, there had been specialists in some places who monopolized research work and suppressed new ideas and new forces. They worked for personal glory and gain and had blind faith in the foreign literature and authorities, thus divorcing themselves from the needs of the masses and from reality. Where such conditions were obtained, the research work was invariably fruitless and inert. But, as a result of the Party's leadership, we have directed research to serve production and the immediate priority tasks, have shattered all the inhibiting ideas of the past as to what could or could not be done by the people's efforts, have launched a mass technical revolution and have practiced large scale cooperation. In this way we have made unprecedented advances in medical research.

The above facts explain why wherever the Party's leadership was strong the health work was carried out well and wherever there was no Party's leadership or deviation from it, however slight, mistakes were made and the work suffered loss. In establishing and strengthening the Party's leadership, the vital link lies in a strong leading core which will resolutely carry out the Party's policies and uncompromisingly fight against bourgeois ideologies. This is a fundamental experience gained by us over the past years.

While the political and ideologies revolution in health work has won decisive victories, it is by no means completed or evenly developed. The political and ideological struggles will continue like waves, with ups and downs. Sometimes they are acute and at other times they are mild. Such struggles will disappear only when the bourgeois political and ideological influences are finally wiped out. Therefore, a long-term task of the medical, pharmaceutical and health fronts is to persevere in the struggle between the socialist and capitalist road and continue with the socialist revolution in politics and ideology.

Criteria of People's health work – All for the masses and large scale mass health movements. Comrade Mao Tse-tung constantly teaches us that health work is a matter involving the birth, aging, sickness and death of all the people of the country, and that health workers should save the dying and heal the sick and wounded in the spirit of revolutionary humanitarianism. He asks us to place on our daily agenda, and find practical solutions for, the diseases that afflict the broad masses of the people. During the Second Revolution Civil War Comrade Mao Tse-tung pointed out that disease was a major enemy of the revolutionary bases and that it must be controlled and finally wiped out. During the Resist America and Aid Korea Movement Comrade Mao Tse-tung called on the people to mobilize, observe sanitation, arrest diseases, raise our health standards and shatter the enemy's germ warfare. In 1956, the Central Committee of the Party and Comrade Mao Tse-tung included in the National Programme for Agricultural Development the task of exterminating the four pests, observing hygiene and eradicating the major diseases as fundamental measures in protecting the people's health and ensuring production. These instructions on health work by the Party's Central Committee and Comrade Mao Tse-tung express their great solicitude for the masses' welfare and whole-hearted dedication to the people's service. Comrade Mao Tse-tung further constantly teaches us to adopt the mass line and mass movements in carrying out health work. "We must tell the masses," he said on one occasion, "to rise and struggle against their own illiteracy, superstitions and unhygienic habits." Early in 1933, he singled out the mass health movements in Ch'angkang hsiang (A township in Hsingkao county, Kiangsi province) for commendation and asked the revolutionary governing body of each hsiang to make it their business to launch large-scale mass health campaigns. The criteria of people's health work are whole-hearted service to the people, and integration of health work with the revolution and construction, with the urgent demands of the masses to exterminate pests and wipe out disease, and with the conscious actions of the broad masses.

With regard to the question as to whom health work should serve and rely upon, we maintain a position fundamentally different from the bourgeois whose policies are not motivated by the needs of the masses. They are totally indifferent to the sufferings of the masses; they harp on the paramountcy of technology, of experts, consider the masses a dull, ignorant drove incapable of grasping technology, and rely only on experts and not on the masses. After, under the Party's leadership, we thoroughly criticized these bourgeois ideologies, health work was able to advance along the way indicated by Comrade Mao Tse-tung. During the past years, the mass line has been greatly developed in health work, and mass health campaigns have brought great results; we have amassed a huge store of experiences which has opened up new vistas for health work in the future.

Extermination of the four pests, observance of the rules of hygiene and elimination of the major diseases are objectives of health work and an important part of our great socialist cultural revolution. Only by organizing wide scale mass health campaigns of extermination of the four pests, observance of the rules of hygiene and elimination of the major diseases can we better realize the policy of prevention first, protect the health of our 600 million people and guarantee production and construction. This in turn will help and reform out-moded customs and habits and transform the world we live in.

Health work must proceed with a view to developing production; it should be closely integrated with and serve production. Under the unified leadership of the Party committees, production and health work must be closely coordinated and planned. The more intense the production, the more attention must we pay to health work; the better the health work is done, the higher will be the production level. This, in a nutshell, is the dialectic unity in the relationship between production and health. Health work concerns every person and every department. By clearly understanding the role of health work in serving production, by closely coordinating health work with production, making it answer the needs of daily life, and by practicing extensive coordination and cooperation, we can enable health work to keep pace with the march of events and continuously leap forward.

Extermination of the four pests, observance of the rules of hygiene and elimination of major diseases have been and will always be carried out by the process of mass campaigns, of thoroughly and extensively mobilizing the masses and continuously raising their consciousness. In fact, educating the masses through mass movements is the most effective way of raising consciousness and increasing their knowledge of hygiene. Once the broad masses become health-conscious and start taking action, health campaigns will be carried out better and more thoroughly. In order to give leadership to the mass health campaigns, we must place reliance on the masses and know their requirements and latent possibilities; we must learn to be in the forefront of their ranks, leading the movement forward; we must place before the masses concrete tasks on the basis of specific local conditions and the most urgent needs of production and daily life; we must put across clearly to the masses all policies and thoroughly carry out ideological work; we must carry out extensive health education and train health work activists. During the movement, it is necessary to boost the advanced aspects of the work, push the lagging aspects, and constantly summarize the experiences gained, thus enabling it to develop in a balanced way and continuously.

Our experiences over the past years have taught us that extermination of four pests must start from residential areas, and gradually spread out until all the areas have been thoroughly covered. Generally the movement for pest extermination and disease-elimination embraces three steps—control, delimit, and eradicate. We have to guide the movement in the spirit of "uninterrupted revolution" and alternate high tempo shock brigade type actions with routine consolidation. It is also important to be thorough and to get at the root of pestilence and disease, and to adopt simultaneously both modern and indigenous methods, both traditional and Western medicine. Further we must guard against rashness as well as slackening. These, we find, are factors that contribute to the smooth and effectual development at each stage of the mass health campaigns.

Medical and pharmaceutical technology must keep pace with the mass health campaigns. It must serve the health movement and the Party's central tasks. Also, medical and pharmaceutical workers must be close to the masses and reality, identifying themselves with the masses and imparting technical knowledge to them. They must also play close attention to inventions and creations by the masses, and continually summarize and improve upon them.

The mass line and mass movements in health work during the past several years have brought forth a set of policies of simultaneous development in health work, which is daily putting into motion more and more positive factors and is producing in our health work greater, better, faster and more economical results. In our future work, the key to further advance is to continue to study and summarize our experiences on simultaneous development in health work, persevere in its application and enhance it.

Yaron: I extract the following summary as for what the Communists envisioned TCM to be: "The criteria for this new medical science are: a) It serves our 600 million people and protects their health; b) It treats the patients as an indivisible entity; c) It is armed with a high degree of dialectical materialism and a still higher degree of science and technology; d) It absorbs the essence of traditional medicine and the advanced achievements of modern science. The study of traditional medicine by western style medical workers is the key to inheriting and developing our medical heritage. We must take all possible measures to carry out thoroughly and extensively the study and systemizing of traditional medicine so as to train highly qualified experts in this field."

Here, Western-style medical workers are key for inheriting and developing the traditional medicine. In a prior article about Tabes Dorsalis, traditional experts selected a certain Shengti formula to participate in the study. How traditional were those traditional experts?

Yun Tieqiao in the 1920s, contrary to Yu Yunxiu and Tan Cizhong, wanted to reform Chinese medicine while maintaining a unique Chinese medicine principle independent of modern medicine. This did not happen with TCM but I believe it should.

UNITY AND COOPERATION BETWEEN TRADITIONAL AND WESTERN MEDICINE IN INHERITING AND ENHANCING OUR MEDICAL LEGACY. For thousands of years our people have relied solely on traditional medicine and pharmacology in combating disease. This medical heritage is a rich treasury, the crystallization of our people's age long fight against disease. We must earnestly systemize and enhance it, integrating it with modern medicine to create our own unique school of medicine. This task has time and again been pointed out by the Party's Central Committee and Comrade Mao Tse-tung. What attitude we adopt towards traditional medicine becomes at once a question of the attitude we adopt towards the needs of our 600 million people and towards uniting the broad masses of traditional medicine workers, a question of mass standpoint and the mass line as well as a question of the correct attitude to take towards our national cultural heritage and towards better developing the medical science of our country. Unity among western and traditional style medical workers, inheritance and enhancement of our medical heritage and creation of our new school of medicine are all important tasks in our health work.

The integration of traditional and Western medicines manifests itself in every aspect of health work. In prevention and treatment, the combination of traditional and Western medicines, each supplementing the other, has enabled us to serve the health of a greater number of people, faster, better and more economically. In pharmaceutics, combination of western and traditional drugs and simultaneous application of indigenous and foreign methods have greatly enhanced our ability to exterminate pest and eliminate diseases. In medical education, the teaching of both traditional and Western medicines and mutual learning among traditional and western style medical workers have raised the level of teaching and techniques. In medical research, the integration of traditional and Western medicine which is of benefit not only to the enhancement of our national medical heritage but also to the development of modern medicine speeds up the creation of a new school of medicine.

On the health front, intense struggles have also taken place during the past several years over the question of whether or not to inherit and develop our medical heritage. Under the Party's leadership, we resolutely criticized the ideology of belittling and refuting traditional medicine and corrected the sectarian discriminations against it. Also, we made determined efforts to strengthen our work in traditional medicine. Since the convening of the All-China Conference of Traditional Medicine and Pharmacy in November 1958 and the *Renmin Ribao* 人民日報 editorial of January 25th, 1959, on *Earnest Implementation of the Party's Policy on Traditional Medicine*, the policy put forth by the Party as regards traditional medicine has been more thoroughly and extensively implemented, and our work in traditional medicine has entered a new stage of development. The unity and cooperation between medical workers of the two schools have been greatly strengthened, and the study of traditional medicine by western style medical workers has become a mass movement. The number currently attending full-time courses has topped the 2,300 mark; needless to say, part-time study is even more widespread. The coordination between traditional and Western medicine has yielded rich results in our effort to exterminate pests and wipe out disease. Where previously, for some diseases, we had no effective methods of cure or prevention, we found them through combining traditional and Western medicine. Work has gone ahead at a rapid pace in the study and systemizing of traditional medicine.

In our work in traditional medicine, we must oppose the national nihilistic ideology of belittling and refuting traditional medicine and also overcome the conservative habit of adhering to obsolete and hide-bound traditions. The main stress, however, should be placed on the former. At the same time, we must also carry out the mass line. The masses should be acquainted with the Party's policy on traditional medicine, for once they understand the policy, the work in traditional medicine will proceed swiftly. In systemizing traditional medicine, we should coordinate the efforts of specialized institutions and the broad masses and in studying traditional medicine we must integrate full-time and part-time study. These are all well tested experiences.

To sum up, the health work in our country, under the close guidance and attention of the Party's Central Committee and Comrade Mao Tse-tung, has developed after a succession of struggles on the political and ideological fronts as to which road to follow. Comrade Mao Tse-tung's guiding principles on health work is a new development of Marxism-Leninism; they point out for New China the most correct path to take in health work.

III

In view of the sustained leap forward in socialist construction, the basic tasks confronting our health work in 1960 are: to better carry out and realize the Party's general line; closely coordinate with industrial and agricultural production; continue launching mass health campaigns with the chief aims of extermination of the four pests, observance of the rules of hygiene and elimination of major diseases; energetically develop and improve the medical and health work in the rural and urban areas and in the mines and factories; and more effectively protect the people's health and guarantee the sustained leap forward in socialist construction.

The mass health campaigns centering on extermination of the four pests, observance of the rules of hygiene and elimination of major diseases have become a movement embracing the whole people. In 1960 we ask that these should be carried out better and more thoroughly, so as to obtain more pest-free counties and districts. We need to further confine and finally wipe out the diseases that constitute a grave menace to the people's health such as schistosomiasis, malaria, ancylostomiasis, filariasis, K'oshan disease, Kaschin-Beck disease. Effective fecal management is a fundamental method of wiping out parasitic diseases, so we should formulate effective systems of fecal control in conjunction with fertilizer collection. Also, we must launch health education drives by utilizing the anti-illiteracy work, school education, and such media as films and skits, to further raise the people's knowledge of hygiene, and help them to form new hygienic habits and customs. By so doing, we shall be establishing a firm groundwork for accomplishing far ahead of schedule the task of wiping out pests and eradicating diseases stipulated in the National Programme for Agricultural Development.

Our current central task is to carry out well the health work in the people's communes. The people's production and mode of life have taken on a higher degree of collectivism. In view of this, we must more effectively implement the policy of "prevention first" and prevent the occurrence and spread of infectious diseases. It is also necessary to strengthen labor protection and health work in the fields, on water conservancy projects and transportation sites. The public dining hall is the center of the commune's collective life. Therefore, improving health work in the dining halls is of great significance not only in protecting the people's health, but also in consolidating the commune. Kindergartens and nurseries involve the care and education of the rising generation and further emancipation of women. They are vitally important matters that concern several hundred millions of our people. We must strengthen leadership in this field, increase the working force, and raise the level of our child care work.

The health protection organization of the people's communes must be energetically developed and steadily improved. At present, the ideal medical care system for commune members, in view of the present level of production and consciousness of the masses, is collective medical care. Under this system, the expenses for medical care are jointly shouldered by the individual members and the commune, and the funds are pooled and used collectively. Expanding and improving the county level hospitals is an important measure in strengthening the health work in the people's communes. To do this, we must first of all strengthen the Party's leadership and then steadily increase the number of highly qualified medical workers, expand basic constructions and increase equipment and facilities, thereby enabling the county level hospitals to assume the role of centers of medical technology and bases for training health cadres.

With the swift advance in industry, large, medium and small enterprises have mushroomed all over the country, which requires that industrial health work must keep pace. The accent of urban health work should be paced on industrial health. For this, it is necessary to strengthen the leadership and organization. All urban medical workers should master preventive and curative techniques in industrial occupational diseases so as to better serve industrial production and the health of the workers.

In order to meet the development of industrial and agricultural production and the people's increasing demand for medical services, reforms must continue in our hospital work. Medical workers must whole-heartedly dedicate themselves to the service of the people and thoroughly rid themselves of the practice of sitting back and waiting for patients to come to them. We must go out from the confines of the hospital, into the mines and mills, into the villages, urban districts, and energetically carry out prevention and treatment. We must foster the communist spirit of going wherever we are needed and doing whatever will benefit the people. We must make our work serve production and the masses by formulating and adopting a variety of systems and methods suited to the needs of collective production and living readily acceptable to the broad masses of the people.

To further advance the great work of the people's health, we must go full strength in training health cadres who are proletarian ideologically and proficient professionally. In implementing the Party's policy of education in the service of proletarian politics and integration of education with productive labor, we must realize the policy of giving unified over-all planning to higher, intermediate and lower grade medical education, coordinating and cooperating on a nationwide scale and following the set of policies of simultaneous development.

This means that medical education must be integrated with productive labor, with the mass health campaigns and with traditional medicine; the efforts of the administrative leadership, the teaching staff and the student body should be coordinated; and education work, medical research and preventive and treatment should be integrated. We must give full scope to the ability of the experts but, at the same time, shatter the vestiges of monopoly of research by them. Efforts must be redoubled in training highly qualified medical workers and physicians. At present, extramural education and county-operated health schools are still weak links in our work which must be greatly strengthened. Hospitals, research institutions, and medical organizations in the industries should extensively undertake to operate extramural schools or even full-time or part-time ones. We must strive to have at least 40% of the county level hospitals open intermediate-grade health schools this year.

In view of the swift development in collective welfare facilities such as nurseries and kindergartens, we must make great efforts to train and raise standards of child care workers, operating child care nursing schools for the training of specialized workers conversant in both child care and health knowledge. Health organizations at all levels should adopt a variety of forms of training health cadres for the people's communes, continually strengthening the communes' health force. During the process of development, however, close attention must be paid to continuously raising the teaching quality. Colleges and schools with facilities should spare no efforts to pave the way for establishing faculties or departments to deal with the advanced sciences, and adopt all effective measures for training teachers in these advanced fields.

The surging progress in our health work demands, more and more every day, that we develop medical science rapidly. To this end, we must earnestly implement the principles of combining "popularization with elevation" and letting "a hundred flowers bloom and a hundred schools contend". We must continue to fight superstition and emancipate the mind. Traditional and Western medicine should be combined and indigenous and modern methods simultaneously developed. Mass movements in technical revolution should be energetically carried out. Medical research should be done under centralized leadership, with over-all planning and coordination.

While priority should be given to topics in advanced science and those specified by the state, research should also be done in connection with our routine work and specialties. Also, research work should be undertaken by medical and pharmaceutical research network across the land. Here we must emphasize the importance of strengthening cooperation between traditional and Western medicine in bringing about a new medical science. The criteria for this new medical science are: a) It serves our 600 million people and protects their health; b) It treats the patients as an indivisible entity; c) It is armed with a high degree of dialectical materialistic viewpoint and a still higher degree of science and technology; and d) It absorbs the essence of traditional medicine and the advanced achievements of modern science. The study of traditional medicine by Western-style medical workers is the key to inheriting and developing our medical heritage. We must take all possible measures to carry out thoroughly and extensively the study and systemizing of traditional medicine so as to train highly qualified experts in this field.

The production and supply of pharmaceutical and biological products must be done efficiently. We should exert our utmost to produce not only what is produced abroad but also new products, not only in adequate quantities but also of highest quality. It is especially important for us to pay close attention to the production of crude drugs and the farms where they are raised. In short, we must make pharmaceutical work coordinate better with the movement to wipe out pests and eliminate diseases.

Our health work is progressing along the brilliant path pointed out to us by Comrade Mao Tse-tung, whose thinking is our compass in all aspects of work. We must seriously study Mao Tse-tung's thinking, arming ourselves with it, to use it in guiding our work. We must continue to criticize and overcome bourgeois ideologies and establish the communistic ideology. We must continue consolidating and strengthening the Party's leadership, enabling the Party's leadership and political and ideological work to permeate every aspect of our work and the ideology of the broad masses of health cadres. We must extensively launch the mass movement to learn from the advanced, achieving a new upsurge of continuous leap forward in health work.

Let us raise high the banner of Mao Tse-tung's thinking, exert greater efforts and, by advancing the great work of the people's health, boldly march forward to new and greater victories.

Article end

[Book] The New Medicine truly is easy

1965 by Zhang Gongrang 張公讓

Published 1965 by China's New Medicine Research Institute, Hong Kong

新醫學實在易　香港：中國新醫學研究院

Yaron: With so many facts it is hard to pinpoint a single dominant event, theory or logic that had the most influence on Chinese medicine scientification. However, one thing changed Chinese medicine forever: the dialectical logic—if it is hot then cool it off; if it is cool then heat it up. This logic, which some say is the ancient Yin Yang, matched perfectly the Marxist dialectical materialism and constructed the core of TCM theory and treatment; it made things appear "physical" and tangible. It removed the ancient Chinese medicine claim that life is connected to heaven or that man is connected to the universe. A patient feeling hot or cold is tangible. Causing a cold person to feel hot is also tangible. Like this, theory and treatment have become tangible and more becoming to a modern scientific logic. Yin Yang, five elements and Zangfu theories all became the physical reality of TCM.

Chinese and Western medicine

Chinese and Western medicines both have their own advantages; Chinese medicine is better with its accumulated experience while Western medicine is better with its theories. Due to scientific research, Western medicine has figured out many mysteries of physiology and pathology. With clinical experience for thousands of years, Chinese medicine so far still has some effective treatments which can't be explained from a scientific angle, but it still fits science; otherwise it would not have a therapeutic effect. Therefore people call it "science of accumulated experience". It will be perfect if we can combine Chinese medical experience with Western medical theories.

Disease observation from a Chinese medicine angle is about human being and life; it's also dynamic and general, while from a Western medical angle it's about things and not about life; it's static and local. Hot and cold treatment is very valuable, and it's based on people's constitution which is divided into different kinds, such as cold, hot, deficient and excessive. According to constitution types, Chinese medicine gives individual and different treatments. The hot and cold treatment seems different from symptomatic and physical treatment. Hot and cold treatment means to heat up if the patient has cold constitution, or to cool down if the patient has hot constitution. It also means to tonify a deficient constitution and reduce an excessive constitution. Basically it brings the unbalanced physiological condition back to balance.

For example, one with weak pulse and low body temperature (metabolic deficiency, which means cold constitution) should be treated with Fuzi 附子 and Ganjiang 乾薑 to heat up, while another one with powerful pulse, high body temperature and extreme thirst (which is hot constitution) should be treated with Bai Hu Tang 白虎湯 to cool down. This is different from etiological therapy in Western medicine, which aims to directly kill bacteria, noting that this kind of treatment is less applicable for patients of weaker constitution. Patients get weaker or even die when Western medicine kills bacteria, while the hot and cold therapeutic treatment brings the patient's physiological condition back to normal (the original balance). Furthermore, the recovery of physiological condition facilitates the immune system to kill bacteria on its own. This is the advantage of Chinese medicine.

Article end

Apply Chairman Mao's teaching and improve even more in service of the workers, peasants and soldiers[454]

Source: *Chinese Medical Journal Foreign Language Publication*, February 1966 Vol. 85, No.2 中華醫學雜誌外文版

Yaron: Coming to the eve of the Cultural Revolution, the extent of merging medicine with ideology reached an extreme. Selecting what will and will not remain in TCM was in constant flux directly related to ideological pressures of that time.

[454] Translation of Jian Kang Bao's 健康報 editorial (slightly abridged), January 1, 1966.

"We should regard Chairman Mao's books as the highest instructions on all aspects of our work. We should creatively study and apply Mao Tse-tung's thinking and, in particular, make the utmost effort to apply his thinking to practice. In the course of transforming the objective world we should also transform our subjective world, so as to promote the revolutionization of both our public health work and public health workers." At this point, TCM and ideology have completely merged into a single entity.

Pages 73–78

In 1965, the people of our country, under the leadership of the Chinese Communist Party and Chairman Mao, by holding aloft the great red banner of Mao Tse-tung's thinking, continued to win great victories on all fronts of our socialist revolution and socialist construction. It was a year during which a very favorable revolutionary situation emerged in the fields of medicine and public health.

During the year, public health branches at all levels resolutely implemented the instructions of the Central Committee of the Chinese Communist Party and Chairman Mao to give priority to medical and public health work in the countryside and took radical measures to carry out the fundamental policy of orientating health service towards the workers, peasants and soldiers. Urban medical and health workers were mobilized to go to rural areas to serve the peasants and train medical and health personnel. The work of prevention and treatment of diseases most harmful to the health of the people was strengthened and a mass patriotic health movement was launched with emphasis on the control of human excreta and improvement of drinking water.

While directing the main attention of our health work to the countryside, we at the same time promoted the revolutionization of our urban medical work and medical workers. In this connection we started to reform medical education and scientific research work and, in active cooperation with the organizations concerned, greatly improved the production and supply of pharmaceuticals and medical equipment needed in the countryside. All this has resulted in remarkable successes. Especially noteworthy is that the broad masses of medical workers have ardently—and with revolutionary enthusiasm—responded to the call of the Party and of Chairman Mao.

A nationwide upsurge to go to the countryside to serve the peasants has started. This is unprecedented in our medical and public health work. Last year, more than

150,000 medical and public health workers in the big and medium-sized cities and county towns organized teams to tour rural areas and mountain regions. Many others went to settle down in the countryside so as to dedicate their efforts to the needs of the peasants. Led by the Party and Government at different levels, these urban medical and public health workers accomplished an enormous amount of work in preventing and treating diseases, training public health personnel and reinforcing rural health units, so that health work could gradually take root in the countryside. As a result, the health of the peasants has been effectively protected and the ties between the Party and the masses have been further strengthened. The peasants hurried to spread the news that "Chairman Mao has sent good doctors here!" The very act of sending city medical and health workers to the countryside demonstrated to the peasants the great concern shown them by the Party and Chairman Mao.

The dispatch of large groups of medical and public health workers to the countryside has not only reinforced the rural health apparatus but also given an impetus to the revolutionization of urban public health work and to that of medical work as a whole. At the same time, it has enabled medical and public health workers to identify themselves more closely with the workers, peasants and soldiers and advance their ideological reform.

These facts have eloquently testified to the correctness of the directives of the Central Committee of the Party and of Chairman Mao. To mobilize the medical and health workers to give service to the 500 million peasants is indeed an extremely important step towards the revolutionization both of our country's public health work and of her public health workers.

Chairman Mao has, all along, taught us to wholeheartedly serve the people, to serve the workers, peasants and soldiers and to serve the laboring people who constitute the overwhelming majority of the population. He said that "the supreme test of the words and deeds of a Communist is whether they conform to the highest interests and enjoy the support of the overwhelming majority of the people." We should always start from this point and never forget it whenever we make plans, do things or grapple with problems.

Chairman Mao has always given explicit instructions concerning the role played by the peasants, who make up over 80% of our country's population, in our revolution and construction and concerning the importance of medical service for the peasants. To orientate our public health work towards the rural areas embodies Chairman Mao's consistent instructions to us and embodies the basic policy of our socialist public health work. It is precisely because we have abided by Chairman Mao's teaching in doing things that such a favorable revolutionary situation, based on our previous achievements, has arisen in our work.

Although the past year has seen great advances, this is only a good beginning. Much more formidable tasks confront us before we can solve, in a practical manner, the medical and public health problems of the 500 million peasants. We will continue to make arrangements for large batches of urban doctors and health workers to go to the countryside on a rotation basis, for urban medical institutions to set up bases in the countryside in order to strengthen the rural health service, and for part of the city personnel to settle down for long periods in the countryside, so that one third of the urban personnel will always be working in rural areas.

Also, utmost efforts should be made to train rural medical and health workers and heighten their skill. The basic medical units at grass root levels should be reorganized and built up. In this way, we can gradually reach the target of having volunteer health workers in every production team, part-time medical workers in every production brigade and from three to five fully-qualified doctors in every commune. When this target has been reached, a relatively complete network of rural medical and public health service will have been formed.

Concurrently with improving rural health work, we should revolutionize our urban public health work and bring about further improvements. All this, of course, cannot be achieved in a short period of time. This year, our country has entered the first year of the Third Five-Year Plan. Based on the continued implementation of the socialist education movement, which will still further enhance the socialist consciousness of the masses, our country's industrial and agricultural production and all construction projects will certainly forge ahead with still greater vigor.

The historic task of creating a new and better socialist countryside is already on the agenda. This situation has provided our work with extremely advantageous conditions. At the same time, it has also put new and higher demands on us. In the coming year, we must continue to resolutely carry out the instructions of the Central Committee of the Party and of Chairman Mao. Our determination should be great, our steps steady and our working method meticulous. On the basis of what we have already achieved, we shall go on to win new and greater victories.

What is great determination? Great determination means to have revolutionary enthusiasm and vigor, the ideology of serving the people wholeheartedly, the class feeling of serving the laboring people who are the overwhelming majority of the population, the lofty ambition to completely transform the poor and blank state of affairs existing in our country's rural medical and public health work. Great determination means daring to go in for revolution, daring to practice, daring to combat difficulties, daring to win victories, daring to do what our predecessors have never done, daring to chart a way well suited to our country's medical and public health work. Great determination means, in the final analysis, doing things in a down-to-earth manner under the guidance of Chairman Mao's teaching. As Chairman Mao directs, so should we do. We should carry out our tasks well and without any reservation. A spirit of this kind is the most valuable quality of a revolutionary.

A deep-going revolution in public health work is needed to fulfil the glorious and arduous task placed on us by the Party and Chairman Mao. This means that we must go on organizing large groups of city medical and public health personnel to go in turns to rural areas and mountain regions, to go on transferring part of the personnel to settle down in the countryside, to completely reform urban public health work. It is inconceivable that this will not meet with obstacles arising from conventional ideas and old habits. It will inevitably be confronted by difficulties of one kind or another. There will be twists and turns. If we are not armed with a thoroughgoing revolutionary spirit, if we do not fully summon up our revolutionary determination and vigor, we are likely to vacillate and hesitate in face of difficulties. If this were so, we would be unworthy of the trust placed in us by the Party and Chairman Mao. Therefore, our determination and vigor should be great and we should have the spirit of surmounting every difficulty to win victory. This will decide whether or not we can, in future, win still greater and better achievements.

To direct the main drive of our public health work towards the countryside and to do genuinely practical work to solve the problems of providing a medical and public health service for the broad peasant masses is an undertaking unprecedented in the history of China and of the rest of the world. It is a long-term strategic policy for our country's public health work. We lack experience in carrying through such a big undertaking. Therefore, we must combine revolutionary vigor with a scientific approach of seeking truth from facts, advance steadily and work meticulously.

What do we mean by advancing steadily? We mean that while we strategically rebuff difficulties, we tactically take full account of them. In the light of existing conditions, we must do more solid work. This concretely means to combine more and faster results with better and more economical results. We must be not only bold but also proficient in revolution. It is necessary to carefully study working methods. Every major reform and construction project should first go through a phase of experimentation, investigation and study. After careful trials, the experiences gained should be summed up and their positive aspects popularized in stages.

Now, the direction of our medical work, i.e., emphasis on the countryside, is clear. However, it is still necessary to solve a series of problems concerning concrete policies and methods before the strategic task can be realized. Only on the basis of serious investigation and study and through summing up of experiences can we solve these problems.

A national conference to discuss rural public health work will be convened in 1966. We hope that health organizations at all levels will make full use of the time before the conference to do thorough preparations and summing up of experiences. Then, on the basis of these experiences, programmes should be mapped out both for a relatively long period of time (e.g., five or ten years) and for one year's concrete work. Once we have acquired adequate experience and have worked out a plan well suited to the existing conditions, we shall be able to see further ahead and be more certain in action. In this way, our work can be planned systematically and still better and faster progress can be made.

What do we mean by meticulous work? Meticulous work means to stress quality and practical usefulness. We should do things in a careful and thoroughgoing manner and discard formalism. We should work perseveringly and meticulously and continue to consolidate and raise our level. In a word, we must always ensure that the quality of work in all fields is progressively improved. Quality and quantity form a dialectical unity. Without quantity there can be no quality to speak of and without quality there can be no quantity. To ensure and raise quality does not mean to ignore quantity. On the contrary, we should strive to obtain quicker results and reap a richer harvest in the pursuit of excellence. The training of rural health workers and the building up of rural health services are major undertakings that directly concern the interests of the peasant masses. We should not set about such things in a reckless manner. It is necessary for us to adopt a careful and responsible attitude and put quality first, only then can our health work pass every trial and test, really take root in the countryside and better serve the peasants.

Great determination, steady advance and careful working method should be welded into one entity. However, the key prerequisite is great determination. It is imperative that we carry out with great determination the instructions of the Central Committee of the Chinese Communist Party and Chairman Mao.

In order to establish rural public health facilities and start to solve the problem of a medical and health service for 600 million people, we should persist in the policy repeatedly taught by Chairman Mao of building the country through hard work and thrift and running every enterprise with industry and frugality by relying mainly on the strength of the masses. It is wrong to depend entirely on the State and to leave everything to be attended to by the Government. While we should reduce the financial burden of the masses, we should not increase the burden of the State or the collective; we should wholeheartedly learn from the revolutionary spirit of self-reliance and hard struggle of the Taohai Production Brigade. We should apply this spirit of industry and frugality in running our health undertakings and solving all problems.

Medical and health work in China is entering a new period of vast development. We must continue to give first place to politics and apply the teaching of Chairman Mao and the Party. Like the People's Liberation Army, we should, in ideological and political work, give first place to the study of Chairman Mao's works. As a corollary to the implementation of the instructions of the Central Committee of the Party and Chairman Mao to stress the rural areas in our health work, a vigorous drive to study Chairman Mao's works in a persistent and profound manner should be launched among all health workers. We should regard Chairman Mao's books as the highest instructions on all aspects of our work. We should creatively study and apply Mao Tse-tung's thinking and, in particular, make the utmost effort to apply his thinking to practice. In the course of transforming the objective world we should also transform our subjective world, so as to promote the revolutionization of both our public health work and public health workers. In this way we will be sure to score ever greater victories in the new year.

Article end

Prelude to the Great March of orientating health work towards the rural areas: Some questions concerning the work of rural mobile medical teams

1966 by Ch´ien Hsin-Chung 錢信忠, Minister of Health, People´s Republic of China

Source: *Chinese Medical Journal Foreign Language Publication*, Vol 85, No 4, April 1966
中華醫學雜誌外文版

Yaron: A Foreign Language Publication, we have kept the linguistic errors.

Ideology turned into a physical reality: "As some comrades have correctly put it, whether or not one makes a detailed calculation of every cent when treating illnesses for peasants is by no means a purely economic problem, but a political problem, a problem that reflects one's class stand. For this reason, many medical teams try to economize in medical expenditures by all sorts of means. Therapies like acupuncture, manipulative treatment and cupping, which require little or no money, are frequently used. Others, in writing prescriptions think hard over the special circumstances of the case so that, often, the medicine costs a few cents only."

The attitude and value placed with Traditional Chinese medicine: "Traditional Chinese medicine should be combined with modern medicine and these rural health workers should master, as part of their basic technique, the simple but effective therapies of traditional Chinese medicine such as acupuncture, moxibustion, manipulation, massage, and other home remedies."

TCM was a cheap and easy kind of remedy similar to home remedy. Most importantly, and here explained well, creating a new kind of affordable and popular medicine to serve cities and countryside was not a short term strategy: "The task of orientating our medical work towards the countryside and of building up a socialist rural health network is a long-term and formidable task with a profound strategic and revolutionary significance. We believe that, so long as we persist in uninterrupted revolution, are proficient in summing up experiences, doggedly march on from one victory to another and are not afraid of hard and bitter struggles, we shall certainly succeed, in not too long a time."

Pages 209–222

The footprints of our mobile medical teams may be found throughout our vast land from the Ch'inghai-Tibetan Plateau to the East China Sea and from the banks of the Heilungchiang River to the Five-Finger Mountains.

Since Spring 1965, large numbers of our health workers have enthusiastically responded to the call of the Central Committee of the Chinese Communist Party and of Chairman Mao, and have organized thousands of mobile medical teams to go deep into rural areas and provide health services for five hundred million peasants. This is both a prelude to the great march of orientating our health work towards the rural areas and a good beginning in the ideological revolutionization of our medical personnel.

HEALTH WORKERS, IN GOING DOWN TO THE COUNTRYSIDE INSPIRE THE MASSES AND ALSO REFORM THEMSELVES

Ever since liberation, in coordination with the current revolutionary and construction tasks, we have organized some medical teams to go to the countryside and to regions inhabited by national minorities where they have won considerable achievements. The present drive, however, has greatly exceeded all previous ones in the large number of people involved, in the wide scope and high technical quality of the service provided and in the great depth of the work done. More important, the vast majority of our health workers have come to understand that our medical and public health work should be directed towards the countryside to serve the peasants and that they should identify themselves with the workers, peasants and soldiers and should reform their own ideology in the course of revolutionary struggle.

Under the leadership of the Party Committees and organs of the People's Government at all levels, the mobile medical teams have, within a short span of time, accomplished an enormous amount of work in the prevention and treatment of disease, and innumerable moving scenes have been enacted.

Showing diligence and economy and improvising in face of the existing poor conditions in the countryside, many team members manifested a highly responsible attitude towards their patients and were able to obtain wonderful successes. To save the life of a patient, they were prepared to neglect sleep and meals, heroically fight for days and nights, and donate their own blood. Undeterred by high mountains, thick forests or dangerous paths, team members would bring medicine to remote mountain regions. Others, on stormy nights, risked their lives in crossing rivers, in order to bring help to mother and child in a difficult labor. They wholeheartedly served the people, cured many commonly-seen diseases in the rural areas, saved many seriously ill patients and restored vision to many blind persons.

Concurrently with treating and preventing disease, our medical teams made energetic efforts to improve the disposal of manure and to purify drinking water. They propagated knowledge of sanitation, trained large batches of volunteer rural health workers for production teams and part-time doctors for production brigades.

The peasants have a high appraisal of the medical teams. Wherever they went, the local people hurried to spread the news that "Chairman Mao has sent good doctors here!" They said: "In the old society, doctors such as you would never have come, even if requested. Now you have come on your own initiative. You have brought medicine to our houses, to our fields and to our bedsides. We owe all this to the good leadership of the Communist Party." Some people cured after long years of blindness or of serious disease were so moved that, with tears in their eyes, they shouted: "Long live Chairman Mao!" The work of the medical teams has vividly demonstrated to the broad masses of peasants the deep concern for their well-being felt by the Party and Chairman Mao, it has fired their enthusiasm in the struggle for production and in the class struggle and has brought still closer the relation between the Party and the masses.

In the course of their work and of participation in the rural socialist education movement, members of the medical teams have deepened their understanding of the present situation of the rural class struggle and have strengthened their class viewpoints. Through close contacts with the peasant masses and by learning from the firm class stand of the poor and lower-middle peasants, their ideology has started to change. A good working style of doing everything for the patient´s benefit and sharing the patient´s anxiety and pain has begun to manifest itself. Some team members have said that "three months stay in the countryside reaps a richer harvest than ten years study". Others have described their change since coming down to the countryside in such words: "Our meals have become more appetizing, our hearts have become warmer, and the paths broader."

The medical teams have embarked on the construction of a permanent rural public health service. They are medical teams that protect the health of the peasants, propaganda teams that popularize the Party's policies and propagate a knowledge of hygiene, and also working teams that reinforce the building of the rural health service. Facts have shown that in order to fundamentally revolutionize both our country's medical and health work and the ideology of our health workers, we must mobilize the medical and health personnel to serve the peasants. Therefore, the organizing of mobile medical teams to tour the countryside is by no means a makeshift measure, but, on the contrary, is a policy to be persisted in over a long period of time.

PERSEVERE IN GIVING THE FIRST PLACE TO POLITICS, TO CREATIVELY STUDYING AND APPLYING CHAIRMAN MAO'S WORKS

The practical work of these months has shown that the mobile medical teams should hold high the red banner of Mao Tse-tung's thinking, give prominence to politics and learn from the People's Liberation Army's "four firsts" and "three-eight" working style.[455] Only thus, can we maintain high revolutionary enthusiasm and fighting spirit and persevere in our task of serving the workers, peasants and soldiers.

Giving prominence to politics means to let Mao Tse-tung's thinking take command of everything. In order to fulfil the historic task of orientating our health work towards the countryside and transforming the health situation in the rural areas and in order to make health work keep pace with the needs of the three revolutionary campaigns of class struggle, struggle for production and scientific experimentation, we must insist on placing Mao Tse-tung's thinking in command. A vigorous upsurge to absorb the essence of Chairman Mao's works should be launched on the public health front. In the struggle against disease, the subjective world must be remoulded simultaneously with the objective world.

The medical teams consist of doctors of all grades, nurses and administrative staff. They differ in age, experience, in their sphere of responsibility and also in their ideology. So long as the medical teams give prominence to politics, professional work will have a reliable guide which will give full play to the initiative of every member

[455] The "four firsts" are: First place must be given to man in handling the relationship between man and weapons, to political work in handling the relationship between political and other work, to ideological work in relation to other aspects of political work and to living ideas in ideological work. With regard to the "three-eight" working style, "three" refers to the three mottoes: "Keep firmly to the correct political orientation", "maintain an industrious and simple style of work" and "be flexible in strategy and tactics"; "eight" refers to eight characters which mean unity, alertness, earnestness and liveliness.

and enable the team as a whole to become a unified collective. In this way, even under difficult conditions, we shall be able to achieve excellent results.

In what way should the mobile medical teams give prominence to politics? We should, first and foremost, understand the great strategic significance of putting the main emphasis on rural health work. The adoption of this revolutionary measure is an essential factor in promoting a new upsurge in agricultural production and in the construction of a new socialist countryside. From the long-term point of view, it is a step in the direction of gradually obliterating the difference between the city and the countryside, between workers and peasants, and between mental and manual labor. Unless team members are aware of this, they will not understand that every part of their work is of revolutionary significance and they will be unable to see the link between their work and the great tasks of socialist revolution and socialist construction. If, however, they are aware of it, they will be far-sighted, full of vigor and ready to dedicate themselves wholeheartedly to the service of the peasants.

In giving prominence to politics, we should unreservedly adopt an outlook of serving the people wholeheartedly. Since the peasants make up the overwhelming majority of the population, to serve the people wholeheartedly must certainly include giving wholehearted service to the peasants and, if politics is to be given due prominence, this must be in the forefront of the mind of every member of the mobile medical teams. Through medical practice in the countryside, members of the medical teams will succeed in establishing a close class feeling with the peasants and they will come to regard service to the vast peasant masses as their greatest happiness and highest glory. All team members should follow the shining examples of Lei Feng and Wang Chieh,[456] learning from their communist spirit, their wholehearted dedication to the revolution and their boundless service to the people.

In giving prominence to politics, medical team members must conscientiously engage in the three revolutionary campaigns, tempering themselves in the course of revolutionary struggle. As their main task, they should do a good job of medical and public health service in the countryside, while closely coordinating with the central tasks set by the Party.

[456] Nationally-known heroes, both of whom were soldiers in the People's Liberation Army who died a martyr's death. Their deeds were widely publicized and inspired millions of people throughout the country.

For instance, during the socialist education movement, they should combine medical work with the mobilization of the masses; in winter and spring when water conservancy work is in full swing, the medical teams must go to the working sites to protect the health of the laborers and to do whatever physical work is suitable for them. They must learn to work among the masses, to understand and to tackle problems with a class viewpoint. By means of medical work, they should propagate the Party's policies, keep in close contact with the masses and fully tap their initiative.

In giving prominence to politics, a fundamental requirement is the creative study and resolute application of Chairman Mao's works to solve practical problems arising in everyday life and as a guide to conduct. A careful study of the instructions of the Central Committee of the Party and Chairman Mao regarding medical and health work should also be made. For the majority of team members, to go to the countryside is a rather severe test. In work and in livelihood, they will inevitably come across difficulties of one kind or another. The rural class struggle will undoubtedly influence them. Under these circumstances, we should always consult Chairman Mao's works for guidance and especially we should try to use Mao Tse-tung's thinking to examine our class stand, viewpoints and methods and to grasp our main ideological problem.

The mobile medical teams in the countryside are confronted with formidable tasks but they are in a very favorable situation for accelerating their revolutionization. They must utilize this favorable situation to the full so as to acquire a deep-going class education and a thorough political training. The experience of many medical teams shows that it is important to solve the following questions.

What should be the correct attitude towards the peasants? Is it to modestly learn from them and to wholeheartedly serve them, or is it to place oneself high above the peasants, to show contempt for them and to regard medical treatment as gifts of grace to them? This is a question of one's standpoint and many team members, since going down to the countryside, have undergone a preliminary change on this cardinal matter. From ignoring the peasants, they have come to keep the peasants in their minds at every moment; from thinking the peasants dirty, rough and boorish, they have come to regard them as respect-worthy and even "cleaner" than intellectuals; from having nothing in common with the peasants, they have developed harmonious and truly intimate feelings with them. Particularly, they have seen with their own eyes that the peasants support the Party and socialism and that they work in the fields day in and day out in order to produce more; that the peasants contribute a great deal to the state. When, by contrast, they examine themselves, they realize that though their own contribution is not so enormous, they live a much better life than the peasants and nevertheless, they are often preoccupied with narrow personal matters. In this way, some team members come to understand more deeply than before that, in many ways, they are inferior to the peasants and that there can be no reason for them to refuse to learn from the peasants. Many of them become aware that they have never taken the needs of the peasants into serious consideration, nor have they ever shown solicitude for the peasants. Some said, with profound emotion: "We cured the physical diseases of the peasants and the peasants cured our ideological diseases", and "Once we have taken the poor and lower-middle peasants to our hearts, we can think of reforming our minds."

What does a correct attitude to the peasants amount to? In going down to the countryside, should we proceed in all cases from the needs of the peasants or should we harbor individualistic designs and assume a perfunctory attitude towards work? This also is a question of cardinal importance. It should be understood that the majority of team members went to the countryside with a correct attitude. Some however had various individualistic motives. For example, some thought only of putting on an act and had no intention of doing earnest and practical work; others cared only for collecting research data and had no heart to serve the peasants; still others deemed it sufficient to spend a few months in the countryside in order to get through with this burdensome task, lacking the will to transform their ideology in the service of the peasants. Medical tours in the countryside include both scientific experimentation and ideological revolution. One must place a strict demand on oneself and must persist in conscientious ideological revolution. Only by so doing, can one gradually get rid of bourgeois individualism and clarify the basic question of whom to serve and how to serve. If, on the other hand, one fails to put a strict demand on oneself, clings to one's individualistic ideas, and works in a sloppy and careless way, this certainly cannot be counted as serving the peasants wholeheartedly, or as transforming one´s ideology through medical practice. A certain chief of the department of general surgery in a hospital from Heilungchiang province went to the rural areas with the idea of performing some operations in order to show off his technique. Once down there, he found that what the peasants needed most was treatment for commonly-seen diseases. After intense ideological struggle and study, he changed his previous ideas. In addition to carefully treating common surgical diseases, he made special visits to public bathrooms to learn how to treat corns from the chiropodists there. He learned basic therapeutic measures from doctors of the departments of otorhinolaryngology, ophthalmology and dental surgery. Many patients were cured by him and all of them acclaimed him as "a good doctor without airs". This illustrates the truth that only after one has rectified one's ideology can one serve the peasants in a correct way.

What should be the attitude of team members towards achievements and praise? The activities of the mobile medical teams in the countryside are frequently welcomed and praised by the masses. In face of praise from the masses, we should cool-mindedly analyze our work in a dialectical way. In this way, we shall be able to find what is lacking in our achievements, gain in vigilance against conceit and impatience, and be stimulated to further efforts to improve our work. Many medical teams realize that, in truth, they owe their achievements to the Party and the masses and that they themselves have merely fulfilled the small contribution required of them; nevertheless they are warmly complimented. This shows, on the one hand, that they have, under the leadership of the Party, made some progress, while on the other hand, it shows that in the past they had done too little in the service of the peasants. They take the masses praise as a stimulus to spur them forward. They invite the poor and lower-middle peasants to discussion meetings and humbly listen to the opinions of the masses. They make it their aim to do an even better job. This is a correct attitude towards achievements and praise.

The experience of these months shows that administrative and political workers must be included in medical teams going to the countryside, if these teams are to become a revolutionized fighting force. Every medical team must include a nucleus of rather strong members to undertake responsibility for political and ideological work. Political and ideological work must be carried out by every comrade in the course of his medical work. In this way, professional work can be integrated with political and ideological work and members of the medical teams, in addition to accomplishing their tasks in preventing and treating diseases and building a rural health service, can have an opportunity to radically transform their ideology. Among the medical teams, the old set of "institution habits" should be discarded and a revolutionized working style and method should be cultivated. We must learn from the People's Liberation Army's spirit that men at all levels, commanders and fighters, are on the same footing. We must develop democracy and solidarity, share the same weal and woe, and stress class feelings. The livelihood and difficulties of members must be taken good care of and, while not exceeding the living standard of the local people, appropriate adjustments in living and working conditions can be made to suit members of different age and physical condition.

ON THE CORRECT HANDLING OF SOME QUESTIONS ARISING AT WORK IN ORDER TO FULLY REALISE THE ROLE OF THE MOBILE MEDICAL TEAMS

In order to fully realise the role of the mobile medical teams, their members should make a serious study of materialist dialectics and correctly handle a series of questions of relationship between different aspects of medical work; namely, the relationship between popularization and the raising of standards; between common and uncommon diseases; between specialization and versatility; between the raising of quality of medical treatment and the need to economize; between prevention and treatment.

With regard to the relationship between popularization and raising of standards in medical and public health work, popularization is the main task of the present time. In so far as the masses are concerned, as Chairman Mao has pointed out to us: "for them the prime need is not 'more flowers on the brocade' but 'fuel in snowy weather'. In present conditions, therefore, popularizing is the more pressing task." Orientating medical and health work towards the countryside is, in effect, a gigantic campaign to popularize public health work. Although the work of the medical teams should accord with the objective possibilities and first solve the most pressing problems confronting the masses, nevertheless, popularization and raising of standards cannot be separated. On the basis of popularization, standards must be raised. Such raising of standards should not blindly copy urban patterns and still less should it uncritically adopt foreign methods. On the contrary, standards should be raised in line with the actual development production of the actual rate improvement of living standards in the countryside. According to the national characteristics and the revolutionary tradition of our country's medical and health work, we should evolve our own set of working methods to run socialist public health work.

The prevention and treatment of common diseases must be combined with prevention and treatment of rare or difficult diseases. Common diseases like parasitic diseases, infectious and endemic diseases are most harmful to the health of the laboring people. Generally speaking, they can be fairly effectively prevented or treated. For this reason, the medical teams together with local health personnel must combine the efforts to prevent and treat these diseases, so as to relieve large numbers of patients of the sufferings and promote production. It is completely incorrect to maintain that since the prevention and treatment of these commonly seen diseases does not require any special skill, they can be neglected by the medical teams. At the same time there are also many difficult diseases in the rural areas and sometimes, owing to lack of timely treatment, some patients originally with simple diseases develop difficult complications. The masses urgently need prevention and treatment of these difficult diseases and a medical team should, in every way open to them, carry out treatment for and research into these diseases.

Specialization should be combined with versatility. To meet the actual needs of the peasant masses, members of the medical teams must train themselves to be versatile. The target should be to learn to prevent and treat all types of common rural diseases and to master commonly used methods of treatment both of traditional Chinese medicine and modern medicine. This policy is all the more necessary in view of the limited scope of the medical teams and the scattered nature of their activities. At the same time, however, attention should be paid to the continuous accumulation of data and summing up of experiences in particular diseases. To the extent that conditions permit, specialized teams for particular aspects of preventive and therapeutic work, or operations teams may be organized in order to upgrade the standard of the work and to solve difficult problems.

In medical and public health work, emphasis should be put on both high quality and economy, between which there is dialectical relationship. The medical teams must develop the spirit of saving one farthing and foster a style of living strictly and practicing economy. We should strive to cure diseases with very little or even with no expenditure. The reason why some peasants delay the treatment of minor ailments, which later on develop into serious ones, is partly due to the economic factor. As some comrades have correctly put it, whether or not one makes a detailed calculation of every cent when treating illnesses for peasants is by no means a purely economic problem, but a political problem, a problem that reflects one's class stand. For this reason, many medical teams try to economise in medical expenditures by all sorts of means. Therapies like acupuncture, manipulative treatment and cupping, which require little or no money, are frequently used. Others, in writing prescriptions think hard over the special circumstances of the case so that, often, the medicine costs a few cents only. A poor peasant from the Anchia commune in Fushen developed cataracts in both eyes. In 1961, he spent more than 100 yuan when he went to a city hospital for cure of his left eye. This time, when the medical team came to his village, he had his right eye cured for a few yuan. The two operations of the same kind were more than 10 times different in price. Many doctors could not conceive of performing operations without a model operating theatre and complete facilities. Through improvisations in face of poor conditions and by breaking through conventions, the medical teams converted thatched cottages and mud houses into operating rooms, made operating tables of doors and bricks, used paraffin lamps and battery torches to replace shadowless lamps and used wicker frames for steaming bread and cooking pots as sterilizers. Operations, big and small, were successfully performed. They did what they previously thought impossible. In this way, they not only made this convenient for the masses and reduced their monetary burden, but they also cultivated the revolutionary spirits of plain living, hard struggle and fulfilling tasks while surmounting every difficulty. It goes without saying that careful attention to cost does not mean in the slightest that the rational use of drugs can be ignored, or that quality medical service can be lowered. On the contrary, we should aim to obtaining economic results with the pursuit of excellence. Economizing of this kind is based on thoroughgoing diagnosis and correct use of drugs, and this calls for a high degree of thoroughness and creativeness on the part of doctors. It is, therefore, an important aspect of technical innovation and technical revolution in medical and public health work.

In order to strengthen preventive work, you must start with therapeutic work and combine one with the other. At the present moment, the most pressing with the broad masses of the peasants is to have their diseases treated. If there is only empty talk about prevention but no practical treatment, the masses can hardly be satisfied. On the other hand if we busy ourselves only with treatment and adopt a passive attitude towards the common preventable diseases, we shall certainly not be displaying a proper sense of responsibility to the people. We advocate that all personnel engaged in therapeutic work should strengthen the awareness of all prevention producing prophylactic work; that all those engaged in public health work could also do some therapeutic work according to the needs of the masses. Therapy without prophylaxis or prophylaxis without therapy are both one-sided and neither is in keeping with the wishes of the people.

ENABLING MEDICAL AND HEALTH WORK TO TAKE ROOT IN THE COUNTRYSIDE-AN IMPORTANT TASK FOR THE MOBILE MEDICAL TEAMS

In order to tackle the medical and health problems of the vast rural areas, the medical teams must entrench themselves and take root in the countryside. Wherever the medical teams go, medical and public health work should gain a firm foothold and flourish.

To this end, the medical team should, under the leadership of the Party and by relying on the masses, carefully accomplish the following tasks:

Firstly, they must energetically prevent and treat especially those diseases which are common in the rural areas, which hinder production and are harmful to the health of the people. An attack on other diseases should follow. We should strive to diagnose and treat disease at the earliest possible stage. In doing so, the masses experience in the prevention treatment of disease should be analyzed and summed up. We should carry out research work to find simple but effective prophylactic and therapeutic methods well-suited to rural conditions. Gradually we can succeed in working out a set of routines for rural medical healthcare, which will raise the quality of medical treatment for common diseases.

Wherever they go, the medical team should invariably investigate the level of local production, living standards and prevalent diseases; they should acquaint themselves with the masses' needs and seek their suggestions. In the prevention and treatment of disease and in the building up of medical service, we must at all times rely on the masses, fully consult with them and give priority to the solution of those problems which need urgent solution in which it is possible to solve.

In activities of the medical teams, the convenience of the masses should be taken into consideration. Methods such as going from village to village from house to house to provide mobile medical treatment fit in with the scattered nature of the habitations in the rural areas, and they are warmly welcome by the peasants. Nevertheless, in order to perform certain operations to treat some difficult cases, a certain degree of concentration of medical resources is necessary. We should also establish therefore, some relatively fixed medical centers in which we should start to work out methods of prevention and treatment for some major diseases.

Our policy is first to treat existing diseases, then to institute prophylactic work and finally consolidate advances gained in area after area, so that, in the interest of the masses, we can more or less eliminate the hazards of these diseases. Medical clinics should also be established in remote inaccessible villages and doctors should regularly attend them to look after the local people and to give them timely and convenient treatment.

At present, we lack knowledge concerning the following questions: what are the characteristics of the onset and development of rural common diseases and what are the most effective methods for the treatment and prevention; how, in the countryside, we effectively eliminate the four pests: flies, rats, mosquitoes and bedbugs and how should we conduct hygiene propaganda; what is the most economical, simple, convenient and effective way to utilize drugs and materials. These are the main obstacles to our satisfactorily meeting with requirements of the peasants and to our taking firm root in the countryside. The medical teams should regard the solution as an important task, and therefore they should closely study the real conditions of production and living standards so as to gradually solve them in a way appropriate to the local conditions.

Secondly we should persistently train medical and health workers for the countryside so as to gradually reach the target of having volunteer health workers in every production team, part-time medical assistance midwives in every production brigade and a few fully qualified doctors in every commune.

To train volunteer health workers and part-time medical assistants is a pressing need in the countryside and, moreover, because of our rural collective economy, it is fully possible to train medical and health personnel of this type. An all round program for the realization of these targets should be worked out including a policy of experimentation, of summing up of experiences gained and of a gradual popularization of the positive aspects of these experiences.

In training rural medical and health personnel, attention should be given to quality, for, if quality is assured, we will certainly be able to turn out a new type of health worker who is both mental and manual worker and he will have both determination and ability to serve the masses in the health field. To do this, it is necessary to combine study with work and to alternate classroom teaching with clinical demonstrations. After a concentrated period of study, trainees should be taken to participate in the medical tours, with the object of consolidating what they've learned in classrooms. Refresher courses at regular intervals and postgraduate classes must be organized. Traditional Chinese medicine should be combined with modern medicine and these rural health workers should master, as part of their basic technique, the simple but effective therapies of traditional Chinese medicine such as acupuncture, moxibustion, manipulation, massage, and other home remedies.

The training of rural medical and public health personnel should develop the revolution tradition cultivated during the Revolutionary war, of training medical workers in a short span of time, and we should, therefore, exert our utmost efforts to shorten study of courses contents and lecture contents. On the other hand, it must also take into consideration existing conditions in the countryside and the needs of the peasants as regards to prevention and treatment of disease. It must make a serious study of both the immediate and long-term requirements, make appropriate arrangements and should never be impatient for successes.

Thirdly, we must improve and reinforce existing rural health organizations. Under the leadership of the party committee, the medical team should coordinate with local organizations to implement Chairman Mao's directive of "unite all medical workers, young and old, of the traditional school and the modern school, and organize solid united front to strive for the development of the people's health work."[457] In the course of improving and building up the rural health units politically, organizationally, and professionally, we should strictly abide by the party's policy of uniting with, educating and reforming the intelligentsia.

The medical teams must regard the rural health workers at the grassroots level as channels through whom they communicate with the masses. They should unite for the modest and learn from them and during joint work with them, they should help them and give them clinical demonstrations and lectures. Short-period training classes in lecture courses may be organized to help them raise the ideological understanding and medical know-how. Both members of the medical teams and health workers at grassroots level should develop their strong points and overcome their shortcomings. They should learn from each other and strengthen the unity. After thoroughgoing investigations of local conditions, the medical teams have an obligation to help local organizations in the allocation training of health workers at the

[457] Chairman Mao Tse-T'ung's directive to the First National Health Conference held in August 1950.

grassroots level. Rural health organization should be run as simply and economically as possible and whole set of working regulations be worked out to suit the convenience of the masses.

Another important aspect of strengthening the building of the rural health service is for experienced doctors and nurses to settle in the countryside apparently and to take root there. In recent years, not a few medical and health personnel and graduates of medical colleges have settled down the countryside without being determined to become politically revolutionary and professionally expert. For instance, many doctors and nurses from the Heart'ao Hospital in Liaoning province have achieved remarkable successes in the medical work. Dr. Ni Li-Chuan of the Shanghai Yench'iao People's Commune has been working in the countryside for seven years and has taken an active part in serving the peasants. In the remote frontier regions of our country, other medical workers are working hard to protect the health of the fraternal national minority peoples and to strengthen national defense. In the wake of the upsurge of rural health work, it is necessary for even more people, who embrace this kind of revolution ambition, to go and take root in the countryside.

Fourthly, we must energetically carryout prophylactic work and improve the hygienic conditions in the rural regions. A fundamental measure to prevent disease is to launch, in coordination with agriculture production and local customs, conditions and experience, a patriotic health movement with emphasis on the disposal of renewal and improvement of drinking water. Only by taking full account of the particular situation in each case, by suiting our actions to the place and conditions and by starting from the actual practice, can we succeed in gaining maximal results. For example, in Tsunhua of Hopei province, Jihchao of Shuniung province and Mienchu of Szechuan province, human and animal manure is under the unified management of the collective. Some people are specially assigned to take charge of the collection, composting and storage of manure and have succeeded in raising the fertility of manure and killing harmful germs and larvae. In the provinces of Hopei, Chekiang, Szechuan, Kwangtung and the suburbs of Shanghai, the local people have been using indigenous methods to install simple running water system by sinking wells and making mechanical water lifting devices. As a result, they are able to supply the masses with clean drinking water. It is very well worthwhile for the medical teams to learn from and popularize such experiences.

Fifthly, we should widely disseminate knowledge of hygiene. On the basis of investigation into common diseases in the locality, the mobile medical teams should utilize the true stories of cured patients to propagandize the etiology and methods of prevention of the disease in question. In the light of the situation in the locality, they can pool the masses' experiences and suggest preventative measures and targets for the patriotic health movement. To disseminate propaganda work, we should use forms which are appreciated by the peasant masses such as loudspeaker broadcasting, theatricals, slides, moving pictures, storytelling, songs and so on and so forth.

Following the orientation of our health work in the countryside, the necessity to revolutionize a show of the other medical work becomes even more pressing. Insofar as our urban medical workers revolutionize, we will be able to make greater efforts in the service of the countryside. The orientation towards the countryside and the organization of medical teams to go to the rural areas have given an impetus to the revolutionisation of our urban medical work. The medical teams, on their return, should further develop the ability and determination to give prominence to politics, study and apply Chairman Mao's works in a creative way, keep in close contact with the masses, wholeheartedly serve the people, practice economy and live thriftily. Thus, the revolutionisation of our urban health work can be promoted enabling the medical work in the cities to be like that in the countryside to assist each other's advance.

The task of orientating our medical work towards the countryside and of building up a socialist rural health network is a long-term and formidable task with a profound strategic and revolutionary significance. We believe that, so long as we persist in uninterrupted revolution, are proficient in summing up experiences, doggedly march on from one victory to another and are not afraid of hard and bitter struggles, we shall certainly succeed, in not too long a time, in transforming the backwardness of our country's rural health work, and in building up a durable rural health organization.

Reference

1. Mao Tse-Tung, *Talks at the Yenan Forum on Literature and Art*, Selected Works, English ed., Vol. 3 page 82, Foreign Languages Press, Peking, 1965.

Article end

A conversation about the motherland medicine[458]

1972

广东中医学院编 by Guangdong TCM College

科学知识普及丛书 (A Part of) A collection of books disseminating scientific knowledge

广东人民出版社 Guangdong People's Press

Published October 1972

Yaron: Springing forward to 1972, after much upheaval in China of different kinds—the Great Leap Forward accompanied by a disastrous famine, political struggles within the Party, decreasing Soviet influence, cultural revolution, prosecutions, educational and labor reform camps, etc, factors leading to a reality where even a single "wrong" word could land a person in labor reform camp indefinitely—we come to a final shape-up of what TCM is (or should be).

The legal struggle for survival against Mr. Science of the 1930s has long faded away. TCM, after shedding all traces of "mysteriousness and feudal thinking", is a national pride. At this point, ancient theories, previously thought of as mysterious and erroneous, are introduced again, but this time around with a modern TCM mindset following a "realistic" dialectical materialism. For example, the meridians' theory is part of the national treasure once more and not imaginary hearsay as was previously thought.

Book begins with:

A Quote from Chairman Mao.

"Our nation has several thousand years of historical heritage. This heritage has its own unique features and its own numerous treasures.

Chinese medicine is a great treasure-house, we must promote it with great effort, improve and enhance it."

---

[458] 谈谈祖国医学

Publisher's preface on first page

In order to promote dialectical materialism and popularize knowledge of natural sciences, we have requested the relevant units and departments to compile this "collection of books disseminating scientific knowledge".

In this collection of works we did our best to adopt a style of popularity and ease of understanding, all along using vivid language. Bringing to the masses of youth, workers, farmers and soldiers some basic knowledge related to physics, mathematics, chemistry, biology, geography, astronomy, meteorology, hygiene, industry and agriculture. We bring this in order to help our comrades to better understand nature, remake nature, in order to serve better the socialist revolution and the building of socialism. However, since our experience is limited, and our skill level limited, during compilation and publication there must be numerous mistakes, we ask our comrades to put forth their precious criticism.

Chapter 1: Mighty medical treasure house: Chinese medicine

Page 1

Our great leader Chairman Mao taught us: "Chinese medicine is a great treasure house. We must promote it with great effort, improve and enhance it." This brilliant guidance of Chairman Mao gives high praise to several thousand years of accumulated treasure by the working people of our nation. At the same time, it strikes with force and repudiates cheaters like Liu Shaoqi 刘少奇 and the like who held "slaving to the West philosophy" and "national nihilism".

We all know that our nation's heritage has long history. Very early on, our forefathers who lived in this land labored with great effort. They worked hard and were brave people, struggling with heavenly and earthly influences as well as oppression by other people. Simultaneously they ever fought the crippling effects of disease. Our nation's medicine is the summary of the struggle of our people over the past several thousand years against disease. This experience, and ensuing theory, has endured time and preserved the health of the people over a long period of time. It gave great contribution to humanity overall. Chinese medicine is a cultural inheritance our forefathers gave us. For the working and accomplishment of the earlier working people of our nation, we should be thankful and feel proud! At the same time, to respect our great leader Chairman Mao, to help the people of our nation and the entire world, we should keep on promoting this piece of inherited treasure.

Page 2

Our nation's earliest medical work: *Neijing* 內經

Because of certain limitations throughout history, of course these theories at times are antiquated. They are not so clear and transparent as modern medicine understanding. At some places it is not accurate, in some places it also incorporates an overtone of feudal superstition. Nonetheless, it stands bright within the overall development of medicine throughout history and can't be wiped out.

Page 4

From acupuncture to the bronze acupuncture model

Acupuncture therapy received attention around the world, shocking the medical world with acupuncture anesthesia; it is a part of our nation's great treasure medical heritage. It is the culmination of a long-term struggle against disease that our nation's working people have endured.

In the 11th century in the Song dynasty, there was a doctor named Wang Weiyi 王惟一 who summarized the acupuncture knowledge up to the Song and took the 300-plus points and the Zangfu 12 meridians and merged them together. This was a great development for the acupuncture points systemization and theory. More notably, under his instruction, the Song government molded two bronze acupuncture statues to serve as learning tools. On the surface of the bronze figures a few hundreds acupuncture points were engraved and then with yellow wax they were sealed off. Inside, it was filled with water. During examinations, the students were told to puncture the statue in the correct points. If punctured correctly, the water will flow; if punctured incorrectly then the needle will not go in. This kind of imagery practice improved greatly the development of medical education and had great practical value. One of the two bronze figures, in the Qing dynasty during the Eight-Power Allied Forces (of 1900), was snatched away by the Japanese imperialists and, until today, is on display in the national museum in Tokyo. From this, one can also see the plundering nature of imperialism.

Pages 5–9

Ma Fu San Formula and mouth-to-mouth resuscitation

In our nation's medicine, external injuries medical knowledge also has great experience. In *The Historical Romance of the Three Kingdoms San Guo Yan Yi* 三国演义, there is a record of the story about the physician Hua Tuo 华陀 who performed "peeling the bone" surgery. This means that external medicine was well developed at that time. Hua Tuo is a famous surgeon of the time. In the second century CE he used Ma Fu San 麻浮散 to administer anesthesia during abdominal surgery. He is the first Chinese doctor to use anesthesia in the entire world. His anesthesia methods were exported to Korea, Japan, Morocco etc nations. In the *World Medical History Book*, it says: "The Arabs' use of anesthetics was probably imported from China." European and American use of anesthesia in medicine only started in the 19th century, a full one thousand six hundred years later.

During our nation's proletariat cultural revolution, by the large number of revolutionary medical personnel from Xuzhou 徐州 Hospital, and under the revolutionary guidance of Chairman Mao, carrying out his brave thoughts, daring to deliver his spirit, inspired by Hua Tuo's Ma Fu San, they performed earnest research into this topic, creating Chinese medicine anesthetics. Chinese medicine anesthetics is today, in many places, better than modern anesthetics. It is only such that in the past "national nihilism" obstructed the development of our nation's medicine and buried it.

In the second century, Hua Tuo not only performed surgery, he also developed something similar to today's heart massage and mouth-to-mouth resuscitation. In the book *Hua Tuo's Spirit-like Prescriptions Hua Tuo Shen Fang* 华陀神方 in rescuing odd diseases we read the following:

> The method of emergency rescue is such: First gently hug around the rope, press up and down on the lying person. One person uses his hand to press on the chest several times. One person pulls the arm and stretches it. If one is stiff, gradually with force bend it and, at the same time, press his abdomen as if allowing it to cook. The Qi comes out from the mouth. (He) breathes and the eyes open. And if it is still not stretched straight, do not strain it, only little by little let him drink gruel, on its own life returns.

In another prescription it says:

> Use a big bag of fried salt, iron with it from the head and throat down to the navel. If it gets cold, replace it—and you cannot stop midway. When his phlegm stops, one uses his mouth against the patient's mouth to water in the Qi; his life will return even faster.

Hua Tuo rescuing methods includes mouth-to-mouth resuscitation and heart massage. This demonstrates that 1,700 years ago, our ancestors already had used techniques similar to what is used today in resuscitation, showing that our ancestors knew of the clinical efficacy of those methods.

Yaron: Switching into ideological propaganda in the midst of an historical narrative. Now, a space is created for the ancient theories to come back with force. There was no shortage of grand fabricated claims to reach this objective: "The comrades of the health branch of the People's Liberation Army division 3016 neared Chairman Mao's invincible thought. They used the new acupuncture to treat successfully numerous cases previously diagnosed as deafness and muteness. They conquered these, previously categorized by the bourgeois medicine as "forbidden" or "incurable" diseases, thereby allowing many deaf and mute patients to hear Chairman Mao's voice, and then they shouted "Chairman Mao lives forever!""

In the feudal society, in order to fool the working class, the ruling class dressed our nation's medicines in a dress of superstition and, on top of that, the craziness and self-indulgence of the ruling class, being closed to others and self-protecting, and not considerate of any scientific evidence, resulted in a gradual developmental slowdown of our nation's medicine. Reaching to the 18th and 19th centuries, it fell behind the European medical sciences.

At the era of half-feudal and half-colonized old China, capitalist landlords ruling class and the nationalist party reactionaries were all subservient, venerated the West and were scared of the West, got polluted with ideas that Chinese medicine is not scientific, it is shamanic, and so they ordered to exterminate Chinese medicine. It caused our nation's medicine to struggle on a path of extermination and suffer great humiliation.

After the birth of new China, with a new attitude of reception towards our nation's medical heritage, there were still two different pathways struggling amongst themselves. There was Chairman Mao's revolutionary line of medical treatment and hygiene, which was to unite Chinese and Western medicine 团结中西医 and transmit and develop further our nation's medical heritage, to take Chinese medicine and herbal knowledge as well as Western medicine and pharmaceutical knowledge and merge them together, in order to create our country's new kind of medical science, new pharmacological science. Our great leader Chairman Mao always attached great importance to our motherland's medical heritage, and often pointed out the need to merge the paths of Western and Chinese medicines into one. However, the renegade, hidden traitor scab Liu Shaoqi 刘少奇 and his gang altogether resisted Chairman Mao's instruction. On the battle-line of medical treatment and hygiene, they propagated with force their revisionism. In the early days right after liberation they claimed: "In the near future Western medicine must replace Chinese medicine." With this, he wanted to use Western medicine to replace Chinese medicine, eradicating Chinese medicine, placing Chinese and Western medicine as opposing entities. This was thoroughly enslaving-to-the-West line of thinking. This kind of biased and strangling attitude caused the organization and development of our motherland's medicine great disturbance.

The great proletariat Cultural Revolution thoroughly destroyed the bourgeois headquarters headed by Liu Shaoqi. It severed Liu Shaoqi's demonic grab of the Health Ministry. It ruthlessly slapped Liu Shaoqi's opposition to the revolution with his revisionism health policy route. It settled the accounts with these few gang members' erroneous acts of biased strangling and humiliating Chinese medicine. Thereby, under the illuminating light of Marxism, Leninism and Mao Zedong thought did Chinese medicine increase its magnificent splendor.

With Chairman Mao's excellent guiding strategy "prepare against war, prepare against natural disasters, for the people" and his glorious "six, two six"[459] guiding instruction, that large numbers of workers, peasants, soldiers and revolutionary medical workers used Chairman Mao's philosophy, guiding their medical experience to overcome one difficulty after the other in medical practice. It produced numerous medical miracles.

---

[459] Mao Zedong heard a report by Qian Xinzhong 钱信忠, Minister of Health at that time, that the majority of medical professionals are concentrated in the cities with only small percentage serving the farmers. He then angrily protested that the Ministry of Health should change its name to "Ministry of City Health". As a result of this angry outburst, immediately new policies went into effect favoring Chinese medicine in the farmlands serving the poor peasants. His outburst took place in June 26th, and thereafter was known as the "six, two six" event.

The comrades of the health branch of the People's Liberation Army division 3016 neared Chairman Mao's invincible thought. They used the new acupuncture to treat successfully numerous cases previously diagnosed as deafness and muteness. They conquered these, previously categorized by the bourgeois medicine as "forbidden" or "incurable" diseases, thereby allowing many deaf and mute patients to hear Chairman Mao's voice, and then they shouted "Chairman Mao lives forever!"

The health workers at the hospital of the People's Liberation Army division 208 used the new acupuncture to conquer another disease which is "incurable" in world's medicine; children night wetting after paralysis. For poor peasants who were born for ironsmith, China Communist Party member comrade Liu Shaoxian 刘绍显 devised the "681 method" to treat Keshan 克山病 disease with great accomplishment, drawing admiration from medical circles around the world. Beijing Chinese Medicine Research Institute members developed further the ancient "golden needle remove obstruction surgery" and, merging it with modern medical methodology, created "needle removal of cataract" and allowed millions of blind people to see again. Also worth mentioning the acupuncture anesthesia success, allowing tens of thousands of patient undergo successfully all kinds of surgeries, which startled the entire world. From all these, one can see the great victory resulting from Chairman Mao's thought. They are all the great victory of Chairman Mao's revolutionary path.

Page 21

Subchapter: Does the human body actually have meridians or not?

Meridians are a theory culminated by our nation's ancient medical doctors, coming out of their constant summary of their practical experience. Even though, to date, from dissecting cadavers and x-rays, one cannot find meridians' evidence, however, from our nation's 2,000-year-old medical work *Neijing*, there are extensive descriptions of the meridians' appearance, functions and acupoints. In addition, a detailed description exists describing where each meridian starts and ends and where it travels through. This description guided several thousand years of medical clinical experience and solved many difficulties. Therefore, one can say that the phenomena of meridians and their workings is objectively observed.

Chairman Mao taught us: "The root of a theory is its practicability, in other words the theory serves the application." After liberation, especially after the Proletariat Cultural Revolution, the entire country's revolutionary medical workers performed research and deliberate discussions, and did many laboratory experiments on the topic, achieving much valuable data.

Yaron: Next, we see the comeback of "scientific" meridians. While not conclusive, it follows the Party line, which makes it desirable.

In order to open up this treasure-house, many medical units in the entire country developed research towards meridians. Methods of investigation and inquiry came in all shapes. Not only did they cover the efficacy of acupuncture therapy and acupuncture anesthesia, but also researched the motherland's ancient medical theories and their essence. Many medical units used modern scientific methods to perform laboratory experiments on humans and animals. Initial stages of research concluded that meridians have a close relationship to the nervous system and body fluids. It is also related to bio-electricity. Even though, up to date, there is no conclusive evidence, however, like our great leader Chairman Mao pointed out, "Humankind has to keep on summarizing their experience, there are discoveries, there are inventions, there are creations, there are advancements." We believe that meridian theory in the near future will conclude with a splendid result.

Page 34

Yaron: The art of TCM is "differentiating syndromes and applying a treatment". TCM medical logic begins with the following excerpt and this is where we conclude our book.

Chapter 5: Chinese medicine guiding principle for differentiation of syndromes: Eight Brocades

---

Mao's quote is in bold print against the rest of the text

Our great leader Chairman Mao taught us:

> **While researching a process of any kind, if there exists a complicated process of two or more conflicts, then one should focus his entire effort on finding the main conflict.**

Each disease has its complex symptomatology. The doctor, using the four diagnostic skills,[460] gathers all this data and weaves it together into a cohesive whole. After analyzing it, he must seek out the main conflict.

End

[460] Seeing, hearing, asking and palpating.

进不能爱人知人，退不能爱身知己，
遇灾值祸，身居厄地，蒙蒙昧昧，蠢若游魂。

哀乎！

趋世之士，驰竞浮华，不固根本，忘躯徇物，
危若冰谷，至于是也。

傷寒論序
張仲景

When advancing they cannot love others and know man, when retreating they cannot love their own body and know their self. When they meet a disaster immediately it becomes a misfortune, their body is always in a dangerous land, in an ignorant state they wriggle like a wandering ghost.

How sorrowful!

The scholar-doctors who rush at modern customs gallop in competition in a flashy manner, they don't solidify the root, [instead] they forget the body and give in to [external] things. It is dangerous like the freezing of grains, it has come to this [situation].

Shang Han Lun Preface
Zhang Zhongjing

Conclusion

If the evolution of life on Earth took place over twenty-four hours then the equivalent point at which humans appeared is within the last five minutes. But just because life has existed for so long up to this point is no guarantee that it will continue—we humans carry a critical responsibility to continue the evolution of life to flourish far into the future, far beyond our own lifetimes.

"TCM" appeared within the last five minutes of Chinese medicine's long evolution. We—Chinese medicine practitioners—carry the responsibility to ensure that Chinese medicine develops from its deep roots through the challenges of modernity and into the future, towards a future where *medicine* equals *life*.

We have a responsibility to research these last five minutes, to uncover the gaps in transmission and determine how to best correct our course. Research in Chinese medicine extends in two directions: backward and forward. Researching backward is examining the ancient literature, theories and techniques, gaining knowledge and skill. Then, through using this knowledge and skill, and within the context of our current reality, we contemplate and investigate it with our hearts and minds, for the benefit of our own generation and the generations to follow—this is researching forward.

The gap that needs to be addressed in this process is Chinese medicine's modern history. Chinese medicine was always influenced by religions and cultures, and by political, social and economic pressures, yet the 20th century was like no other. Mr. Science triumphed all over the world, diminishing old religions, folklore and primitive medical arts. Chinese medicine faced, for the first time in history, imminent extinction.

As a result, Chinese medicine underwent "scientification"—a selection process with the aim of creating a new, "science-like" medicine. In addition, disturbingly, it was subjugated to ideological selection. The final product was "TCM", a medical system that is now widely practiced throughout the entire world.

If we can recognize TCM for what it is—a standardized system of medicine with its origins in Chinese, Western and Soviet medical theory, using herbs and acupuncture as therapeutic tools—then we can appreciate this system for what it has delivered thus far. More importantly, however, we can then exercise our current condition of political freedom, material wellbeing and global connectedness to research together

Chinese medicine principle, in a very grounded way, to discover what it means for medical practice in the 21st century.

It is time for *Chinese Medicine Liberation*.

Modern science, art, religion and other subjects can assist us in researching the essence of Chinese medicine forward into the future. Chinese medicine is concerned with human life being part of nature and the universe; it talks about understanding life as part of the big picture and it treats health as part of life. If we research Chinese medicine forward, maintaining this principle, then it remains Chinese medicine regardless of specific treatment techniques.

In fact, the artificial dichotomy we create—Western medicine versus Chinese medicine—revolves around this. When or if Western medicine will see a person as part of nature, life as part of the universe, being connected in space and time to the physical surrounding and the life that came before me to the life that will come after me, then Chinese and Western medicines will simply and naturally become as one, having no difference in principle. There will be need for neither forced merging nor ideological coercion. There will be one complete understanding of life and medicine.

Until this time comes, Chinese medicine must maintain its own principle. We must be able to research backward and research forward without obstacle, without a gap in medical wisdom and logic.

Practitioners are often drawn to the practice because of the depth of Chinese philosophy, the ability to give patients an alternative worldview of their illness experience and then to offer effective treatments. Even the promise of being able to deliver miraculous treatments is often a motivation to study and practice Chinese medicine.

In my personal journey as a practitioner, starting with TCM like everyone else, I found myself increasingly frustrated with the materialistic view and set about to really examine the ancient texts and find out what it was that they were getting at. Maybe the real treasure is not so readily apparent because it requires that we open our minds and hearts and discover what it means to be alive, what it means to treat and what it means to heal.

Now, when I see patients, I find myself feeling great responsibility for their wellbeing. Of course, in the past, I wished the patient well too. I wanted to help them with their pains and aches and I wanted them to be healthy. However, and despite the good intention, what was missing for me was true understanding of health. I asked myself, what does it mean to be alive, how is the Heart connected to life, what is the importance of ancestry and descendants. The TCM explanations I received always revolved *around* the Chinese medicine principle without ever *touching* it. I therefore dedicated my life to finding the *Chinese medicine principle of life* by researching backward and forward, in order to bring a deeper and more proper cure to patients, so our medicine contributes to society where Western medicine still cannot, to make our medicine useful.

I called this the Hunyuan principle, a circular motion depicting a living person in which one recharges, then separates—reaching out to nature—and unifies with nature in order to recharge. This continuous cyclical motion is carried from my ancestors to my offspring, propelling my life between them, a motion connected to natural cyclical phenomena around me and driven by my Heart's separation and unification movement.

Thus, my Chinese medicine practice became an act of service to Chinese medicine life principle.

Dr Yaron Seidman

Acknowledgements

A special thanks goes to all the wonderful practitioners, scholars and institutions who have contributed to our *Chinese Medicine Liberation* effort. Special acknowledgement and heartfelt recognition for outstanding editing work we give to Tristin McLaren for tirelessly helping us fix the manuscript.

Our gratitude for helping with, and commenting on, translations from Chinese goes to Pedro Albuquerque, Gloria Yang, Yim Wing Man, Tam Judy Pui Sum, Siu Sheung Yuen and Tang Lok See. Our sincere thanks for helping with English literature goes to Tristin McLaren, Aharon Henderson, Emily Horning, Alex Kolaczynski, Eric Grose, Lisa Sloane, Sebastian Ruppel, Clare Arvidsson, David Trevino, Jennifer Spain, Stephanie Swanson, Kamini Patel and Susan Søndergaard. Our endless gratitude goes to Harvard University Yenching Library and Yale University Sterling Memorial Library for providing us materials for this research.

In addition, we would like to thank the many practitioners who volunteered to read this gigantic manuscript and provide us with comments and suggestions; to all of you: thank you!

Last but not least we thank Sean Hsiang-lin Lei 雷祥麟 for reviewing our manuscript, contributing a spot-on foreword and inspiring us through many personal communications about this manuscript.

Images

Several images in this book are credited to Mr Paul Goux. Mr Goux is the great grand uncle of Geneviève Le Goff of California USA, Chinese medicine practitioner and fellow of the Hunyuan Research Institute. Mr Goux was a veterinarian and a colonel in the French cavalry, "Colonel-Veterinaire de la Cavalerie", at the turn of the 20th century. He traveled widely and Genevieve Le Goff's mother, Elizabeth Zveguintzoff, has preserved albums of his photography from that time from China, Singapore, Ceylon, India, Saudi Arabia with bedouins and so on. The China pictures are from around 1900, at the time of the Boxer revolt and the Tientsin battle. During the Tientsin battle Mr Goux was wounded and left for dead. A Native medicine doctor found him, saw that he was alive and brought Mr Goux back to his home. Mr Goux recalls having acupuncture needles through his legs, and under the care of the doctor his gangrene was healed. The captions that appear in this book were hand written by Mr Goux on the back of the original photos.

The authors are very grateful to Mme Zveguintzoff for sharing these images. For permission to reproduce any images credited to Mr Paul Goux, please request directly to Geneviève Le Goff.

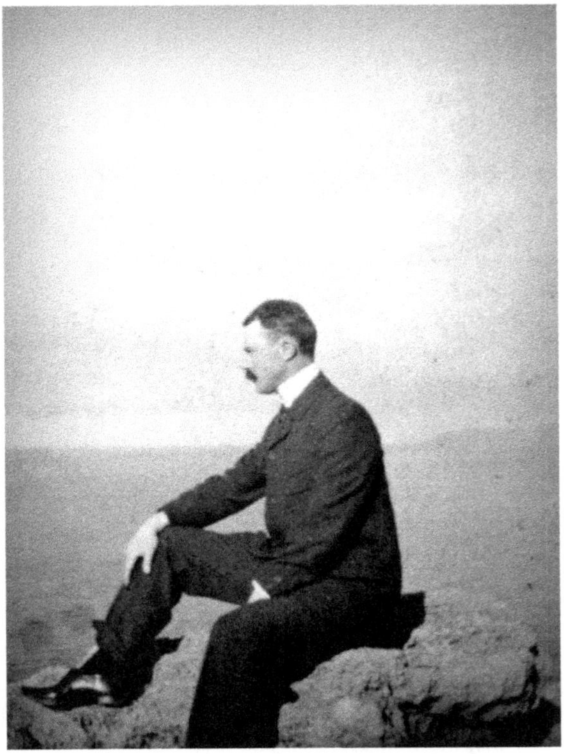

Mr Paul Goux at Oran in 1904.

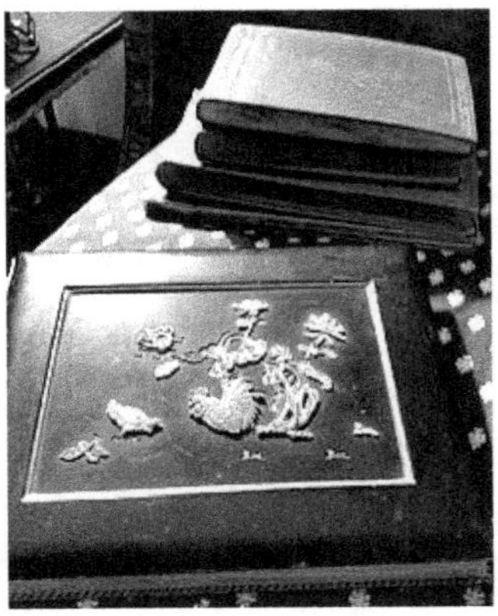

Mr Paul Goux's photo albums, preserved by Mme Elizabeth Zveguintzoff.

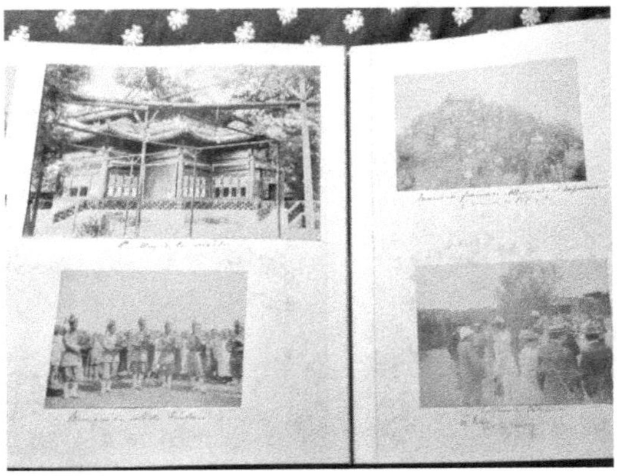

Mr Paul Goux's album of Summer Palace and Imperial Lakes.

Appendix 1

Table of Contents for *Compilation of Discussions about Chinese Medical Education* 中醫教育討論集

Excerpt end. In this compilation there is a break in page sequence; page 12 jumps to page 367.

Appendix 2

Cover photo detail

Following are portraits of the Shanghai Medical College graduating class of 1929.

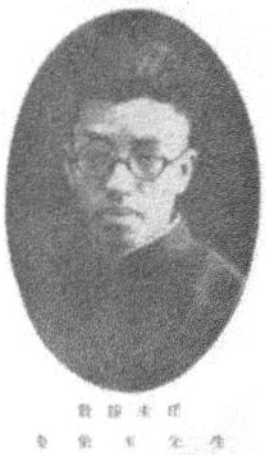

Academic dean,
Mr. Qin Bowei

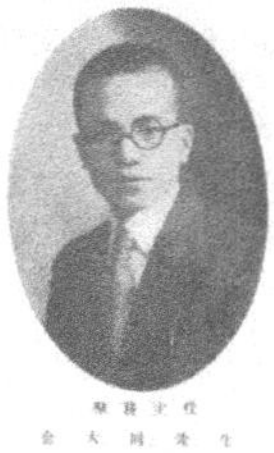

Public affairs director,
Mr. Yu Datong

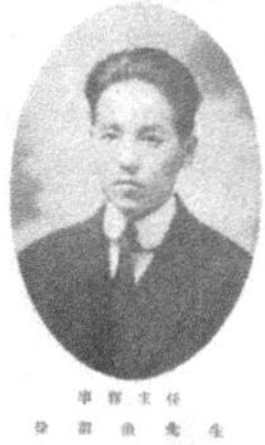

General affairs director,
Mr. Xu Weiyu

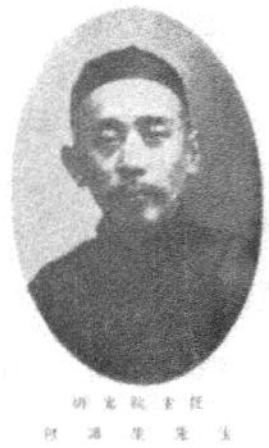

Graduate school director,
Mr. Bao Shisheng

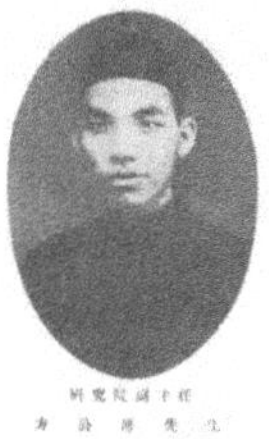

Graduate school vice-director,
Mr. Fang Gongpu

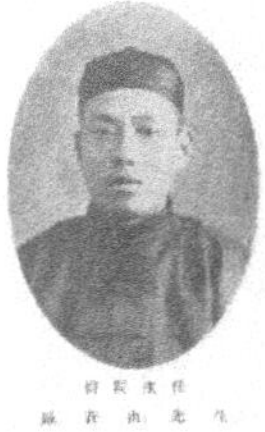

Hospital director
Mr. Yan Cangshan

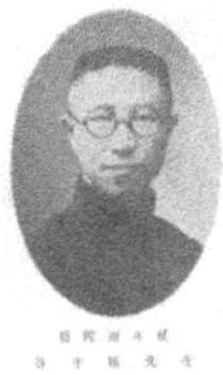

Hospital vice-director,
Mr. Xu Banlong

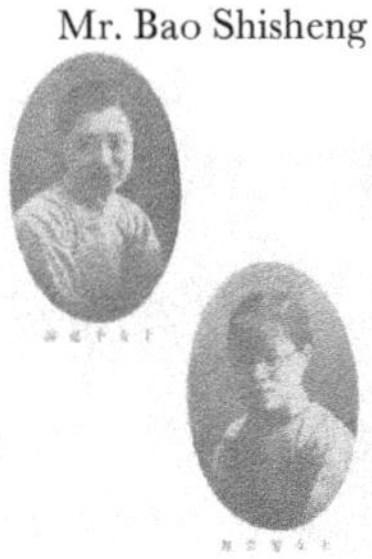

Miss Xie Feiyu
Miss Jing Yunfang

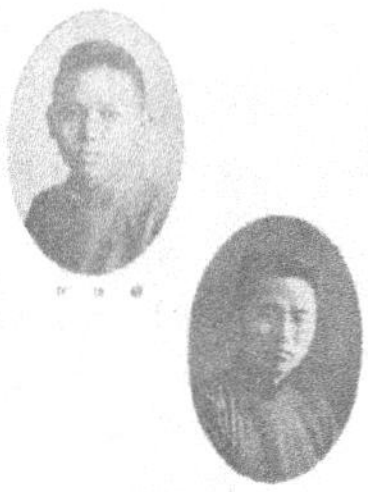

Wang Ruchun
Tai Jiali

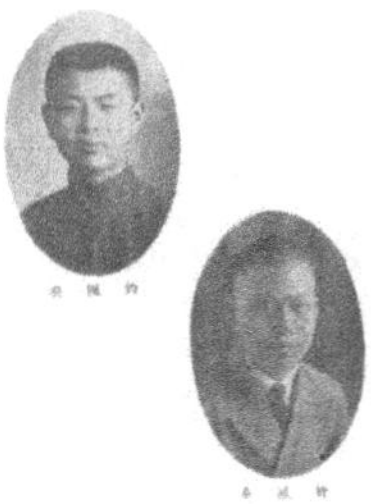

Wu Guojun
Yu Fengzhi

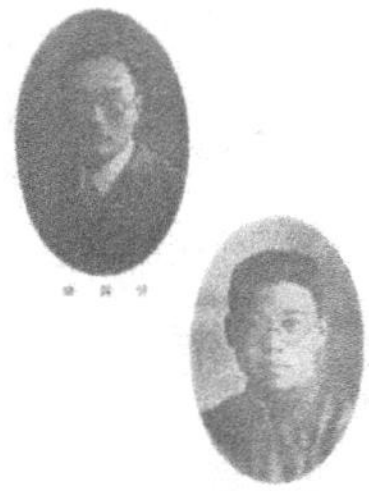

Yao Xihan
Xu Renlong

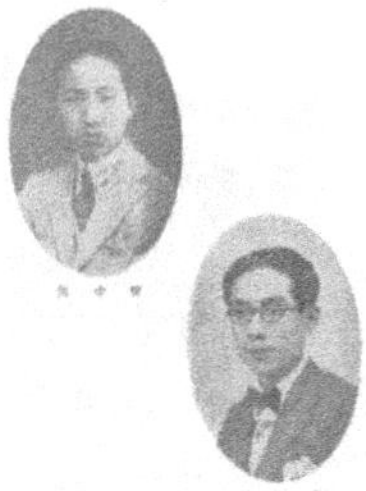

Chen Zhongquan
Ma Shizhi

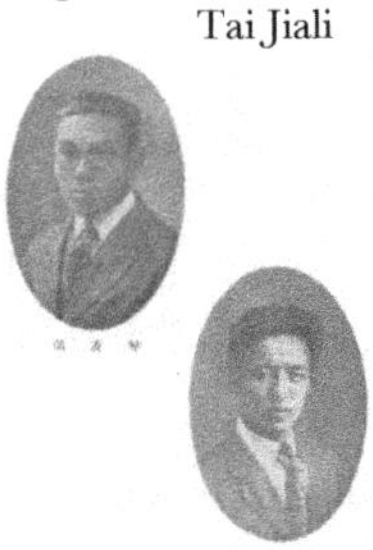

Zhang Youqin
Zhang Hanjie

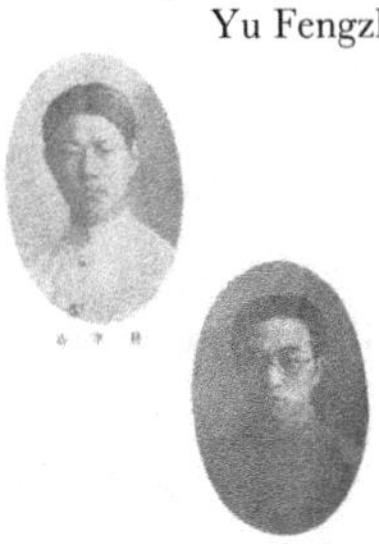

Xu Shengeng
Huang Yiding

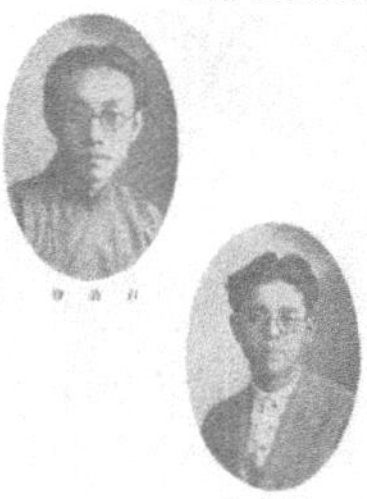

Qian Gongbai
Han Guoyong

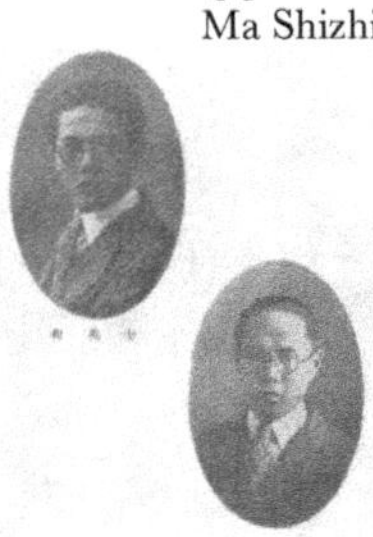

Gu Zhaokui
Gu Yinglong

Other titles by Dr Yaron Seidman

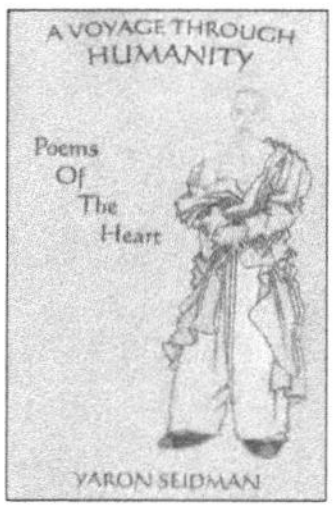

A Voyage Through Humanity: Poems of the Heart (2001)

Yaron Seidman brings in his book a new level of understanding for cultivation practice through Daoist poetry. This book is a must for any practitioner who seeks a level beyond the physical in Taijiquan and Qigong.

http://ChineseClassics.org/hunyuan4.html

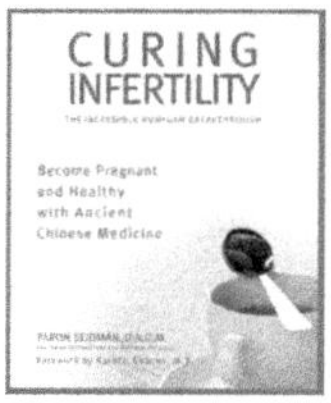

Curing Infertility: The Incredible Hunyuan Breakthrough (2010)

Using ancient Chinese medicine to cure infertility and improve health, renowned practitioner Yaron Seidman demonstrates how patients can use the Hunyuan Method to dramatically increase their ability to conceive in a healthy, natural way.

http://www.CuringInfertility.org

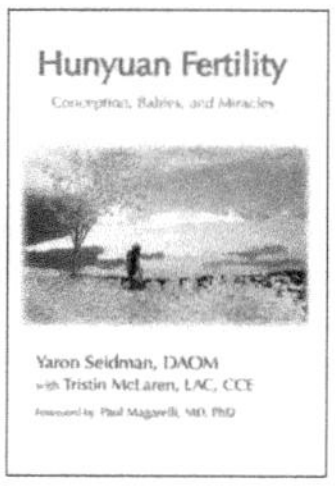

Hunyuan Fertility: Conception, Babies, and Miracles (2012)

IVF specialist and president of Pacific Coast Reproductive Society, Paul C Magarelli, MD, Ph.D. writes in the book's foreword: "Hunyuan is a song with many notes that sound discordant until the words, meanings and intentions fuse. It is not a How To book of treating fertility nor is it giving words that will rock your world. It simply pleads for us to return to what we know, know from the heart and not the mind. It begs in impassioned terms for individuals to contemplate, live simply, sleep, follow the natural patterns of spring, summer, fall and winter and act with "upright" intention. Simple and to the point—NOT! I was curious, defensive, and critical of this work and then it happened… I understood." [Co-authored with Tristin McLaren]

http://HunyuanFertility.com

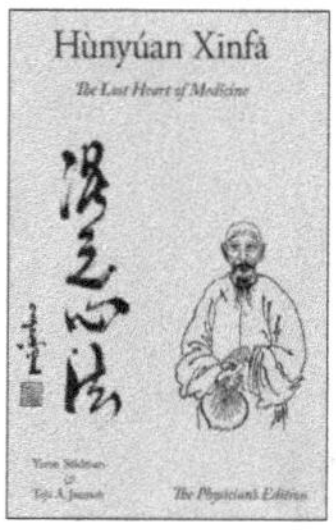

Hunyuan Xinfa: The Lost Heart Of Medicine (2013)

Hunyuan Xinfa is a book from the Heart. The authors, Dr Yaron Seidman and Teja A. Jaensch, present an investigation into the human Heart, revealing a method of healing never seen before. In this practical and profound exploration, the authors reach numerous breakthroughs in the understanding of Natural Character and the Heart, how to comprehend health and disease, and how to approach medicine from a point of Center.

http://www.HeartCultivation.com

About the Hunyuan Research Institute

The Hunyuan Research Institute was founded in the USA by Dr. Yaron Seidman D.A.O.M., drawing Chinese medicine practitioners from around the world who together develop and uphold the life principle of Chinese medicine. Today, local Hunyuan Research Institutes spring forth in countries all around the world, bringing the message of Hunyuan medicine to practitioners and patients on every continent.

The purpose of Hunyuan is to re-establish Chinese medicine as a life principle medicine, a medicine that can supplement and better the modern materialistic view of healthcare, disease and remedies.

Fellows of the Institute now include senior Chinese medicine practitioners who have been practicing TCM for decades, senior Western medicine doctors, new graduates from TCM schools, other professionals and lay people who want to learn and understand more about their own life and health.

Hunyuan medicine is deeply rooted in the Chinese medicine classics, but it is neither limited to nor confined by them. Hunyuan medicine involves researching forward and developing life principle in order to reach the deepest understanding of why and how we live, the source of disease and the best approach to remedy it.

In a world where a new "connectedness to nature" consciousness is developing, the Hunyuan Research Institute finds itself on the forefront of remaking a materialistic TCM into a life medicine; a Hunyuan medicine.

Websites:

http://www.ChineseClassics.org

http://www.HunyuanInstitute.com

http://www.Hunyuan.org

www.ingramcontent.com/pod-product-compliance
Lightning Source LLC
LaVergne TN
LVHW062241200926
848484LV00006B/1587
9780989167932